AIDS AND
RESPIRATORY MEDICINE

AIDS AND RESPIRATORY MEDICINE

Edited by

Alimuddin Zumla BSc MB ChB MSc PhD FRCP

Director, Academic Infectious Diseases Unit
Department of Medicine
University College London Medical School
Honorary Consultant in Infectious Diseases
Camden and Islington Community Health Services NHS Trust
London, UK

Visiting Professor
Department of Medicine
University of Zambia School of Medicine
Lusaka, Zambia

Margaret Johnson MD FRCP

Consultant Physician
Department of Respiratory Medicine
The Royal Free Hospital
London, UK

Robert Miller MB FRCP

Senior Lecturer/Honorary Consultant Physician
Department of Sexually Transmitted Diseases
Division of Pathology and Infectious Diseases
University College London Medical School
Honorary Consultant Physician
Camden and Islington Community Health Services NHS Trust
London, UK

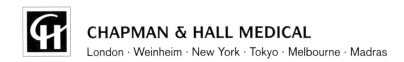

CHAPMAN & HALL MEDICAL

London · Weinheim · New York · Tokyo · Melbourne · Madras

Published by Chapman & Hall, 2–6 Boundary Row, London SE1 8HN, UK

Chapman & Hall, 2–6 Boundary Row, London SE1 8HN, UK

Chapman & Hall GmbH, Pappelallee 3, 69469 Weinheim, Germany

Chapman & Hall USA, 115 Fifth Avenue, New York NY 10003, USA

Chapman & Hall Japan, ITP-Japan, Kyowa Building, 3F, 2-2-1 Hirakawacho, Chiyoda-ku, Tokyo 102, Japan

Chapman & Hall Australia, 102 Dodds Street, South Melbourne, Victoria 3205, Australia

Chapman & Hall India, R. Seshadri, 32 Second Main Road, CIT East, Madras 600 035, India

First edition 1997

© 1997 Chapman and Hall

Typeset in 10/12 Palatino by Keyset Composition, Colchester, Essex

Printed in Great Britain at The University Press, Cambridge

ISBN 0 412 60140 0

A catalogue record for this book is available from the British Library

Library of Congress Catalog Card Number: 96-86531

∞ Printed on acid-free text paper, manufactured in accordance with ANSI/NISO Z39.48-1992 (Permanence of Paper).

CONTENTS

CONTRIBUTORS

PROFESSOR P. ARMSTRONG
Professor of Diagnostic Radiology
St Bartholomew's Hospital Medical College
West Smithfield
London EC1A 7BE
UK

PROFESSOR C. CHINTU
Dean and Professor of Paediatrics
University of Zambia School of Medicine
University Teaching Hospital
PO Box 50110
Lusaka
ZAMBIA

PROFESSOR J. CHRÉTIEN
International Union Against Tuberculosis
    and Lung Disease
68 Boulevard Saint-Michel
Paris 75006
FRANCE

DR J.H. DARBYSHIRE
Head and Senior Lecturer
MRC HIV Clinical Trials Centre
Mortimer Market Centre
UCLMS
London
UK

DR K.M. DE COCK
Senior Lecturer
Department of Clinical Sciences
London School of Hygiene and Tropical
    Medicine
Keppel Street
London WC1E 7HT
UK

PROFESSOR P. DEE
Professsor of Radiology
University of Virginia Health Services
Charlottesville
Virginia
USA

DR A.S. DENTON
Registrar
Department of Radiotherapy
Royal Free Hospital
Pond Street
London NW3 2QG
UK

DR G. DESAI
Senior Lecturer and Consultant Surgeon
University of Zambia School of Medicine
University Teaching Hospital
PO Box 50110
Lusaka
ZAMBIA

PROFESSOR D.A. ENARSON
International Union Against Tuberculosis
    and Lung Disease
68 Boulevard Saint-Michel
Paris 75006
FRANCE

PROFESSOR H.W. FARBER
Associate Professor of Medicine
Pulmonary Center
Boston University School of Medicine
USA

DR D. GIBB
Senior Lecturer in Epidemiology/Honorary
  Consultant Paediatrician
Epidemiology and Biostatistics Unit
Institute of Child Health
30 Guilford Street
London WC1N 1EH
UK

DR C.F. GILKS
Senior Lecturer
Liverpool School of Tropical Medicine
Pembroke Place
Liverpool L3 5QA
UK

DR P. GODFREY-FAUSSETT
Senior Lecturer
London School of Hygiene and Tropical
  Medicine
Keppel Street
London WC1E 7HT
UK

PROFESSOR R. HAY
Professor of Cutaneous Medicine
Dermatology Department
UMDS
Guy's Hospital
St Thomas's Street
London SE1 9RT
UK

DR M.A. JOHNSON
Consultant Physician
Department of Respiratory Medicine
The Royal Free Hospital
Pond Street
London NW3 2QG
UK

DR M.C.I. LIPMAN
Senior Registrar
Department of Respiratory Medicine
The Royal Brompton Hospital
Sydney Street
London SW3 6NP
UK

DR A.S. MALIN
Clinical Lecturer
Department of Clinical Sciences
London School of Hygiene and Tropical
  Medicine
Keppel Street
London WC1E 7HT
UK

PROFESSOR K.P.W.J. McADAM
Director
Medical Research Council (UK)
  Laboratories
Faraja
PO Box 273
Banjul
THE GAMBIA
West Africa

A. McMICHAEL
Director
Molecular Immunology Group
Institute of Molecular Medicine
John Radcliffe Hospital
Headington
Oxford OX3 9DU
UK

DR R.F. MILLER
Department of Sexually Transmitted
  Diseases
Division of Pathology and Infectious
  Diseases
UCLMS
Mortimer Market Centre
Mortimer Market, off Capper Street
London WC1E 6AU
UK

DR P.P. NUNN
Global Tuberculosis Programme
World Health Organization
CH-1211 Geneva 27
SWITZERLAND

DR M.J. O'DOHERTY
Consultant Physician
Departments of Nuclear Medicine,
Haemophilia and General Medicine
St Thomas's Hospital
Lambeth Palace Road
London SE1 7EH
UK

DR B.S. PETERS
Head of Academic Unit and Senior Lecturer
  in Genitourinary Medicine and HIV
Department of Genitourinary Medicine
UMDS
St Thomas's Hospital
Lambeth Palace Road
London SE1 7EH
UK

DR A. POZNIAK
Senior Lecturer in Genitourinary Medicine
Department of Genitourinary Medicine
King's College Hospital Medical School
15–22 Caldecot Road
London SE5 9RS
UK

DR M.C. RAVIGLIONE
Medical Officer
Global Tuberculosis Programme
World Health Organization
CH-1211 Geneva 27
SWITZERLAND

PROFESSOR G.A. ROOK
Department of Bacteriology
UCLMS
Windeyer Building
46 Cleveland Street
London W1P 6DB
UK

DR S. ROWLAND-JONES
MRC Senior Fellow
Molecular Immunology Group
Institute of Molecular Medicine
John Radcliffe Hospital
Headington
Oxford OX3 9DU
UK

PROFESSOR J.J. SAUKKONEN
Associate Professor of Medicine
Pulmonary Center
Room K-603
80 East Concord Street
Boston MA 02118
USA

DR M. SCHRAPPE
Klinik I für Medizin
Universität zu Köln
Josef-Stelzmann-Str. 9
D-50924 Köln
GERMANY

PROFESSOR T.F. SCHULZ
Professor of Genitourinary Medicine
University of Liverpool
Daulby Street
Liverpool L69 3BX
UK

DR G.M. SCOTT
Consultant Microbiologist
University College Hospital
Department of Clinical Microbiology
Grafton Way
London WC1E 6AU
UK

DR M. SHARLAND
Consultant in Paediatric Infectious Diseases
Paediatric Infectious Diseases Unit
St George's Hospital
Cranmer Terrace
London SW17 0RE
UK

DR M.F. SPITTLE
Consultant Oncologist
The Middlesex Hospital
Mortimer Street
London
W1A 8AA
UK

DR J.L. STANFORD
Head of Department
Department of Bacteriology
UCLMS
Windeyer Building
46 Cleveland Street
London W1P 6DB
UK

PROFESSOR E. TSHIBWABWA-TUMBA
Associate Professor of Diagnostic Radiology
University of Zambia School of Medicine
University Teaching Hospital
PO Box 50110
Lusaka
ZAMBIA

DR A.E. WAKEFIELD
Royal Society University Research Fellow
Molecular Infectious Diseases Group
Department of Paediatrics
Institute of Molecular Medicine
John Radcliffe Hospital
Headington
Oxford OX3 9DU
UK

DR A. ZUMLA
Director
Academic Infectious Disease Unit
Department of Medicine
UCLMS
The Windeyer Building
46 Cleveland Street
London W1P 6DB
UK

PREFACE

In the 15 years of the acquired immunodeficiency syndrome (AIDS) pandemic much has been learnt about its natural history and complications. It is clear that the lung is a major target organ both for the human immunodeficiency virus (HIV), and a wide array of infectious and non-infectious pulmonary complications. A great deal of information on the epidemiology, microbiology, immunology, clinical features, diagnosis and management of these pulmonary complications has accumulated during the past 15 years. Given the enormous explosion in information, it is now timely to bring together this knowledge in this 25-chapter volume on AIDS and respiratory medicine.

The contributors to this volume are prominent epidemiologists, doctors, microbiologists and scientists from Europe, USA and Africa. Professors Chrétien and Enarson give a masterful account of the epidemiology of lung complications of HIV. Drs Zumla, Rowland-Jones and Professor McMichael give a detailed summary of the lung immune responses to HIV. They outline normal lung defenses and discuss the consequences of HIV infection on them. The pulmonary radiological features of HIV and its complications as seen in the USA and Europe are illustrated by Professors Armstrong and Dee and this is compared and contrasted by Professor Tshibwabwa-Tumba who brings together his vast experience of chest X-rays in AIDS patients from Central Africa. Drs O'Doherty and Miller deal with the uses, and potential applications, of nuclear medicine in imaging of the chest in AIDS patients. Detailed coverage of *Pneumocystis carinii* pneumonia is given by Drs Wakefield and Miller (molecular biology) and Drs Lipman and Johnson (prophylaxis and treatment). We do not apologize for devoting five chapters to tuberculosis, which has recently been declared a global emergency by the World Health Organization: Drs Raviglione and Nunn (epidemiology); Drs Malin and De Cock (clinical features in adults); Professor Chintu and Dr Zumla (pediatric TB); Dr Godfrey-Faussett (diagnosis and molecular biology); Drs Darbyshire and Scott (management). Dr Pozniak gives an excellent overview of atypical mycobacteria in AIDS. Other pulmonary infectious complications are comprehensively described by Dr Gilks (acute bacterial infections); Dr Desai (empyema thoracis); Professor Hay (fungal infections); and Dr Peters (parasitic infections). The clinical features of pulmonary Kaposi's sarcoma are reviewed by Drs Denton and Spittle while Professor Schulz brings us up to date with the etiology and pathogenesis of Kaposi's sarcoma. Lymphomas of the lung are outlined by Dr Schrappe and lymphocytic interstitial pneumonitis by Professor Farber. Sinusitis and sinus disease are covered by Drs Zumla and Miller and pulmonary disease in children with HIV by Drs Gibb and Sharland. Dr Stanford and Professor Rook discuss the potential of immunotherapy for TB and HIV and Dr Malin and Professor McAdam outline the more urgent research priorities.

It is our hope that this book, with international contributors bringing together experience from Europe, USA and Africa, will be of educational value to all health workers who are currently engaged in the management of AIDS patients worldwide.

A. Zumla, M. Johnson, R.F. Miller (Editors)

FOREWORD

Although the initial very rapid increase in the AIDS epidemic in the developed world has now slowed, it still produces very considerable morbidity in these countries and is a leading cause under the age of 40 in many of them. The pandemic remains virtually unchecked in many countries of the developing world and, worryingly, large increases in the number of cases are being reported from some Asian countries. Thus it remains true that HIV infection is one of the major health problems affecting the world.

The HIV virus replicates at a staggering rate with 10^{11} viral particles being produced and destroyed each day. This is associated with the disappearance and re-creation of 10^9 T helper cells and while for many years the production rate of these cells keeps pace with their destruction, eventually the numbers of these cells fall and there are other changes in the immune system which leave patients susceptible to opportunistic infections which are the hallmark of AIDS. The commonest single organ to be involved in such infection is the lung where, in addition to the widely recognized *Pneumocystis carinii* pneumonia, a variety of other bacteria, viruses and fungi also cause disease. Not only is a clear understanding of these diseases important for the management of HIV-infected patients but understanding the pathogenetic processes potentially gives unique insight into host–parasite interactions in the lung.

The management of patients with AIDS has developed very rapidly and most large units managing considerable numbers of patients have adopted a multidisciplinary approach to care. As the volume of new literature on HIV infection each year is enormous, it is not possible for any clinician to keep abreast of all new aspects of treatment. Thus volumes such as this one are important and timely, and provide an excellent source to update clinicians and others with an interest in HIV management on current thoughts about pathogenesis, presentation, treatment and further directions for research.

Brian Gazzard
London, 1996

EPIDEMIOLOGY OF LUNG COMPLICATIONS IN PATIENTS WITH AIDS

Jacques Chrétien and Donald A. Enarson

INTRODUCTION

The study of the distribution and determinants of disease in a human population (epidemiology) forms the basis for our understanding of disease and of the interventions necessary to prevent and control it. The distribution of disease is usually described by person, place and time. This chapter will discuss the complications of the lung (other than tuberculosis, which will be dealt with in subsequent chapters) during the clinical course of infection with the human immunodeficiency virus (HIV) and its ultimate outcome, AIDS, and will discuss the factors associated with their development in such patients.

The chapter will commence with a discussion of general aspects of complications in the course of HIV infection, go on to discuss complications related to the lungs, the specific conditions causing lung complications, their distribution in the population by person, place and time and the determinants of such complications, including level of immunity, the environment, the type of immune suppression and the clinical course of HIV infection.

COMPLICATIONS: GENERAL ASPECTS

Progressive immunosuppression associated with HIV infection is a continuous process and complications related to this infection vary during the course of the infection. The greatest proportion of such complications affecting the lungs are due to infectious agents. Complications due to other conditions are less common and information concerning their epidemiology is very limited. Information concerning the epidemiology of lung complications is available mostly from industrialized countries; there is much less information on complications other than tuberculosis, from developing countries. Out of necessity, this chapter will focus predominantly on infectious complications and those, by and large, in industrialized countries.

COMPLICATIONS RELATED TO OPPORTUNISTIC INFECTIONS

Some of the opportunistic infections in AIDS patients cause disease in the individual by reactivation of latent infections which the individual had previously contracted. It is

AIDS and Respiratory Medicine. Edited by A. Zumla, M.A. Johnson and R.F. Miller. Published in 1997 by Chapman & Hall, London. ISBN 0 412 60140 0

therefore important to distinguish between 'infection' (which implies that the person harbors the agent, often in a latent stage) and 'disease' (in which the individual develops an illness related to the agent).

A review of the English-language literature from 1985 to 1993 concerning diseases due to opportunistic infectious agents in patients with AIDS in the USA and Europe identified the following agents as causes of serious conditions in order of the frequency of their occurrence: *Pneumocystis carinii*, cytomegalovirus, *Mycobacterium avium*-complex, *Toxoplasma gondii*, *Cryptococcus neoformans*, and *Mycobacterium tuberculosis* (Gallant, Moore and Chaisson, 1994). The cumulative probability of these conditions over 2 years following enrollment into a cohort study in the USA was 0.40 for *P. carinii* pneumonia, 0.22 for cytomegalovirus, 0.18 for *M. avium*-complex and approximately 0.04 each for toxoplasmosis, cryptococcosis and tuberculosis (Chaisson *et al.*, 1992a,b; Gallant *et al.*, 1992; Moore *et al.*, 1992).

At a conference at the National Institutes of Health in Bethesda, Maryland, which addressed the problem of management of infectious complications in AIDS patients, it was noted that serious disease due to opportunistic infections rarely develops until the CD4$^+$ lymphocyte count in peripheral blood declines to below 200 cells per cubic millimeter (Lane, 1994). These 'late' events in the clinical course of HIV infection are the cause of death in AIDS patients in 80% of cases. The conference noted that, before the routine use of prophylaxis, *P. carinii* pneumonia occurred in 80% of North American patients.

COMPLICATIONS INVOLVING THE LUNGS

From 1982 to 1988, a series of 119 episodes of pneumonia were documented at the National Institutes of Health in 100 patients with HIV infection in whom CD4$^+$ counts had been obtained (Masur *et al.*, 1989). There were 49 episodes of pneumonia due to *P. carinii*, 8 of cytomegalovirus pneumonia, 2 episodes of cryptococcal pneumonia, one of pneumonia due to *M. avium*-complex and 41 of nonspecific pneumonia without an identifiable infectious agent.

The Prospective Study of Pulmonary Complications of HIV Infection (Wallace *et al.*, 1993) was commenced in 1988 in 6 cities in the United States of America (San Francisco, Los Angeles, Detroit, Chicago, Newark and New York City). In this study, 1353 persons (1116 initially HIV positive and 165 HIV negative) were followed for 18 months to determine the nature of respiratory complications in the group. The majority of episodes in those HIV positive were upper respiratory infections (with an attack rate of 30.8%), bronchitis being next in frequency (16.0%), pulmonary infections next (10.3%, as compared with an attack rate of 1.2% in those not HIV infected) with other pulmonary conditions (neoplasms, nonspecific pneumonias and miscellaneous pulmonary events) much less common (1.6%). The most frequent infectious lung complications were bacterial pneumonia (4.8%), *P. carinii* (3.9%), nontuberculosis mycobacteria (1.1.%), *M. tuberculosis* (0.9%), *C. neoformans* (0.5%), cytomegalovirus (0.3%), *Histoplasma capsulatum* (0.1%), *herpes simplex* virus (0.1%), and *T. gondii* (0.1%). Nonspecific pneumonitis was next most common as a group (0.7%), and neoplasms were encountered much less frequently, including Kaposi's sarcoma (0.2%) and carcinoma (0.3%).

H. capsulatum (Minamoto and Armstrong, 1990) and *Coccidioides immitis* (Ampel, Dols and Galgiani, 1993) have been shown to be important pathogens giving rise to lung complications of HIV infection in geographic areas where they are endemic. *Streptococcus pneumoniae* (Janoff *et al.*, 1992) and *Haemophilus influenzae* (Steinhart *et al.*, 1992) are noted to cause pneumonia more frequently in association with AIDS.

The direct involvement of the lung by HIV infection has been noted to be responsible for deterioration of lung function (Meltzer *et al.*, 1993), although, at present, there is insufficient information available to clearly determine its frequency, trend or determinants.

SPECIFIC LUNG COMPLICATIONS

Bacterial pneumonia caused by pathogens similar to those causing community-acquired pneumonia in the general population is seen with increased frequency in those with HIV infection and in AIDS patients (Murray and Mills, 1990). A series of 59 patients with AIDS or advanced HIV infection in Massachusetts was followed over a 44 month period (Witt, Craven and McCabe, 1987); 14 of these patients had 21 episodes of community-acquired pneumonia and 7 had 8 episodes of nosocomial pneumonia. Community-acquired pneumonia was most commonly due to *Str. pneumoniae* (10 other agents). These episodes were noted early in the clinical course of the HIV infection, and were often recurrent, with disease caused by the same organism despite adequate treatment.

A review of the English-language literature concerning *Str. pneumoniae* (Janoff *et al.*, 1992) identified this agent as the most frequent cause of invasive bacterial respiratory disease in individuals with HIV infection in the reports reviewed. Most such infections (71% of evaluable episodes) preceded the AIDS-defining illness, with a rate ratio for incidence of bacteremia due to *Str. pneumoniae* of greater than 100 in AIDS patients as compared with the general population in San Francisco (Redd *et al.*, 1990). The serotype distribution of bacteria causing invasive disease was similar for those with or without HIV infection. In another study of individuals with AIDS, the attack rate of pneumonia due to *Str. pneumoniae* was estimated to be over five times higher than that in the general population (Polsky *et al.*, 1986).

A registry-based study of the occurrence of invasive *H. influenzae* in San Francisco indicated that, of 17 cases, 7 had AIDS and 9 had HIV infection without AIDS with a rate ratio of 5.4 and 1.5 for *H. influenzae* and *H. influenzae* type b respectively in AIDS patients as compared with those merely HIV-infected (Steinhart *et al.*, 1992). Most cases (Janoff *et al.*, 1992) had septicemia, and there were 5 cases with pneumonia (3 of 7 with AIDS and 2 of 9 with HIV infection).

Prior to 1981, *P. carinii* was seen infrequently and only in patients with immune suppression. The organism was first recognized as the cause of an outbreak in a human population in the 1950s when it was identified in a group of small children with malnutrition in Europe (Gajdusek, 1957). Although disease due to these organisms is distinctly uncommon, virtually all children in the population are believed to be infected with *P. carinii* by the age of four years (Menwissen *et al.*, 1977; Kovacs *et al.*, 1988). Transmission is usually by aerosol (Hughes, 1982) and evidence of horizontal transmission exists from community outbreaks (Watanabe *et al.*, 1965; Singer *et al.*, 1975). In adult patients infected with HIV, $CD4^+$ cell levels in the peripheral blood are very low by the time *P. carinii* is observed to cause disease (Masur *et al.*, 1989).

A prospective study (the Multicenter AIDS Cohort Study (Phair *et al.*, 1990)) of 1665 homosexual/bisexual men without AIDS and without prophylaxis against *P. carinii* reported an attack rate over 48 months of 10.1% for new episodes of *P. carinii* pneumonia. Those at greatest risk were those who entered the study with $CD4^+$ counts in the peripheral blood of less than 200 cells per cubic millimeter. There was a linear, inverse, relationship between $CD4^+$ cell count at entry to the study and the duration of time to the first episode of pneumonia.

Cytomegalovirus is an almost universal infection of asymptomatic, sexually active homosexual men (Mintz *et al.*, 1983), causing serious disease in 40% of homosexual men with AIDS (Drew, 1992). Much lower prevalence rates, approximating those in the general population, are reported in other groups of individuals with HIV infection (intravenous drug users and hemophiliacs) (Brodie, Drew and Maayan, 1984).

A prospective study of complications in 1002 AIDS patients treated with zidovudine in the USA (the Zidovudine Epidemiology Study Group (Gallant *et al.*, 1992)) indicated a high probability of development of disease (2-year actuarial risk of 15%) due to cytomegalovirus. However, manifestations occurred primarily in the eyes, gastrointestinal tract, and brain with no important impact noted on the lungs. It is estimated that at least 7.4% of AIDS patients in San Francisco have complications related to cytomegalovirus whereas, in only 1.2% of AIDS patients, was disease due to cytomegalovirus the AIDS-defining event (Jacobson and Mills, 1988). Cytomegalovirus was the causative agent in 17% of patients presenting with symptomatic pneumonia, while in only 4% it was the sole pathogen isolated (Murray *et al.*, 1984). Other reports suggest that cytomegalovirus is a co-infection along with other pathogens with only a trivial impact on the clinical course of the patient (Jacobson and Mills, 1988). Latent infection with cytomegalovirus was noted to be associated with an accelerated clinical course of HIV in hemophiliacs in the United Kingdom (Webster *et al.*, 1989).

Mycobacteria other than tuberculosis and leprosy are common in the environment but their occurrence varies with geography and climatic conditions. From a survey of cutaneous sensitivity to the Battey antigen (related to *M. avium*), the distribution of this infection was shown to be largely restricted to the south and southeast states of the USA (Edwards *et al.*, 1969), although the organism is known to be present in the environment in all states. Lung disease in those not immunocompromised usually occurs in those with damaged lungs. In individuals infected with HIV, while disease due to such bacteria is very frequent, it is usually a disseminated illness without specific lung involvement (Horsburgh, 1991) (see Chapter 14).

There is a varying preponderance of species of non-tuberculous mycobacteria which are associated with disease in humans: *M. avium* is more commonly isolated in AIDS patients whereas *Mycobacterium intracellulare* and *Mycobacterium scrofulaceum* are more commonly isolated in those with mycobacterial disease who are not immunosuppressed, such as small children with lymphadenitis (Gruthertz *et al.*, 1989).

A prospective study in Texas of 1006 persons infected with HIV (Nightingale *et al.*, 1992) indicated a cumulative incidence of disease due to *M. avium*-complex of 21% at 12 months and 43% at 24 months. Another cohort study of 1020 persons with AIDS and HIV infection treated with zidovodine from centers in Baltimore, Los Angeles, Chicago, San Diego, Washington, San Francisco, Atlanta, Houston, New York, Bethesda and Research Triangle Park identified a 2-year actuarial risk of 19% (Chaisson *et al.*, 1992b). Another study of 972 in Atlanta defined an incidence of 23% over one year (Havlik *et al.*, 1992).

The most common causes of systemic fungal disease in North America, *H. capsulatum*, *C. immitis* and *C. neoformans*, are also the most likely fungi to cause lung complications in North American AIDS patients. Although other fungi, notably *Aspergillus fumigatus* and related species, are ubiquitous in the environment and are important pathogens in patients on immunosuppressive therapy, they are uncommon as causes of disease in AIDS patients. *C. neoformans* in AIDS patients usually presents as meningoencephalitis with only a small number (4 out of 106 in a series from San Francisco) presenting with only pneumonia (Chuck and Sande, 1989). In about one-half of such patients presenting with pneumonia, the disease was the initial manifestation of AIDS.

H. capsulatum and *C. immitis* are highly circumscribed geographically, but in endemic areas, a high proportion of the population carried latent infection with these organisms. A map of the distribution of latent infection with *H. capsulatum*, based upon a survey of histoplasmin cutaneous sensitivity in naval recruits in the USA from 1958–65 (Edwards *et al.*, 1969), indicates a distribution virtually restricted to the valleys of the Ohio and Mississippi rivers. *C. immitis* is present in specific geographic areas in the southwestern USA.

By 1990, only 140 cases of histoplasmosis associated with AIDS had been reported in the literature (Minamoto and Armstrong, 1990). The uncommon occurrence of this complication may reflect the concentration of HIV infection in the coastal areas of the USA and not in the heartland where exposure to *H. capsulatum* is encountered. It also suggests that the mechanism of development of disease is new infection with prompt dissemination; only 3 of the 140 cases were reported among American-born persons without current residence or travel history related to endemic areas. Although lung involvement is frequently noted among AIDS patients with histoplasmosis, it is usually without specific characteristics and is overshadowed by the disseminated illness which universally occurs.

A cohort study of 170 individuals infected with HIV living in an area endemic for *C. immitis* (Ampel, Dols and Galgiani, 1993) indicated a cumulative incidence of 25% at 41 months of follow-up. The probability of developing active coccidioidomycosis was not associated with a history of previous active disease or with the length of residence in the area suggesting that disease might have been due to recent, rather than latent, infection. Coccidioidomycosis is the third most common presentation of AIDS in endemic areas, following *P. carinii* pneumonia and esophageal candidiasis (Galgiani and Ampel, 1990).

Pulmonary Kaposi's sarcoma usually occurs in the advanced stages of AIDS (Tirelli, Franceschi and Carbone, 1994). Very little further information has been published concerning epidemiological aspects of Kaposi's sarcoma involving the lung. The same is true for other malignancies, such as lymphomas and carcinomas as well as for the effect of HIV infection itself on the lung.

DISTRIBUTION OF DISEASE

PERSONS

The association of conditions causing infectious lung complications of AIDS together with personal characteristics is summarized in Table 1.1.

Age

Among adult patients, *M. avium*-complex is not related to age in HIV infected persons in some studies (Nightingale *et al.*, 1992; Gallant *et al.*, 1992) but in others it is more common in younger as compared with older patients (Horsburgh and Selik, 1989; Havlik *et al.*, 1992), suggesting recent infection; *H. capsulatum* predominantly affects young adults (Wheat *et al.*, 1981); rates for community-acquired pneumonia in persons not infected with HIV increase with age but rate ratios for pneumonia in HIV-infected do not (Caiaffa, Graham and Vlahov, 1993) (that is to say, rates rise with age in both HIV-infected and uninfected persons but the rate of rise with age is the same in both groups although the attack rate is higher in HIV-infected persons).

Gender

P. carinii pneumonia is less common in women than in men as the presenting episode and as an intercurrent illness in Rhode Island (Carpenter *et al.*, 1989). Disease due to *M. avium*-complex, without predispos-

Table 1.1 Personal determinants of opportunistic infections in persons infected with the human immunodeficiency virus

Condition/agent	Age	Gender	Race	Group	SES	Other
P. carinii		men		homosexual		
Cytomegalovirus				homosexual	low	
C. neoformans		men	white			diabetes
H. capsulatum	young		black			
C. immitis		men	non-white			diabetes
Non-tuberculous mycobacteria						
Bacterial pneumonia	old	women		IVDU	low	

Note: references concerning the association are given in the text.
SES, socio-economic status;
Group, epidemiologic category associated with risk of transmission of HIV infection;
IVDU, intravenous drug use.

ing factors, is more common in elderly women in some studies (Prince *et al.*, 1989) whereas it is reported to be more common in men in others (O'Brien, Geiter and Snider, 1987); *M. avium*-complex in HIV infected groups is unrelated to gender in the USA (Nightingale *et al.*, 1992; Chaisson *et al.*, 1992b; Havlik *et al.*, 1992) and occurs as an AIDS-defining illness with the same frequency in men and in women in Australia (Australian HIV Surveillance Report, 1994). *C. neoformans* is more common in men as compared with women (Moellering and Drutz, 1989). *C. immitis* presents as a disseminated disease more frequently in men as compared with women (Drutz and Catanzaro, 1978). Women are more likely than men to have bacterial pneumonia (Greenberg *et al.*, 1992).

Race

M. avium-complex without antecedents is more commonly observed in white women (Prince *et al.*, 1989); it is not related to race in persons with HIV infection in a number of studies (Nightingale *et al.*, 1992; Chaisson *et al.*, 1992b; Havlik *et al.*, 1992) although has been noted to be less frequently observed in

hispanics in one (Horsburgh and Selik, 1989). *C. neoformans* is more common in whites than in other races in the USA (Moellering and Drutz, 1989). *H. capsulatum* attack rates are higher in blacks than in other races (Wheat *et al.*, 1981). Dissemination of *C. immitis* is seen more commonly in blacks and filipinos than in other groups in the USA (Drutz and Catanzaro, 1978).

Epidemiologic category

Among those infected with HIV, *M. avium*-complex is not associated with any particular risk group for transmission of HIV infection (Chaisson *et al.*, 1992b; Havlik *et al.*, 1992). The prevalence of cytomegalovirus infection and of disease related to it is extraordinarily high in homosexual men (Jordan *et al.*, 1984; Gallant *et al.*, 1992) as compared with other groups. Intravenous drug users have an increased risk of pneumonia due to *Str. pneumoniae* as compared with other transmission risk groups (Selwyn *et al.*, 1988).

In the Prospective Study of Pulmonary Complications of HIV Infection (Wallace *et al.*, 1993), intravenous drug users were significantly more likely to suffer from bacterial pneumonia (rate ratio 3.0) as compared with homosexual/bisexual individuals, while the latter group were more likely to experience infection with *P. carinii* (rate ratio 2.9).

Both Kaposi's sarcoma and non Hodgkin's lymphoma are much more common in male homosexuals than in other groups, with lymphoma being also more common in hemophiliacs than in intraveneous drug users.

Socio-economic status

The prevalence of infection with cytomegalovirus is higher in persons with lower socio-economic status (Jordan *et al.*, 1984). Bacterial community-acquired pneumonia is more likely to occur in HIV infected persons with a low socio-economic status (Stoneburner *et al.*, 1988) with a documented excess risk for *Str. pneumoniae* associated with living in urban slums and in developing countries (Caiaffa, Graham and Vlahov, 1993).

Concomitant medical conditions

Disease related to *C. neoformans* and dissemination of *C. immitis* is more frequently observed in diabetics (Drutz and Catanzaro, 1978; Moellering and Drutz, 1989). Disease due to *M. avium*-complex is observed more frequently in those with previously damaged lungs in those not infected with HIV (Wolinsky, 1992), although there is no evidence of a similar association in those with HIV infection.

PLACE

In a study of homosexual men (Hoover *et al.*, 1991), there was a geographic variation in the distribution of *P. carinii* pneumonia as the AIDS-defining event with proportions, in order, highest in Pittsburgh (54%) followed by Chicago (51%), Baltimore (48%) and Los Angeles (43%). There was a relationship (with a lag period) between the seasonal peaks and troughs for upper respiratory infections and the first episodes of *P. carinii* pneumonia, suggesting to the authors the possibility of person to person transmission of *P. carinii* infection.

There is a marked geographic variation in distribution of infection with *M. avium*-complex (Wolinsky, 1992). Areas with a high prevalence of infection include the southeastern USA (Edwards *et al.*, 1969) and Sweden (Lind *et al.*, 1991). Geographic variation is also noted in the occurrence of disease due to *M. avium*-complex in individuals with AIDS, with the following prevalences observed in the USA. Rates, in order of frequency, are: 7.8% in northeast states, 7.1% in midwest states, 7% in southern states, 4.5% in the great lakes area, 4.4% in west coast states, 3.9% in eastern states and in southeast states (Horsburgh and Selik, 1989). Such disease is distinctly uncommon in Uganda (Okello *et al.*, 1990) and in Burundi (Kamanfu *et al.*, 1993). Serotypes 4 and 8 are most common in the USA and these differ from patients without AIDS and with environmental isolates (Crawford and Bates, 1986; Hampson *et al.*, 1989).

As previously noted, the systemic fungal infections *H. capsulatum* and *C. immitis* have distinctly circumscribed geographic areas. Disease due to *C. immitis* in AIDS patients appears to be associated with residence at the time of disease (Ampel, Dols and Galgiani, 1993) suggesting recent infection with progressive disease.

Table 1.2 illustrates the distribution of AIDS-defining illnesses in selected countries in 1992: Australia (Australian HIV Surveillance Report, 1994), the United States of America (Fleming *et al.*, 1993), France (Réseau national de Santé publique, 1994) and Denmark (Smith and Orholm, 1990). This comparison is complicated by some variation in the definition of an AIDS-defining illness and differences in diagnostic approach in

Table 1.2   Opportunistic infections reported as AIDS-defining illnesses in selected countries

	Geographic location			
Agent/condition	Australia	USA	France	Denmark
P. carinii pneumonia	187 (29)	13,754 (51)	1201 (25)	40 (49)
Aspergillus	0 (0)	0 (0)	0 (0)	0 (0)
Other fungi	0 (0)	3,154 (12)	0 (0)	18 (22)
Mycobacteria	42 (7)	3,469 (13)	147 (3)	2 (2)
Other bacteria	0 (0)	186 (1)	0 (0)	1 (1)
Cytomegalovirus	79 (12)	1,026 (4)	299 (6)	3 (3)
Other viruses	35 (5)	748 (3)	83 (2)	0 (0)

Note: references for data sources are given in the text.

Table 1.3   Etiologic agents responsible for opportunistic infections in consecutive patients with lung disease presenting to a major referral hospital in Burundi (from Kamanfu *et al.* (1993))

Condition/agent	HIV-negative n = 80	HIV-positive n = 222
P. carinii pneumonia	0 (0)	11 (5)
Aspergillus species	0 (0)	0 (0)
Other fungi	0 (0)	1 (<1)
Mycobacteria	39 (49)	109 (49)
Other bacteria	32 (40)	79 (36)
Cytomegalovirus	0 (0)	0 (0)
Other viruses	0 (0)	0 (0)

various locations among AIDS patients. The year 1992 was selected to minimize differences in the standards of an AIDS-defining illness. The particular countries were selected to minimize differences in diagnostic facilities. Nevertheless, quite remarkable differences appear in the proportions of conditions giving rise to an AIDS case definition in the various countries. Australia and France are similar to one another (as are the USA and Denmark) in the occurrence of *P. carinii* pneumonia and of fungal infections (predominantly *C. neoformans*) as the AIDS-defining events. The occurrence of *M. avium*-complex is most striking in the USA,

whereas disease related to cytomegalovirus is more frequently reported in Australia. The 'paucity' of total events in Australia and France is explained by the occurrence of other AIDS-defining conditions in those locations (in France, in 1992, 16% of events were Kaposi's sarcoma, 13% esophageal candidiasis and 16% cerebral toxoplasmosis; a similar distribution was seen in Australia, except for a lower proportion of cases with cerebral toxoplasmosis, 6% of AIDS-defining conditions).

The situation in SubSaharan Africa, as illustrated in a study from Bujumbura, Burundi (Kamanfu *et al.*, 1993) is quite different (Table 1.3). In this prospective, etiologic study of patients presenting with lung disease to a large referral hospital, the types of lung diseases observed were quite different from those seen in industrialized countries, with the greatest proportion being community-acquired pneumonia and tuberculosis, whether or not the patient was infected with HIV. All cases with mycobacterial disease had disease due to *M. tuberculosis*, both in those infected or not with HIV, with a small excess of cases due to *P. carinii* in those infected with HIV but little other difference in the distribution of etiologic agent.

TIME

In the previously noted prospective study of homosexual men (Hoover *et al.*, 1991), there was a temporal variation in the occurrence of *P. carinii* pneumonia in relation to HIV infection. At this point in the study, there were 916 HIV seropositive participants and 2161 who were seronegative. The study identified a seasonal peak (May–June) and trough (November–December) in those in whom *P. carinii* pneumonia was the initiating event of an AIDS diagnosis, in contrast with those in whom other illnesses were the AIDS-defining event in whom there was no seasonality.

In the USA the occurrence of disseminated nontuberculosis mycobacterial infection in AIDS patients has steadily risen from 5.9% in late 1987 to 7.6% in late 1990 (Horsburgh, 1991; Wolinsky, 1992; Caiaffa, Graham and Vlahov, 1993). This increase is partly related to improved case detection but may also be related to increased survival of patients due to treatment of their underlying illness.

There has been a sharp decline in the occurrence of Kaposi's sarcoma in association with AIDS in many places (Beral *et al.*, 1990; Serraino *et al.*, 1992), possibly due to an increasing proportion of risk groups other than male homosexuals among patients with AIDS.

KEY DETERMINANTS OF OPPORTUNISTIC LUNG INFECTIONS

LEVEL OF IMMUNITY

The level of immune suppression as measured by the peripheral blood $CD4^+$ count, is the key predictor of the type of clinical condition due to opportunistic infections in the individual infected with HIV: coccidioidomycosis occurs at a level of $CD4^+$ count less than 250 (Ampel, Dols and Galgiani, 1993); *P. carinii* pneumonia is seen at counts less than 200 (Phair *et al.*, 1990; Horsburgh, 1991); *M. avium*-complex (Nightingale *et al.*, 1992; Chaisson *et al.*, 1992b), cytomegalovirus and coccidioidomycosis are seen at levels less than 60 (Gallant *et al.*, 1992). Tuberculosis and community-acquired pneumonia appear at an early stage in the clinical course of HIV infection. In identifying other independent determinants related to opportunistic infections in persons infected with HIV, it is essential to know the $CD4^+$ count.

The Prospective Study of Pulmonary Complications of HIV Infection (Wallace *et al.*, 1993) identified a statistically signficant association between the level of $CD4^+$ count at entry into the study and the risk of development of pulmonary infections (rate ratio 4.2 for those below 250 cells per cubic millimeter as compared with those at 250 or above). The significant excess was observed for *P. carinii* (rate ratio 11.9) and for bacterial pneumonia (rate ratio 3.1). The excesses of neoplasms (rate ratio 5.0) and for idiopathic pneumonitis (rate ratio 1.7) were not statistically significant as the number of cases was very small.

A study from Australia (Gillieatt *et al.*, 1992) comparing the mode of presentation in those who presented 'early' in the course of their HIV-related condition with those who presented 'late' found a much higher proportion of late presenters with *P. carinii* pneumonia (66% of cases as compared with

35% of early presenters) and a lower proportion of those with opportunistic illnesses due to other agents such as *T. gondii, M. avium*, cytomegalovirus and *C. neoformans*. The authors, however, attributed this to the impact of preventive therapy for *P. carinii*.

THE ENVIRONMENT

As noted above in the discussion concerning specific infectious agents associated with complications of AIDS, the type of lung disease which occurs depends, to some extent, upon the prevalence and type of pathogens in the environment in which the person with HIV infection or with AIDS lives. This has been clearly shown for complications due to *H. capsulatum* and for *C. immitis*.

The geographic differences in occurrence of *M. avium*-complex cannot be so easily explained. Indeed, the virtual absence of such complications in Africa is definitely not related to the absence of the pathogen in the environment, although it may relate to the mode of exposure to the pathogen (for example, through water supply systems which are quite different in Africa as compared with industrialized countries), or to the point in the clinical course of HIV infection at which the patient presents to the health service (in Africa, patients may present at an earlier stage with tuberculosis or community-acquired pneumonia as compared with patients in the USA, in whom the extent of immune suppression may be considerably more advanced before a serious complication intervenes). Moreover, the distribution of infection with *M. avium*-complex in the USA does not appear to correspond with the frequency with which disease due to this organism is reported as an AIDS-defining event.

The differences in attack rates of *P. carinii* pneumonia in various cities of the USA (with higher rates in cities in the interior and lower rates in coastal cities) is possibly associated with seasonal transmission which is affected by climate.

The association of community-acquired pneumonia with low socio-economic level, including residence in low income countries, probably reflects the level of the carrier rate of common pathogens associated with community-acquired pneumonia in such populations (Montgomery *et al.*, 1990).

TYPE OF IMMUNOSUPPRESSION

Table 1.4 illustrates the occurrence of lung disease due to opportunistic infections in patients treated with immune suppressive therapy for the management of hematological malignancies, giving a comparison of those studies of patients with and without bone marrow transplant as a part of the treatment (Miller, 1995). All patients underwent lung biopsy for determination of the cause of their lung condition. The pattern of infectious lung complications in those without bone marrow transplant is similar, to some degree, with that in AIDS patients in the USA with the exception of increased proportions of cases related to *A. fumigatus*, cytomegalovirus and to bacteria other than mycobacteria, all of which are more common in the patients treated for malignancies. The situation is entirely different for those undergoing bone marrow transplant, in whom there is a striking predominance of cytomegalovirus. The differences and similarities among the groups might be related to the type of immune suppression, in particular the duration of the immune suppression and the rate at and extent to which severe degrees of immune suppression develop.

THE CLINICAL COURSE OF HIV INFECTION

Because the nature of lung complications is closely associated with the level of immune suppression associated with HIV infection, anything which will prolong or shorten the clinical course of HIV infection (and its

Table 1.4 Etiologic agents of opportunistic infections causing lung disease in patients undergoing treatment for hematologic malignancies, determined from lung biopsies

Agent/condition	No bone marrow transplant (144 episodes in 360 patients)	Bone marrow transplant (151 episodes in 230 patients)
P. carinii pneumonia	54 (38)	9 (6)
A. fumigatus	10 (7)	14 (9)
Other fungi	16 (11)	4 (3)
Mycobacteria	3 (2)	0 (0)
Other bacteria	33 (23)	24 (16)
Cytomegalovirus	27 (19)	94 (62)
Other viruses	1 (1)	6 (4)
Multiple agents	22 (15)	19 (13)

associated immune status) will change the nature of the lung complications encountered. Unquestionably, the survival of AIDS and HIV-infected patients is changing in relation to treatment of complications associated with the disease and to prophylaxis being used to prevent such complications. The further extension of prophylactic measures will undoubtedly change the situation even further. As this occurs, those complications with a longer clinical course (such as lymphomas and carcinomas) and those related to lower levels of immune function will increase in frequency and certain other conditions which are amenable to preventive treatment (such as tuberculosis and *P. carinii* pneumonia) will become less evident.

The use of active and preventive treatment and of prophylaxis will change the natural history of HIV infection as well, particularly in relation to those complications which have been shown to shorten the clinical course of HIV infection.

CONCLUSION

Lung complications in HIV infection and AIDS due to opportunistic infections are common and clinically important. The type of complication encountered is closely associated with the level of immune deficiency related to HIV infection and varies, to some extent, with the environment in which the infected person lives. Many of the conditions are treatable and some are preventable. Finally, infection and disease with some of these agents may adversely affect the clinical course of HIV infection.

Up to the present time, most epidemiologic investigations of lung complications of HIV infection and of AIDS have been largely descriptive with a poorly developed analytic component (the testing of hypotheses related to etiology, clinical course and related risk factors). Future studies need to become more analytical to focus upon such risk factors in order to target such interventions as are presently known to have a beneficial effect and to identify aspects of the clinical course of the disease which might give a clue to its management and (hopefully) its eventual cure.

REFERENCES

Ampel, N.M., Dols, C. and Galgiani, J.N. (1993) Coccidioidomycosis during human immunodeficiency virus infection: results of a prospective study in a coccidioidal endemic area. *Am. J. Med.*, **94**, 235–40.

Australian HIV Surveillance Report (1994) National Centre for HIV Epidemiology and Clinical Research. Cases of AIDS by AIDS-defining condition and sex, cumulative to 31 December

1993, and for two previous yearly intervals. p. 14.

Beral, V., Perterman, A.T., Berkelman, R.L. and Jaffe, H.W. (1990) Kaposi's sarcoma among persons with AIDS: a sexually transmitted infection? *Lancet*, **335**, 123–8.

Brodie, H.R., Drew, W.L. and Maayan, S. (1984) Prevalence of Kaposi's sarcoma in AIDS patients reflects differences in rates of cytomegalovirus infection in high risk groups. *AIDS Memo*, **1**, 12–15.

Caiaffa, W.T., Graham, N.M.H. and Vlahov, D. (1993) Bacterial pneumonia in adult populations with human immunodeficiency virus (HIV) infection. *Am. J. Epidemiol.*, **138**, 909–22.

Carpenter, C.C.J., Mayer, K.H., Fisher, A. *et al.* (1989) Natural history of acquired immunodeficiency syndrome in women in Rhode Island. *Am. J. Med.*, **86**, 771–5.

Chaisson, R.E., Keruly, J., Richman, D.D. and Moore, R.D. (1992a) *Pneumocystis* prophylaxis and survival in patients with advanced human immunodeficiency virus infection treated with zidovudine. The Zidovudine Epidemiology Study Group. *Arch. Intern. Med.*, **152**, 2009–13.

Chaisson, R.E., Moore, R.D., Richman, D.D. *et al.* (1992b) Incidence and natural history of *Mycobacterium avium*-complex infections in patients with advanced human immunodeficiency virus disease treated with zidovudine. *Am. Rev. Respir. Dis.*, **146**, 285–9.

Chuck, S.L. and Sande, M.A. (1989) Infections with *Cryptococcus neoformans* in the acquired immunodeficiency syndrome. *N. Engl. J. Med.*, **321**, 794–9.

Crawford, J.T. and Bates, J.H. (1986) Analysis of plasmids in *Mycobacterium avium-intracellulare* isolates from persons with acquired immunodeficiency syndrome. *Am. Rev. Respir. Dis.*, **134**, 650–61.

Drew, W.L. (1992) Cytomegalovirus infection in patients with AIDS. *Clin. Infect. Dis.*, **14**, 608–15.

Drutz, D.J. and Catanzaro, A. (1978) Coccidioidomycosis: state of the art. *Am. Rev. Respir. Dis.*, **117**, 559–85; 727–71.

Edwards, L.B., Acquaviva, F.A., Livesay, V.T. *et al.* (1969) An atlas of sensitivity to tuberculin, PPD-B, and histoplasmin in the United States. *Am. Rev. Respir. Dis.*, **99**, 1–132.

Fleming, P.L., Cieslelski, C.A., Byers, R.H. *et al.* (1993) Gender differences in reported AIDS-indicative diagnoses. *J. Infect. Dis.*, **168**, 61–7.

Gajdusek, D.C. (1957) *Pneumocystis carinii* – etiologic agent of interstitial plasma cell pneumonia of premature and young infants. *Pediatrics*, **19**, 543.

Galgiani, J.N. and Ampel, N.M. (1990) Coccidioidomycosis in human immunodeficiency virus-infected patients. *J. Infect. Dis.*, **162**, 1165–9.

Gallant, J.E., Moore, R.D., Richman, D.D. *et al.* (1992) Incidence and natural history of cytomegalovirus disease in patients with advanced human immunodeficiency virus disease treated with zidovudine. The Zidovudine Epidemiology Study Group. *J. Infect. Dis.*, **166**, 1223–7.

Gallant, J.E., Moore, R.D. and Chaisson, R.E. (1994) Prophylaxis for opportunistic infections in patients with HIV infection. *Ann. Intern. Med.*, **120**, 932–44.

Gillieatt, S.J., Mallal, S.A., French, M.A.H. and Dawkins, R.L. (1992) Epidemiology of late presentation of HIV infection in Western Australia. *Med. J. Austral.*, **157**, 117–8.

Greenberg, A.E., Thomas, P.A., Landesman, S.H. *et al.* (1992) The spectrum of HIV-1-related disease among outpatients in New York City. *AIDS*, **6**, 849–59.

Guthertz, L.S., Damsker, B., Bottone, E.J. *et al.* (1989) *Mycobacterium avium* and *Mycobacterium intracellulare* infections in patients with and without AIDS. *J. Infect. Dis.*, **160**, 1037–41.

Hampson, S.J., Portaels, F., Thompson, J. *et al.* (1989) DNA probes demonstrate a single highly conserved strain of *Mycobacterium avium* infecting AIDS patients. *Lancet*, **1**, 65–8.

Havlik, J.A., Horsburgh, C.R., Metchock, B. *et al.* (1992) Disseminated *Mycobacterium avium* complex infection: clinical identification and epidemiologic trends. *J. Infect. Dis.*, **165**, 577–80.

Hoover, D.R., Graham, N.M.H., Bacellar, H. *et al.* (1991) Epidemiologic patterns of upper respiratory illness and *Pneumocystis carinii* pneumonia in homosexual men. *Am. Rev. Respir. Dis.*, **144**, 756–9.

Horsburgh, C.R., Selik, R.M. (1989) The epidemiology of nontuberculous mycobacterial infection in the acquired immunodeficiency syndrome (AIDS). *Am. Rev. Respir. Dis.*, **139**, 4–7.

Horsburgh, C.R. (1991) *Mycobacterium avium* complex infection in the acquired immunodeficiency syndrome. *N. Engl. J. Med.*, **324**, 1332–8.

Hughes, W.T. (1982) Natural mode of acquisition of *de novo* infection with *Pneumocystis carinii*. *J. Infect. Dis.*, **145**, 842–8.

Jacobson, M.A. and Mills, J. (1988) Serious cytomegalovirus disease in the acquired immunodeficiency syndrome (AIDS). *Ann. Intern. Med.*, **108**, 585–94.

Janoff, E.N., Breiman, R.F., Daley, C.L. and Hopewell, P.C. (1992) Pneumococcal disease during HIV infection: epidemiologic, clinical and immunologic perspectives. *Ann. Intern. Med.*, **117**, 314–24.

Jordan, M.C., Jordan, G.W., Stevens, J.G. *et al.* (1984) Latent herpesviruses of humans. *Ann. Intern. Med.*, **100**, 866–80.

Kamanfu, G., Mlika-Cabanne, N., Girard, P.-M. *et al.* (1993) Pulmonary complications of human immunodeficiency virus infection in Bujumbura, Burundi. *Am. Rev. Respir. Dis.*, **147**, 658–63.

Kovacs, J.A., Halpern, J.L., Swan, J.C. *et al.* (1988) Identification of antigens and antibodies specific for *Pneumocystis carinii*. *J. Immunol.*, **140**, 2023–31.

Lane, H.C., moderator. (1994) Recent advances in the management of AIDS-related opportunistic infections. *Ann. Intern. Med.*, **120**, 945–55.

Lind, A., Larsson, L.O., Bentzon, M.W. *et al.* (1991) Sensitivity to sensitins and tuberculin in Swedish children. I. A study of schoolchildren in an urban area. *Tubercle*, **72**, 29–36.

Masur, H., Ognibene, F.P., Yarchoan, R. *et al.* (1989) CD4 counts as predictors of opportunistic pneumonias in human immunodeficiency virus (HIV) infection. *Ann. Intern. Med.*, **111**, 223–31.

Meltzer, M.S., Kornbluth, R.S., Hansen, B. *et al.* (1993) HIV infection of the lung. Role of virus-infected macrophages in the pathophysiology of pulmonary disease. *Chest*, **103**, 103–8S.

Meuwissen, J.H.E., Tauber, I., Leeuwenberg, A.D. *et al.* (1977) Parasitologic and serologic observations of infection with *Pneumocystis* in humans. *J. Infect. Dis.*, **136**, 43–9.

Miller, R.R. (1995) Pulmonary diseases in the immunocompromised host, in (eds W.M. Thurlbeck and A.M. Churg), *Pathology of the Lung* 2nd edn, Thieme Medical, New York, pp. 349–364.

Minamoto, G. and Armstrong, D. (1990) Fungal infections in AIDS: Histoplasmosis and coccidioidomycosis, in *The Medical Management of AIDS* (eds M.A. Sande and P.A. Volberding),

WB Saunders, Philadelphia, pp. 280–90.

Mintz, L., Drew, W.L., Miner, R.C. and Braf, E.H. (1983) Cytomegalovirus infections in homosexual men: an epidemiologic study. *Ann. Intern. Med.*, **98**, 326–9.

Moellering, R.C. and Drutz, D.J. (eds) (1989) Systemic fungal infections: diagnosis and treatment II. *Infect. Dis. Clin. North Am.*, **3**, 1–133.

Montgomery, J.M., Lehmann, D., Smith, T. *et al.* (1990) Bacterial colonization of the upper respiratory tract and its association with acute lower respiratory tract infections in highland children of Papua New Guinea. *Rev. Infect. Dis.*, **12**, S1006–16.

Moore, R.D., Keruly, J., Richman, D.D. *et al.* (1992) Natural history of advanced HIV disease in patients treated with zidovudine. The Zidovudine Epidemiology Study Group. *AIDS*, **6**, 671–7.

Murray, J.F., Felton, C.P., Garay, S.M. *et al.* (1984) Pulmonary complications of the acquired immunodeficiency syndrome: report of a National Heart, Lung and Blood Institute Workshop. *N. Engl. J. Med.*, **310**, 1682–8.

Murray, J.F. and Mills, J. (1990) Pulmonary infectious complications of human immunodeficiency virus infection. *Am. Rev. Respir. Dis.*, **141**, 1356–72.

Nightingale, S.D., Byrd, L.T., Southern, P.M. *et al.* (1992) Incidence of *Mycobacterium avium-intracellulare* complex bacteremia in human immunodeficiency virus-positive patients. *J. Infect. Dis.*, **165**, 1082–5.

O'Brien, R.J., Geiter, L.J. and Sindre, D.E. (1987) The epidemiology of nontuberculous mycobacterial diseases in the United States. *Am. Rev. Respir. Dis.*, **135**, 1007–14.

Okello, D.O., Sewankambo, N., Goodgame, R. *et al.* (1990) Absence of bacteremia with *Mycobacterium avium-intracellulare* in Ugandan patients with AIDS. *J. Infect. Dis.*, **162**, 208–10.

Phair, J., Munoz, A., Detels, R. *et al.* (1990) The risk of *Pneumocystis carinii* pneumonia among men infected with human immunodeficiency virus type 1. *N. Engl. J. Med.*, **322**, 161–5.

Polsky, B., Gold, J.W.M., Whimbey, E. *et al.* (1986) Bacterial pneumonia in patients with the acquired immunodeficiency syndrome. *Ann. Intern. Med.*, **104**, 38–41.

Prince, D.S., Peterson, D.D., Steiner, R.M. *et al.* (1989) Infection with *Mycobacterium avium* complex in patients without predisposing conditions. *N. Engl. J. Med.*, **321**, 863–8.

Redd, S.C., Rutherford, G.W., Sande, M.A. *et al.* (1990) The role of human immunodeficiency virus infection in pneumococcal bacteremia in San Francisco residents. *J. Infect. Dis.*, **162**, 1012–17.

Réseau national de Santé publique. (1994) Surveillance du Sida en France. *Bull Epidémio Hebdo*, **45**, 214.

Selwyn, P.A., Feingold, A.R., Hartel, D. *et al.* (1988) Increased risk of bacterial pneumonia in HIV-infected intraveneous drug users without AIDS. *AIDS*, **2**, 267–72.

Serraino, D., Franceschi, S., Tirelli, U. and Monfardini, S. (1992) The epidemiology of acquired immunodeficiency syndrome and associated tumours in Europe. *Annals of Oncology*, **3**, 595–603.

Singer, C., Armstrong, D., Rosen, P.P. *et al.* (1975) *Pneumocystis carinii* pneumonia: A cluster of eleven cases. *Ann. Intern. Med.*, **82**, 772–7.

Smith, E. and Orholm, M. (1990) Trends and patterns of opportunistic diseases in Danish AIDS patients 1980–1990. *Scand. J. Infect. Dis.*, **22**, 665–72.

Steinhart, R., Reingold, A.L., Taylor, F. *et al.* (1992) Invasive *Haemophilus influenzae* infections in men with HIV infection. *JAMA*, **268**, 3350–2.

Stoneburner, R.L., Des Jarlais, D.C., Benezra, D. *et al.* (1988) A larger spectrum of severe HIV-1-related disease in intravenous drug users in New York City. *Science*, **242**, 916–9.

Tirelli, U., Franceschi, S. and Carbone, A. (1994) Malignant tumours in patients with HIV infection. *Br. Med. J.*, **308**, 1148–53.

Wallace, J.M., Rao, A.V., Glassroth, J. *et al.* (1993) Respiratory illness in persons with human immunodeficiency virus infection. *Am. Rev. Respir. Dis.*, **148**, 1523–9.

Watanabe, J.M., Chinchinian, H., Weitz, G. *et al.* (1965) *Pneumocystis carinii* pneumonia in a family. *JAMA*, **193**, 685.

Webster, A., Cook, D.G., Emery, V.C. *et al.* (1989) Cytomegalovirus infection and progression towards AIDS in haemophiliacs with human immunodeficiency virus infections. *Lancet*, **2**, 63–5.

Witt, D.J., Craven, D.E. and McCabe, W.R. (1987) Bacterial infections in adult patients with the acquired immune deficiency syndrome (AIDS) and AIDS-related complex. *Am. J. Med.*, **82**, 900–6.

Wheat, L.J., Slama, T.G., Eitzen, H.E. *et al.* (1981) A large outbreak of histoplasmosis: clinical features. *Ann. Intern. Med.*, **94**, 331–7.

Wolinsky, E. (1992) Mycobacterial diseases other than tuberculosis. *Clin. Infect. Dis.*, **15**, 1–12.

Alimuddin Zumla, Sarah Rowland-Jones and Andrew McMichael

INTRODUCTION

Infection with the human immunodeficiency virus (HIV) results in a wide spectrum of clinical illness from the rapidly fatal to the chronically indolent. Cohort studies of HIV type-1 (HIV-1) infected individuals in the USA and Europe place the median time for HIV-1 infection to the development of the acquired immunodeficiency syndrome (AIDS) at approximately 8 to 10 years (Schrager *et al.*, 1994). AIDS can occur in as little as 2–4 months (Isaksson *et al.*, 1988) while some infected individuals have remained healthy for more than 12 years (Lifson *et al.*, 1991). The outcome of the progressive deterioration of the immune system that occurs in the majority of patients infected with HIV is clinically apparent disease, manifest with either severe and persistent constitutional signs and symptoms or an opportunistic infection or neoplasm.

Published literature on AIDS suggests that the lung is one of the most common organs involved in patients with AIDS worldwide (Murray *et al.*, 1984; Clumeck *et al.*, 1984; Biggar, 1986; Meduri and Stein, 1992; Sei *et al.*, 1994). Postmortem studies have shown the lung to be affected in up to 90% of AIDS patients (Neidt and Schinella, 1985; Afessa *et al.*, 1992). The lung is a dominant site for development of a variety of infectious (both opportunistic and non-opportunistic)

(Table 2.1), and non-infectious (Table 2.2) complications of infection with HIV. This broad spectrum of disease seen is consequential upon the local and systemic immunodeficiency induced by HIV.

The immunopathogenesis of HIV is not yet fully understood and is a subject of intense study (Pantaleo *et al.*, 1994; Levy, 1993, 1994; Coffin, 1995; Pantaleo and Fauci, 1995a, b). The profound immunosuppression that occurs at the terminal stages of the disease usually marks the end stage of immunopathogenic events that began at the time of the primary infection when the virus disseminated through the lymphoid organs and continued through clinically latent, but microbiologically active, stages of infection (Pantaleo *et al.*, 1993; Levy, 1993; Pantaleo and Fauci, 1995b). During this process, host defenses are gradually made defective by the relentless progression of HIV infection (Beck and Shellito, 1989; Rankin *et al.*, 1988; Pantaleo and Fauci, 1995a; Coffin, 1995). This chapter gives an introduction to normal lung defenses and details an overview of the published immune responses to HIV with particular emphasis on pulmonary studies.

NORMAL LUNG DEFENSES

During the past decade there has been an explosive growth of information on the complexities of the human immune

AIDS and Respiratory Medicine. Edited by A. Zumla, M.A. Johnson and R.F. Miller. Published in 1997 by Chapman & Hall, London. ISBN 0 412 60140 0

Table 2.1   Lung infectious complications of HIV

Parasites	Bacteria	Fungi	Viruses
Pneumocystis carinii	*Mycobacterium tuberculosis*	*Cryptococcus neoformans*	Cytomegalovirus
Toxoplasma gondii	*Salmonella* spp	*Histoplasma capsulatum*	*Herpes simplex* virus
Cryptosporidium spp	*Legionella* spp	*Candida albicans*	*Varicella zoster* virus
Microsporidium spp	*Nocardia asteroides*	*Coccidiodes immitis*	Epstein-Barr virus
Leishmania spp	*Listeria monocytogenes*	*Aspergillus* spp	HHV-6
Strongyloides spp	*Mycobacterium avium* complex		JC virus
	Streptococcus pneumoniae		Respiratory
	Haemophilus influenzae		syncytial virus
	Staphylococcus aureus		?HHV-8 (KSAHV)
	Klebsiella spp		
	Pseudomonas aeruginosa		
	Enterobacter spp		
	Listeria spp		
	Branhamella catarrhalis		
	Rochalimaea (Bartonella) spp		
	Rhodococcus equi		
	Mycoplasma pneumoniae		

(Compiled from Gottlieb, 1984; Brady *et al.*, 1984; Blaser and Cohn, 1986; Gold, 1987; Cook, 1987; Rankin *et al.*, 1988; Beck and Shellitto, 1989; Chaisson, 1989; Zumla, 1991, 1992; Cohn, 1991; Meduri and Stein, 1992; Agostini *et al.*, 1993; Weber *et al.*, 1993.)

Table 2.2   Non-infectious lung manifestations associated with HIV infection

Tumors	Idiopathic conditions
Kaposi's sarcoma	Lymphoid interstitial pneumonitis (LIP)
B cell lymphoma	Non-specific interstitial pneumonia (NIP)
Bronchogenic carcinoma	Diffuse infiltrative CD8$^+$ lymphocytosis syndrome
	(Lymphocytic alveolitis)
	Lymphocytic bronchiolitis

(Compiled from: Gottlieb, 1984; Grieco and Chinoy-Acharya, 1985; Guillon *et al.*, 1988; Murray *et al.*, 1987.)

response, its regulation, and its role in disease pathogenesis (Paul, 1994). The lung has several strategies to avoid or contain infection (Zumla and James, 1991; Reynolds, 1994; Lipscomb, 1995). The antigen deposited in the lung encounters non-specific, immune and non-immune, responses and is also translocated to the lung associated lymph nodes where a specific immune response is produced. The immune response in lung tissue augments the combination of anatomical barriers, mechanical mechanisms, chemical substances, immunoglobulins, and cellular components. The mucosal surface changes along the airways; the nares and the oropharynx are lined with stratified squamous epithelium, while from the nasal turbinates and the upper trachea down to the respiratory bronchioles, a pseudostratified, columnar, ciliated epithelium with mucus secreting goblet cells exists. In the periphery of the airways the epithelial layer becomes thinner and less stratified. The cell layer flattens in the terminal air sacs and over the alveolar surface and blends into a single layer of epithelium of type 1 pneumocytes, interspersed with type 2 pneumocytes. Present on the alveolar surface are free moving, phagocytic cells and lymphocytes. Lymphocytes and plasma cells are also distributed in the submucosa and lamina propria. Elements of systemic immunity are often brought in to reinforce local lung mechanisms.

LYMPHOCYTES

A foreign substance which manages to penetrate the local defense mechanisms of an individual (skin, cilia, mucous membrane, secretions) will encounter macrophages and two populations of circulating lymphocytes: T and B cells. In the normal lung lymphocytes make up 10% of all effector cells (Hunninghake *et al.*, 1979). The distribution of lymphocyte subtypes is similar to that in the blood although there are relatively more T than B cells. Approximately 7% of the airway T cells are natural killer (NK) cells (Robinson *et al.*, 1984). In children, the CD4/CD8 ratio of lung lymphocytes may be slightly lower than that of adults (Ratjen *et al.*, 1995).

T LYMPHOCYTES

T lymphocytes utilize the T cell antigen receptor (TcR) to recognize antigen presented in association with human leukocyte antigen (HLA) class I and class II molecules by antigen presenting cells (Royer and Reinherzel, 1987). Two distinct subpopulations of T lymphocytes exist: helper (CD4 or T4 or Th) and cytotoxic cells (CD8 or T8 or Ts). The functions, interactions and relationships of these cells are interrelated and complex. In general, CD4 subsets signal B lymphocytes to proliferate and differentiate into antibody producing cells, whereas CD8 cells exert a cytotoxic function. Stimulated T cells produce interleukin-2 (IL-2) and acquire receptors for IL-2, causing clonal expansion of antigen-specific CD4 cells. Activated T cells produce a variety of soluble mediator lymphokines to fan the immune response. Apart from the interleukins, they include macrophage, chemotactic and migration inhibition factors, α-interferon, collagen stimulating factor, and growth inhibitory and cytotoxic factors. What T cells recognize and the mechanism by which they see it continues to be a subject of intense study (Marx, 1988, 1995).

The CD4 cells are involved in a spectrum of immune responses at the poles of which two distinct cell type responses may occur (Mosmann and Coffman, 1989; Mosman *et al.*, 1991; Romagnani, 1991). The pro-inflammatory response, known as the 'Th-1 type response', is made up of production of cytokines such as IL-2, interferon-gamma (IFN-γ) and tumor necrosis factor-beta (TNF-β), and in general it promotes cell-mediated responses such as delayed hypersensitivity and macrophage activation. The anti-inflammatory response, known as the 'Th-2 type response', involves cytokines such as IL-4, IL-5, IL-6 and this occurs in association with the generation of antibodies, especially IgG1 and IgE, and allergic responses. Cross-regulation of the Th-type responses may occur *in vivo* and one type of response may dominate in certain infectious disease states (Bretscher *et al.*, 1993). Th0 patterns of cytokine secretion have also been described (Firestein *et al.*, 1993) which include both Th1 and Th2 cytokine profiles and these are thought to represent uncommitted CD4[+] cell populations.

B LYMPHOCYTES

B lymphocytes, responsible for humoral immunity, synthesize five major immunoglobulin classes (IgG, IgA, IgM, IgD, IgE) which form the pool of circulating antibodies (Bird, 1988). Poor humoral immunity, absolute or functional, is associated with recurrent or chronic pulmonary disease and increased susceptibility to respiratory tract infections (Polmar, 1976). T lymphocytes interact closely with B cells. Interleukin-4, which is produced by Th-2 type CD4 cells, acts on activated B lymphocytes possessing IL-4 receptor and induces their proliferation. Antibodies defend the body in several ways. They may combine with antigen and fix complement leading to antigen lysis. Antibody may neutralize microorganisms and their products; or opsonization may occur when phagocytosis is enhanced by coating of bacteria with specific antibody. IgG and IgA are present in the mucosa of the respiratory tract, alveolar epithelium and respiratory secretions (Reynolds, 1988). Approximately 90% of IgA is in the dimerous form. Secretory IgA (sIgA) is synthesized by plasma cells in the bronchial mucosa (Bell *et al.*, 1981). It is a dimer (300 000 daltons) whereas serum IgA is a monomer. Local plasma cells polymerize two 7S monomers of IgA; and a J chain glycoprotein, also made by plasma cells, acts as linkage. Secretory component, made by local epithelial cells, combines with it to form sIgA, which transports more readily across the mucosa into bronchial secretion. It anchors bacteria, neutralizes respiratory viruses, and with the help of lysozyme and complement promotes phagocytosis.

NATURAL KILLER CELLS (NK CELLS)

These are the third class of lymphocytes (non-T, non-B) which do not have the conventional T-cell antigen receptors on their surfaces (Granger *et al.*, 1988). NK cells can lyse a variety of targets in the absence of prior sensitization and do not require MHC antigens on target cells. NK cells can combine with the FcIgG-type IIIA receptor (CD16) cellular antigens and activation causes release of cytokines such as IFN-γ, TNF and granulocyte-macrophage colony

stimulating factor (GM-CSF) (Hiserodt *et al.*, 1982; Lotzova and Herberman, 1986).

MACROPHAGES

Macrophages are derived from peripheral blood monocyte which as a result of pathogen invasion, migrate to site of localization of pathogen, phagocytose and process the antigen in an attempt to directly kill pathogens or scavenge inhaled particles (Gordon *et al.*, 1995). They are also important in effector cell function. Pulmonary macrophages are phenotypically and functionally diverse (Lipscomb *et al.*, 1995). Macrophages modulate activity of other immune responses through secretion of cytokines and presentation of antigen to T cells. Macrophages secrete an enormous number of substances (over a hundred) and mediators (Nathan *et al.*, 1987). These provide important signalling functions to other immune cells. Macrophages are particularly active against organisms which have an intracellular phase during infection such as viruses, fungi, mycobacteria, brucella, and toxoplasma.

In the normal lung there are approximately 80 effector cells per alveolus (Crapo *et al.*, 1982). These cells are located within the alveolar interstitium and on the alveolar epithelial surface. More than 90% of these are alveolar macrophages with a lifespan of months to years. Interstitial macrophages, when compared to alveolar macrophages, also exhibit size, functional and phenotypic differences (Lipscomb *et al.*, 1995). In contrast to alveolar macrophages, there have been very few studies on the role of interstitial, pleural and intravascular lung macrophages.

Although macrophages can replicate in the normal lung, most are derived from blood monocytes that migrate through the alveolar walls. Alveolar macrophages migrate to the site of antigen deposition in the lung following chemotaxis and utilize their phagocytic mechanisms to engulf the organism. Their phagocytic ability is enhanced by the presence of opsonins, but depressed by hypoxia, intoxication with ethanol, and by cigarette smoke and HIV-1. After internalization, microorganisms may be killed by macrophages through a variety of mechanisms including generation of toxic oxygen metabolites ('respiratory burst and release of free oxygen radicals'). When activated they release a variety of mediators relevant to inflammatory and immune processes. Activation of the macrophage by immune or non-immune opsonins or by the complement cascade stimulates them to produce chemotactic factors, including protein factors, and leukotrienes (LT) such as LTB4, and complement components. These recruit PMNs from the circulating and marginating pools. They generate complement which amplifies host defenses and mediates immune mechanisms in the lung. Antibody-dependent cellular cytotoxicity (ADCC) is an important mechanism by which monocytes recognize and lyse target cells. Macrophages play an important role in antigen recognition and presentation of antigens to T lymphocytes in association with its own major histocompatibility complex (MHC) class I and II products. Together with T cells, B cells and NK cells, the cell-to-cell interplay is a crucial pulmonary defense mechanism.

DENDRITIC CELLS

Pulmonary dendritic cells originate from the bone marrow and are phenotypically heterogeneous (Lipscomb *et al.*, 1995). Dendritic cells in the lung may play an important role in initiating local immunity (Holt, 1993). The role of dendritic cells in priming naive T cells is increasingly being recognized. Lung dendritic cells constitutively express pan T, NK cells, B cell and CD54 and CD58 molecules. It remains to be determined whether antigen presented by pulmonary dendritic cells is more likely to result in Th1 or Th2-type T cell responses in the lungs.

MAST CELLS

Mast cells express membrane receptors for IgE that signal self degranulation. They generate and release histamine, leukotrienes, proteases and eosinophilic chemotactic factors, platelet activating factors, prostaglandins (PGD2 and PGF2) (Paul, 1994).

POLYMORPHONUCLEAR LEUKOCYTES (PMNs)

These cells are present in small numbers in the normal lung (1% of all cells), being sequestered in interstitial areas and marginated in capillaries. The mobilization of inflammatory cells and phlogistic factors from the intravascular component into the lung is important for effective host defense (Reynolds, 1994; Lipscomb, 1995). Phagocytes (macrophages, monocytes, polymorphonuclear leukocytes) reach the site of invasion by chemotaxis where, with the aid of opsonins and complement, they phagocytose and dispose of foreign particles and organisms. Impairment of function includes poor chemotaxis, intrinsic cellular defects and abnormal opsonization. The polymorphonuclear neutrophil is assumed to be the principal responding cell in the inflammatory focus. Like the macrophage, it utilizes chemotaxis, phagocytosis, and subsequent generation of nitric oxide and toxic metabolites to eliminate pathogens. Other inflammatory conditions elicit a response of the eosinophils (as in parasitic infections, allergen-induced asthma or other lung diseases). Several different chemotactic molecules are required for the selective attraction of these cells (Donabedian and Gallin, 1983). The role and relative importance of chemotactic factors in pulmonary diseases have been reviewed by Fantone and Ward (1983). Opsonic activity requires intact receptor sites, and neutrophil attachment to the organism at the Fab site of the opsonizing antibody.

OPSONINS

The role of immune opsonins focuses on the requirements for IgG subclasses to bind to the membrane surface of alveolar macrophages and on specific kinds of antibody contained within the respective subclasses. Alveolar macrophages have cell surface receptors for IgG and complement. Among the IgG subclasses there are differences in the extent of avidity for Fc gamma receptors. In the alveolar lining fluid are several substances such as surfactant (Benson *et al.*, 1983) and fibronectin that act as opsonins. Surfactant has anti-staphylococcal and anti-pneumococcal activity. Palmitoyl lysophosphatidylcholine which represents a component of surfactant seems to be the most active fraction. Fibronectin fragments (which originate from plasma, fibroblasts or macrophages) enhance non-immune opsonin phagocytosis by macrophages. The fragments are thought to work by interacting with the trypsin-sensitive membrane receptor on the macrophage, which is the putative complement C3b receptor (Proctor, 1987). Fibronectin is present on cell surfaces where it may limit pathogen adherence. Although AIDS patients appear to have normal plasma levels of fibrinectin (Ogden *et al.*, 1988), the amount present in the airways is not known.

COMPLEMENT

Complement components including factor B have been identified in lung lavage fluids. Both the alternative and direct pathways of complement activation are important in immunity against microbial antigens (Hunninghake *et al.*, 1979).

HUMAN LEUKOCYTE ANTIGENS (HLA)

Molecules of the HLA system are found on the membranes of cells and are intimately associated with antigen presentation and interaction with the T cell receptor (McDevitt,

1980). The HLA system is a series of closely linked genes which occur on the short arm of the 6th chromosome in the region termed the major histocompatibility complex (MHC). The A, B and C loci code for class I antigens, which are cell surface glycoproteins found on all nucleated cells. The D locus codes for class II cell surface antigens which are expressed on restricted populations of cells, particularly macrophages, B cells, some activated T cells and vascular endothelial cells. The immune regulatory capacity of MHC can theoretically affect susceptibility to infection, the rate of disease progression and disease outcome (Hill, 1992).

IMMUNE RESPONSES TO HIV

The central immunological events which consequently lead to development of AIDS are (1) infection with HIV of CD4$^+$ cells, particularly T lymphocytes, dendritic cells and macrophages; (2) an early and progressive functional impairment of CD4 cell function; and (3) a decline in the number of CD4$^+$ T lymphocytes. The exact mechanism for this is not understood although it has been speculated that it may be due to binding of free gp120 to the CD4 molecule. There is also an early defect in the antigen-presenting function of dendritic cells and macrophages which probably impairs the ability to make immune responses to new antigens. The mechanisms of regulation of viral replication and by which immunodeficiency is manifest are areas of intense research (Levy, 1993, 1995; Safrit *et al.*, 1994; Coffin, 1995; Wain-Hobson, 1995; Finkel *et al.*, 1995; Pantaleo and Fauci, 1995a). During the acute phase of HIV infection a viremia is seen with high levels of infectious HIV particles in plasma. It is now known that HIV-1 enters the lung early in the course of infection (Sei *et al.*, 1994) and infects pulmonary cells (Agostino, 1993; Clarke *et al.*, 1995). A wide variety of host immune responses to HIV occur following infection (Table 2.3). As part of the general immune response,

Table 2.3 Human immune responses to HIV

Humoral immune responses
1. Neutralizing antibodies to:
    HIV envelope glycoprotein gp120
        – V3 loop (principal neutralizing domain)
        – V2 region
        – CD4-binding domain
        – carbohydrate moieties
        – conformational epitope
    HIV envelope glycoprotein gp41

2. ADCC (Antibody dependent cell-mediated cytotoxicity)
    NK cells and monocytes involved in ADCC via
        – IgG1 against gp120
        – IgG1 against gp41

3. Enhancing antibodies
    complement and Fc-mediated responses

4. Complement-fixing anti-HIV antibodies
    lysis via neutralizing and non-neutralizing antibodies

Cell-mediated immune responses
1. Cytotoxic natural killer cell activation
    non-MHC restricted killing of HIV-infected target cell
2. CD4$^+$ lymphocyte responses
    Th1 and Th2 immunoregulatory responses
3. CD8$^+$ lymphocyte cytotoxic responses
    MHC restricted killing of HIV-infected target cell
4. Macrophage activation
    increased cytokine production
    enhanced antigen presenting capacity
    enhanced ADCC

(Compiled from Lane *et al.*, 1984; Bonavida *et al.*, 1986; Plata *et al.*, 1987; Walker *et al.*, 1987; Agostino *et al.*, 1993; Nixon *et al.*, 1991; Autran *et al.*, 1991, 1988; Levy *et al.*, 1993; Fauci, 1993; Clerichi and Shearer, 1993; Pantaleo *et al.*, 1993; Meltzer *et al.*, 1993; McMichael and Walker, 1994; Coffin, 1995.)

both humoral and cell-mediated protective responses are evoked at time of initial infection (Pantaleo *et al.*, 1993, 1994, 1995; Rosenberg and Fauci, 1990). Much of this information has been obtained from studies of immune cells from peripheral blood and enlarged lymph nodes. Over the past few years efforts at studying immune responses have shifted to the actual site of pathology to unravel the immune mechanisms operating in affected organs and to ascertain the role of

HIV-1 in the functional dysregulation of local and systemic host defenses.

LUNG IMMUNE RESPONSES DURING HIV-1 INFECTION

Due to technical limitations, immunologic studies relating to the lungs of HIV patients have been restricted to cell populations, fluid and tissue obtained at bronchoscopy (Beck and Shellito, 1989; Clarke *et al.*, 1995). These studies have provided valuable insight into the role of lung defense mechanisms in patients infected with HIV and results of these studies are summarized here. Several factors explain some of the varying and conflicting data that have been published. It is prudent to note that conclusions about lung-specific immune function based on lavaged cell populations are difficult to interpret. Bronchoalveolar lavage (BAL) collects samples of single subsegmental areas and does not sample the lung as a whole. This does not provide information on the state of the upper or lower airways. Furthermore, cells within pulmonary interstitial spaces are difficult to access. Comparisons of the results between various series are confounded by the use of different methods for reporting quantitative yields of cellular populations which are themselves dependent on technique, volume of lavage fluid instilled and returned, and on the processing of the sample. Reporting of data has also been varied and has been expressed as relative percentage of cells; concentration of cells per unit of returned lavage volume, or total cells in the entire lavage volume. For example, several studies on the total cell yield at BAL from AIDS patients at the time of clinical pneumonia have drawn different results, such as the same number of cells (Wallace *et al.*, 1984; Young, *et al.*, 1985; Moore *et al.*, 1987), or cells per unit volume (White *et al.*, 1985) as compared to healthy controls; increased in AIDS patients as compared to normal controls (Venet *et al.*, 1985), or in AIDS patients with *Pneumocystis carinii* pneumonia (PCP) compared with AIDS or HIV-infected patients without PCP (Spragg *et al.*, 1987; Smith *et al.*, 1988).

HIV-1 and the lung

At postmortem it has been shown that the predominant infected cell in the lung is the alveolar macrophage (Donaldson *et al.*, 1994). HIV-1 RNA has been identified in lung tissues of patients with AIDS and HIV isolated from BAL fluid (Chayt *et al.*, 1986; Ziza *et al.*, 1985) suggesting that HIV-1 may play a direct role in mediating pulmonary dysfunction. Virus is rarely isolated from BAL in patients with blood CD4$^+$ counts of 300/mm^3 (Jeffrey *et al.*, 1991; Clarke *et al.*, 1993a, 1993b).

The mode by which HIV-1 gains access to the lung is not clear. It is likely that HIV-1 gets into the lung through several different ways (1) by HIV-1 infected peripheral blood monocytes entering the lung and differentiating into resident alveolar macrophages (Agostini *et al.*, 1993; Clarke *et al.*, 1993); (2) by migration of circulating CD4$^+$ infected T lymphocytes into the lung; (3) by HIV-1 crossing the alveolar-capillary membrane as a free extracellular virion and subsequently infecting pulmonary lymphocytes and macrophages. Genetic analysis of HIV-1 proviral DNA recovered from blood monocytes and alveolar macrophages isolated from 8 patients showed varied V3 and V4 loop region sequences of HIV-1 isolates from both cell types (Nakata *et al.*, 1994). This study suggested that the cell populations in blood and lung were being infected with HIV-1 separately. HIV-1 has been isolated from BAL in several studies (Dean *et al.*, 1988; Lebargy *et al.*, 1994). Existing data suggest that the isolation of HIV from BAL reflects the extent of trafficking of lymphocytes into the lung from peripheral blood.

HIV-1 host cellular range

While the major target cell for HIV is the CD4 lymphocyte, HIV is not solely lymphotropic. Cell culture studies have shown the presence of HIV in several tissues (Levy, 1993). A variety of human cells are susceptible to infection with HIV and the extent of infection varies according to cell type and also expression of CD4. In the lungs, HIV infection has been shown to occur in the pulmonary fibroblasts, T and B lymphocytes, macrophages, NK cells, eosinophils, monocytes and dendritic cells (Plata *et al.*, 1990; Dolei *et*

Table 2.4 HIV-induced T and B lymphocyte dysfunction

T cell defects
  decrease in number of CD4$^+$ T cells
  decreased mitogen-induced responses
  decreased cytokine production
  decreased ability to induce immunoglobulin production from B cells
  decreased IL-2 receptor expression
  decreased HLA-restricted cytotoxic responses
  defective natural killer cell (NK) activity

B cell defects
  increased B cell activation
  hypergammaglobulinemia
  decreased mitogen-induced immunoglobulin secretion

(Compiled from: Heagy *et al.*, 1984; Creemes *et al.*, 1985; Bonavido *et al.*, 1986; Rosenberg and Fauci, 1987; Joly *et al.*, 1989; Clerichi *et al.*, 1989; Gruters *et al.*, 1990; Fauci, 1993; Levy, 1993; Pantaleo *et al.*, 1993; Pantaleo *et al.*, 1994; Coffin, 1995.)

al., 1988; Levy, 1994). It is not clear whether type I and type II pneumocytes or bronchial epithelial cells are susceptible to infection with HIV.

Lymphocyte responses in the lung in HIV infection

Throughout the course of HIV infection, there is an increase in the number of lymphocytes that can be found in BAL fluid (Rankin, 1988; Young *et al.*, 1985; Wallace *et al.*, 1984; White *et al.*, 1985), and the majority of these are of the CD8$^+$ phenotype (Bernard *et al.*, 1984; Young *et al.*, 1985; Wallace *et al.*, 1984; Venet *et al.*, 1985). The percentage of CD4$^+$ T cells in BAL compared to peripheral blood is decreased and since there is an increase in the absolute numbers of lymphocytes, the total CD4 quantity may be low, normal or elevated (Young *et al.*, 1985, Venet *et al.*, 1985). Infection with HIV in the lung results in infiltration of pulmonary parenchyma and peribronchial and interstitial spaces with lymphocytes and plasma cells (Rubenstein *et al.*, 1986; Ettensohn *et al.*, 1988; Solal-Celigny, 1985) in AIDS patients without identifiable pulmonary infections has been described. This is particularly common in pediatric AIDS.

CD4 lymphocyte responses

Although there is clear evidence of a functional defect in populations of CD4$^+$ lymphocytes taken from the peripheral blood of people with HIV infection (Table 2.4) (Beck and Shellito, 1989; Levy, 1993; Coffin, 1995), function of lung CD4$^+$ cells has not been well studied, although it seems likely that they would show a similar functional defect. Studies with human T cell clones have shown that CD4 lymphocytes, although sensitive to infection by HIV, can also exhibit cytotoxic activity of HIV-infected targets (Orentas *et al.*, 1990; Zarling *et al.*, 1990). Functional and phenotypic evidence for a selective loss of memory T cells in asymptomatic HIV-infected patients has been described (Van Nossell *et al.*, 1990). Since the majority of lung CD4$^+$ T cells are of the memory phenotype (Saltini *et al.*, 1990), this may explain the decrease in CD4$^+$ T cells and may occur earlier in the lung than in the blood.

It has been suggested that cytokines from Th1 and Th2 CD4$^+$ lymphocytes play an immunoregulatory role in HIV infection and can affect progression to AIDS. Clonal proliferation of CD4 lymphocytes in response to antigens, and elaboration of cytokines such as IFN-γ and IL-2 are reduced by HIV infection (Clerici et al., 1989). The ability of HIV to promote a Th1 to Th0 shift and replicate preferentially in Th2 and Th0 cells has also been suggested (Maggi et al., 1994). Clerici and Shearer (1993), using their results from longitudinal studies of CD4$^+$ T cell responses in HIV-infected patients and HIV-exposed but seronegative donors, proposed that Th1-type immunity (probably stimulated by exposure to low doses of HIV), was more likely to be of value in controlling and, exceptionally, clearing HIV infection. They suggested that development of disease would be associated with the development of a dominant Th2 pattern of immunity. Their findings have been disputed by some authors (Maggi et al., 1994; Graziosi et al., 1994) and confirmed by others (Meyaard et al., 1994). The relative importance of Th-type responses in HIV infection remain controversial and are currently subjects of intense study (Clerici and Berzofsky, 1994; Montaner and Gordon, 1995). The effects of Th2 cytokines on macrophage function and viral replication in macrophages are also not clear (Montaner and Gordon, 1995). A clinical trial evaluating the role of CD4$^+$ T cell cytokine IL-2 in restoring the immune function in HIV-infected patients has been carried out (Kovacs et al., 1995). It was shown that intermittent courses of IL-2 can improve some of the immunologic abnormalities associated with HIV infection in patients with a peripheral blood CD4 count of >200 cells/mm^3. Data on the effects of IL-2 therapy on lung immune responses are not available. Changes in T cell subsets and in T cell and macrophage cytokine profiles in the lung, and their relationship to development of opportunistic infections, require further definition.

Cytotoxic T-lymphocyte (CTL) responses in the lung

Accumulating lines of evidence suggest that circulating CD8$^+$ HIV-specific CTL play a key role in the control of HIV replication during the asymptomatic period of HIV infection (reviewed by Rowland-Jones and McMichael, 1993; McMichael and Walker, 1994). Their appearance within a few days of acute infection coincides with the clearance of virus from the circulation (Koup et al., 1994), several weeks before the appearance of neutralizing antibody (Ariyoshi et al., 1992). Their levels are high through the asymptomatic period (a single HIV-specific clone may account for up to 1% of circulating lymphocytes (Moss et al., 1995), and inversely correlate with viral load (Ariyoshi et al., 1995). Vigorous HIV-specific activity is a particular feature of the immune response to HIV in a group of long-term non-progressors (Pantaleo et al., 1994). The decline in detectable CTL activity late in HIV infection is not fully explained, but often precedes the development of disease (Carmichael et al., 1993). Cytotoxic T-cells recognize short fragments of viral antigen, in the form of 8–11 amino acid peptides processed from HIV proteins in the infected cell, and this allows them to respond to what may often be conserved viral epitopes (McMichael and Walker, 1994). In other viral infections such as influenza, virus-specific CTLs are associated with viral clearance, and although this not been unequivocally shown to occur for HIV infection, a number of studies have shown HIV-specific Th-1 and cytotoxic T-cell responses in apparently uninfected and seronegative people exposed to HIV infection (reviewed in Rowland-Jones and McMichael, 1995). HIV-specific CTL are known to secrete a number of cytokines when they encounter their target cell (Jassoy et al., 1993): in addition to the known cytokines, such as TNF and interferon-gamma, a proportion of CD8$^+$

cells produce a so-far-unidentified substance which potently suppresses HIV replication in *in vitro* systems (Mackewicz and Levy, 1992).

One of the first descriptions of HIV-specific CTL came from BAL fluid in patients with lymphocytic alveolitis (Plata *et al.*, 1987): these cells were able to kill HIV-infected alveolar macrophages, leading to speculation that, although circulating and lymphoid-associated CTL may be beneficial, in other organs such as the lung (Autran *et al.*, 1988) and CNS (Jassoy *et al.*, 1992), they may be responsible for disease. The majority of lymphocytes found in BAL are CD8$^+$ and have the phenotype of CTL (Bernard *et al.*, 1984; Agostini *et al.*, 1990). In the early stages of HIV infection a peripheral blood lymphocytosis is seen due to expansion of the CD8 cytotoxic T lymphocyte population (Autran *et al.*, 1991). This lymphocytosis is more pronounced in the lung and the CD4/CD8 ratio in the lung is lower than peripheral blood (Wallace *et al.*, 1984; Gellene *et al.*, 1984; Young *et al.*, 1985; Jensen *et al.*, 1991). Although a mild lymphocytic alveolitis can be detected in the majority of asymptomatic patients with no respiratory symptoms, vigorous HIV-specific CTL activity is confined to patients with lymphoid interstitial pneumonitis (LIP) (Autran *et al.*, 1990), an HIV-related disorder frequently observed before the onset of opportunistic infections. There is a correlation between the extent of BAL HIV-specific CTL activity and lung epithelial permeability (Meignan *et al.*, 1990). Patients without LIP show only a mild CD8$^+$ lymphocytic infiltration, without cytolytic activity. However, in the LIP patients, there is a progressive decline in HIV-specific CTL activity which precedes the onset of opportunistic infections (Autran *et al.*, 1990).

A study by Saukkonen and colleagues (1993) examined the T cell subsets in BAL from 6 HIV-seropositive patients and 8 healthy volunteers and showed that HIV-posi-tive subjects had a lymphocytosis and lower CD4/CD8 ratios than normal subjects. Significant increases in CD8$^+$ CD28$^-$ cells in the lungs of HIV-positive patients were seen. The HIV infection did not appear to directly downmodulate CD28 expression. Increased numbers of CD28$^-$ T cells may be the result of immunological activation or expansion of a pre-existing CD28$^-$ subset. It was inferred that absence of CD28 surface expression on T cells from HIV-positive patients may have significant immunological consequences: decreased proliferative potential of T cells, with reduced ability to generate cytotoxic or helper T cells, T cell anergy resulting from T cell receptor/CD3 complex activation in the absence of CD28 co-stimulation, increased susceptibility to activation-induced apoptosis and reduction of Th1 cell cytokine production.

In addition to classical HLA-restricted CTL, a second population of CD8$^+$ cells has been described in BAL fluid. These cells express CD57, and appear to be able to regulate and suppress the activity of specific CTL (Joly *et al.*, 1989) as well as NK cell activity (Autran *et al.*, 1991). The mechanism of suppression appears to be by means of a soluble factor (Sadat-Sowti *et al.*, 1991), and the increase in CD57$^+$ CD8$^+$ cells with disease progression correlates with the disappearance of detectable HIV-specific CTL activity in BAL from patients with AIDS (Sadat-Sowti *et al.*, 1994). Recent studies of patients with the acute HIV syndrome show major oligoclonal expansions in peripheral blood of CD8$^+$ T cells with a restricted set of variable domain Vβ-chain T-cell receptor families and HIV-specific cytotoxicity (Pantaleo *et al.*, 1994; Pantaleo and Fauci, 1995b). No information on the T cell receptor gene usage of lung lymphocytes is available to date.

HIV infection of macrophages

The macrophage itself is a target for HIV infection (Stevenson and Gendelman, 1994)

Table 2.5 Effects of HIV on lung macrophages

Macrophage function	Effect on lung macrophage
Chemotaxis	reduced
Phagocytosis	decreased
Intracellular killing	normal
Superoxide production	normal
Monocyte dependent T-cell proliferation	reduced
Fc receptor function	reduced
C3 receptor-mediated clearance	reduced
ADCC	unknown
Antigen presentation	unknown
Cytokine production	
IL-1	
resting	normal
stimulated	increased
TNF-α	
resting	increased
TGF-β, IL-6, GM-CSF	increased
MHC expression	decreased

(Compiled from Smith *et al.*, 1984; Poli *et al.*, 1985; Holt *et al.*, 1986; Weiss *et al.*, 1989; Beck and Shellito, 1989; Musher *et al.*, 1990; Twigg *et al.*, 1989, 1994; Cox *et al.*, 1990; Levy, 1993; Agostini *et al.*, 1993; Clarke *et al.*, 1995; Coffin, 1995; Montaner and Gordon, 1995.)

and a potential source of virus dissemination. Pulmonary macrophages (Salahuddin *et al.*, 1986) from both AIDS patients and normal healthy donors are susceptible to infection with HIV-1 infection *in vitro*. Infection of the pulmonary macrophage can occur through phagocytosis of HIV particles or through attachment to the CD4 receptor on the macrophage surface. Some investigators have reported that certain isolates of HIV display a specific tropism for macrophages or for CD4 cells. HIV grown from lung or brain tissue from infected individuals grows much more readily in macrophages than do standard laboratory strains (Gartner *et al.*, 1986). The complex interplay between macrophages and HIV (Table 2.5) is an important one since macrophages appears to be relatively refractory to the cytopathic effects of HIV-1 and may serve as a major reservoir for the virus as well as a means of delivering the virus to other tissues.

HIV production and macrophages

Spontaneous production of HIV-1 has been detected in primary pulmonary macrophage cultures from AIDS patients, suggesting that these cells are targets for infection *in vivo*. However, the absolute load of HIV-1 in alveolar macrophages or any other tissue macrophage and its correlation with cellular function and stage of disease are unknown.

Recently Sierra-Madero *et al.* (1994) studied the levels of HIV-1 in lymphocytes and monocytes from the blood and pulmonary alveoli of 14 patients with HIV infection. HIV-1 was undetectable or low in blood monocytes and alveolar macrophages among asymptomatic individuals. Among subjects with AIDS, there was a significant increase of HIV-1 in alveolar macrophages but not in blood monocytes. Furthermore, alveolar macrophages but not blood monocytes expressed increased levels of LPS-stimulated mRNA for TNFα, IL-1β, IL-6, during both early and late stages of HIV-1 infection regardless of virus load. This suggests that alveolar macrophages may serve as a reservoir for virus in the late stages of disease and yet contribute to immunopathogenesis of lung disease in both early and late stages through increased cytokine production.

Macrophage–HIV relationship

There are important differences in the outcome of HIV infection of monocytes/macrophages as compared to CD4 lymphocytes. HIV infection of macrophages appears to be persistent and does not result in significant cell death or the syncytia formation that occurs after infection of CD4 cells (Rosenberg and Fauci, 1993). Since macrophages develop highly productive infection it has been suggested that they serve as reservoirs for virus during infection with HIV (Meltzer et al., 1990). The effects of HIV on macrophage function have been extensively studied and a summary of the functional studies is given in Table 2.5 above. The pathogenic significance of HIV-infection in macrophages is not as clear as for T-lymphocytes. HIV-1 is less cytopathic to macrophages infected *in vitro* than to T cells. The HIV-infected macrophage serves as a reservoir for virus and HIV-induced defects in their functional activity may be responsible for the increased likelihood of opportunistic infections (reviewed by Cook, 1987a). HIV-infected pulmonary macrophages expressing viral antigen have been shown to be targets for lysis by HIV-specific cytotoxic T lymphocytes and may be responsible for induction of inflammatory reactions in the lungs of HIV-infected individuals (Plata *et al.*, 1987).

Macrophage numbers

Decreased numbers of circulating HLA-DR$^+$ monocytes (Heagy *et al.*, 1984) have been described in patients with AIDS. The absolute numbers of macrophages in AIDS patients who have pulmonary infections compared to normal controls and those in AIDS patients without PCP appear unchanged (Wallace *et al.*, 1984; Young *et al.*, 1985; White *et al.*, 1985; Venet *et al.*, 1985). Generally, results of BAL studies in AIDS patients have revealed decreased percentages of lavaged alveolar macrophages which are the result of proportional increases in other cell populations in lavage fluid. However, when reported as absolute concentrations rather than percentages, the numbers of lavaged macrophages are not different from control values (Wallace *et al.*, 1984; Young *et al.*, 1985; White *et al.*, 1985; Venet *et al.*, 1985).

Macrophage function

While macrophage numbers appear unchanged, the clinical pulmonary infections associated with AIDS suggest that macrophage function is abnormal. Macrophage-monocyte chemotaxis, phagocytosis and killing are reported to be defective in patients with AIDS (Smith *et al.*, 1984). Tissue macrophages are important for killing of intracellular organisms such as *Mycobacterium tuberculosis* and *Cryptococcus neoformans*. The increased prevalence of intracellular pathogens in HIV-infected patients implies that this cellular function is impaired. Alveolar macrophages from AIDS patients with pneumonia have decreased phagocyte activity (Musher *et al.*, 1990). While it is not prudent to extrapolate data obtained from peripheral blood monocytes or monocyte-derived macrophages to that of alveolar macrophages, data on lung macrophages in HIV-infected patients are accumulating. Alveolar macrophages serve as phagocytes and regulators of specific immune responses. Alveolar macrophages express surface HLA molecules but are poor antigen-presenting cells in normal people and suppress T cell responses (Holt *et al.*, 1986; Meyaard *et al.*, 1993). Other studies have found that the antimicrobial function of peripheral blood monocytes is intact in patients with AIDS (Murray *et al.*, 1984; Washburn *et al.*, 1985). Monocyte incubation *in vitro* with human gamma interferon reconstitutes HLA-DR-positivity to near normal levels (Heagy *et al.*, 1984) and incubation with cytokines or interferon enhances antimicrobial activity (Murray *et al.*, 1987). In HIV infection alveolar macrophages demonstrate enhanced antigen presenting capacity and increased IL-1 and IL-6 production *in vitro* when compared to cells from normal volunteers (Twigg *et al.*, 1989, 1994).

Macrophages and cytokines

The effect of HIV on the production of cytokines by alveolar macrophages remains controversial (Montaner and Gordon, 1995). Several studies have shown that alveolar macrophages in BAL from HIV-infected patients release these cytokines spontaneously or in response to LPS from infectious organisms. It is possible that early in HIV infection there is activation of alveolar macrophages leading to cytokine production and paradoxical activation of HIV replication with a later loss of alveolar macrophage activating cytokines such as IFNγ. Alveolar macrophages amplify immune responses through production of IL-1 and TNFα, IL-6, GM-CSF, IL-8 and MIP1-α (Millar *et al.*, 1991). Alveolar macrophages from HIV-1 infected individuals at all stages of disease have been shown to express macrophage inflammatory protein-1 alpha (MIP-1α) which is chemotactic on activated blood CD8[+] T cells (Denis *et al.*, 1994). MIP-1α levels in HIV *in vitro* correlate with intensity of CD8[+] alveolitis (Denis *et al.*, 1994). While these responses may be beneficial in the defense against HIV and other infectious organisms, cytokines such as TNFα, IL-1, and IL-6 can potentially activate HIV replication by actions on the NFkB promoter (Osborn *et al.*, 1989; Poli *et al.*, 1990) and may increase propagation of HIV in the

lung. TGFβ is also produced by alveolar macrophages in HIV infection (Twigg *et al.*, 1989). Some studies show that alveolar macrophages from HIV-1-infected patients produce increased levels of IL-1 and TNFα (Weiss *et al.*, 1989; Millar *et al.*, 1991) while others show that production of these cytokines is decreased (Cox *et al.*, 1990; Gupta *et al.*, 1987). Increased levels of IL-10 and IL-6 have been shown to be produced by HIV-1 infected alveolar macrophages (Twigg *et al.*, 1992). Increased levels of IL-8, IL-10 and IL-12 by alveolar macrophages is found in BAL fluid of asymptomatic HIV-1 positive individuals and those with non-specific interstitial pneumonitis. Patients with *Pneumocystis carinii* pneumonia show increased levels of IL-8 and IL-10 but not IL-12 (Denis and Ghadiran, 1994). Cytokines may be directly toxic to pulmonary epithelium and activate neutrophils and this may contribute to alveolar capillary leak seen in PCP. Corticosteroids have been shown to be beneficial adjunct therapy in the treatment of PCP (Bozette *et al.*, 1990) and patients with PCP receiving steroids show decrease in production of IL-1β and TNFα (Zheng *et al.*, 1993). Alveolar macrophages from AIDS patients undergoing diagnostic broncho-scopy respond normally to lymphokines including recombinant IFN-γ by inhibiting replication of *Toxoplasma gondii* and *Chlamydia psittaci* (Murray *et al.*, 1985). The role of macrophage derived IL-10 in inhibiting Th1 and Th2 cell cytokine production (Hsich *et al.*, 1992; Montaner and Gordon, 1995) or IL-12 with switching Th1 IFNγ production remains to be studied in lung HIV infection.

Antibodies to HIV antigens

It is recognized that systemic humoral immune response is abnormal in patients with AIDS. B lymphocyte abnormalities described in association with HIV infection are summarized in Table 2.4. Most studies of neutralizing antibody sites on HIV indicate at least six regions of the HIV viral envelope that are involved (Broliden *et al.*, 1992). The clinical relevance of the neutralizing antibodies remains uncertain and their effect in controlling viral spread following infection is not clear. Serum IgA is elevated in HIV-infected patients and may correlate with progression to AIDS (Lefrere *et al.*, 1988). Circulating IgA1 subclass immune complexes have been demonstrated in a subpopulation of AIDS patients (Lightfoot *et al.*, 1985; Jackson *et al.*, 1988) and whether a parallel production of IgA2 from the respiratory mucosa occurs is not known. Quantitation of immunoglobulins sampled by BAL has shown that patients with AIDS have significant increases in IgG and IgA but not IgM (Young *et al.*, 1985) and it appears that the IgA is a mixture of local production by plasma cells and transudation from the intravascular space.

POLYMORPHONUCLEAR LEUKOCYTES

Impairment of polymorphonuclear leukocyte function in patients with AIDS is well described (Lazzarin *et al.*, 1986; Nielson *et al.*, 1986). Patients with AIDS have an increased susceptibility to pulmonary pyogenic infections. The role of granulocytes in HIV lung pathology is unclear (Agostini *et al.*, 1992). Increase in the mean concentration or percentage of PMNs (Wallace *et al.*, 1984; Young *et al.*, 1985; White *et al.*, 1985, Venet *et al.*, 1985) obtained at BAL of AIDS patients compared to normals have been reported. Neutrophils from AIDS patients have decreased bactericidal activity against *Staphylococcus aureus* and decreased phagocytosis of *Candida albicans* (Ellis *et al.*, 1988). Chemotactic properties of neutrophils have also been shown to be decreased in HIV-infected asymptomatic patients (Rollides *et al.*, 1990). C3b receptors have been found to be reduced in stimulated neutrophils from AIDS patients (Tausk and Gigli, 1990). A small subset of AIDS patients demonstrate increased numbers of neutrophils in BAL

(Young *et al.*, 1985; Venet *et al.*, 1985) although no consistent association with a particular pathogen exists (Wallace *et al.*, 1984). GM-CSF and IL-8 are chemotactic to neutrophils and eosinophils and have been demonstrated in BAL fluid from AIDS patients with PCP (Lipschik *et al.*, 1993). Increased neutrophil counts in BAL from subjects with PCP carry a poor prognosis (Mason *et al.*, 1989), and BAL eosinophilia may also accompany PCP (Sample *et al.*, 1990).

NATURAL KILLER CELL

NK cells are a major component of cellular immunity and they kill virus-infected cells in a non-MHC restricted manner. However, this cell type function is deficient in HIV-infected persons (Sirianni *et al.*, 1990).The number of circulating NK cells in AIDS patients has been reported as normal but other studies have shown a decrease of this cell population with disease progression (Creemes *et al.*, 1985). The defect appears to be the trigger for release of the cytotoxic factors for target cell lysis (Bonavida *et al.*, 1986). IL-2 supplementation can partially restore cytolytic function, suggesting that the underlying problem is that of a lack of T-cell signaling.

DENDRITIC CELLS

Lung dendritic cells appear to form a dense network in the lung (Holt, 1989) and these may become infected with HIV, leading to alteration of accessory signals or antigen presentation (Knight and Macatonia, 1991; Helbert *et al.*, 1993). As a consequence, incoordination of T lymphocyte responses may occur and this requires further investigation.

HLA STUDIES

The immune response genes of the major histocompatibility complex (MHC) are known to contribute both to susceptibility to, and the natural history of several infectious diseases

(Hill, 1992). The immune regulatory capacity of MHC could theoretically affect susceptibility to HIV infection; the rate of disease progression and the eventual outcome (Mann *et al.*, 1993). The role of MHC in HIV pathogenesis has recently been comprehensively reviewed by Mann *et al.* (1994). Most studies on MHC and HIV come from the USA and Europe and the potential contribution to the outcome of HIV infection of polymorphism in the immune response genes of the MHC has not given clear results. This is probably due to the small scale of studies so far published and the mixed populations studied where the allele frequencies in control groups may not be known with certainty (Kaslow and Mann, 1994). The most consistent findings have been associations with rapid progression to disease of the HLA-1, B8, DR3 haplotype (Kaslow *et al.*, 1990; Steele *et al.*, 1988; Mallal *et al.*, 1990; Cameron *et al.*, 1990) and its southern European equivalent HLA-B35 (Itescu *et al.*, 1992; Sahmoud *et al.*, 1993; Klein *et al.*, 1994). Other associations include HLA-B62 with symtomatic primary infection, HLA-DR1 with Kaposi's sarcoma, and the presence of syncytium-inducing HIV variants with HLA-DQ2 (Klein *et al.*, 1994). Susceptibility to HIV infection has been associated with HLA-B51 (Fabio *et al.*, 1992). Resistance to HIV infection in a European study was associated with HLA-B52 and HLA-B44 (Fabio *et al.*, 1992) and with HLA-A28, HLA-B18 and HLA-DR13 in a cohort of highly HIV-exposed but apparently HIV-negative Nairobi prostitutes (Plummer *et al.*, 1993). A $CD8^+$ lymphocytic host response in HIV-1 known as 'diffuse infiltrative lymphocytosis' (DILS) has been associated with HLA-DR5 (Itescu *et al.*, 1990). In this syndrome, a $CD8^+$ T cell lymphocytosis is accompanied by extensive infiltration of the lungs and salivary glands (Itescu *et al.*, 1992).

HIV-INDUCED IMMUNODEFICIENCY

Efficient pulmonary host defenses against infection involve the concerted actions of mechanical, humoral, cellular and mucosal mechanisms. These are apparently rendered ineffective in patients with AIDS. The extent of cytopathology produced by a variety of HIV-1 and HIV-2 strains differs substantially (summarized by Levy, 1993). The exact mechanism by which HIV infection results in the loss of immune function remains unknown. While there is little consensus on the mechanism of $CD4^+$ T cell loss it is generally thought to be the primary determinant of the observed immunodeficiency and a good marker for both the rate and stage of disease progression (Sheppard *et al.*, 1993). HIV-1 may deplete alveolar lymphocytes and alveolar macrophages by cytolysis mediated by 3 mechanisms: (1) cytotoxic $CD8^+$ T cell-mediated cytolysis; (2) direct virus-mediated cytolysis; (3) synytium mediated cytolysis (Agostini *et al.*, 1993; Agostini *et al.*, 1994). However, the defects are more complicated than the simplistic view that initially emerged of a gradual decline in T helper lymphocytes. While the case definition for AIDS relies on $CD4^+$ cell quantitation it is no longer tenable that the intervening infections are related solely to lymphopenia (Mukadi *et al.*, 1993).

LYMPHOCYTIC INTERSTITIAL PNEUMONITIS

A lymphocytic alveolitis which can lead to LIP occurs in 60% of HIV-1 infected adults at any stage of disease (Guillon *et al.*, 1988; Rankin *et al.*, 1988). The pathogenesis of LIP remains unknown. Non-specific interstitial pneumonitis occurs in between 10–38% of HIV-seropositive patients with pulmonary symptoms (Suffredini *et al.*, 1987). Histology of pulmonary tissue shows interstitial inflammation with a mixed mononuclear cell infiltration. A small lymphocytic infiltrate of the alveolar septa with an absence of vasculitis or granuloma occurs (Teirstein and Rosen, 1988). BAL reveals significant lymphocytosis with 25–75% of total cells recovered having a CD8 phenotype (Solal-Celigny *et al.*, 1985). The lymphocytes are predominantly HIV-specific CD8$^+$ cytotoxic T cells and the early stage at which these CD8$^+$ T cells can be detected in the lung further suggests that early infection of the lung occurs by HIV- 1 (Plata *et al.*, 1987; Autran *et al.*, 1988). Cytotoxic T cell activity was also reported in HIV infection in children (Buseyne *et al.*, 1993) and this may be important in disease progression and development of LIP.

CLINICAL CONSEQUENCES OF HIV-INDUCED LUNG IMMUNE DYSFUNCTION

The pathological manifestations of infection with any of the two human immunodeficiency viruses, HIV-1 and HIV-2, once symptoms and signs develop, are similar (Clavell *et al.*, 1987). As a consequence of infection with HIV, persistent, quantitative, and progressive functional depression within the CD4 lymphocyte subset and other immunological abnormalities occurs and renders the patient more prone to developing a variety of infections and neoplasms (Murray *et al.*, 1984; Meduri and Stein, 1992; Sei *et al.*, 1994).

Infectious complications

The lung is an early and most frequent target of opportunistic and pathogenic infections in AIDS. Table 2.1 lists the infectious agents frequently seen causing lung pathology in patients with HIV infection. In general, intracellular pathogens are consequential upon defects in macrophage-T cell axis of the immune response while infections with pyogenic organisms are due to the secondary defects in neutrophils and the humoral responses. Progressive decline in numbers of CD4 lymphocytes in the blood is associated with development of select opportunistic infections, some of which manifest when

circulating CD4 counts are between 250 and 200/μl or less than 20% of the total number of lymphocytes. In general, this progressive decline in CD4 counts is associated with development of clinically evident infections caused by virulent organisms which are usually kept at bay by cell-mediated immune responses. However, tuberculosis may occur over a wide range of peripheral blood CD4 counts (Mukadi *et al.*, 1992; Ainslie *et al.*, 1992; Martin *et al.*, 1995). An increased risk of pneumonia due to encapsulated organisms such as *Streptococcus pneumoniae* or *Haemophilus influenzae* occurs presumably due to a secondary deficiency in humoral response. As CD4 count decreases to less than 200/μl, opportunistic pathogens such as *Pneumocystis carinii*, cytomegalovirus and atypical mycobacteria supervene to cause clinical significant infections. Parasitic diseases are endemic in parts of the tropics but there is no convincing evidence that their prevalence or incidence is increasing due to the HIV epidemic. Furthermore the high prevalence of parasitic infection in the tropics makes it hard to determine whether a particular infection arises because of HIV-induced immunodeficiency or not. Potentially invasive parasites which can affect the lung, *Entamoeba histolytica* and *Strongyloides stercoralis*, are closely associated with immunosuppression of cell-mediated immunity, yet these have not been reported as major clinical problems in HIV-infected patients from Africa despite the high prevalence of these two parasites in these populations (Lucas, 1988; Zumla and Croft, 1992).

Non-infectious complications

Table 2.2 lists the non-infectious complications of infection with HIV. Kaposi's sarcoma, B cell lymphoma and bronchogenic carcinoma have all been associated with HIV infection. Subsequent chapters in this book deal with the wide array of infectious and non-infectious pulmonary complications which cause enormous morbidity and mortality in HIV-infected individuals worldwide.

REFERENCES

Afessa, B., Greaves, W., Gren, W. *et al.* (1992) Autopsy findings in HIV-infected inner city patients. *J. AIDS*, **5**, 132–36.

Agostini, C., Poletti, V., Zambello, R. *et al.*, (1988) Phenotypical and functional analysis of bronchoalveolar lavage lymphocytes in patients with HIV infection. *Am. Rev. Respir. Dis.*, **138**, 1609–15.

Agostini, C., Zambello, R. and Trentin, L. (1990) Cytotoxic events taking place in the lungs of patients with HIV-1 infection. *Am. Rev. Respir. Dis.*, **142**, 516–20.

Agostino, C., Trentin, L., Zambello, R. *et al.* (1992) Release of granulocyte-macrophage colony-stimulating factor by alveolar macrophages in the lung of HIV-1 infected patients. *J. Immunol.*, **149**, 3379–85.

Agostino, C., Tentrin, L., Zambello, R. and Semenzato, G. (1993) HIV-1 and the lung: Infectivity, pathogenic mechanisms, cellular immune responses taking place in the lower respiratory tract. *Am. Rev. Respir. Dis.*, **147**, 1038–49.

Agostino, C. and Semenzato, G. (1994) Does analysis of bronchoalveolar lavage fluid provide a tool to monitor disease progression or to predict survival in patients with HIV-1 infection? *Thorax*, **49**, 848–51.

Ainslie, G.M., Solomon, J.A. and Bateman, E.D. (1992) Lymphocyte and lymphocyte subset numbers in blood and bronchoalveolar lavage and pleural fluid in various forms of human pulmonary tuberculosis at presentation and during recovery. *Thorax*, **47**, 513–18.

Ariyoshi, K., Harwood, E., Chiengsong-Popov, R. and Weber, J. (1992) Is clearance of HIV-1 viraemia at seroconversion mediated by neutralising antibodies? *Lancet*, **340**, 1257–8.

Ariyoshi, K., Cham, F., Berry, N. *et al.* (1995) HIV-2-specific CTL activity is inversely related to proviral load. *AIDS*, **9**, 555–59.

Autran, B., Sadat-Sowti, B., Hadida, F. *et al.* (1991) HIV-specific CTL against alveolar macrophages: specificities and down-regulation. *Res. Virol.*, **142**, 113–18.

Autran, B., Maynaud, C., Raphael, M. *et al.* (1988) Evidence for cytotoxic T lymphocyte alveolitis in human immunodeficiency virus infected patients. *AIDS*, **2**, 179–83.

Autran, B., Plata, F. and Debre, P. (1991) MHC-restricted cytotoxicity against HIV. *J. AIDS*, **4**, 361–68.

Beck, J.M. and Shellito, J. (1989) Effects of human immunodeficiency virus on pulmonary host defenses. *Sem. Respir. Infect.*, **4**, 75–84.

Bell, D.Y., Haseman, J.A., Spock, A. *et al.* (1981) Plasma proteins of the bronchoalveolar surface of lungs of smokers and non-smokers. *Am. Rev. Respir. Dis.*, **124**, 72–79.

Benson, B.J., Dobbs, L.G. and Ansfield, M.J. (1983) Immunopharmacology of lung surfactant, in *Immunopharmacology of the Lung: Lung Biology in Health and Disease* series (ed. H.H. Newball) Executive ed. C. LenFant. Marcel Dekker, New York.

Bernard, A., Gay-Belille, V., Amiot, M. *et al.* (1984) A novel human leucocyte differentiation antigen: monoclonal antibody anti-D44 defines a 28Kd molecule present on immature haematological cells and a subpopulation of mature T cells. *J. Immunol.*, **132**, 2345–53.

Biggar, R.J. (1986) The clinical features of HIV infection in Africa. *Lancet*, **ii**, 1453–54.

Bird, P. (1988) Structure and function of antibody molecules, in *B Lymphocytes in Human Disease*. (ed. G. Bird and J. Calvert) Oxford Medical Publishers, Oxford.

Bowen, D.L., Lane, H.C. and Fauci, A.S. (1985) Immunopathogenesis of the acquired immunodeficiency syndrome. *Ann. Intern. Med.*, **103**, 704–709.

Bonavida, B., Katz, J. and Gottleib, M. (1986) Mechanism of defective NK cell activity in patients with acquired immunodeficiency syndrome (AIDS) and AIDS related complex. *J. Immunol.*, **137**, 1157–63.

Borrow, P., Lewicki, H., Hahn, B.H. *et al.* (1994) Virus-specific CD8+ cytotoxic T-lymphocyte activity associated with control of viremia in primary human immunodeficiency virus type 1 infection. *J. Virol.*, **68**, 6103–10.

Brady, E.M., Margolis, M.L. and Korzeniowski, O.M. (1984) Pulmonary cryptosporidiosis in the acquired immunodeficiency syndrome. *JAMA*, **252**, 89–90.

Bretscher, P.A., Wei, G., Menon, J.N. and Bielefeldt-Ohmann, H. (1992) Establishment of stable, cell-mediated immunity that makes "susceptible" mice resistant to *Leishmania major*.

Science, **257**, 539–42.

Broliden, P.A., von Gegerfelt, A., Clapham, P. *et al.* (1992) Identification of human neuralization-inducing regions of the human immunodeficiency virus type-1 envelope glycoproteins. *Proc. Natl. Acad. Sci.*, **89**, 461–65.

Carmichael, A., Jin, X., Sissons, P. and Borysiewicz, L. (1993) Quantitative analysis of the human immunodeficiency virus type 1 (HIV-1)-specific cytotoxic T lymphocyte (CTL) response at different stages of HIV-1 infection: differential CTL response to HIV-1 and Epstein-Barr virus in late disease. *J. Exp. Med.*, **177**, 249–56.

Cameron, P.U., Mallal, S.A., French, M. and Dawkins, R.L. (1990) MHC genes influence the outcome of HIV infection. *Human Immunol.*, **29**, 282–95.

Chayt, K.J., Harper, M.E., Merselle, L.M. *et al.* (1986) Detection of HTLV-III RNA in lungs of patients with AIDS and pulmonary involvements. *JAMA.*, **256**, 2356.

Chaisson, R.E. (1989) Bacterial pneumonia in patients with HIV infection. *Sem. Respir. Infect.*, **4**, 133–38.

Clarke, J.R., Krishnan, V., Bennett, J. *et al.* (1990) Detection of HIV-1 in human lung macrophages using polymerase chain reaction. *AIDS*, **4**, 1133–36.

Clarke, J.R., Taylor, I.K., Flemming, J. *et al.* (1993) Relation of HIV-1 in bronchoalveolar lavage cells to abnormalities of lung function and to the presence of *Pneumocystis* pneumonia in HIV-1 seropositive patients. *Thorax*, **48**, 1222–26.

Clarke, J.R., Taylor, I.K., Fleming, J. *et al.* (1993) The epidemiology of HIV-1 infection of the lung in AIDS patients. *AIDS*, **7**, 555–60.

Clarke, J.R., Williamson, J.D. and Mitchell, D.M. (1993) The biological properties of HIV-1 isolates from the lung: relationship to disease progression. *Am. Rev. Respir. Dis.*, **147**, A1001.

Clarke, J.R., Coker, R. J., Harris, J.R. and Mitchell, D.M. (1994) Rapidly evolving HIV-1 infection in the lung of AIDS patients. *Lancet*, **344**, 679–80.

Clarke, J.R., Robinson, D.S., Coker, R.J. *et al.* (1995) Role of human immunodeficiency virus within the lung. *Thorax*, **50**, 56.

Clavell, F., Mansinho, K., Chamaret, S. *et al.* (1987) Human immunodeficiency virus type-2 infection associated with AIDS in West Africa. *New. Engl. J. Med.*, **316**, 1180–85.

Clerichi, M. and Shearer, G.M. (1993) A TH1-TH2 switch is a critical step in the aetiology of HIV infection. *Immunol. Today*, **14**, 107–11.

Clerici, M. and Berzofsky, J.A. (1994) Cellular immunity and cytokines in HIV infection. *AIDS*, **8**, S175–S182.

Clerici, M. and Shearer, G. (1994) The Th1-Th2 hypothesis of HIV infection: new insights. *Immunol. Today*, **15**, 575–581.

Clumeck, N., Sonnet, J., Taelman, H. and Mascart-Lemone, F. (1984) Acquired immunodeficiency syndrome in African patients. *New. Engl. J. Med.*, **310**, 492–97.

Coffin, J.M. (1995) HIV population dynamics *in vivo*: implications for genetic variation, pathogenesis, and therapy. *Science*, **267**, 483–89.

Cohn, D.L. (1991) Bacterial pneumonia in the HIV-infected patient. *Infect. Dis. Clin. N. Am.*, **5**:3, 485–504.

Cook, G.C. (1987) Opportunistic parasitic infections associated with the acquired immunodeficiency syndrome (AIDS): parasitology, clinical presentation, diagnosis and management. *Quart. J. Med.*, New Series, **65**:248, 967–83.

Cox, R.A., Anders, G.T. and Cappelli, P.J. (1990) Production of tumour necrosis factor alpha and interleukin-1 by alveolar macrophages from HIV-1 infected persons. *AIDS Res. Hum. Retroviruses.*, **6**, 431–41.

Crapo, J.D., Barry, B.E., Gehr, P. *et al.* (1982) Cell number and cell characteristics of the normal human lung. *Am. Rev. Respir. Dis.*, **126**, 332–37.

Creemers, P.C., Stark, D.E. and Boyko, W.J. (1985) Evaluation of natural killer activity in patients with persistent and generalized lymphadenopathy and acquired immunodeficiency syndrome. *Clin. Immunol. Immunopathol.*, **36**, 141–50.

Dolei, A., Serra, C., Arca, M.V. and Toniola, A. (1992) Acute HIV-1 infection of $CD4^+$ human lung fibroblasts. *AIDS*, **6**, 232–34.

Dean, W.C., Golden, J.A., Evans, L. *et al.* (1988) Human immunodeficiency virus recovery from bronchoalveolar lavage fluid in patients with AIDS. *Chest*, **93**, 1176–79.

Denis, M. and Ghadirian, E. (1994) Alveolar macrophages from subjects infected with HIV-1 express macrophage inflammatory protein-1 (MIP-1): contribution to the $CD8^+$ alveolitis. *Clin. Exp. Immunol.*, **96**, 187–92.

Denis, M. and Ghadirian, E. (1994) Dysregulation of IL-8, IL-10 and IL-12 release by alveolar macrophages from HIV-type-1 infected subjects. *AIDS Res. Hum. Retroviruses*, **10**, 12, 1619–27.

Donabedian, H. and Gallin, J.I. (1983) Neutrophil dysfunction and lung disease in *Immunopharmacology of the Lung*. (ed. H.H. Newball), Marcel Dekker, New York.

Donaldson, Y.K., Bell, J.E., Holmes, E.C. *et al.* (1994) *In vitro* distribution and cytopathology of variants of human immunodeficiency virus type 1 showing restricted sequence variability in the V3 loop. *J. Virol*, **68**, 59991–60005.

Ellis, M., Gupta, S., Galant, S. *et al.* (1988) Impaired neutrophil dysfunction in patients with AIDS or AIDS-related complex: a comprehensive evaluation. *J. Infect. Dis.*, **158**, 1268–76.

Ettensohn, D.B., Mayer, K.H., Kessimian, N. *et al.* (1985) Lymphoid interstitial pneumonitis in acquired immune deficiency syndrome-related complex. *Am. Rev. Respir. Dis.*, **131**, 956–60.

Fabio, G., Scorza, R., Lazzarin, A. *et al.* (1992) HLA-associated susceptibility to HIV-1 infection. *Clin. Exp. Immunol.*, **87**, 20–3.

Fantone, J.C. and Ward, P.A. (1983) Chemotactic Mechanisms in the Lung. 243–272, in *Immunopharmacology of the lung*. (ed. H.H. Newman), Marcel Dekker, New York.

Fauci, A.S. (1993) Immunopathogenesis of HIV infection. *J. AIDS*, **6**, 655–62.

Finkel, T.H., Tudor-Williams, G., Banda, N.K. *et al.*, (1995) Apoptosis occurs predominantly in bystander cells and not in productively infected cells of HIV- and SIV-infected lymph node. *Nature Medicine*, **1**, 2, 129–33.

Firestein, G.S., Roeder, W.D., Laxer, J.A. *et al.* (1988) A new murine CD4$^+$ T-cell subset with an unrestricted cytokine profile. *J. Immunol.* **143**, 518.

Gellene, R.A., Stover, D., Gebhard, D. *et al.* (1984) Analysis of cellular content and T lymphocyte subsets in bronchoalveolar lavage of the acquired immunodeficiency syndrome. *Clin. Res.*, **32**, 429A.

Gendelman, H.E., Baca, L.M., Husayni, H. *et al.* (1990) Macrophage-HIV interaction: viral isolation and target cell tropism. *AIDS*, **4**, 221–28.

Gold, J.W.M. (1988) Infectious complications in patients with HIV infection. *AIDS*, **2**, 327–34.

Gordon, S., Clarke, S., Greaves, D. and Doyle, A. (1995) Molecular immunobiology of macrophages: recent progress. *Curr. Opin. Immunol.*, **7**, 24–33.

Gottlieb, M.S. (1984) Pulmonary disease in the acquired immunodeficiency syndrome. *Chest*, **112**, 357–82.

Granger, D.L. and Hobbs, M.M. (1988) Do natural killer cells help protect us from disease caused by fungi? *Am. Rev. Respir. Dis.*, **138**, 510–11.

Graziosi, C., Pantaleo, G., Gantt, K.R. *et al.* (1994) Lack of evidence for the dichotomy of Th1 and Th2 predominance in HIV-infected individuals. *Science*, **265**, 248–52.

Grieco, M.H. and Chinoy-Acharya, P. (1985) Lymphocytic interstitial pneumonia associated with the acquired immunodeficiency syndrome. *Am. Rev. Respir. Dis.*, **131**, 952–55.

Gruters, R.A., Terpstra, F.G., DeJong, R. *et al.* (1990) Selective loss of T cell functions in different stages of HIV infection. *Eur. J. Immunol.*, **20**, 1039–45.

Guillon, J.-M., Autran, B., Denis, M. *et al.* (1988) Human immunodeficiency virus related lymphocytic alveolitis. *Chest*, **94**, 1264–69.

Gupta, S., Vayuvegula, B., Ruhling, M. and Thornton, M. (1987) Interleukin 1 and interleukin-2 production in the acquired immunodeficiency syndrome (AIDS) and AIDS-related complex. *J. Clin. Lab. Immunol.*, **22**, 113–16.

Heagy, W., Kelly, V.E., Storm, T.B. (1984) Decreased expression of human class II antigens on monocytes from patients with acquired immune deficiency syndrome. *J. Clin. Invest*, **74**, 2089–96.

Helbert, M.R., L'age-Stehr, J. and Mitchison, N.A. (1993) Antigen presentation, loss of immunological memory and AIDS. *Immunol. Today*, **14**, 340–43.

Hiserodt, J.C., Britvan, L.J. and Targan, S.R. (1982) Characterisation of the cytolytic mechanism of human nature killer cells (NK) lymphocyte: resolution into binding, programming and killer cell-independent steps. *J. Immunol.*, **129**, 1782–87.

Hill, A.V.S. (1992) HLA and infection. *J. Royal Coll. Phys.*, **26**, 11–16.

Hoffenbach, A., Langlade-Demoyen, P., Dadaglio, G. *et al.* (1989) Unusually high frequencies of HIV-specific cytotoxic T lymphocytes in humans. *J. Immunol.*, **142**, 452–57.

Holt, P.G., Schon-Hegrad, M.A., Phillips, M.J. and McMenamin, P.G. (1989) Ia-positive dendritic cells form a tightly meshed network within human airway epithelium. *Clin. Exp. Allergy*, **19**, 597–601.

Holt, P.G. (1993) Regulation of antigen presenting cell function(s) in lung and airway tissues. *Eur. Respir. J.*, **6**, 120–29.

Holt, P.G. (1986) Down-regulation of immune responses in lower respiratory tract: the role of alveolar macrophages. *Clin. Exp. Immunol.*, **63**, 261–70.

Hunninghake, G.W., Gadek, J.E., Kawanami, O. *et al.* (1979) Inflammatory and immune processes in the human lung in health and disease: Evaluation by bronchoalveolar lavage. *Am. J. Pathol.*, **97**, 149–206.

Isaksson, B., Albert, J., Chiodi, F. *et al.* (1988) AIDS two months after primary human immunodeficiency virus infection. *J. Infect. Dis.*, **158**, 866–68.

Itescu, S., Brancato, L.J., Buxbaum, J. *et al.* (1990) A diffuse infiltrative CD8 lymphocytosis syndrome in HIV infection: a host immune response associated with HLA-DR5. *Ann. Intern. Med.*, **112**, 3–10.

Itescu, S. and Winchester, R. (1992) Diffuse infiltrative lymphocytosis syndrome: a disorder occurring in HIV-1 infection that may present as a sicca syndrome. *Rheum. Dis. Clin. N. Am.*, **18**, 683–97.

Itescu, S., Mathur, W.U., Skovron, M.L. *et al.* (1992) HLA-B35 is associated with accelerated progression to AIDS. *J. AIDS*, **5**, 37–45.

Itescu, S., Dalton, J., Zhang, H.Z. and Winchester, R. (1993) Tissue infiltration in a CD8 lymphocytosis syndrome associated with human immunodeficiency virus-1 infection has the phenotypic appearance of an antigenically driven response. *J. Clin. Invest.*, **91**, 2216–25.

Jassoy, C., Harrer, T., Rosenthal, T. *et al.* (1993) Human immunodeficiency virus type 1-specific cytotoxic T lymphocytes release gamma interferon, tumour necrosis factor alpha (TNF-alpha), and TNF-beta when they encounter their target antigens. *J. Virol.*, **67**, 2844–52.

Jassoy, C., Johnson, R.P., Navia, B.A. *et al.* (1992) Detection of a vigorous HIV-1-specific cytotoxic T lymphocyte response in cerebrospinal fluid from infected persons with AIDS dementia complex. *J. Immunol.*, **149**, 3113–19.

Jenson, B.N., Lisse, I.M., Gerstoff, J. *et al.* (1991) Cellular profiles in bronchoalveolar lavage fluid of HIV-infected patients with pulmonary symptoms: relation to diagnosis and prognosis. *AIDS*, **5**, 527–33.

Jeffrey, A.A., Israel-Beit, D., Andrieu, J.M. *et al.* (1991) HIV isolation from pulmonary cells derived from bronchoalveolar lavage. *Clin. Exp. Immunol.*, **85**, 488–92.

Joly, P., Guillon, J.-M., Mayaud, C. *et al.* (1989) Cell-mediated suppression of HIV-specific cytotoxic T lymphocytes. *J. Immunol.*, **143**, 2193–98.

Just, J., Louie, L. and Norams, E. (1992) Genetic risk factors for perinatally acquired HIV-1 infection. *Paediatr. Perinatal Epidemiol.*, **6**, 215–24.

Kaslow, R.A., Duquesnoy, R., van Raden, M. *et al.* (1990) A1,Cw7,B8,DR3 HLA antigen combinations associated with rapid decline of T-helper lymphocytes in HIV-1 infection. *Lancet*, **i**, 927–30.

Kovacs, J.A., Baseler, M. and Dewar, R.J. (1995) Increases in CD4 T lymphocytes with intermittent course of IL-2 in patients with human immunodeficiency virus infection. *N. Engl. J. Med.*, **332**, 567–75.

Kaslow, R.A. and Mann, D.L. (1994) The role of the MHC in HIV infection – ever more complex? *J. Infect. Dis.*, **169**, 1332–3.

Kaslow, R.A., Duquesnoy, R., VanRaden, M. *et al.* (1990) A1, Cw7, B8, DR3 HLA antigen combination associated with rapid decline of T-helper lymphocytes in HIV-1 infection. A report from the Multicenter AIDS Cohort Study. *Lancet*, **335**, 927–30.

Klein, M.R., Keet, I.P., D'Amaro, J. *et al.* (1994) Associations between HLA frequencies and pathogenic features of human immunodeficiency virus type 1 infection in seroconverters from the Amsterdam cohort of homosexual men. *J. Infect. Dis.*, **169**, 1244–9.

Knight, S.C. and Macatonia, S.E. (1991) Effect of HIV on antigen presentation by dendritic cells and macrophages. *Res. Virol.*, **142**, 123–8.

Koup, R.A., Safrit, J.T., Cao, Y. *et al.* (1994) Temporal association of cellular immune responses with the initial control of viremia in primary human immunodeficiency virus type 1 syndrome. *J. Virol.*, **68**, 4650–5.

Lane, H.C., Masur, H., Edgar, L.C. *et al.* (1984) Abnormalities of B cell activation and immunoregulation in patients with the acquired immunodeficiency syndrome. *N. Engl. J. Med.*, **309**, 453–58.

Landay, A., Schade, S.Z., Takefman, D.M. *et al.* (1993) Detection of HIV-1 provirus in bronchoalveolar lavage cells by polymerase chain reaction. *J. AIDS*, **6**, 171–75.

Lazzarin, A., Uberti-Fobba, C., Galli, M. *et al.* (1986) Impairment of polymorphonuclear leukocyte function in patients with acquired immune deficiency syndrome and with lymphadenopathy syndrome. *Clin. Exp. Immunol.,* **65**, 105–11.

Lebargy, F., Branellee, A., Deforges, L. *et al.* (1994) HIV-1 in human alveolar macrophages from infected patients is latent in vivo but replicates after in vitro stimulation. *Am. J. Respir. Cell. Mol. Biol.,* **10**, 72–78.

Levy, J.A. (1993) Pathogenesis of human immunodeficiency virus infection. *Microbiol Rev.,* **57**, 1, 183–289.

Levy, J.A. (1995) HIV research: a need to focus on the right target. *Lancet,* **345**, 1619–21.

Lifson, A.R., Buchbinder, S.P., Sheppard, H.W. *et al.* (1991) Long-term human immunodeficiency virus infection in asymptomatic homosexual and bisexual men with normal CD4$^+$ lymphocyte counts: immunologic and virologic characteristics. *J. Infect. Dis.,* **163**, 959–65.

Lipschik, G.Y., Doerfler, M.E., Kovacs, J.A. *et al.* (1993) Leukotriene B4 and interleukin-8 in human immunodeficiency virus related pulmonary disease. *Chest,* **104**, 763–69.

Lipscomb, M.F., Bice, D.E., Lyons, R. *et al.* (1995) The regulation of pulmonary immunity. *Adv. Immunol.,* **59**, 369–455.

Louie, L.G., Newman, B. and King, M.C. (1991) Influence of host genotype on progression to AIDS among HIV-infected men. *J. AIDS,* **4**, 814–18.

Lucas, S. (1988) Aids in Africa – clinicopathological aspects. *Trans. Roy. Soc. Med.,* **82**, 801–2.

Mackewicz, C. and Levy, J.A. (1992) CD8$^+$ cell anti-HIV activity: nonlytic suppression of virus replication. *AIDS Res. Hum. Retroviruses,* **8**, 1039–50.

Maggi, E., Mazezetti, M., Ravina, A. *et al.* (1994) Ability of HIV to promote a Th1 to Th0 shift and replicate preferentially in Th2 and Th0 cells. *Science,* **265**, 244–48.

Mallal, S., Cameron, P.U., French, M.A.H. and Dawkins, R.L. (1990) MHC genes and HIV infection. *Lancet,* **335**, 1591–92.

Mann, D., Carrington, M., O'Donnell, M. *et al.* (1993) Selected HLA class I and II alleles are associated with relative rates of disease progression in HIV-infection. IX International Conference on AIDS and/IV STD World Congress, Berlin, June 1993: (Abstract WS-AO7-6).

Mann, D.L., Carrington, M.N. and Kroner, B.L. (1994) The human MHC and HIV-1 pathogenesis. *AIDS,* **8** (suppl. 1), S53–S60.

Martin, D.J., Sim, J.G., Sole, G.J. *et al.* (1995) CD4$^+$ lymphocyte count in African patients co-infected with human immunodeficiency virus and tuberculosis. *J. AIDS Hum. Retrovirol.,* **8**, 4, 386–91.

Marx, J. (1988) What T cells see and how they see it. *Science,* **242**, 863–65.

Marx, J. (1995) The T cell receptor begins to reveal its many facets. *Science,* **267**, 459–60.

Mason, G.R., Hashimoto, C.H., Dickman, P.S. *et al.* (1989) Prognostic implications of bronchoalveolar lavage neutropenia in patients with *Pneumocystis carinii* pneumonia and AIDS. *Am. Rev. Respir. Dis.,* **139**, 1336–42.

McDevitt, H.O. (1980) Regulation of the immune response by the major histocompatibility system. *N. Engl. J. Med.,* **303**, 514–17.

McMichael, A.J. and Walker, B.D. (1994) Cytotoxic T lymphocyte epitopes: implications for HIV vaccines. *AIDS,* **8** (suppl. 1), S155–73.

Miedema, F., Petit, A.J., Terpstra, F.G. *et al.* (1988) Immunological abnormalities in human immunodeficiency virus (HIV)-infected asymptomatic homosexual men. HIV affects the immune system before CD4$^+$ T helper cell depletion occurs. *J. Clin. Invest.,* **82**, 1908–14.

Miedema, F., Tersmette, M. and van Lier, R.A. (1990) AIDS pathogenesis: a dynamic interaction between HIV and the immune system. *Immunol. Today,* **11**, 293–7.

Meignan, M., Guillon, J.M., Denis, M. *et al.* (1990) Increased lung epithelial permeability in HIV-infected patients with isolated cytotoxic T-lymphocytic alveolitis. *Am. Rev. Respir. Dis.,* **141**, 1241–48.

Meduri, G.U. and Stein, D.S. (1992) Pulmonary manifestations of the acquired immunodeficiency syndrome. *Clin. Infect. Dis.,* **14**, 98–113.

Meltzer, M.S., Skillman, D.R., Hoover, D.L. *et al.* (1990) Macrophages and the human immunodeficiency virus. *Immunol. Today,* **11**, 217–23.

Meltzer, M.S., Kornbluth, R.S., Hansen, B. *et al.* (1993) HIV infection of the lung: role of virus-infected macrophages in the pathophysiology of pulmonary disease. *Chest,* **103**, 1035–85.

Meyaard, L., Schuitemaker, H. and Miedema, F. (1993) T-cell dysfunction in HIV infection: anergy due to defective antigen presenting cell function? *Immunol. Today,* **14**, 161–63.

Meyaard, L., Otto, S.A., Keet, I.P.M. *et al.* (1994) Changes in cytokine secretion patterns of CD4$^+$

T-cell clones in HIV infection. *Blood*, **12**, 4262–68.

Millar, A.B., Millar, R.F., Foley, N.M. *et al.* (1991) Production of TNFα by blood and lung mononuclear phagocytes from patients with human immunodeficiency virus related lung disease. *Am. J. Respir. Cell. Mol. Biol.*, **5**, 144–8.

Montaner, L.J. and Gordon, S. (1995) Th2 down-regulation of macrophage HIV-1 replication. *Nature*, **267**, 538–39.

Moore, S., Kenyan, C., Cryzan, S. *et al.* (1987) A comparison of bronchoalveolar lavage cells in organ recipients with AIDS. *Am. Rev. Respir. Dis.*, **135**, A169.

Mosmann, T.R. and Coffman, R.L. (1989) Heterogeneity of cytokine secretion patterns and functions of helper T cells. *Adv. Immunol.*, **46**, 111–47.

Mosmann, T.R., Schumacher, J.H., Street, N.F. *et al.* (1991) Diversity of cytokine synthesis and function of mouse CD4$^+$ T cells. *Immunol. Rev.*, **123**, 209–29.

Mosmann, T.R. (1994) Cytokine patterns during the progression to AIDS. *Science*, **265**, 193–4.

Moss, P.A.H., Rowland-Jones, S.L., Frodsham, P.M. *et al.* (1995) Persistent very high frequency of HIV-specific CTL in peripheral blood of infected donors. *Proc. Natl. Acad. Sci., USA*, **92**, 5773–7.

Mossman, T.R. (1994) Cytokine patterns during the progression to AIDS. *Science*, **265**, 193–4.

Mukadi, Y., Perriens, J.H., St. Louis, M.E. *et al.* (1993) Spectrum of immunodeficiency in HIV-1 infected patients with pulmonary tuberculosis in Zaire. *Lancet*, **342**, 143–6.

Murray, J.F., Felton, C.P., Goray, S.M. *et al.* (1984) Pulmonary complications of the acquired immunodeficiency syndrome: a report of a National Heart, Lung and Blood workshop. *N. Engl. J. Med.*, **310**, 1682–5.

Murray, J.F., Garray, S.M., Hopewell, P.C. *et al.* (1987) Pulmonary complications of the acquired immunodeficiency syndrome. An update. *Am. Rev. Respir. Dis.*, **135**, 504–9.

Murray, H.W., Gellere, R.A., Libby, D.M. *et al.* (1985) Activation of tissue macrophages from AIDS patients: *in vitro* response of AIDS alveolar macrophages to lymphokines and interferon-gamma. *J. Immunol.*, **5**, 2374–7.

Musher, D.M., Watson, D.A., Nickelson, D. *et al.* (1990) The effect of HIV infection on phagocytosis and killing of *Staphylococcal aureus* by human pulmonary macrophages. *Am. J. Med. Sci.*, **299**, 158–63.

Nathan, C.F. (1987) Secretory products of macrophages. *J. Clin. Invest.*, **79**, 319–26.

Niedt, G.W. and Schinella, R.A. (1985) Acquired immunodeficiency syndrome: clinicopathological study of 56 autopsies. *Arch. Pathol. Lab. Med.*, **109**, 727–34.

Nielson, H., Kharazmi, A. and Faber, V. (1986) Blood monocyte and neutrophil functions in the acquired immune deficiency syndrome. *Scand. J. Immunol.*, **24**, 291–96.

Nixon, D.F. and McMichael, A.J. (1991) Cytotoxic T cell recognition of HIV proteins and peptides. *AIDS*, **5**, 1049–59.

Ogden, D.M., Fischer, H.E. and Liu, F.J. (1988) Plasma fibronectin values in patients with the acquired immunodeficiency syndrome (AIDS) and AIDS-related complexes. *Am. J. Clin. Pathol.*, **90**, 293–6.

Orentas, R.J., Hildreth, J.E.K., Obah, E. *et al.* (1990) Induction of CD4$^+$ human cytolytic T cells specific for HIV-infected cells by a gp160 subunit vaccine. *Science*, **248**, 1234–37.

Osborn, L., Kunkel, S. and Nabel, G.J. (1989) Tumour necrosis factor-α and interleukin-1 stimulate the HIV enhancer by activation of the NFkB transcription factor. *Proc. Natl. Acad. Sci. USA*, **86**, 2336–40.

Pantaleo, G., DeMaria, A., Koenig, S. (1990) CD8$^+$ T lymphocytes of patients with AIDS maintain normal broad cytolytic function despite the loss of human immunodeficiency virus-specific cytotoxicity. *Proc. Natl. Acad. Sci. USA*, **87**, 4818–24.

Pantaleo, G., Graziosi, C. and Fauci, A. (1993) The immunopathogenesis of human immunodeficiency virus infection. *N. Engl. J. Med.*, **328**, 5, 327–35.

Pantaleo, G., Menzo, S., Vaccarezza, M. *et al.* (1994) Studies in subjects with long-term non-progressive HIV infection. *New Engl. J. Med.*, **332**, 209–16.

Pantaleo, G., Demarest, J.F., Soudeyns, H. *et al.* (1994) Major expansion of CD8$^+$ T cells with a predominant Vβ usage during primary immune response to HIV. *Nature*, **370**, 463–67.

Pantaleo, G. and Fauci, A.S. (1995a) Apoptosis in HIV infection. *Nature Medicine*, **2**, 1, 118–20.

Pantaleo, G. and Fauci, A.S. (1995b) New concepts in the pathogenesis of HIV infection. *Ann. Rev. Immunol.*, **13**, 487–512.

Plata, F., Autran, B., Martins, L.P. and Wain-

Hobson, S. (1987) Aids virus specific cytotoxic T lymphocytes in lung disorders. *Nature*, **328**, 348–51.

Plata, F., Garcia-Pons, F., Ryter, A. *et al.* (1990) HIV-1 infection of lung alveolar fibroblasts and macrophages in humans. *AIDS Res. Hum. Retroviruses*, **6**, 979–86.

Plummer, F. A. *et al.* (1993) IXth International Conference on AIDS, 1993.: Abstract WS-A07-3, 1993.

Paul, W.E. (1994) *Fundamental Immunology*. 3rd edn, Raven Press, New York.

Perlo, S., Jalowayski, A.A., Durand, C.M. and West, J.B. (1975) Distribution of red and white cells in the alveolar walls. *J. Appl. Physiol.*, **38**, 117–24.

Poli, G., Bressler, P., Kinter, A. *et al.* (1990) Interleukin-6 induces HIV expression in infected monocytic cells alone and in synergy with tumour necrosis factor-α by transcriptional and post-transcriptional mechanisms. *J. Exp. Med.*, **172**, 151–8.

Polmar, S.H. (1976) Immunodeficiency and pulmonary disease. Chapter 10 in *Immunologic and Infectious Reactions in the Lung*. (eds. C.H. Kirkpatrick and H.Y. Reynolds). Marcel Dekker, New York.

Polsky, B., Gold, J.W.M. and Whimbey, E. (1986) Bacterial pneumonia in patients with the acquired immunodeficiency syndrome. *Ann. Intern. Med.*, **404**, 38–41.

Proctor, R.A. (ed.) (1987) Fibronectin and the pathogenesis of infections. *Rev. Infect. Dis.*, **9**. Suppl 4, S317–S430.

Ratjen, F., Bredendiek, M., Zheng, L. *et al.* (1995) Lymphocyte subsets in bronchoalveolar lavage fluid of children without bronchopulmonary disease. *Am. J. Respir. Care Med.*, **152**, 174–8.

Rankin, J.A., Collman, R. and Daniele, R.P. (1988) Acquired immune deficiency syndrome and the lung. *Chest*, **94**, 1, 155–64.

Reynolds, H.Y. (1994) Normal and defective respiratory host defenses, in *Respiratory Infections, Diagnosis and Management*. Raven Press, New York, Chapter 1, pp. 1–34.

Reynolds, H.Y. (1987) Lung inflammation: normal host defense or a complication of some diseases? *Ann. Rev. Med.*, **38**, 295–323.

Reynolds, H.Y. (1988) Subject review: Immunoglobulin G and its function in the human respiratory tract. *Mayo. Clin. Proc.*, **63**, 161–74.

Robinson, B.W.S., Pinkston, P. and Crystal, R.G. (1984) NK cells are present in the normal human lung but are functionally impotent. *J. Clin. Invest.*, **74**, 942–54.

Robinson, D.S., Sun, Y., Taylor, I.K. *et al.* (1994) Evidence for a Th1-like bronchoalveolar T cell subset and predominance of IFNγ gene activation in pulmonary tuberculosis. *Am. Rev. Respir. Dis.*, **149**, 989–93.

Rollides, E., Mertins, S., Eddy, J. *et al.* (1990) Impairment of neutrophil chemotactic and bacterial function in children infected with HIV-type-1 and partial reversal after *in vitro* exposure to granulocyte-macrophage-colony stimulating factor. *J. Pediatr.*, **117**, 331–540.

Romagnani, S. (1991) Human Th1 and Th2 subsets: doubts no more. *Immunol. Today*, **12**, 256–8.

Rose, R.M., Krivine, A., Pikston, P. *et al.* (1991) Frequent identification of HIV-1 DNA in bronchoalveolar lavage cells obtained from individuals with the acquired immunodeficiency syndrome. *Am. Rev. Respir. Dis.*, **143**, 850–4.

Rosenberg, Z.F. and Fauci, A.S. (1989) The immunopathogenesis of HIV infection. *Adv. Immunol.*, **47**, 377–431.

Rowland-Jones, S. and McMichael, A. (1993) Cytotoxic T lymphocytes in HIV infection. *Sem. Virol.*, **4**, 83–94.

Rowland-Jones, S.L. and McMichael, A.J. (1995) Immune responses in HIV-exposed seronegatives: have they repelled the virus? *Curr. Opin. Immunol.*, **7**, 448–55.

Royer, H.D. and Reinherz, E.L. (1987) T lymphocytes: ontogeny, function and relevance to clinical disorders. *N. Engl. J. Med.*, **317**, 8, 1136–42.

Rubenstein, A., Marecki, R., Silverman, B. *et al.* (1986) Pulmonary disease in children with acquired immune deficiency syndrome and AIDS-related complex. *J. Pediatr.*, **108**, 498–503.

Sadat-Sowti, B., Parrot, A., Quint, L. *et al.* (1994) Alveolar CD8+ CD57+ lymphocytes in human immunodeficiency virus infection produce an inhibitor of cytotoxic functions. *Am. J. Respir. Crit. Care. Med.*, **149**, 927–80.

Sadat-Sowti, B., Debre, P., Idziorek, T. *et al.* (1991) A lectin-binding soluble factor released by CD8+ CD57+ lymphocytes from AIDS patients inhibits T cell cytotoxicity. *Eur. J. Immunol.*, **21**, 737–41.

Safrit, J.T., Andrews, C.A., Zhu, T. *et al.* (1994) Characterization of human immunodeficiency virus type 1-specific cytotoxic T lymphocyte clones isolated during acute seroconversion: recognition of autologous virus sequences within a conserved immunodominant epitope. *J. Exp. Med.*, **179**, 463–72.

Sahn, S.A. (1988) State of the art: the pleura. *Am. Rev. Respir. Dis.*, **138**, 184–234.

Salahuddin, S.Z., Rose, R.M. and Groopman, J.E. (1986) Human T-lymphotropic virus type III infection of human alveolar macrophages. *Blood*, **68**, 281–4.

Sahmoud, T., Laurian, Y., Gazengel, C. *et al.* (1993) Progression to AIDS in French haemophiliacs: association with HLA-B35. *AIDS*, **7**, 497–500.

Samle, S., Chernoff, D.N., Lenahan, G.A. *et al.* (1990) Elevated serum concentrations of IgE antibodies to environmental antigens in HIV-seropositive male homosexuals. *J. Allergy Clin. Immunol.*, **86**, 876–80.

Saukkonen, J.J., Kornfeld, H. and Berman, J.S. (1993) Expansion of a $CD8^+$ $CD28^-$ cell population in the blood and lung of HIV-positive patients. *J. AIDS*, **6**, 1194–204.

Scrager, L.K., Young, J.M., Fowler, M.G. *et al.* (1994) Long-term survivors of HIV-infection: definitions and research challenges. *AIDS*, **8**, Suppl 1, S95–S108.

Sei, S., Kleiner, D.E., Kopp, J.B. *et al.* Quantitative analysis of viral burden in tissues from adults and children with symptomatic human immunodeficiency virus type 1 infection assessed by polymerase chain reaction. *J. Infect. Dis.*, **170**, 325–33.

Shearer, G.M. and Clerici, M. (1992) T helper cell immune dysfunction in asymptomatic HIV-seropositive individuals: the role of Th1-Th2 cross regulation, in *Regulation and Functional Significance of T-cell Subsets* (ed. R.L. Coffman), Karger, Basel, 21–43.

Sheppard, H.W., Lang, W., Ascher, M.S. *et al.* (1993) The characterisation of non-progressors: long term HIV-1 infection with stable CD4 T cell levels. *AIDS*, **7**, 1159–66.

Sierra-Madero, J.G., Toosi, Z., Hom, D.L. *et al.* (1994) Relationship between load of virus in alveolar macrophages from human immunodeficiency virus-type-1 infected persons, production of cytokines and clinical status. *J. Infect. Dis.*, **169**, 18–27.

Sirriani, M.C., Tagliaferri, F. and Auti, F. (1990) Pathogenesis of the natural killer cell deficiency in AIDS. *Immunol. Today*, **11**, 81–2.

Smith, Rl, El Sadr, W.M. and Lewis, M.L. (1988) Correlation of bronchoalveolar lavage cell populations with clinical severity of *Pneumocystis carinii* pneumonia. *Chest*, **92**, 60–4.

Smith, P.D., Ohura, K., Masur, H. *et al.* (1984) Monocyte function in the acquired immune deficiency syndrome. *J. Clin. Invest.*, **74**, 2121–28.

Solal-Celigni, P., Couderc, L.J., Herman, D., *et al.* (1985) Lymphoid interstitial pneumonitis in AIDS-related complex. *Am. Rev. Respir. Dis.*, **131**, 956–60.

Sprag, R.G., Smith, R.M. and Harrell, J.H. (1987) Evidence of lung inflammation in patients with AIDS and *Pneumocystis carinii* pneumonia. *Am. Rev. Respir. Dis.*, **135**, A169.

Spry, C.J.F. (1988) Parasitic Diseases: Chapter 10 in *Eosinophils – A Comprehensive Review and Guide to the Scientific and Medical Literature*. Oxford University Press, Oxford.

Stanley, S.K. and Fauci, A.S. (1993) T cell homeostasis in HIV infection: Part of the solution or part of the problem? *J. AIDS*, **6**, 142–3.

Steel, C.M., Ludlam, C.A., Beatson, D. *et al.* (1988) HLA haplotype Al B8 DR3 as a risk factor for HIV-related disease. *Lancet*, **1**, 1185–8.

Stevenson, M. and Gendelman, H.E. (1994) Cellular and viral determinants that regulate HIV-1 infection in macrophages. *J. Leuco. Biol.*, **56**, 278–88.

Suffredini, A.F., Ognibene, F.P., Lack, E.E. *et al.* (1987) Non-specific interstitial pneumonitis: a common cause of pulmonary disease in AIDS. *Ann. Intern. Med.*, **107**, 7–13.

Tausk, F. and Gigli, I. (1990) The human C3b receptor: function and role in human disease. *J. Invest. Dermatol.*, **94**, 1451–5.

Teirstein, A.S. and Rosea, M.J. (1988) Lymphoid interstitial pneumonitis. *Clin. Chest Med.*, **94**, 195–6.

Trentin, L., Garbisi, S., Zambello, R. *et al.* (1992) Spontaneous production of interleukin-6 by alveolar macrophages from human immunodeficiency virus type-1-infected patients. *J. Infect. Dis.*, **166**, 731–37.

Twigg, H.L., Iwamoto, G.K. and Soliman, D.M. (1992) Role of cytokines in alveolar macrophage accessory cell function in HIV-infected individuals. *J. Immunol.*, **149**, 1462–69.

Twigg, H.L., Lipscomb, M.F., Yoffe, B. *et al.* (1989) Enhanced accessory cell function by alveolar macrophages from patients infected with the human immunodeficiency virus: potential role for depletion of CD4$^+$ cells in the lung. *Am. J. Respir. Cell. Mol. Biol.*, **1**, 391–400.

Twigg, H.L. and Soliman, D.M. (1994) Role of alveolar macrophage-T cell adherence in accessory cell function in human immunodeficiency virus-infected individuals. *Am. J. Respir. Cell. Mol. Biol.*, **11**, 138–46.

Twigg, H.L., Soliman, D.M. and Spain, B. (1994) Impaired alveolar macrophage accessory cell function and reduced incidence of lymphocytic alveolitis in HIV-infected patients who smoke. *AIDS*, **8**, 611–18.

Venet, A., Clarel, F., Israel-Biet, D. *et al.* (1985) Lung in acquired immunodeficiency syndrome: infections and immunological status assessed by bronchoalveolar lavage. *Bull. Eur. Physiopathol. Respir.*, **21**, 535–43.

Wain-Hobson, S. (1995) Virological mayhem. *Nature*, **373**, 102.

Walker, B.D., Chakrabarti, S., Moss, B. *et al.* (1987) HIV-specific cytotoxic T lymphocytes in seropositive individuals. *Nature*, **328**, 345–8.

Wallace, J.M., Barbers, R.G., Oishi, J.S. and Prince, H. (1984) Cellular and T-lymphocyte subpopulation profiles in bronchoalveolar lavage fluid from patients with AIDS and pneumonitis. *Am. Rev. Respir. Dis.*, **130**, 786–94.

Wasserman, K., Subklewe, M., Pothof, G. *et al.* (1994) Expression of surface markers on alveolar macrophages from symptomatic patients with HIV infection as detected by flow cytometry. *Chest*, **105**, 1324–34.

Weber, R., Kuster, H., Visvesvara, G.S. *et al.* (1993) Disseminated microsporidiosis due to *Encephalitozoon hellem*: Pulmonary colonization, microhaematuria, and mild conjunctivitis in a patient with AIDS. *Clin. Infect. Dis.*, **17**, 415–19.

Wei, X., Gosh, S.K., Taylor, M.E. *et al.* (1995) Viral dynamics in human immunodeficiency virus type-1 infection. *Nature*, **373**, 117–22.

Weiss, L., Haefner-Cavaillon, N., Laude, M. *et al.* (1989) HIV infection is associated with spontaneous production of interleukin-1 *in vivo* and with abnormal release of IL-1 *in vitro*. *AIDS*, **3**, 695–9.

White, D.A., Gellen, R.A. and Gupta, S. (1985) Pulmonary cell populations in the immunosuppressed patient. Bronchoalveolar lavage findings during episodes of pneumonitis. *Chest*, **88**, 352–9.

Young, K.R., Jnr., Rankin, J.A., Naegel, G.P. *et al.* (1985) Bronchoalveolar lavage cells and proteins in patients with acquired immunodeficiency syndrome. *Ann. Intern. Med.*, **103**, 522–33.

Zarling, J.M., Ledbetter, J.A., Sias, J. *et al.* (1990) HIV-infected humans but not chimpanzees, have circulating cytotoxic T lymphocytes that lyse uninfected CD4$^+$ cells. *J. Immunol.*, **144**, 2992–8.

Zheng, B.H. and Eden, F. (1993) Effect of corticosteroids on IL-1 and TNFα release by alveolar macrophages from patients with AIDS and *Pneumocystis carinii* pneumonia. *Chest*, **104**, 751–5.

Zumla, A., James, D.G. (1991) Lung immunology in the tropics in *Lung Disease in the Tropics*, (ed. O.P. Sharma) Marcel-Dekker, New York, pp. 1–65.

Zumla, A. and Croft, S. (1992) Chemotherapy and immunity of parasitic infections in AIDS patients. *Parasitology*, **105**, S93–S101.

Ziza, J.-M., Brun-Vizinet, F., Venet, A. *et al.* (1985) Lymphadenopathy-associated virus isolated from bronchoalveolar lavage fluid in AIDS-related complex with lymphoid interstitial pneumonitis. *N. Engl. J. Med.*, **313**, 183.

Peter Armstrong and Paul Dee

PULMONARY INFECTIONS IN AIDS

Chest imaging plays a key role in the management of patients with HIV infection. Usually, its role is to detect the presence of pulmonary disease and to assess its extent, severity and response to treatment, but sometimes chest imaging strongly suggests a specific diagnosis.

PNEUMOCYSTIS CARINII INFECTION

The chest radiograph is abnormal in over 90% of patients with *Pneumocystis carinii* pneumonia. The most common radiographic presentation is widespread opacity of the lung parenchyma. In the early stages there is a fine reticular pattern which subsequently progresses to confluent air space filling (Delorenzo *et al.*, 1987) (Figures 3.1 and 3.2). The apparent 'interstitial' radiographic pattern is illusory, since *P. caranii* pneumonia is pre-eminently an alveolar process (Weber, Askin and Dehner, 1977). Ordinarily, the radiographic consolidation is symmetrical without any zonal predominance, though perihilar predominance is a frequent feature. Air-bronchograms may be visible within the consolidated areas. *P. carinii* pneumonia may progress to a picture resembling adult respiratory distress syndrome with extensive whiteout of major portions of lung (Figure 3.3). Focal or asymmetric consolidation may occur (Figure 3.4). Patients receiving aerosol-ized pentamidine show an increased tendency to develop focal parenchymal opacity particularly in the upper lung zones (Figure 3.5). (Chaffey *et al.*, 1990; Edelstern and McCabe, 1990). It has been suggested that uneven distribution of aerosolized particles within the lung is responsible for this upper zone predominance (O'Doherty *et al.*, 1990).

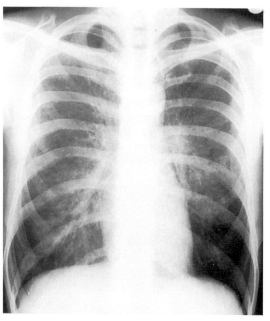

Fig. 3.1 *Pneumocystis carinii* pneumonia. A chest radiograph taken early in the course of the pneumonia shows hazy, confluent shadowing radiating from the hila into the lungs. The periphery of the lungs is relatively spared.

AIDS and Respiratory Medicine. Edited by A. Zumla, M.A. Johnson and R.F. Miller. Published in 1997 by Chapman & Hall, London. ISBN 0 412 60140 0

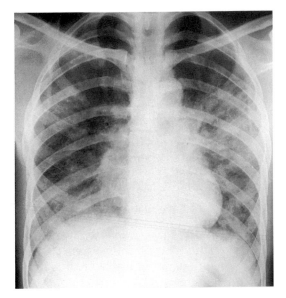

Fig. 3.2 In this case of *Pneumocystis carinii* pneumonia the consolidation is widespread, though still patchy. The shadowing involves both the perihilar and peripheral portions of the lungs. Note the absence of pleural effusions despite extensive pulmonary involvement.

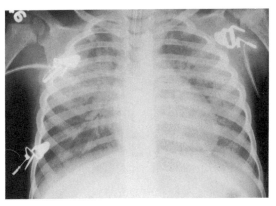

Fig. 3.3 *Pneumocystis carinii* pneumonia in a four-year-old child. The consolidation in this case is widespread and severe. Air bronchograms are visible. The pneumonia was so severe that endotracheal ventilation was required.

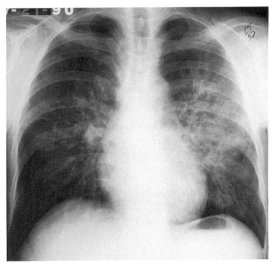

Fig. 3.4 *Pneumocystis carinii* pneumonia showing asymmetrical consolidation, substantially more severe on the left than the right. On both sides, however, the pulmonary shadowing radiates out from the hilar regions.

Pneumatoceles (thin-walled air spaces in the lung) have been noted with increasing frequency (Figure 3.6). Pneumothorax is a frequent complication (Beers, Sohn and Swartz, 1990). The pathophysiology of the pneumatoceles is debated but the balance of evidence suggests that aerosolized pentamidine is the provoking factor, possibly by causing a more indolent fibrotic or granulomatous response to *P. carinii* infection (Kuhlman *et al.*, 1989; Feuerstein *et al.*, 1990).

Other variant radiographic appearances of *P. carinii* pneumonia may be seen and often cause diagnostic confusion, notably isolated spherical pneumonia, cystic disease, bilateral apical disease resembling tuberculosis, pulmonary nodulation and cavitation (Milligan *et al.*, 1985; Delorenzo *et al.*, 1987; Bleiweiss *et al.*, 1988; Klein *et al.*, 1988).

Extrapulmonary dissemination may be present (Cohen and Stoeckle, 1991; Lubat *et al.*, 1990). Pleural effusions and hilar or mediastinal adenopathy are encountered from time to time (Horowitz *et al.*, 1993).

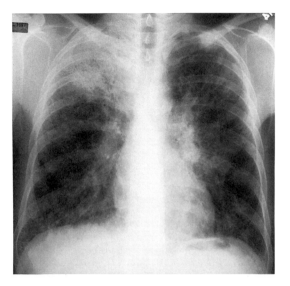

Fig. 3.5 *Pneumocystis carinii* pneumonia showing marked upper zone predominance. Prophylactic aerosolized pentamidine was used prior to the development of the pneumonia. The consolidation in this case shows an unusual degree of asymmetry.

Computed tomography may demonstrate amorphous cloud-like calcification in the involved nodes as well as calcifications in liver, spleen, kidneys and adrenals (Groskin, Massi and Randall, 1990; Radin *et al.*, 1990). Only rarely is such calcification dense enough to be visualized on plain radiographs.

A normal chest radiograph does not exclude *P. carinii* pneumonia. Gallium-67 scintigraphy (Reiss and Golden, 1990) is a highly sensitive method of determining the presence of diffuse opportunistic infections of the lungs. A normal Ga-67 scan excludes *P. carinii* pneumonia with 90% certainty. However, the specificity is low: many different opportunistic infections can result in positive scans. Other potential causes of a positive gallium-67 scan, such as lymphoma and lymphocytic interstitial pneumonia, are unlikely however to be associated with a normal chest radiograph. Thin section (high-resolution) CT scanning may show diffuse al-

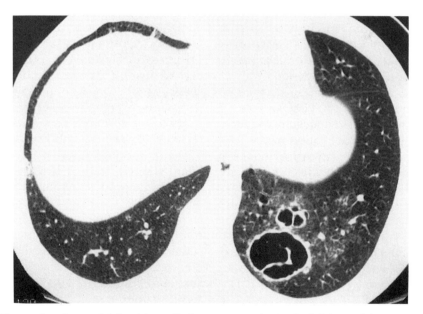

Fig. 3.6 CT scan showing multiple, thin-walled pneumatoceles in the left lower lobe in an AIDS patient with *Pneumocystis carinii* pneumonia (PCP). Such cysts are particularly well seen on CT scanning. Note the ground-glass shadowing, due to PCP, adjacent to the pneumatoceles.

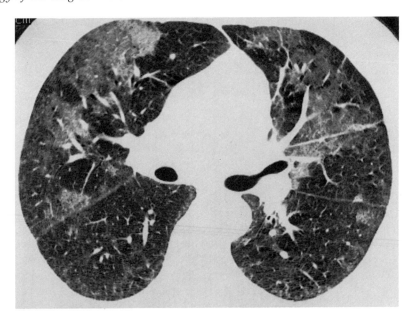

Fig. 3.7 High-resolution (thin-section) CT scan in a patient with *Pneumocystis carinii* pneumonia. This scan was taken at a time when the plain chest radiograph was still normal. The sign of patchy ground-glass shadowing is particularly well demonstrated in this example.

veolar opacity in patients due to *P. carinii* pneumonia in the presence of a normal or questionably abnormal chest radiograph (Figure 3.7) (Bergin *et al.*, 1990; Moskovic, Miller and Pearson, 1990; Richards *et al.*, 1996), but Ga-67 may be superior to CT in detecting the earliest changes of *P. carinii* pneumonia (Tumeh *et al.*, 1992). The CT scan shows ground-glass opacity in the early stages and denser consolidation in the later stages. The term 'ground-glass opacity' refers to a hazy density, through which the pulmonary vessels can be clearly identified. With denser consolidation the blood vessels and the consolidation are equally dense and the vessels cannot be separately distinguished. Air-bronchograms, a sign of air-space filling, are particularly well seen on CT scans.

TUBERCULOUS INFECTION

Tuberculosis in HIV-infected individuals is usually a reactivation of previously acquired

disease (Pitchenik and Rubinson, 1985). It particularly affects intravenous drug abusers in deprived inner cities and immigrants from third-world countries (Chaisson and Slutkin, 1989; Selwyn *et al.*, 1989). The tubercle bacillus, because of its innate virulence, strikes at levels of immunocompromise at which resistance to organisms such as *Pneumocystis carinii* or *Mycobacterium avium*-complex is retained (Barnes, Le and Davidson, 1993).

The pathophysiology of tuberculosis is often directly related to the degree of immunocompromise although it may occur across a wide spectrum of CD4 counts. With lesser degrees of immunocompromise, tuberculin reactivity may be retained and tuberculous pulmonary infection will usually be of the classical cavitary variety involving the apico-posterior segments of the upper lobes and the superior segments of the lower lobes. Lymphadenopathy is not a feature (Chaisson and Slutkin, 1989). However, as the immunocompromise worsens, the individual becomes anergic to tuberculin and the normal granulomatous response to the tubercle bacillus is dampened or even absent (Hill *et al.*, 1991). Lymphadenopathy is a prominent, even dominant, feature and dissemination throughout the lungs as well as systemic spread are both common (Pitchenik and Rubinson, 1985).

As the immunocompromise worsens hilar and mediastinal lymphadenopathy becomes more frequent. The incidence varies substantially in different series, varying from 33–82%, presumably reflecting differing patient population groups (Colebunders *et al.*, 1989; Suster *et al.*, 1986; Saks and Posner, 1992). Focal parenchymal consolidation and cavitation are less common in this group of patients, but there is a greater tendency to disseminated involvement of the lungs or miliary spread (Saks and Posner, 1992). The chest film may be normal even in the face of systemic dissemination of tuberculosis (Suster *et al.*, 1986; Hill *et al.*, 1991).

Tuberculous infection in severely immunocompromized patients is poorly contained. Not only is systemic dissemination common, but direct intrathoracic spread of disease is more pronounced than in classical tuberculosis. Thus, pleural effusions are common and infection may spread to mediastinal nodes and then involve the esophagus resulting in bronchoesophageal fistulae (de Silva, Stoopack and Raufmah, 1990; Hill *et al.*, 1991; Saks and Posner, 1992). Tuberculosis may involve the pericardium resulting in pericardial effusions. Endobronchial involvement is another feature of tuberculosis in AIDS (Wasser, Shaw and Talavera, 1988).

As previously indicated, worsening immunocompromise in HIV-infected individuals alters the clinical features of tuberculosis quite profoundly. It should be realized, however, that this alteration is a continuum without defined thresholds or borders. The trend is towards a form of tuberculosis akin to the conventional primary form of tuberculosis, with hilar and mediastinal lymphadenopathy becoming an increasingly dominant feature (Greenberg *et al.*, 1994). However, the virulent spread of tuberculosis both locally and systemically in HIV-infected individuals is quite unlike anything found in classical primary tuberculosis.

NON-TUBERCULOUS MYCOBACTERIAL INFECTIONS IN AIDS

Unlike infection with *M. tuberculosis*, the atypical mycobacteria infect patients with a severe degree of immunocompromise: in effect, established AIDS (Chaisson and Hopewell, 1989). In HIV-positive individuals, *M. avium-intracellulare* species (MAI) are the responsible organisms in at least 95% of cases of atypical mycobacteriosis. There is evidence to suggest that the main portal of entry for the organisms is the gastrointestinal tract (Horsburgh *et al.*, 1991). Enteritis caused by MAI is much more frequent than overt pulmonary disease, and mesenteric and retroperitoneal lympadenopathy is a frequent finding (Hawkins *et al.*, 1986). This is a radically different pattern from that seen with atypical mycobacterioses in non-immunocompromised individuals where primary pulmonary involvement is virutally the rule and disseminated disease is exceptionally rare.

An immuno-competent individual with atypical mycobacterial infection usually shows an indolent fibrocavitary process in the lung with no evidence of lymphadenopathy or dissemination. In some patients, especially in older women, there may be widespread bronchiectasis with peribronchial opacities, which are often nodular in shape (Hartman, Swensen and Williams, 1993). The AIDS patient on the other hand develops a fulminant form of disease with pronounced lymphadenopathy extending widely outside the thorax.

On chest radiographs, the dominant

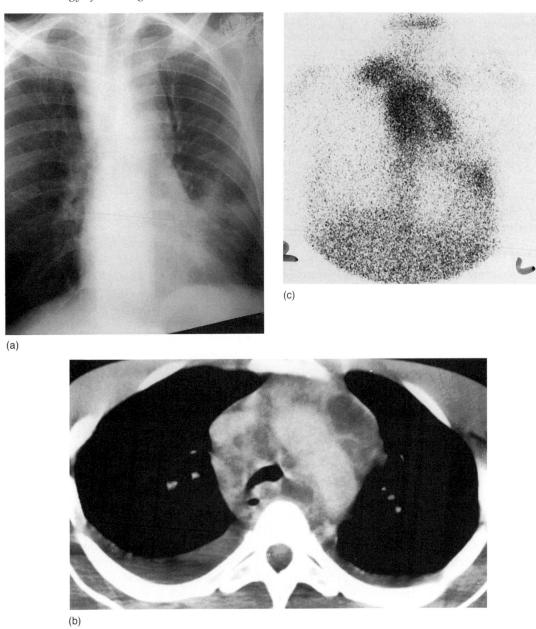

(c)

(a)

(b)

Fig. 3.8 Intrathoracic atypical mycobacterial infection disease in a patient with AIDS. (a) The plain chest radiograph shows a small focus of pulmonary infection in the lingula and massive enlargement of lymph nodes in the upper half of the mediastinum. (b) The CT scan (taken following intravenous contrast-enhancement) shows greatly enlarged lymph nodes in all mediastinal compartments. Note that the nodes show low density centres and enhancing rims, a sign that is rare in conditions other than mycobacterial infections. (c) The ^{67}Ga radionuclide scan shows increased activity in the enlarged lymph nodes and in the lingular consolidation.

feature is hilar and mediastinal lymphadenopathy (Figure 3.8). CT scans show that the lymph node enlargement frequently involves the abdomen, the neck and the axillae. The enlarged nodes often show a low attenuation center with a thin margin that enhances following intravenous contrast injection (Figure 3.8b) (Miller, 1994). The lungs may appear normal or may show non-specific focal consolidation. Some patients show more diffuse, nodular or patchy consolidation with or without associated lymphadenopathy (Tenholder, Moser and Tellis, 1988). Pleural involvement is uncommon. Bronchiectasis may be seen but much less frequently than in non-immunocompromised patients with diffuse disease (Hartman, Swensen and Williams, 1993). Cavitation is rare. Endobronchial lesions have been identified in a few patients, presumably incriminating the airways as a portal of entry in these patients (Packer, Cesanio and Williams, 1988; Mehle *et al.*, 1989).

NON-TUBERCULOUS BACTERIAL INFECTIONS

The usual organisms responsible for community-acquired pneumonia in HIV-infected individuals are encapsulated organisms such as *Streptococcus pneumoniae*, *Haemophilus influenzae*, and *Moraxella* species. In other words, the same organisms as in the population at large, but with four times the prevalence. The radiographic findings correspond to those found in the non-HIV infected population, namely single or multiple segmental or lobar areas of consolidation. There is a greater tendency for HIV-infected individuals to show multilobar involvement. Pleural effusions frequently accompany the pneumonia and on occasion may progress to empyema. In general, the clinical onset of bacterial pneumonia is more abrupt and the leukocyte count higher. Some

20% of AIDS patients with bacterial infection show widespread pulmonary shadowing indistinguishable from *P. carinii* pneumonia (Amorosa *et al.*, 1990). Alternatively, *P. carinii* pneumonia may co-exist with bacterial pneumonia.

VIRAL PULMONARY INFECTION

The prevailing consensus is that viral infections are an infrequent cause of pneumonia in HIV-infected persons. Cytomegalovirus is the commonest virus to be incriminated. On chest radiographs, viral pneumonias may cause a diffuse parenchymal opacity, often indistinguishable from non-cardiogenic edema (Murray and Mills, 1990), or focal, sometimes rounded, consolidation. The shadowing may be coarse, giving a reticular or even a slightly reticulonodular character. Pleural effusions and lymphadenopathy are not seen. CT scanning may show ground-glass attenuation or dense consolidation, which may appear similar to pulmonary nodules, as well as bronchiectasis and interstitial reticular shadowing (McGuiness *et al.*, 1994). Gallium-67 citrate scanning in CMV infection may be helpful if, in addition to diffuse low grade uptake in the lungs, there is uptake in the eyes, adrenals and esophagus and persistent uptake in the colon (Vanarthos *et al.*, 1992).

HIGHER BACTERIA AND FUNGI

Although *Nocardia asteroides* may infect otherwise healthy individuals, infection is most frequent in immunosuppressed patients. The appearances in the chest are varied. The series of Feigin (1986) and Kramer and Uttamchandani (1990) each included 21 patients and are broadly comparable in their findings, even though Feigin's series did not include AIDS patients. Lobar or multilobar consolidations, often extensive, are the commonest manifestation. Solitary or multiple, irregular, ill-defined, mass-like densities are also frequent. Cavitation and pleural effusions occur in one-third to two-thirds of cases. The pulmonary involvement may be more diffuse with nodular or reticulonodular opacities. Hilar and mediastinal lymph node enlargement occurs in up to one-third of patients. Progression of the disease is rapid and the mortality in AIDS patients is high.

Candida organisms, usually *C. albicans*, are a frequent finding on mucous membranes in AIDS patients. The mere recovery of the organism is, therefore, not sufficient to incriminate it as an infective agent in patients with pneumonia: tissue invasion should be demonstrated histologically. Pulmonary candidiasis, when it occurs, is a late manifestation of HIV infection and, therefore, may be submerged by AIDS-related malignancies and other infections.

Cryptococcosis is the most common fungal infection in AIDS patients in the United States. Cryptococcal meningitis is more common than cryptococcal pneumonia, but the two conditions so frequently coexist that the presence of an associated meningitis is a strong clue to the cause of pneumonia (Chuck and Sande, 1989). Cryptococcal pneumonia in immunocompromised patients, particularly AIDS patients, differs from the pneumonia found in nonimmunocompromised patients in that the infection is less contained (Chechani and Kamholz, 1990; Miller, 1990). Thus, nodular parenchymal consolidations are less common; the usual finding is a more ill-defined focal or diffuse air space filling process (Figure 3.9). Cavitation and pleural effusions are features of cryptococcal pneumonia in AIDS patients, and hilar and mediastinal adenopathy is a frequent finding. Miliary cryptococcosis has been described in an AIDS patient (Douketis and Kesten, 1993).

Histoplasmosis is an extremely common infective condition in large areas of the United States, although almost unknown in

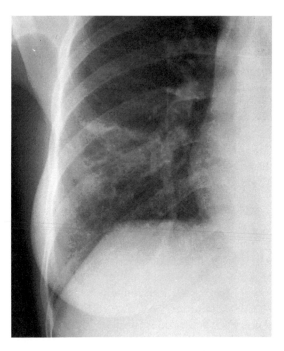

Fig. 3.9 *Cryptococcus neoformans* infection of the lung. The plain chest radiograph shows ill-defined consolidation in the right lower zone.

Europe. It is surprising, given its prevalence, that it is not a more common opportunistic infection in AIDS patients. Histoplasmosis in AIDS patients is almost invariably a widely disseminated process involving bone marrow, liver, spleen, adrenals, lungs, brain and meninges (Wheat *et al.*, 1990). Even in the presence of established infection the chest radiograph is normal in some 40–50% of cases (Wheat *et al.*, 1990; Conces *et al.*, 1993). The chest radiographs, when abnormal, show evidence of diffuse disease ranging from miliary nodulation through coarser reticulonodular opacities to more extensive air space opacification. Pleural effusions are uncommon and lymphadenopathy, ordinarily a striking feature of histoplasmosis, is also very uncommon. Wheat and colleagues (Wheat *et al.*, 1990) found lymphadenopathy in only 3–5% of their cases and in cases from the literature.

Coccidioidomycosis is another relatively common fungal infection in AIDS patients in the US, with an incidence approximately one-fifth that of histoplasmosis. Only 30% of patients have chest radiographic abnormalities (Fish *et al.*, 1990): usually diffuse shadowing ranging from miliary nodulation to reticulonodular opacities (Bronnimann *et al.*, 1987). Isolated cavitary masses may be seen. Lymphadenopathy is uncommon and pleural effusions are not a feature.

Pulmonary aspergillosis is a relatively rare complication of AIDS (Denning *et al.*, 1991). The *Aspergillus* species of fungi, most commonly *A. fumigatus*, may cause pneumonia in AIDS patients, usually in the terminal stages of the disease.

Blastomycosis is a rare cause of pulmonary disease in AIDS patients. Blastomycosis frequently involves the skin and biopsy of a skin lesion can provide the diagnosis. Blastomycosis may be disseminated, particularly to the central nervous system, and in these cases diffuse miliary or reticulonodular shadowing may be seen. Otherwise lobar consolidation or multiple focal opacities are the main features. Cavitation may occur and pleural effusions and lymphadenopathy are described.

PROTOZOAL PULMONARY INFECTION

Toxoplasma gondii, *Cryptosporidium* spp and *Strongyloides stercoralis* infection may be encountered in HIV-infected individuals (Goodman and Schnapp, 1992; Makris *et al.*, 1993). These parasites ordinarily involve extrapulmonary sites, most commonly the brain and meninges or the gastrointestinal tract. Pulmonary involvement ascribed to these parasites is very rare and the diagnosis inevitably relies on identifying parasites in lung tissue. In the limited number of cases described, the pulmonary opacity has tended to be diffuse and variably described as alveolar, nodular or interstitial in character.

INTRATHORACIC NEOPLASMS IN AIDS

KAPOSI'S SARCOMA

The lungs have been found to be involved in some 20–40% of patients with disseminated Kaposi's sarcoma diagnosed during life (Garay *et al.*, 1987), but the incidence at autopsy may be much higher (Lemlick, Schwam and Lebwohl, 1987). Pulmonary Kaposi's sarcoma appears to be rare in the absence of cutaneous involvement (Lemlick, Schwam and Lebwohl, 1987). Involvement of the tracheobronchial tree is relatively frequent but parenchymal involvement may occur in the absence of endobronchial disease.

Pulmonary Kaposi's sarcoma is frequently associated with pulmonary infections. There is, therefore, a variable pattern of disease shown on chest radiographs. The chest radiograph may be normal in the presence of Kaposi's sarcoma diagnosed by biopsy or autopsy (Davis *et al.*, 1987; Miller *et al.*, 1992).

In focal Kaposi's sarcoma the resultant segmental or lobar opacities are usually due to the tumor itself although endobronchial Kaposi's sarcoma may result in atelectasis or post-obstructive pneumonia (Naidich *et al.*, 1989). Radiographically, widespread disease is the most frequent pattern and there is a pronounced tendency to perihilar predominance reflecting a bronchocentric distribution of the lesions (Davis *et al.*, 1987; Sivit, Schwartz and Rockoff, 1987) (Figure 3.10). The pattern of involvement on chest radiographs may be broadly divided into linear interstitial shadowing and nodular or coalescing mass-like shadowing. The linear interstitial pattern reflects infiltration of the pulmonary parenchyma, not too dissimilar to lymphangitis carcinomatosa. The nodular or mass-like pattern is produced by widespread often coalescing foci of tumour. A characteristic feature of the radiographic patterns is that the appearances do not show day-to-day changes as do pulmonary edema or oppor-

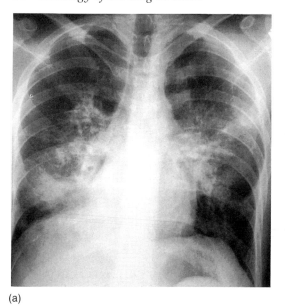
(a)

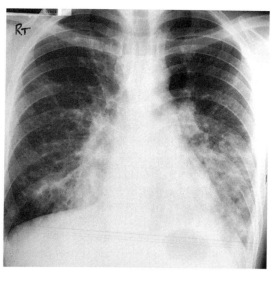
(b)

Fig. 3.10 Two patients with Kaposi's sarcoma of the lung. Both patients show a typical mixture of consolidation and mass-like or nodular lesions. The perihilar (bronchocentric) distribution is more obvious in (a) than (b).

tunistic infections. Pleural involvement is frequent: pleural effusions are commonly bilateral and may on occasion be large (Figure 3.11). Hilar and mediastinal adenopathy is seen in 25–60% of cases in some series.

Computed tomography may strongly suggest the diagnosis of pulmonary Kaposi's sarcoma (Naidich *et al.*, 1989) in those cases when the lesions show a clear peribronchial and perivascular distribution (Figure 3.12). The pulmonary densities may be either distinctly nodular or may merge into conglomerate densities. High CT attenuation of the lesions after contrast enhancement has been described in a large proportion of cases (Herts *et al.*, 1992), presumably reflecting the pronounced hypervascularity of Kaposi lesions. Wolff, Kuhlman and Fishmann (1993) noted CT evidence of extrapulmonary disease, lytic bone lesions or soft tissue masses in the chest wall in more than 50% of patients with Kaposi's sarcoma.

Radionuclide studies can be helpful al-

though it is not certain whether they are cost effective. Thallium-201 chloride scanning either alone or in sequence with gallium 67-citrate scanning can help separate Kaposi's sarcoma from neoplastic or inflammatory processes (Lee *et al.*, 1991). Kaposi's sarcoma along with a variety of neoplasms is thallium avid, whereas inflammatory processes are not. Gallium scanning can help distinguish Kaposi's sarcoma from lymphoma: lymphoma shows avid uptake of gallium, whereas Kaposi's sarcoma shows little or no uptake.

INTRATHORACIC LYMPHOMA IN AIDS

Pulmonary lymphoma associated with HIV infection is usually a high-grade B cell non Hodgkin's lymphoma (Ahmed *et al.*, 1987; Lowenthal *et al.*, 1988; Kaplan *et al.*, 1989). Non Hodgkin's lymphoma in an individual infected with HIV is accepted as a diagnostic criterion for AIDS. AIDS-related non

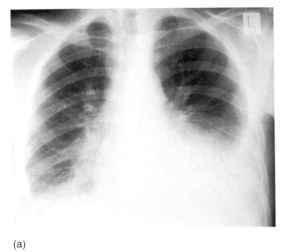

(a)

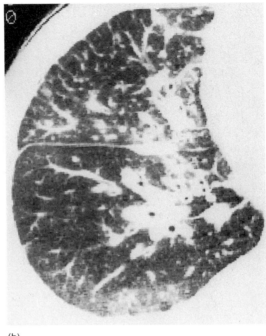

(b)

Fig. 3.11 Kaposi's sarcoma. (a) Plain chest radiograph showing bilateral pleural effusions. The pulmonary lesions cannot be identified on this film. (b) CT scan in the same patient. This section through the right middle and lower lobes shows numerous nodular opacities surrounding the more centrally located airways and thickening of the interlobular septa at the extreme periphery of the middle lobe.

Hodgkin's lymphoma usually presents with widely disseminated disease and virtually all cases show extranodal disease. AIDS-related lymphoma often occurs late in the course of AIDS and most patients die as a result of opportunistic infections rather than as a direct result of their lymphoma (Knowles *et al.*, 1988; Lowenthal *et al.*, 1988). The incidence of pulmonary involvement by lymphoma in HIV-infected individuals has varied widely from zero to 30%. Primary pulmonary involvement is very uncommon (Poelzleitner *et al.*, 1989).

The main radiographic findings in AIDS-related lymphoma are pleural effusions (usually bilateral), lymphadenopathy and pleural or intrapulmonary masses, all of which may occur together or in isola-tion (Blunt and Padley, 1995). Pulmonary parenchymal disease may be either focal or diffuse. Focal lung disease is usually nodular or mass-like and the lesions may be single or multiple (Poelzleitner *et al.*, 1989; Sider *et al.*, 1989; Blunt and Padley, 1995). The pulmonary masses are frequently peripherally located and may show cavitation (Blunt and Padley, 1995). A noteworthy feature is that the mediastinal lymph nodes are frequently normal in size in patients with AIDS-related lymphoma of the lung or pleura (Sider *et al.*, 1989; Blunt and Padley, 1995).

Diffuse shadowing may show an interstitial or alveolar pattern. The radiographic and CT findings can, therefore, readily be confused with opportunistic infection or with Kaposi's sarcoma.

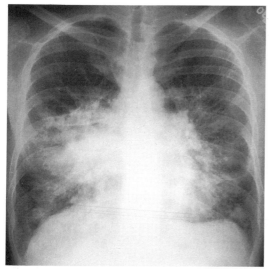

(a)

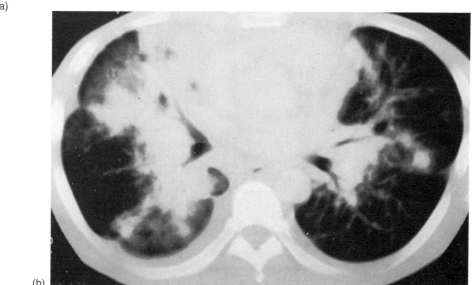

(b)

Fig. 3.12 Kaposi's sarcoma. (a) Plain chest radiograph. (b) CT scan. The bronchocentric distribution of disease is well shown in this patient. The CT scan shows that the opacities are predominantly due to nodular-shaped masses centered on the major airways.

Lymphoproliferative disorders of the lung

Individuals infected with HIV may develop lymphocytic and monocytic infiltration of the airways and pulmonary parenchyma. The process appears unrelated to any infective agent, except possibly to HIV itself (Travis, Fox and Devaney, 1992) or more remotely to the Epstein-Barr virus (Fackler *et al.*, 1985). The lymphoproliferative disorders can be subdivided into lymphocytic interstitial pneumonitis (LIP), non-specific interstitial pneumonitis (NSIP), lymphocytic alveolitis, lymphocytic bronchiolitis, and pulmonary lymphoid hyperplasia, although there is overlap between these conditions.

Lymphocytic interstitial pneumonitis (LIP)

HIV infection is associated with a striking increase in the incidence of LIP, particularly in children, and the occurrence of LIP in an HIV-infected individual under 13 years of age is an accepted diagnostic criterion for AIDS (Centers for Disease Control, 1987).

In LIP, there is infiltration of the peribronchial and interstitial tissues of the lung by mature polyclonal lymphocytes, plasma cells, and immunoblasts (Kradin and Mark, 1983). The pleura, the blood vessels, and the endobronchial tissues are spared. Although LIP is essentially a diffuse interstitial process, nodular masses resulting from coalescence of areas of alveolar air space obliteration may develop and may, on occasion, be quite large.

Oldham *et al.* (1989) subdivided the radiographic findings seen in LIP into 3 basic types: diffuse fine reticular infiltrates; diffuse reticulonodular infiltrates with nodules up to 2 cm in diameter; and diffuse reticulonodular infiltrates with larger patchy areas of air space consolidation (Figure 3.13). All three types show a pronounced tendency to basal predominance (Morris *et al.*, 1987; Lin *et al.*, 1988). Pleural effusions are not a feature. If enlarged lymph nodes are present an alternative diagnosis such as lymphoma or tuberculosis should be considered. A small number of patients have been noted on CT to have bronchiectasis in association with LIP (Amorosa *et al.*, 1992; Berdon *et al.*, 1993). Lymphocytic interstitial pneumonia tends to wane as the patient deteriorates and more sinister complications develop. Some children may have peripheral lymphadenopathy and salivary gland enlargement. Gallium scanning may show increased uptake in the salivary glands, as well as the lungs, indicating a parallel lymphoproliferative process (Ganz *et al.*, 1988; Rosenberg, Joffe and Itescu, 1992; Schif, Kabat and Kamoni, 1987). Other potential causes of increased gallium uptake in the lungs, such as *Pneumocystis carinii* pneumonia or lymphoma, do not show increased activity in the salivary glands.

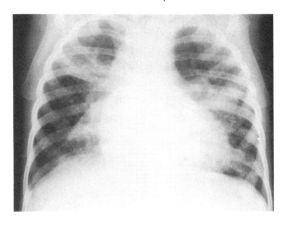

Fig. 3.13 Lymphocytic interstitial pneumonitis in a three-year-old child with AIDS. The widespread reticulo-nodular shadows which have coalesced to form confluent shadows in several areas of the lung are well shown.

Non-specific interstitial pneumonitis (NSIP)

Non-specific interstitial pneumonitis is a form of interstitial pneumonitis resembling drug-induced diffuse alveolar damage. In HIV-infected individuals, no causal agent has been identified, although there has been speculation that HIV itself may be responsible (White and Matthay, 1989; Travis, Fox and Devaney, 1992). It is evident that NSIP can be very difficult to distinguish from LIP clinically, histologically and radiologically. The chest radiographs may be normal but some patients show diffuse reticular or reticulo-nodular shadowing (Simmons *et al.*, 1987). Gallium scans are usually normal or only weakly positive reflecting, perhaps, the relatively mild mononuclear cell infiltration (Ognibene *et al.*, 1988).

Lymphocytic alveolitis, lymphocytic bronchiolitis, and pulmonary lymphoid hyperplasia

Hyperplasia of normal lymphoid foci in the bronchial tree, so-called bronchial-associated lymphoid tissue, may result in mild obstructive lung disease associated with generalized lymphadenopathy. The hyperplastic lymphoid tissue may reach the threshold of radiographic visibility as fine nodular or miliary shadowing with basal predominance (Ettensohn *et al.*, 1988; Guillon *et al.*, 1988).

REFERENCES

Ahmed, T., Wormser, G.P., Stahl, R.E. *et al.* (1987) Malignant lymphomas in a population at risk for acquired immune deficiency syndrome. *Cancer*, **60**, 719–23.

Amorosa, J.K., Miller, R.W., Laraya-Cuasay, L. *et al.* (1992) Bronchiectasis in children with lymphocytic interstitial pneumonia and acquired immune deficiency syndrome. Plain film and CT observations. *Pediatric Radiology*, **22**, 603–7.

Amorosa, J. K., Nahass, R.G., Nosher, J.L. *et al.*, (1990) Radiologic distinction of pyogenic pulmonary infection from *Pneumocystis carinii* pneumonia in AIDS patients. *Radiology*, **175**, 721–4.

Barnes, P.F., Le, H.Q. and Davidson, P.T. (1993) Tuberculosis in patients with HIV infection. *Medical Clinics of North America*, **77**, 1369–90.

Beers, M.F., Sohn, M. and Swartz, M. (1990) Recurrent pneumothorax in AIDS patients with pneumocystis pneumonia. *Chest*, **98**, 266–70.

Berdon, W.E., Mellins, R.B., Abramson, S.J. *et al.* (1993) Pediatric HIV infection in its second decade – the pediatric HIV infection in its second decade – the changing pattern of lung involvement. Clinical, plain film and computed tomographic findings. *Radiologic Clinics of North America*, **31**, 453–63.

Bergin, C.J., Wrath, R.L., Berry, G.J. *et al.* (1990) *Pneumocystis carinii* pneumonia: CT and HRCT observations. *Journal of Computer Assisted Tomography*, **14**, 756–9.

Bleiweiss, I. J., Jagirdar, J. S., Klein, M. J. *et al.* (1988) Granulomatous *Pneumocystis carinii* pneumonia in three patients with the acquired immunodeficiency syndrome. *Chest*, **94**, 580–3.

Blunt, D.M. and Padley, S.P.G. (1995) Radiographic manifestation of AIDS-related lymphoma of the thorax. *Clinical Radiology*, **50**, 607–612.

Bronnimann, D.A., Adem, R.D., Galgiani, J.N. *et al.* (1987) Coccidioidomycosis in the acquired immunodeficiency syndrome. *Annals of Internal Medicine*, **106**, 372–9.

Centers for Disease Control. (1987) Revision of the case definition of acquired immunodeficiency syndrome – United States. *MMWR*, **36**, 1–15.

Chaffey, M.H., Klein, J.S., Gamsu, G. *et al.* (1990) Radiographic distribution of *Pneumocystis carinii* pneumonia in patients with AIDS treated with prophylactic inhaled pentamidine. *Radiology*, **175**, 715–9.

Chaisson, R.E. and Hopewell P.C. (1989) Mycobacteria and AIDS mortality. *American Review of Respiratory Disease*, **139**, 1–3.

Chaisson, R.E. and Slutkin, G. (1989) AIDS commentary: Tuberculosis and human immunodeficiency virus infection. *Journal of Infectious Diseases*, **159**, 96–100.

Chechani, V. and Kamholz, S.L. (1990) Pulmonary manifestations of disseminated cryptococcosis in patients with AIDS. *Chest*, **98**, 1060–6.

Chuck, S.L. and Sande, M.A. (1989) Infections with *Cryptococcus neoformans* in the acquired immunodeficiency syndrome. *New England Journal of Medicine*, **321**, 794–9.

Cohen, O.J. and Stoeckle, M.Y. (1991) Extrapulmonary *Pneumocystis carinii* infections in the acquired immunodeficiency syndrome. *Archives of Internal Medicine*, **151**, 1205–14.

Colebunders, R. L., Ryder, R. W., Nzilambi, N. *et al.* (1989) HIV infection in patients with tuberculosis in Kinshasa, Zaire. *American Review of Respiratory Disease*, **139**, 1082–5.

Conces, D.J., Stockberger, S.M., Tarber, R.D. *et al.* (1993) Disseminated histoplasmosis in AIDS: Findings on chest radiographs. *American Journal of Radiology*, **160**, 15–9.

Davis, S.D., Henschke, C.I., Chamides, B.K. *et al.* (1987) Intrathoracic Kaposi's sarcoma in AIDS patients: radiographic–pathologic correlation. *Radiology*, **163**, 495–500.

Delorenzo, L.J., Huang, C.T., Maguire, G.P. *et al.* (1987) Roentgenographic patterns of *Pneumocystis carinii* pneumonia in 104 patients with AIDS. *Chest*, **91**, 323–7.

Denning, D.W., Follansbee, S.E., Scolaro, M. *et al.* (1991) Pulmonary aspergillosis in the acquired immunodeficiency syndrome. *New England Journal of Medicine*, **324**, 654–62.

de Silva, R., Stoopack, P.M. and Raufman, J.P. (1990) Esophageal fistulas associated with mycobacterial infection in patients at risk for AIDS. *Radiology*, **174**, 449–53.

Douketis, J.D and Kesten, S. (1993) Miliary pulmonary cryptococcosis in a patient with the acquired immunodeficiency syndrome. *Thorax*, **48**, 402–3.

Edelstern, H. and McCabe, R.E. (1990) Atypical presentations of *Pneumocystis carinii* pneumonia in patients receiving inhaled pentamidine prophylaxis. *Chest*, **98**, 1366–9.

Ettensohn, D.B., Mayer, K.H., Kessimian, N. *et al.* (1988) Lymphocytic bronchiolitis associated with HIV infection. *Chest*, **93**, 201–2.

Fackler, J.C., Nagel, J.E., Adler, W.H. *et al.* (1985) Epstein-Barr virus infection in a child with acquired immunodeficiency syndrome. *American Journal for Diseases of Children*, **139**, 1000–4.

Feigin, D.S. (1986) Nocardiasis of the lung: Chest radiographic findings in 21 cases. *Radiology*, **159**, 9–14.

Feuerstein, I.M., Archer, A., Peuda, J.M. *et al.* (1990) Thin-walled cavities, cysts, and pneumothorax in *Pneumocystis carinii* pneumonia: Further observations with histopathologic correlation. *Radiology*, **174**, 697–702.

Fish, D.G., Ampel, N.M., Galgiani, J.N. *et al.* (1990) Coccidioidomycosis during human immunodeficiency virus infection. A review of 77 patients. *Medicine*, **69**, 384–91.

Ganz, W.I., Serafini, A.N., Ganz, S.S. *et al.*, (1988) Diagnostic pattern of Ga-67 uptake in lymphocytic interstitial pneumonia. *Journal of Nuclear Medicine*, **29**, 887–8.

Garay, S.M., Belenko, M., Fazzine, E. *et al.* (1987) Pulmonary manifestations of Kaposi's sarcoma. *Chest*, **91**, 39–43.

Goodman, P.C. and Schnapp, L.M. (1992) Pulmonary toxoplasmosis in AIDS. *Radiology*, **184**, 791–3.

Greenberg, S.D., Frager, D.F., Suster, B.S. *et al.* (1994) Active pulmonary tuberculosis in patients with AIDS: spectrum of radiographic findings (including a normal appearance). *Radiology*, **193**, 115–19.

Groskin, S.A., Massi, A.F. and Randall, P.A. (1990) Calcified hilar and mediastinal lymph nodes in an AIDS patient with *Pneumocystis carinii* infection. *Radiology*, **175**, 345–60.

Guillon, J.M., Autran, B., Denis, M. *et al.* (1988) Human immunodeficiency virus-related lymphocytic alveolitis. *Chest*, **94**, 1264–70.

Hartman, T.E,. Swensen, S.J. and Williams, D.E. (1993) *Mycobacterium avium-intracellulare* complex: Evaluation with CT. *Radiology*, **187**, 23–6.

Hawkins, C.C., Gold, J.W.M., Whimbery E. *et al.*

(1986) *Mycobacterium avium* complex infections in patients with the acquired immunodeficiency syndrome. *Annals of Internal Medicine*, **105**, 184–8.

Herts, B.R., Megibow, A.J., Birnbaum, B.A. *et al.* (1992) High-attenuation lymphadenopathy in AIDS patients: significance of findings at CT. *Radiology*, **185**, 777–81.

Hill, A.R., Premkumar, S., Brustein, S. *et al.* (1991) Disseminated tuberculosis in the acquired immunodeficiency syndrome era. *American Review of Respiratory Disease*, **144**, 1164–70.

Horowitz, M.L., Schiff, M., Samuels, J. *et al.* (1993) *Pneumocystis carinii* pleural effusion. Pathogenesis and pleural fluid analysis. *American Review of Respiratory Disease*, **148**, 232–4.

Horsburgh C.R., Havlik J.A., Ellis D.E. *et al.* (1991) Survival of patients with acquired immune deficiency syndrome and disseminated *Mycobacterium avium* complex infection with and without antimycobacterial chemotherapy. *American Review of Respiratory Disease*, **144**, 557–9.

Kaplan, L.D., Abrams, D.I., Feigal, E. *et al.* (1989) AIDS-associated non-Hodgkin's lymphoma in San Francisco. *Journal of the American Medical Association*, **261**, 719–24.

Klein, J.S., Warnock, M., Webb, W.R. *et al.* (1988) Cavitating and noncavitating granulomas in AIDS patients with pneumocystis pneumonia. *American Journal of Radiology*, **152**, 753–4.

Knowles, D.M., Chamulak, G.A., Subar, M. *et al.* (1988) Lymphoid neoplasia associated with the acquired immunodeficiency syndrome (AIDS): The New York University Medical Center experience with 105 patients (1981–1986). *Annals of Internal Medicine*, **108**, 744–53.

Kradin, R.L. and Mark, E.J. (1983) Benign lymphoid disorders of the lungs with a theory regarding their development. *Human Pathology*, **14**, 857–67.

Kramer, M.R. and Uttamchandani, R.B. (1990) The radiographic appearance of pulmonary nocardiasis associated with AIDS. *Chest*, **98**, 382–5.

Kuhlman, J.E., Knowles, M.C., Fishman, E.K. *et al.* (1989) Premature bullous damage in AIDS: CT diagnosis. *Radiology*, **173**, 23–6.

Lee, V.M., Fuller, J.D., O'Brien, M.J. *et al.* (1991) Pulmonary Kaposi sarcoma in patients with AIDS: Scintigraphic diagnosis with sequential thallium and gallium scanning. *Radiology*, **180**, 409–12.

Lemlick, G., Schwam, L. and Lebwohl, M. (1987) Kaposi's sarcoma and acquired immunodeficiency syndrome: Postmortem findings in twenty-four cases. *Journal of the American Academy of Dermatology*, **16**, 319–25.

Lin, R.Y., Gruber, P.J., Saunders, R. *et al.* (1988) Lymphocytic interstitial pneumonitis in adult HIV infection. *New York State Journal of Medicine*, **88**, 273–6.

Lowenthal, D.A., Strauss, D.J., Campbell, S.W. *et al.* (1988) AIDS-related lymphoid neoplasia. The Memorial Hospital experience. *Cancer*, **61**, 2325–37.

Lubat, E., Megibow, A.J., Bulthazar, E.J. *et al.* (1990) Extrapulmonary *Pneumocystis carinii* infections in AIDS: CT findings. *Radiology*, **174**, 157–60.

Makris, A.N., Sher, S., Bertolic, C. *et al.* (1993) Pulmonary strongyloidiasis: an unusual opportunistic pneumonia in a patient with AIDS. *American Journal of Radiology*, **161**, 545–7.

McGuiness, G., Scholes, J.V., Garay, S.M. *et al.* (1994) Cytomegalovirus pneumonitis: spectrum of parenchymal CT findings with pathological correlation in 21 AIDS patients. *Radiology*, **192**, 451–9.

Mehle, M.E., Adamo, J.P., Mehta, A.C. *et al.* (1989) Endobronchial *Mycobacterium avium*-intracellulare in a patient with AIDS. *Chest*, **96**, 119–200.

Miller, R.F., Tomlinson, M.C., Cottrill, C.P. *et al.* (1992) Bronchopulmonary Kaposi's sarcoma in patients with AIDS. *Thorax*, **47**, 721–5.

Miller, W.T. (1994) Spectrum of pulmonary nontuberculous mycobacterial infection. *Radiology*, **191**, 343–50.

Miller, W.T., Edelman, J.M. and Miller, W.T. (1990) Cryptococcal pulmonary infection in patients with AIDS: Radiographic appearance. *Radiology*, **175**, 725–8.

Milligan, S.A., Stulbarg, M.S., Gamsu, G. *et al.* (1985) *Pneumocystis carinii* pneumonia radiograpically simulating tuberculosis. *American Review of Respiratory Disease*, **132**,1124–8.

Morris, J.C., Rosen, M.J., Marchevsky, A. *et al.* (1987) Lymphocytic interstitial pneumonia in patients at risk for the acquired immune deficiency syndrome. *Chest*, **91**, 63–7.

Moskovic, E., Miller, R. and Pearson, M. (1990) High resolution computed tomography of *Pneumocystis carinii* pneumonia in AIDS. *Clinical Radiology*, **42**, 239–43.

Murray, J.F. and Mills, J. (1990) Pulmonary infectious complications of human immunodeficiency virus infection. *American Review of Respiratory Disease*, **141**, 1356–72.

Naidich, D.P., Tarras, M., Garay, S.M. *et al.* (1989) Kaposi's sarcoma: CT-radiographic correlation. *Chest*, **96**, 723–8.

O'Doherty, M.J., Thomas, S.H., Page, C.J. *et al.* (1990) Does inhalation of pentamidine in the supine position increase deposition in the upper part of the lung? *Chest*, **97**, 1343–8.

Ognibene, F.P., Masur, H., Rogers, P. *et al.* (1988) Non specific interstitial pneumonitis without evidence of *Pneumocystis carinii* in asymptomatic patients infected with human immunodeficiency virus (HIV). *Annals of Internal Medicine*, **109**, 874–9.

Oldham, S.A.A., Castillo, M., Jacobson, F.L. *et al.* (1989) HIV associated lymphocytic interstitial pneumonia: Radiologic manifestations and pathologic correlation. *Radiology*, **170**, 83–7.

Packer, S.J., Cesario, T. and Williams, J.H. (1988) *Myobacterium avium* complex infection presenting as endobronchial lesions in immunosuppressed patients. *Annals of Internal Medicine*, **109**, 389–93.

Pitchenik, A.E. and Rubinson, H.A. (1985) The radiographic appearance of tuberculosis in patients with the acquired immuno deficiency syndrome (AIDS) and pre-AIDS. *American Review of Respiratory Disease*, **131**, 393–6.

Poelzleitner, D., Huebsch, P., Mayerhofer, S. *et al.* (1989) Primary pulmonary lymphoma in a patient with the acquired immune deficiency syndrome. *Thorax*, **44**, 438–9.

Radin, D.R., Baker, E.L., Klatt, E.C. *et al.* (1990) Visceral and nodal calcification in patients with AIDS-related *Pneumocystis carinii* infection. *American Journal of Radiology*, **154**, 27–31.

Reiss, T.F. and Golden, J. (1990) Abnormal lung gallium-67 uptake preceding pulmonary physiologic impairment in an asymptomatic patient with *Pneumocystis carinii* pneumonia. *Chest*, **97**, 1261–3.

Richards, P.J., Riddell, L., Reznek, R.H. *et al.* (1996) High resolution computed tomography in HIV patients with suspected *Pneumocystis carinii* pneumonia and a normal CXR. *Clinical Radiology*, **51**, 689–94.

Rosenberg, Z.S., Joffe, S.A. and Itescu, S. (1992) Spectrum of salivary gland disease in HIV-infected patients: characterization with Ga-67 citrate imaging. *Radiology*, **184**, 761–4.

Saks, A.M. and Posner, R. (1992) Tuberculosis in HIV positive patients in South Africa: a comparative radiological study with HIV negative patients. *Clinical Radiology*, **46**, 387–90.

Schif, R.G., Kabat, L. and Kamoni, N. (1987) Gallium scanning in lymphoid interstitial pneumonitis of children with AIDS. *Journal of Nuclear Medicine*, **28**, 1915–9.

Selwyn, P.A., Hartell, D., Lewis, V.A. *et al.* (1989) A prospective study of the risk of tuberculosis among intravenous drug users with human immunodeficiency virus infection. *New England Journal of Medicine*, **320**, 545–50.

Sider, L., Weiss, A.J., Smith, M.D. *et al.* (1989) Varied appearance of AIDS-related lymphoma in the chest. *Radiology*, **171**, 629–32.

Simmons, J.T., Suffredini, A.F., Lack, E.E. *et al.* (1987) Non specific interstitial pneumonitis in patients with AIDS: Radiologic features. *American Journal of Roentgenology*, **149**, 265–8.

Sivit, C.J., Schwartz, A.M. and Rockoff, S.D. (1987) Kaposi's sarcoma of the lungs in AIDS: Radiologic-pathologic analysis. *American Journal of Roentgenology*, **148**, 25–8.

Suster, B., Akerman, M., Orenstein, M. *et al.* (1986) Pulmonary manifestation of AIDS: review of 106 episodes. *Radiology*, **16l**, 87–93.

Tenholder, M.F., Moser, R.J. and Tellis, C.J. (1988) Mycobacteria other than tuberculosis: pulmonary involvement in patients with acquired immunodeficiency syndrome. *Archives of Internal Medicine*, **148**, 953–5.

Travis, W.D., Fox C.H. and Devaney, K.O. (1992) Lymphoid pneumonitis in 50 adult patients infected with the human immunodeficiency virus: lymphocytic interstitial pneumonitis versus nonspecific interstitial pneumonitis. *Human Pathology*, **25**, 529–41.

Tumeh, S.S., Belville, J.S., Pugatch, R. *et al.* (1992) Ga-67 scintigraphy and computed tomography in the diagnosis of *Pneumocystis carinii* pneumonia in patients with AIDS. A prospective comparison. *Clinical Nuclear Medicine*, **17**, 387–94.

Vanarthos, W.J., Ganz, W.I., Vanarthos, J.C. *et al.* (1992) Diagnostic uses of nuclear medicine in AIDS. *Radiographics*, **12**, 731–49.

Wasser, L.S., Shaw, G.W. and Talavera, W. (1988) Endobronchial tuberculosis in the acquired immunodeficiency syndrome. *Chest*, **94**, 1240–4.

Weber, W.R., Askin, F.B. and Dehner, L.P. (1977) Lung biopsy in *Pneumocystis carinii* pneumonia: A histopathologic study of typical and atypical features. *American Journal of Clinical Pathology*, **67**, 11–9.

Wheat, L.J., Connolly-Stringfield, P.A., Baker, R.L. *et al.* (1990) Disseminated histoplasmosis in the acquired immune deficiency syndrome: Clinical findings, diagnosis and treatment, and review of the literature. *Medicine*, **69**, 361–74.

White, D.A and Matthay, R.A. (1989) Noninfectious pulmonary complications of infection with the human immunodeficiency virus. *American Review of Respiratory Disease*, **140**, 1763–87.

Wolff, S.D., Kuhlman, J.E. and Fishmann, E.K. (1993) Thoracic Kaposi sarcoma in AIDS: CT findings. *Journal of Computer Assisted Tomography*, **17**, 60–2.

PULMONARY RADIOLOGICAL FEATURES OF AIDS IN THE TROPICS

4

E. Tshibwabwa-Tumba

INTRODUCTION

In patients with the acquired immunodeficiency Syndrome (AIDS) the lung is one of the major organs to be involved, both in developed and developing countries (Murray and Mills, 1990; Rubin *et al.*, 1991; Coulomb *et al.*, 1992; Castro, 1995; Perriens *et al.*, 1995). In the USA and Europe, the usefulness of radiological imaging by chest X-rays and computerized axial tomography (CT) of the chest has been shown to be invaluable in the diagnosis and management of AIDS patients (Coulomb *et al.*, 1992; Chapter 3). While radiological investigations of the lungs in resource-poor tropical countries are restricted to chest X-rays, they provide useful information in the detection of pulmonary disease and in the assessment of response to specific treatment.

The frequency of pulmonary clinical manifestations and their associated radiological features in HIV-infected patients in the tropics may differ from those found in patients in the USA and Europe. Several reasons which may account for these differences may include: prevalence of background microbial flora; degree of immunodeficiency; nutritional status; and HLA types. Several lung diseases such as tuberculosis (Nunn *et al.*, 1993, Mukadi *et al.*, 1993), pyogenic pneumonias (Amorosa *et al.*, 1990; Daley, 1991; Chapter 14), and Kaposi's sarcoma (Kaplan *et al.*, 1988; Lee *et al.*, 1991) are common manifestations of HIV-infection although cryptococcosis and *Pneumocystis carinii* pneumonia (PCP) are increasingly being recognized. Apart from extensive studies on tuberculosis in adults (Elliott, Lou and Tembo, 1990; Nunn *et al.*, 1993; Saks and Posner, 1992), there is a paucity of literature from developing countries on the interpretation and usefulness of radiology in the management of HIV-associated pulmonary complications. This chapter summarizes chest X-ray and clinical data obtained from a 4-year (1990–94) retrospective study of 2500 black African adults (15 to 48 years of age) and 300 children (8 months to 6 years) with a diagnosis of AIDS (defined by the CDC criteria, 1987) as seen consecutively by the author from 3 large hospitals in Central Africa (1) The University Teaching Hospital, Lusaka, Zambia; (2) Sendwe General Hospital, Lubumbashi, Zaire; (3) Mama Yemo Hospital, Kinshasa, Zaire (Table 4.1).

INFECTIOUS COMPLICATIONS

TUBERCULOSIS

Tuberculosis is one of the most important opportunistic infection in HIV-infected individuals and has been declared a global emergency by the World Health Organiza-

AIDS and Respiratory Medicine. Edited by A. Zumla, M.A. Johnson and R.F. Miller. Published in 1997 by Chapman & Hall, London. ISBN 0 412 60140 0

Table 4.1 Chest X-ray findings of 2500 adults and 300 children with AIDS presenting at 3 major hospitals in Central Africa

	Adults	*Children*	*Total*
Pulmonary TB	963 (38.5%)	101 (33.6%)	1064 (38%)
PCP	784 (31.3%)	72 (24%)	856 (30.6%)
Pyogenic infection	215 (8.6%)	46 (15.3%)	261 (9.3%)
Kaposi's sarcoma	252 (10.1%)	28 (9.3%)	280 (10%)
B-cell lymphoma	243 (9.7%)	38 (12.6%)	281 (10%)
LIP	27 (1.1%)	10 (3.3%)	37 (1.3%)
Other	16 (0.6%)	5 (1.7%)	21 (0.8%)

tion (Raviglione *et al.*, 1995). Several studies from Sub-Saharan Africa have documented the impact of HIV on TB and illustrate associated changes in presentation seen on chest radiographs in many cases (Colebunders *et al.*, 1989; Nunn *et al.*, 1993; Elliot, Luo and Tembo, 1990; Williame, 1988; Long *et al.*, 1991; Kassim *et al.*, 1995). These studies have drawn attention to the fact that HIV-related tuberculosis presents with atypical clinical and radiological changes which are more dramatic in some cases and not in others. A similar picture is being seen in the USA (Buckner *et al.*, 1991; Huebner and Castro, 1995).

An increased incidence of adenopathy, pleural effusions, and abnormal parenchymal changes but less cavitary disease is seen in HIV-infected patients (Pitchenik and Rubinson, 1985). It appears that the severity of presentation in TB patients is not related to the degree of immunosuppression as evidenced by low $CD4^+$ lymphocyte counts (Mukadi *et al.*, 1993). Factors responsible for these differences are currently being studied. In a comparative radiological study of 61 HIV-positive South African TB patients with 50 HIV-negative TB patients, Saks and Posner (1992) found that chest X-rays of the HIV-positive group showed significantly higher percentage of hilar lymphadenopathy (50% vs 8%), pleural effusions (38% vs 20%), and miliary (8% vs 0%) or interstitial changes

(11% vs 4%). Cavitation (38% vs 82%) and atelectasis (31% vs 82%) were less common in the seropositive group than in the seronegative group.

In our series 1064 patients out of 2800 patients studied had pulmonary TB (963 were adults and 101 were children). Radiological findings were similar to those seen by Saks and Posner (1992) from South Africa. In 68% of adult cases the classic appearance of upper zone cavitating, fibrotic pulmonary TB, was not present. Other common findings were lobar consolidation (Figure 4.1), middle or lower involvement (Figure 4.2), hilar and paratracheal enlarged lymph nodes (Figure 4.3), and absence of cavities within pulmonary lesions. Pleural effusions were common X-ray findings in adults (74 out of 963). Pleural effusions (Figure 4.4) have been documented by several studies to be closely associated with HIV infection (Elliott, Luo and Tembo, 1990) in adults but not with HIV infection in children (Chintu and Zumla, 1995).

The remaining 32% of our adult cases showed classical chest X-ray features of TB (Leung *et al.*, 1992). Differential diagnoses which were considered before bacteriological confirmation was obtained were PCP, Kaposi's sarcoma, and community-acquired pneumonias. As has been observed by Chintu and Zumla (1995), HIV-infected children may have more serious disease but

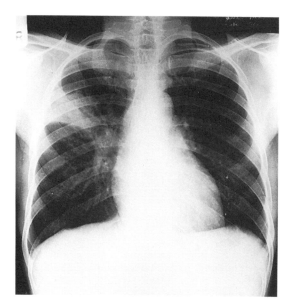

Fig. 4.1 Right upper lobe anterior axillary segment consolidation of tuberculosis is seen on the posteroanterior chest radiograph in a 15-year-old HIV patient with acid-fast bacilli in the sputum, confirmed on culture.

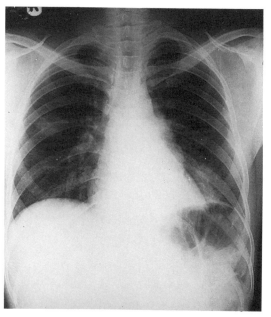

Fig. 4.3 Postero-anterior view of the chest in a 34-year-old HIV patient shows left hilar adenopathy and patchy infiltrates at the left base. The diagnosis of respiratory tuberculosis was made on culture of acid-fast bacilli from broncho-alveolar lavage fluid.

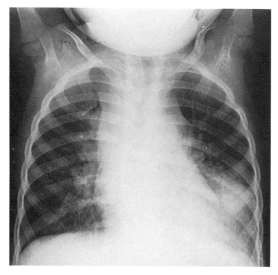

Fig. 4.2 Anteroposterior view of the chest in a 3-year-old HIV patient with tuberculosis shows alveolar consolidation involving the lower lobe of the left lung. Note evidence of ancillary hilar adenopathy and absence of cavities within the lesion.

there appear to be no significant atypical changes on chest X-rays as seen in adults. Despite the atypical appearance of TB in HIV-infected adults, it is generally recognized that TB should be a prime consideration in HIV-infected individuals in developing and developed countries (Buckner *et al.*, 1991).

PYOGENIC CHEST INFECTIONS

The list of organisms causing pneumonia in HIV-infected individuals has been reviewed by Gilks (Chapter 14). In this series, pyogenic chest infections were seen in 215 out of 2500 adults (8.6%) and 46 out of 300 children (15.3%). Chest X-ray findings were similar to those observed in other studies from Africa (Gilks *et al.*, 1994; Amorosa *et al.*, 1990; Witt, Craven and McCabe, 1987). Lobar consolida-

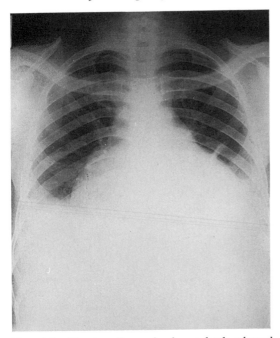

Fig. 4.4 Chest radiograph shows both pleural and pericardial effusion in a 44-year-old HIV patient. This pattern was also present on echocardiography and epigastric ultrasound of the patient.

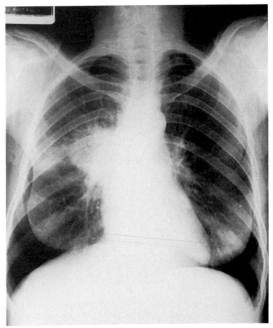

Fig. 4.6 Round infiltrate in a patient with *Streptococcus pneumoniae* is evident on the posteroanterior chest radiograph. The diagnosis was made in the presence of bacterial pathogens in blood and sputum cultures.

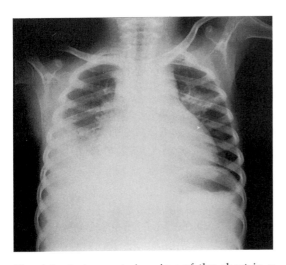

Fig. 4.5 Anteroposterior view of the chest in a 4-year-old child with AIDS shows bilateral infiltrates and a right-sided pleural effusion. *Streptococcus pneumoniae* was found in pleural fluid and blood culture.

tion was the most frequent finding and was seen in 91 out of 215 adults and 26 out of 46 children with bacterial chest infection. Other findings included bilateral nodules in 54 out of 215 adults and 20 out of 46 children (Figure 4.5), round infiltrates in 41 adults out of 215 (Figure 4.6) and pleural effusion in 21 out of 215 (Figure 4.7). While several features of pyogenic chest infections are common with TB and PCP, the presence of localized consolidation or round infiltrates may suggest a pyogenic etiology.

PNEUMOCYSTIS CARINII PNEUMONIA

Pneumocystis carinii pneumonia (PCP) was initially thought to be a rare manifestation of AIDS in Africa (Elvin *et al.*, 1989; Carme *et al.*, 1991; Abouya *et al.*, 1992). Data emerging from Central Africa about the significance of PCP have yielded conflicting evidence

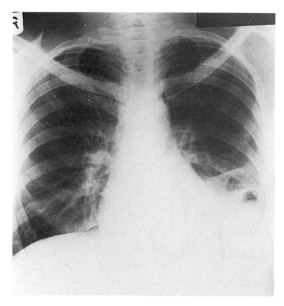

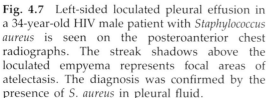

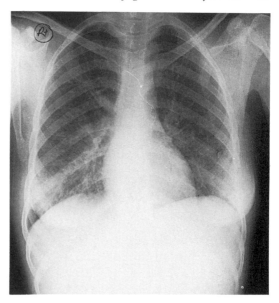

Fig. 4.7 Left-sided loculated pleural effusion in a 34-year-old HIV male patient with *Staphylococcus aureus* is seen on the posteroanterior chest radiographs. The streak shadows above the loculated empyema represents focal areas of atelectasis. The diagnosis was confirmed by the presence of *S. aureus* in pleural fluid.

Fig. 4.8 Posteroanterior view of the chest in a 22-year-old female patient demonstrates fine reticulo-nodular interstitial pattern throughout both lung bases. *Pneumocystis carinii* were seen on examination of induced sputum.

(Machiels and Urban, 1992; Atzori *et al.*, 1993; Russian and Kovacs, 1995) with more recent studies documenting PCP occurring at a significant frequency (Malin *et al.*, 1995). In our series, PCP was the second commonest infectious complication of HIV seen in the lungs. 784 out of 2500 adults reviewed had PCP as diagnosed by examination of sputum obtained by induction of sputum (620 cases) and of bronchoalveolar lavage fluid (164 cases). The most common radiological feature seen (60% cases) in these patients was diffuse bilateral, fairly symmetrical interstitial shadowing (Figure 4.8). Other radiographic changes included localized areas of homogeneous consolidation (Figure 4.9), pulmonary nodules (Figure 4.10), thin-walled cavities (Figure 4.11), pneumothorax and cavitating nodules. These radiological features are similar to those seen in developed countries (De Lorenzo, Huang and Maguin, 1987; Afessa *et al.*, 1988; Mayaud and Carette, 1989; Sandhu and Goodman, 1989; Feuerstein *et al.*, 1990). While inhaled pentamidine prophylaxis or treatment was not prescribed, upper lobe shadowing resembling pulmonary tuberculosis (Figure 4.12) was also seen in 20 cases.

NON-INFECTIOUS CAUSES

Pulmonary Kaposi's Sarcoma

This AIDS-defining condition has been reviewed by Denton and Spittle (Chapter 18). In this series from Zambia and Zaire 280 patients with clinically suspected Kaposi's sarcoma (KS) with cutaneous KS and absence of infectious etiology (252 adults and 28

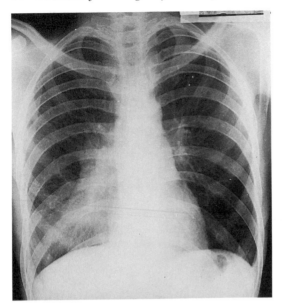

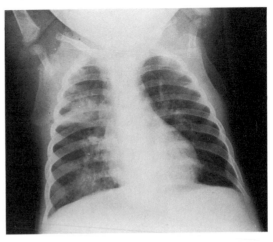

Fig. 4.10 Anteroposterior chest radiograph of a 27-month-old child with *Pneumocystis carinii* pneumonia demonstrating patchy alveolar infiltrates in the right upper lobe and coarse nodular interstitial infiltrates in the right lower lobe.

Fig. 4.9 Posteroanterior chest radiograph shows consolidation in the medial segment, right lower lobe in a patient with *Pneumocystis carinii* pneumonia.

children) underwent chest X-rays. Pulmonary KS was confirmed by bronchoscopy and histopathological examination in 70 adult cases. Among these, chest X-ray features varied from a normal chest X-ray (3 out of 70), nodular opacities associated with hilar adenopathy (35 out of 70) (Figure 4.13), alveolar or interstitial infiltrates (16 out of 70) (Figure 4.14) and pleural effusion (7 out of 70). These radiological features are similar to those seen in the USA and Europe (Meduri *et al.*, 1986) and are indistinguishable from those described in the sections on TB and PCP and they only provide additional supportive evidence to the diagnosis.

B cell lymphoma

The data on pulmonary B cell lymphoma in HIV-infected individuals in Africa are scanty. Studies from the USA and Europe have described it as an aggressive systemic tumour (Zeigler *et al.*, 1984; Lee *et al.*, 1991;

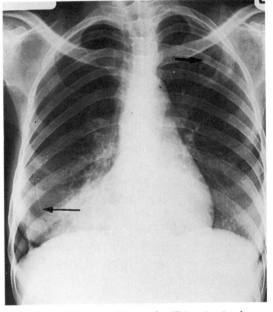

Fig. 4.11 Chest radiograph (PA view) shows interstitial infiltrates at both lung bases, right-sided pneumothorax (thin arrows) and left upper lobe thin-walled cavities (thick arrow) in *Pneumocystis carinii* pneumonia.

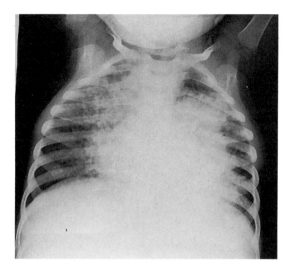

Fig. 4.12 Anteroposterior chest radiograph of a 4-year-old child demonstrates patchy alveolar infiltrates of *Pneumocystis carinii* pneumonia in both lungs, predominantly in the upper lobes. These nodules resemble those of reactivation of tuberculosis.

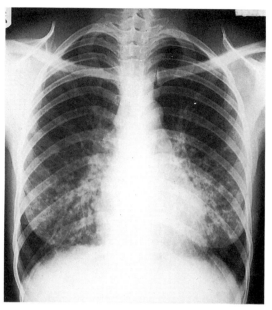

Fig. 4.13 Chest radiograph demonstrates bilateral opacities in the lower lobes and perihilar region. Postmortem section of the left lung demonstrated infiltration by Kaposi's sarcoma in the hilar and perihilar region.

Coulomb *et al.*, 1992; Sider *et al.*, 1989; Chapter 20) with chest X-ray findings similar to that of TB, KS and PCP. The diagnosis is difficult since the clinical presentation and radiographic findings are not specific. In our series there were 281 proven cases of thoracic lymphoma (221 cases by cytologic examination of pleural fluid and 60 by transthoracic needle biopsy). Chest X-ray findings were pleural effusion (84 out of 281), pulmonary nodules (79 out of 281, 40 of whom had associated pleural effusion) and reticular lung disease (39 out of 281) (Figures 4.15–4.17). The latter may be confused with PCP or lymphoid interstitial pneumonitis (LIP) and the former with lung metastasis. Hilar and mediastinal adenopathy were seen in 43 out of 281 cases.

Lymphoid interstitial pneumonitis

This entity was initially described by Carrington and Liebow (1966) in immunocompromised patients prior to the AIDS

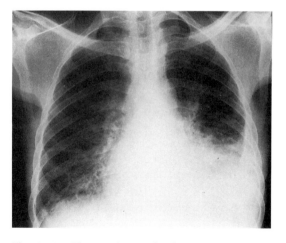

Fig. 4.14 Chest radiograph of a 35-year-old HIV-positive man. Interstitial and alveolar areas of increased opacity are seen at both pulmonary bases as well as a moderate left-sided pleural effusion. A violaceous nodule on the perineum was noted, and biopsy confirmed that it was Kaposi's sarcoma. No opportunistic infection was found in the sputum and at thoracocentesis.

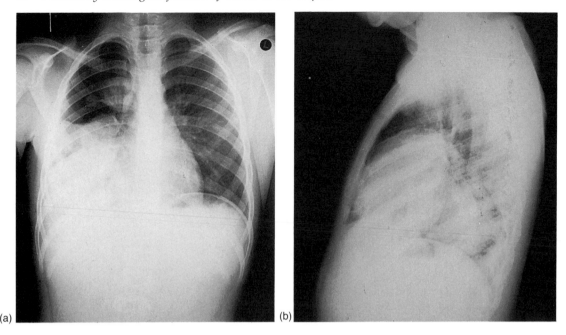

Fig. 4.15 Posteroanterior (a) and lateral (b) chest radiographs show several ill-defined nodules in the right lower lobe and two well-defined nodules in the middle upper lobes. The 38-year-old male HIV patient had biopsy proved lymphoma involvement of the chest and peripheral adenopathy.

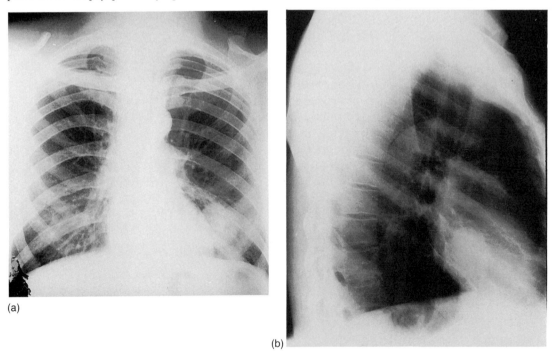

Fig. 4.16 Posteroranterior (a) and lateral (b) chest views depict one well-defined pulmonary nodule in the left lower lobe. The lungs are otherwise clear. This lesion was at first thought to be a metastasis to the lung from an extra-thoracic primary tumour. The diagnosis of pulmonary lymphoma in this 48-year-old HIV male patient was made by means of transthoracic needle aspiration biopsy.

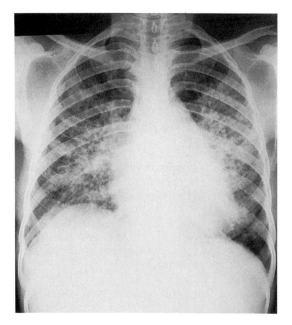

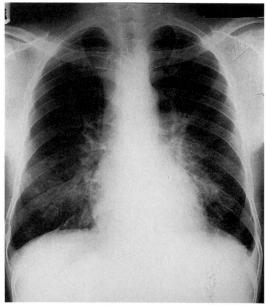

Fig. 4.17 Chest radiograph shows coarse bilateral reticulonodular infiltrates in the middle of the lower zones. This pulmonary disease was thought to represent *Pneumocystis carinii* pneumonia. After repeated negative sputum bronchoscopy studies, transthoracic needle aspiration confirmed the diagnosis of lymphoma.

Fig. 4.18 Posteroanterior chest radiograph of the right lung base and of the left perihilar region shows fine reticular interstitial infiltration corresponding to lymphoid interstitial pneumonia. Biopsy findings in this adult HIV patient confirmed the diagnosis of LIP in this patient who had no concomitant evidence of opportunistic infection or neoplasm.

pandemic. It is characterized by a diffuse infiltration of lung interstitium with a polymorphic mixture of lymphocytes becoming radiologically visible as fine reticular interstitial infiltration (Figure 4.18) (Grieco and Chinoy-Acharya, 1985; Oldham *et al.*, 1989; Chapter 21). In our series 27 out of 2500 adult patients and 10 out of 300 children showed changes of LIP on chest X-ray.

CONCLUSIONS

As has been observed in the USA and Europe, a wide spectrum of infectious and non-infectious complications of HIV are seen in Central Africa. While differences in the frequency of presentation of these illnesses are seen, as more information from Africa emerges, it is becoming apparent that conditions described commonly in developed countries are also seen frequently in the tropics. Although the chest X-ray findings of many of these conditions are often indistinguishable from each other it provides additional supportive data to clinical findings to aid diagnosis and monitor clinical progress with initiation of treatment.

ACKNOWLEDGMENTS

The author gratefully acknowledges the assistance of Abou Moussa, UNHCR representative to Zambia, and Catherine Gondwe for secretarial assistance.

REFERENCES

Abouya, Y., Beaumal, A., Lucas, S. *et al.* (1992) *Pneumocystis carinii* pneumonia. An uncommon cause of death in African patients with AIDS. *Trans. Roy. Soc. Med. Hyg.*, **145**, 617–20.

Afessa, B., Green, W., Williams, W. *et al.* (1988) *Pneumocystis carinii* pneumonia complicated by lymphadenopathy and pneumothorax. *Arch. Intern. Med.*, **148**, 2651–4.

Amorosa, J., Nahass, R., Noshar, J. and Gocke, D. (1990) Radiological distinction of pyogenic pulmonary infection from *Pneumocystis carinii* pneumonia in AIDS patients. *Radiology*, **175**, 721–4.

Atzori, C., Bruno, G., Chichimo, G. *et al.* (1993) *Pneumocystis carinii* pneumonia and tuberculosis in Tanzanian patients infected with HIV. *Trans. Roy. Soc. Trop. Med. Hyg.*, **87**, 55–56.

Buckner, C.B., Leithiser, R.E., Walker, C.W. and Allison, J.W. (1991) Changing epidemiology of tuberculosis and other bacterial infections in the United States: Implications for the radiologist. *Am. J. Radiol.*, **156**, 255–64.

Carrington, C.B. and Liebow, A.A. (1966) Lymphocytic interstitial pneumonia (abstr). *Am. J. Pathol.*, **48**, 36a.

Castro, K.G. (1995) Tuberculosis as an opportunistic disease in persons infected with human immunodeficiency virus. *Clin. Infect. Dis.*, **21**, suppl 1:S66–S71.

Carme, B., Mboussa, J., Andzin, M. *et al.* (1991) *Pneumocystis carinii* is rare in AIDS in Central Africa. *Trans. Roy. Soc. Trop. Med. Hyg.*, **85**, 80.

Chintu, C. and Zumla, A. (1995) Childhood tuberculosis and infection with the human immunodeficiency virus. *J. Roy. Coll. Phys.*, **29**, 92–4.

Colebunders, R., Ryder, R., Nzilambi, Z. *et al.* (1989). HIV infections with patients with tuberculosis in Kinshasa, Zaire. *Am. Rev. Respir. Dis.*, **139**, 1082–85.

Coulomb, M., Ferret, G., Leclerco, P. *et al.* (1992) L'imagerie des principales manifestations respiratoires du sujet infect par le virus de l'immunodeficience humaine. *Feuillets de Radiologie*, **32**, 463–84.

Daley, C.L. (1991) Pyogenic bacterial pneumonia in the acquired immunodeficiency syndrome. *J. Thorac. Imaging*, **6**, 36–42.

De Lorenzo, L., Huang, C. and Maguin, G. (1987) Roentegenographic pattern of *Pneumocystis carinii* pneumonia in a 104 patients with AIDS. *Chest*, **91**, 323–27.

Elliott, A., Luo, N., and Tembo, G. (1990) Impact of HIV on tuberculosis in Zambia: a cross-sectional study. *B. Med. J.*, **301**, 412–15.

Elvin, K., Lumbwe, C.M., Luo, N.P. *et al.* (1989) *Pneumocystis carinii* is not a major cause of pneumonia in HIV-infected patients in Lusaka, Zambia. *Trans. Roy. Soc. Trop. Med. Hyg.*, **83**, 553–55.

Feurstein, I., Archer, A., Pluda, J. *et al.* (1990) Thin-walled cavities, cyst and pneumothorax in pneumonia: further observation with histopathological correlation. *Radiology*, **174**, 697–702.

Grieco, M.H. and Chinoy-Acharya, P. (1985) Lymphocytic interstitial pneumonia associated with the acquired immune-deficiency syndrome. *Am. Rev. Respir. Dis.*, **131**, 952–55.

Huebner, R.E. and Castro, K.G. (1995). The changing face of tuberculosis. *Annu. Rev. Med.*, **46**, 47–55.

Kaplan, L., Hopwell, P.H., Joffe, H. *et al.* (1988) Kaposi's sarcoma involving the lung in patients with the immunodeficiency syndrome. *J. AIDS*, **1**, 23–30.

Kassim, S., Sassan-Morokro, M., Ackah, A. *et al.* (1995) Ten year follow-up of persons with HIV-1 and HIV-2 associated pulmonary tuberculosis treated with short course chemotherapy in West Africa. *AIDS*, **9**, 1185–91.

Lee, V., Fuller, J., O'Brien, M. *et al.* (1991) Pulmonary Kaposi sarcoma in patients with AIDS: scintigraphic diagnosis with sequential thallium and gallium scanning. *Radiology*, **180**, 409–12.

Leung, V., Muller, N., Pineda, P. *et al.* (1992) Primary tuberculosis in childhood: radiographic manifestations. *Radiology*, **182**, 87–91.

Long, R., Maycher, B., Scalcini, M. *et al.*, (1991) The chest roentgenogram in pulmonary tuberculosis patients seropositive for HIV type 1. *Chest*, **99**, 123–27.

Machiels, G. and Urban, M.I. (1992) *Pneumocystis carinii* as a cause of pneumonia in HIV-infected patients in Lusaka, Zambia. *Trans. Roy. Soc. Trop. Med. Hyg.*, **86**, 399–400.

Machiels L. (1992) *Pneumocystis-carinii* as a cause of pneumonia in HIV infected patients in Lusaka, Zambia. *Trans. Roy. Soc. Trop. Med. Hyg.*, **86**(4), 399–400.

Malin, A.S., Gwanzura, L.K.Z., Klein, S. *et al.* (1995) *Pneumocystis carinii* pneumonia in Zimbabwe. *Lancet*, **346**, 1258–62.

Mayaud, C. and Carette, M.F. (1989) Les nouveaux aspects radiologiques des pneumocystoses: un defi diagnostic pour le pneumologue. *Rev. Pneumol. Clin.*, **45**, 97–8.

Meduri, G.U., Stover, D.E., Lee, M. *et al.* (1986) Pulmonary Kaposi sarcoma in the acquired immune deficiency syndrome: clinical, radiographic, and pathological manifestations. *Am. J. Med.*, **81**, 11–18.

Murray, J.F. and Mills, J. (1990) Pulmonary infections complication of human immunodeficiency virus infection. Part 11: *Am. Rev. Respir. Dis.*, **141**, 1582–98.

Mukadi, Y., Perriens, J.H., St. Louis. M.E. *et al.* (1993) Spectrum of immunodeficiency in HIV-1 infected patients with pulmonary tuberculosis in Zaire. *Lancet*, **342**, 143–6.

Nunn, P., Gathua, S., Kibuga, D. *et al.*(1993) The impact of HIV on resource utilization by patients with tuberculosis in a tertiary referral hospital, Nairobi, Kenya. *Tuber Lung Dis.*, **74**, 273–9.

Nunn, P. (1991) HIV-associated pulmonary tuberculosis. *Africa Health*, **14**, 10–11.

Oldham, S., Castillo, M., Jacobson, F. *et al.* (1989) HIV-associated lymphocytic interstitial pneumonia: radiological manifestations and pathological correlation. *Radiology*, **170**, 83–7.

Perriens, J.H., St Louis, M.E., Mukadi, Y.B. *et al.* (1995) Pulmonary tuberculosis in HIV-infected patients in Zaire: a controlled trial of treatment for either 6 months or 12 months. *N. Engl. J. Med.*, **332**, 779–84.

Pitchenik, A. and Rubinson, H. (1985) The radiographic appearance of tuberculosis in patients with the acquired immunodeficiency syndrome (AIDS) and pre-AIDS. *Am. Rev. Respir. Dis.*, **131**, 393–6.

Raviglione, M.C., Snider, D.E. and Kochi, A. (1995) Global epidemiology of tuberculosis. Morbidity and mortality of a worldwide epidemic. *JAMA*, **273**, 220–26.

Rubin, S. (ed). (1991) Thoracic Manifestations of AIDS. *J. Thorac. Imaging*, **6**, 1–86.

Russian, D. and Kovacs, J.A. (1995) *Pneumocystis carinii* in Africa: an emerging pathogen? *Lancet*, **346**, 1242–3.

Saks, A.M. and Posner, R. (1992) Tuberculosis in HIV positive patients in South Africa: a comparative radiological study with HIV negative patients. *Clin. Rad.*, **46**, 387–90.

Sandhu, J. and Goodman, L. (1989) Pulmonary cysts associated with *Pneumocystis carinii* pneumonia in patients with Aids. *Radiology*, **173**, 33–35.

Sider, L., Weiss, A., Smith, M. *et al.* (1989) Varied appearance of AIDS-related lymphoma in the chest. *Radiology*, **171**, 629–32.

Williame, J. (1988) Tuberculosis and anti-HIV seropositivity in Kinshasa, Zaire. *Ann. Soc. Belg. Med. Trop.*, **68**, 165–7.

Witt, D., Craven, D. and McCabe, W. (1987) Bacterial infections in adult patients with the acquired immune deficiency syndrome (AIDS) and AIDS-related complex. *Am. J. Med.*, **82**, 900–6.

Ziegler, J., Beckstead, J., Volberding, P. *et al.* (1984) Non-Hodgkin's lymphoma in 90 homosexual men. *New Engl. J. Med.*, **311**, 565–70.

NUCLEAR MEDICINE AND THE CHEST IN AIDS

5

Michael J. O'Doherty and Robert F. Miller

INTRODUCTION

The lung is frequently involved by the infections and malignant complications of progressive immunodeficiency induced by the human immunodeficiency virus (HIV). This chapter focuses on the role of nuclear medicine in aiding the clinician in the identification of intrathoracic infection and malignancy.

Despite the widespread use of antibiotic prophylaxis in the prevention of *Pneumocystis carinii* pneumonia (PCP), this is still the most common chest infection. The difficulty for the clinician is to devise a strategy to distinguish between this and other infections of the lung which may produce similar clinical presentations. The pyogenic bacterial pneumonias are being seen with increasing frequency (Chapter 14) (Pitkin *et al.*, 1993; Chien *et al.*, 1992). Patients present with nonspecific symptoms of cough, breathlessness, fever, thoracic pain and occasionally hemoptysis. Often there are few clinical signs and further investigation is necessary in order to make a diagnosis. The chest radiograph may show abnormal parenchymal infiltrates, pleural disease, tumor or lymphadenopathy. However the chest radiograph may be normal when disease processes are at their earliest stage and probably most amenable to outpatient therapy. Similarly, the use of the more expensive ways of assessing intrathoracic disease, such as the presence of lymphadenopathy by CT or MRI, are largely dependent on abnormal increases in size.

Patients with PCP now frequently present early in the course of the disease and up to 15% of patients will have a normal or atypical chest radiograph. It is therefore necessary to consider which further tests may help define the site or nature of the disease process. The variety of chest radiographic appearances associated with PCP have been outlined in Chapter 3.

The role of nuclear medicine imaging techniques (described below) is to direct the clinician down an appropriate management path, particularly in patients who have normal or atypical chest radiographs. Whilst none of these nuclear medicine tests are specific for a particular infection, the high sensitivity of the tests is often of great use in directing further investigation and management and should be part of a diagnostic strategy. In addition, since some of the methods described also survey the entire body, other pathologies may be identified.

It is important to bear in mind that this group of patients may experience any of the disease processes in immune competent people, as well as opportunistic infections or tumors associated with HIV infection.

AIDS and Respiratory Medicine. Edited by A. Zumla, M.A. Johnson and R.F. Miller. Published in 1997 by Chapman & Hall, London. ISBN 0 412 60140 0

The role of nuclear medicine in thoracic AIDS focuses on:

1. detection of inflammation/infection;
2. localization of tumor and assessment of dissemination;
3. assessment of drug delivery.

DETECTION OF INFLAMMATION/INFECTION

Inflammation and infection may occur in any area of the body and may involve multiple sites, especially in the case of intravenous drug users. In non HIV-positive patients infection would normally be assessed using labeled leukocytes; in the lung, however, ^{67}Ga is the most appropriate agent. The use of leukocytes labeled with either ^{99m}Tc exametazime or ^{111}In oxine or tropolone can be effected using donor leukocytes rather than autologous cells, or by using agents that can be labeled from manufacturers' kits, e.g. antigranulocyte antibodies, polyclonal antibodies or human immunoglobulin IgG. An alternative nonspecific method of examining inflammation in the lung is to use aerosolized ^{99m}Tc DTPA as a reflection of lung permeability. Infiltration of the sternum with mycoses or bone involvement in bacillary angiomatosis (Baron *et al.*, 1990) would be investigated more appropriately with bone scanning. The radionuclides/radiopharmaceuticals used are discussed below.

^{67}Ga citrate

This agent has been in use since the late 1960s/early 1970s for imaging inflammation and infection. Gallium is a cyclotron-generated radionuclide with a physical half-life of 78 hours. The principal gamma emissions used for imaging are the 93, 184 and 296 keV; all three photopeaks are used to increase the sensitivity of the acquisition. The ability to detect where gallium accumulates is dependent on the amount of gallium in the abnormal tissue, the depth of the lesion and the background activity. Thus uptake in the thorax where in individuals without infection or tumor physiological accumulation of gallium is low, makes this region suitable for imaging with gallium. Scans are usually performed at 24 and 48 hours after injection of 150–200 MBq of gallium-67, although attempts have been made to scan earlier. Tomographic imaging has predominantly been used when malignant or lymph node infection is suspected and for this 400 MBq of gallium-67 is injected which will allow later imaging and larger accumulation within the abnormal sites. Tumeh and colleagues (Tumeh *et al.*, 1987) demonstrated that the sensitivity for detection of lymphoma within the chest can be increased from 66% with planar imaging to 96% with tomography. This higher dose also allows delayed imaging to be performed at 5–7 days, which may also improve lesion-to-background appearance.

Gallium is distributed throughout the body into bone, bone marrow, liver and kidneys. Lacrimal, salivary, nasopharyngeal and genital activity are seen as well as accumulation in bowel and spleen which is highly variable. Breast uptake is also found particularly during the menarche and lactation. The bowel uptake presents large difficulties in the interpretation of scans in the abdomen.

The mechanism for localization in normal or abnormal tissue is not understood, but theories range from binding to transferrin receptors on cell surfaces or to lactoferrin within leukocytes, or to bacteria on siderophores, or direct permeation into the tissues. In non-HIV related lung conditions the uptake of ^{67}Ga is thought to be due to neutrophil accumulation of gallium (Hunninghake *et al.*, 1981). In HIV-infected patients where the neutrophil count may be low, the gallium is found predominantly in the supernatant of lavage fluid at 24 hours after injection and yet this accumulation is not related to the transferrin concentration.

Also the neutrophil content of the lavage fluid is not related to the intensity of gallium accumulation (Smith, Berkowitz and Lewis, 1992). This suggests that either most of the gallium is trapped in the interstitium or there is some other cause of the leak into the alveolar space.

Gallium is the agent of choice in a number of countries for the investigation of pulmonary pathology and in particular PCP. The pattern of uptake in the chest may broadly be classed as normal, focal nodal accumulation, focal parenchymal lung accumulation, focal accumulation in soft tissues including the myocardium and diffuse pulmonary parenchymal uptake.

Gallium scanning is easy to perform; however, unless an individual department has the radionuclide in stock then there is the potential for a delay whilst the order is placed (1–2 days) and the scans are most commonly performed at 24 and 48 hours after injection into the patient. This has prompted the development of protocols for quantifying lung/liver count rate ratios at 4 hours following injection (Cordes *et al.*, 1989). In this study Cordes and colleagues showed that the counts/pixel ratio for the lung to liver were similar at 4, 24, 48 and 72 hours in patients with PCP with the ratio at 4 hours being 1.05 whereas those patients without PCP had ratios of approximately 0.7. This ratio was similar at 24 hours. The use of a scoring system comparing uptake in the liver with the lung is open to error, particularly in those patients with disease of the liver where the uptake may be very low, for example in patients with the effects of hepatitis B or C disease (Figure 5.1).

Patients with PCP classically show diffuse distribution throughout both lung fields, such that a negative cardiac silhouette is seen (Bitran *et al.*, 1987; Kamer *et al.*, 1987) but a variety of scan appearances can be seen (Miller, 1990; Palestro, 1994). Uptake in the lung can be graded (Table 5.1); if this accumulation is equal to or higher than that

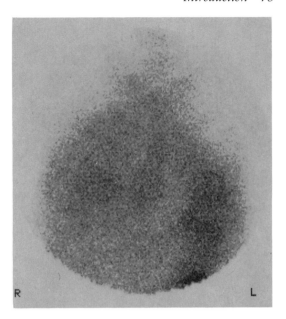

Fig. 5.1 ^{67}Gallium lung scan in a patient with liver dysfunction due to hepatitis C induced cirrhosis and *Pneumocystis carinii* pneumonia. Note the reduced hepatic uptake and the slight increase in lung uptake.

in the liver and is diffuse, a confident diagnosis of diffuse lung disease can be made and the probability of this being due to PCP is high. Low uptake however does not exclude the diagnosis and in the context of an abnormal CXR this low uptake often carries a worse prognosis (Bitran *et al.*, 1987). Uptake is highly variable and four examples are shown in Figure 5.2a–d. The sensitivity and specificity of ^{67}Ga are 80–90% and 50–74% respectively (Tumeh *et al.*, 1992), rising to 100% in those patients with a normal chest X-ray (Tuazon *et al.*, 1985). The other important point is that the negative predictive value for pulmonary pathology is high (91%) (Woolfenden *et al.*, 1987) when both the CXR and the gallium scan are normal.

Difficulties with gallium accumulation in lung parenchyma arise when the classical diffuse distribution is not seen. These

Table 5.1 Grading system used in defining gallium-67 uptake in the lung

Grade	Gallium accumulation	Likelihood of lung pathology
0	Normal	Low (if the CXR is normal)
1	Less intense than rib accumulation	Equivocal significance
2	Accumulation equal to or greater than marrow but less than liver	Pathology present
3	Accumulation equal to or greater than liver	Pathology present

unusual distributions may be seen increasingly with widespread use of nebulized pentamidine for prophylaxis, against PCP, such that bilateral upper lobe uptake can occur (Bradburne *et al.*, 1989). These appearances may also be seen in miliary mycobacterial infection with a diffuse lung accumulation and/or high accumulation in the upper lobes (Figure 5.3a–c). Indeed, a variety of non-infectious conditions may cause a diffuse intrapulmonary accumulation of gallium, including sarcoidosis, various drugs (bleomycin, amiodarone), pulmonary vasculitis, fibrosing alveolitis, lymphocytic and nonspecific interstitial pneumonitis. Diffuse distribution has also been reported in HIV-positive patients who were smokers and had no respiratory symptoms (Stafianakis *et al.*, 1989), although this observation has not been repeated by others (Rosso *et al.*, 1992).

The pattern of distribution within the lung and in other tissues may indicate the possible pathologic process and the differential diagnosis. Possible patterns of uptake include a diffuse lung uptake with symmetrical increased parotid accumulation which may suggest lymphocytic interstitial pneumonitis (Ganz *et al.*, 1988). This pattern is seen with sarcoidosis which is very uncommon in HIV-infected individuals, PCP associated with benign cystic hyperplasia of the

parotid or occasionally with cytomegalovirus (CMV) infection. The association of lung accumulation and increased bowel or eye accumulation may suggest CMV as a unifying disease process. Other possible patterns of diffuse lung accumulation of gallium associated with lymph node accumulation may suggest atypical mycobacterial infection, or could be indicative of an alveolitis associated with lymphoma. A diffuse lung accumulation of gallium has also been seen in HIV-infected children with lymphoid interstitial pneumonitis (Schiff *et al.*, 1987; Zuckier, Ongseng and Goldbarb, 1988) and also in adults with pneumonitis (Ognibene *et al.*, 1988).

Bacterial pneumonia may present with cough and pyrexia and a normal CXR, yet gallium imaging will show focal accumulation in either a lobar or multilobar distribution (Figure 5.4a,b). If accumulation is focal in the lung and/or is associated with bone involvement, then atypical fungal infection or lymphoma should be considered in the differential diagnosis.

Other anatomical areas that can be imaged with gallium include the myocardium and pericardium. Cardiac problems associated with HIV include cardiomyopathy, myocarditis, Kaposi's sarcoma, metastatic lymphoma, pericarditis and endocarditis. Unexpected increased accumulation in the

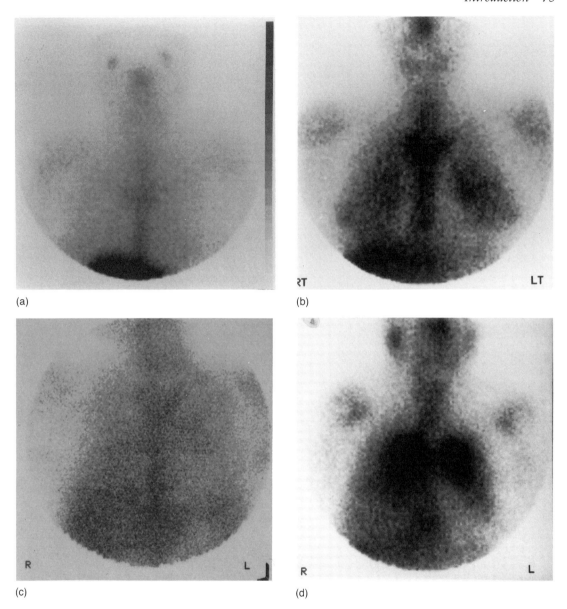

(a)

(b)

(c)

(d)

Fig. 5.2 ^{67}Gallium lung scans (anterior view) from four patients with *Pneumocystis carinii* pneumonia. There is highly variable uptake ranging from (a) normal; (b) less than marrow uptake; (c) to the clear definition of a negative cardiac silhouette (uptake almost equivalent to the marrow but less than the liver); or (d) high diffuse uptake equivalent to or greater than the liver.

heart indicates further investigation is necessary; this appearance has been reported in myocarditis (Cregler *et al.*, 1990). A normal scan however will not exclude a myocarditis.

The major advantage of gallium imaging is that the whole body can be studied and therefore other unsuspected disease processes may be discovered. Gallium ac-

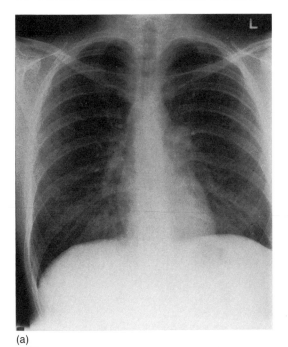

(a)

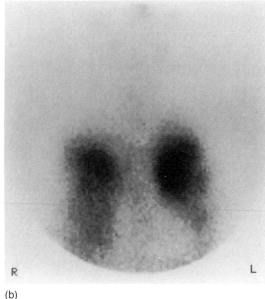

(b)

Fig. 5.3 ^{67}Gallium scan appearances in a patient with a normal CXR (a) when the scan was requested (for weight loss). (b) The scan appearances show higher uptake in the apices of the lung but diffuse uptake through the rest of the lung in a patient on nebulized pentamidine. The ^{99m}Tc DTPA transfer did not indicate PCP. The chest radiograph appearances subsequent to the scan in (b) showed a diffuse abnormality (c) and a diagnosis of atypical mycobacterial infection was made at bronchoscopy.

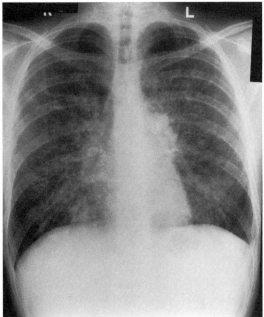

(c)

cumulation in regional lymph nodes within the chest is consistent with lymphoma, *Myobacterium avium intracellulare*, persistent generalized lymphadenopathy, *Pneumocystis carinii* infection or other infective processes (Figure 5.5). Nodal uptake may also be scaled according to whether the intensity is similar to the liver uptake when it is more likely to

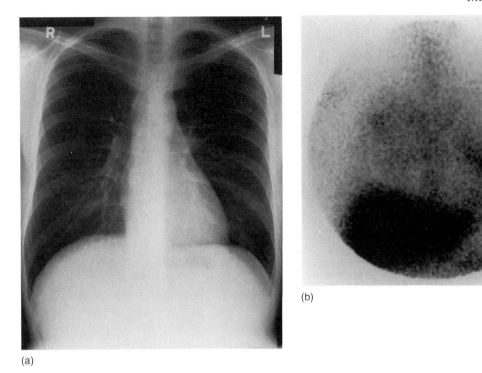

(b)

(a)

Fig. 5.4 (a)^{67}Gallium scan appearance in a patient with pneumococcal chest infection. The chest radiograph appearances were normal at the time of the scan. (b) There is increased accumulation of ^{67}gallium in the right upper lobe and the left lower lobe.

represent mycobacterial infection, lymphoma or other infection rather than follicular hyperplasia, although this is not invariable (Podzamczer *et al.*, 1990). Gallium undoubtedly has a role in the investigation of a pyrexia of unknown origin, when there are no specific localizing features, thus directing further investigation to a specific site.

Polyclonal/monoclonal antibodies

The use of antibodies for the localization of infection and inflammation has an advantage over leukocyte imaging because preparations are available in kit form. The disadvantage of using indium-111 as the radionuclide is that it is not a radionuclide that can be produced on site and therefore has to be

ordered especially for the labeling procedure. Animal and human studies have shown localization of ^{111}In polyclonal antibodies (^{111}In HIgG) in lungs infected with PCP (Fischman *et al.*, 1991; Ruben *et al.*, 1989a, b). Polyclonal antibodies are obtained from pooled serum and thus have to meet blood transfusion criteria and be negative for HIV, hepatitis B and C. Imaging for ^{111}In HIgG is performed after injecting 37 MBq of activity. In a study of 51 patients (Buscombe *et al.*, 1993) with either bacterial infection or PCP a focal pattern of uptake of ^{111}In HIgG was found in bacterial infections and a diffuse pattern in patients with PCP. If the patients had a mixed infection then both focal and diffuse appearances were seen. Diffuse accumulation was seen even in those

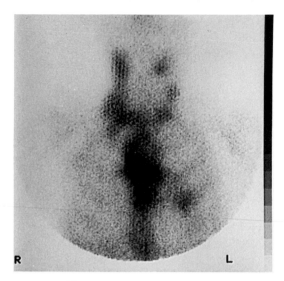

Fig. 5.5 [67]Gallium scan appearance in a patient who presented with sweats, breathlessness and tiredness associated with a mild cough. The scan shows widespread uptake in multiple lymph nodes in the mediastinum, hilum and cervical regions. The appearances were those of non Hodgkin's lymphoma.

patients with PCP who had a normal chest radiograph. Negative scans were found in five patients with Kaposi's sarcoma and three with intrapulmonary lymphoma. This study had a 100% sensitivity for identifying pulmonary infection compared with a previous study by the same group (Buscombe, 1990) when ^{99m}Tc labeled HIgG was used. Here the sensitivity for identifying pulmonary infection was only 33%; this was thought to be due to blood pool activity within the thorax obscuring infection-related accumulation at 24 hours but not at 48 hours. Therefore the longer half-life of indium-111 allows later images to be performed once blood pool activity has diminished and so detects more areas of infection. The appearances in other diffuse parenchymal diseases are not yet known but it is likely that diffusely abnormal scans would result. Imaging with ^{111}In labeled HIgG has similar disadvantages to imaging with gallium because images and

therefore diagnosis is delayed to 48 hours and does require a delivery of a non-stock radionuclide.

A recent report of a monoclonal antibody imaging technique for PCP raises the possibility of a more specific test for this infection (Goldenberg *et al.*, 1994). This technique involves raising a monoclonal antibody against a surface antigen of human *Pneumocystis carinii* in mice and then producing the Fab' fragment for direct labeling with [99m]Tc. The labeled Fab' fragment was then infused into the patients (approximately 1110 MBq): images could be obtained at 2–5 hours but those obtained at 24 hours provided the most reliable results. These studies were performed on 16 patients with presumptive or definite diagnosis of PCP, all of the definite diagnoses had moderate to severe disease (pO_2 mmHg 41–81) with chest radiograph abnormalities. The technique raises the interesting possibility of its use in extrapulmonary disease detection but has not addressed the more relevant issues of whether there will be uptake in the lungs of patients with mild disease or normal chest radiographs. It is possible that the increased permeability of the pulmonary endothelium to proteins of this size in severe disease is due to a nonspecific protein leak and therefore will not have the sensitivity and specificity of 85.7 and 86.7% respectively quoted for these 16 patients. The study by Goldenberg *et al.* does indicate that therapy for PCP can be given without affecting the result since images were positive even when performed 28 days after the initiation of PCP treatment; this may mean that the test may be of no help in follow-up studies and this question needs to be resolved.

Leukocyte imaging

Although inflammation can be detected using ^{99m}Tc and ^{111}In human immunoglobulin or gallium, other methods are used to localize inflammation/infection elsewhere in the body such as ^{111}In or ^{99m}Tc autologous labeled leukocytes or donor leukocytes. This technique requires specialist equipment to perform the leukocyte labeling and the whole labeling procedure takes approximately one-and-a-half-hours. Finneman and colleagues (Finneman *et al.*, 1989) performed a comparative study of gallium and ^{111}In leukocyte scanning in 36 patients with AIDS, in which gallium identified 44% of the abnormalities and the leukocytes 78%. Leukocyte scans were positive in sinusitis, bacterial chest infection and colitis, whereas gallium identified patients with lymph node disease and PCP. These data suggest that gallium should be used for suspected PCP and lymphatic causes of pyrexia (mycobacterial infection, lymphoma, etc.), whereas leukocyte scans should be used for all other causes. Using autologous leukocytes involves a small risk to the staff performing the labeling. Since these patients may be neutropenic, staff will need to handle large volumes of blood in the labeling procedure and thus increase the risk to themselves of contamination. An alternative is to use donor leukocytes. This technique has been shown to be safe and effective at demonstrating abnormal areas of infection/inflammation using either ^{111}In oxine or ^{99m}Tc exametazime as the label, albeit in a small number of patients (O'Doherty *et al.*, 1990). Donor cells are obtained from individuals of the same blood group who are CMV and hepatitis C negative and labeled in the normal way.

It should be noted that in the investigation of possible thoracic infection, leukocyte imaging is inferior to gallium scanning.

Lung ^{99m}Tc DTPA transfer

This method has been used for many years to assess the integrity of the pulmonary epithelium and is abnormal in a range of disease processes. The measurement is related to the permeability of the lung epithelium to molecules of various sizes. In the case of ^{99m}Tc DTPA (diethylenetriaminepentaacetate) any process which causes disruption of the alveolar and respiratory bronchiole epithelium will increase this permeability.

The permeability is measured in terms of either a half-time of transfer (expressed in minutes) or a clearance rate (expressed as a %/minute reduction in initial activity). The use of the technique has been described in PCP and other lung infections by a number of groups (Rosso, 1992; O'Doherty *et al.*, 1987, 1989; Leach *et al.*, 1991; Van der Wall *et al.*, 1991; Robinson *et al.*, 1991). Lung ^{99m}Tc DTPA transfer (permeability, clearance) relies on the inhalation for 1–2 minutes of an aerosol of ^{99m}Tc DTPA with the particle size being approximately 1 micron or less. The rate of removal from the lungs is measured using a gamma camera positioned either posteriorly or anteriorly with the data being acquired dynamically. Acquisition time (from 20 to 60 minutes) varies from centre to centre but from the resultant time–activity curves, the half-time or clearance rate (with or without background correction) can be derived.

Some groups have measured the rate of transfer or permeability over the first 7 minutes of acquisition and others have measured over a longer time period, 30–40 minutes. Results from the different methods are similar for normal nonsmokers and smokers because the removal is a single exponential and mean half-times of 60 minutes and 20 minutes (0.8%/minute and 2.5%/minute) are recorded for the two groups respectively. However, if measurements are limited to the first 7 minutes, the descriptive appearance of the curve may be missed. The appearance of a biphasic curve with a rapid first component (half-time < 4 minutes (12.5%/minute)) is the hallmark of an alveolitis (Figure 5.6a/6b). The most likely cause of an alveolitis and hence the biphasic pattern (in HIV-positive patients) is still PCP, but other causes of this pattern include CMV infection, lymphocytic intersti-

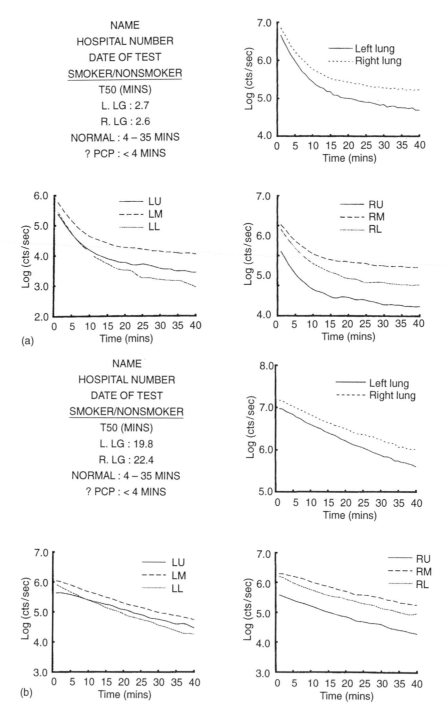

Fig. 5.6 Lung ^{99m}Tc DTPA transfer in a patient who presented with breathlessness and a normal CXR. *Pneumocystis carinii* pneumonia was diagnosed. The transfer curves are shown (a) at presentation and (b) after three weeks' outpatient treatment with high dose co-trimoxazole. The curves are biphasic in the whole lung (LL = left lung; RL = Right lung) and the lung thirds (L = left; R = right: U = upper third by height; M = middle third; L = lower third). The transfer times are for the first component of this biphasic curve. The curves become monoexponential with successful therapy.

Step 1

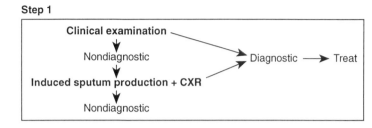

Step 2

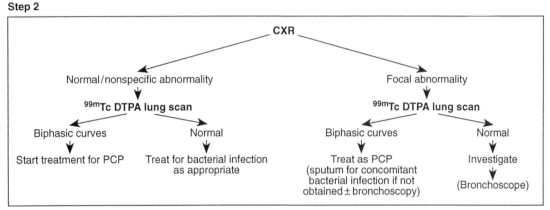

CXR mediastinal abnormality - Gallium scan
Note: Failure of response to therapy requires bronchoscopy and further sputum

Fig. 5.7 Suggested algorithm for the investigation of a patient who is HIV-antibody-positive and has breathlessness. Step 1 is the early investigation of the patient, step 2 is the investigation path using radionuclide techniques. Depending on the availability of sputum induction and scanning the step 2 algorithm may be instituted before or after a CXR has been obtained as part of step 1.

tial pneumonitis and nonspecific interstitial pneumonitis. The test has a high sensitivity and specificity, in this patient population for PCP, but false negative results may occur (Leach *et al.*, 1991). False negative results usually show an abnormally fast transfer/permeability rate, but not with a typical biphasic pattern and therefore further investigation (induced sputum examination or bronchoscopy) is suggested rather than initiation of treatment for PCP. Occasionally, a biphasic curve can be found in heavy smokers with HIV infection in the absence of an alveolitis and therefore it is suggested that baseline scans are performed in all smokers (authors' experience). Transfer times are not biphasic in other bacterial infections (with the exception of *Legionella pneumophila*) (O'Doherty *et al.*, 1989). Rosso *et al.* (1992)

have demonstrated that using only the first 7 minutes of the time activity curve the clearance rate for PCP is higher than for other pulmonary conditions. The biggest area of overlap was in patients who had a cytotoxic lymphocytic alveolitis.

The ^{99m}Tc DTPA technique has a higher sensitivity than gallium scanning (92% compared with 72%) for infectious pulmonary complications (Rosso *et al.*, 1992). This difference is more marked for patients with normal chest radiographs and normal blood gases. A normal chest radiograph and a normal DTPA clearance virtually exclude pulmonary infection/inflammation requiring therapy.

An algorithm for the optimum use of ^{99m}Tc DTPA, CXR and gallium scanning in the investigation of the breathless HIV-positive

Table 5.2   Gallium-67 scanning and the lung

CXR appearance	Gallium scan appearance	Probable diagnosis
Normal CXR	Normal gallium scan	Suggests no abnormality (but DTPA more sensitive screening test)
	Abnormal	See below
Abnormal CXR	Diffuse	PCP
		Alveolitis of other cause
		Mycobacterium avium intracellulare (MAI)
	Diffuse + nodes	Likely MAI or
	Patchy + nodes	lymphoma + opportunistic disease
	No uptake	Kaposi's sarcoma (KS) (but all diagnoses can be negative)
	Lobar or discrete areas of uptake	Infection or lymphoma (*Note*: including infected KS)
	Diffuse lung + gastrointestinal uptake + eye uptake	CMV

patient is shown in Figure 5.7 and Table 5.2. A chest radiograph and ^{99m}Tc DTPA scan will differentiate patients who have essentially normal lungs from those who have an alveolitis or another infection. Decisions about treatment of patients with an alveolitis depends on the prevalence of the causes of an alveolitis and whether empirical therapy is administered or further investigation is undertaken. Gallium imaging may allow specific identification as suggested in Table 5.2 but it should be remembered that the scan may show no uptake in all of the conditions discussed.

A variety of conditions affect ^{99m}Tc DTPA transfer, some of which may be found in patients with HIV, e.g. interstitial lung disease (fibrosing alveolitis, radiation pneumonitis, sarcoidosis) (Rinderknecht *et al.*, 1980; Wells *et al.*, 1993), 'crack' cocaine use (Susskind *et al.*, 1993), adult respiratory distress syndrome (Mason *et al.*, 1985). More recently Pertechnegas (which is generated from Technegas by the addition of oxygen)

has been used to assess patients with HIV infection and respiratory symptoms (Monaghan *et al.*, 1991). This imaging technique appears to convey little advantage over ^{99m}Tc DTPA.

LOCALIZATION OF TUMOR AND ASSESSMENT OF DISSEMINATION

Tumors particularly associated with HIV infection include non Hodgkin's lymphoma and Kaposi's sarcoma (KS). The presence of tumor within mediastinal lymph nodes (not KS) may be detected using gallium or ^{18}F-FDG (fluorodeoxyglucose). These agents also have the advantage of delineating the extent of disease throughout the patient. In addition they are capable of detecting disease in normal-sized lymph nodes and thus direct further investigation. There are at present immense difficulties in imaging Kaposi's' sarcoma both in the lung and elsewhere in the body.

Kaposi's sarcoma represents a major challenge to the nuclear medicine clinician. Gallium is not taken up into this lesion (Kramer *et al.*, 1987; Woolfenden, 1987; Davis *et al.*, 1987) and is of use in the presence of an abnormal chest radiograph when the absence of gallium accumulation is consistent with KS. If there is accumulation in the region of known KS in the lungs then this would indicate a dual pathology and the need for further investigation. Currently the only agent that may localize in Kaposi's sarcoma is thallium-201 (Lee *et al.*, 1988, 1991). Skin lesions have been localized as have lesions in lymph nodes and lung. Uptake of thallium in KS is not predictable and therefore is not reliable clinically. As thallium is actively excreted into bowel, gastrointestinal KS lesions may be missed. The technique may be used to localize a lymph node for biopsy. It is not known however whether thallium is taken up in persistent generalized lymphadenopathy or only tumor-involved lymph nodes. There is a clear need for other agents to be assessed in this regard.

Lymphoma does accumulate both gallium and ^{18}F-FDG and imaging with either agent will allow the extent of disease throughout the body to be defined (Figure 5.8a–e); ^{18}FDG has lower bowel accumulation than gallium. Both agents do have false positive results with accumulation seen in lymph nodes involved by infection and in persistent generalized lymphadenopathy (see earlier section on ^{67}Ga).

Positron emission tomography (PET) is a powerful quantitative imaging technique which is capable of displaying many problems of intrathoracic biochemistry. Positron emitting radionuclides (carbon-11, oxygen-15, nitrogen-13 and fluorine-18) are formed into biologically active compounds and are administered intravenously. The radionuclides have a very short half-life compared with conventional nuclear medicine radionuclides and therefore centers using these have a cyclotron 'on site' to produce them. The positron emitters when administered into the body as ^{18}F fluorodeoxyglucose or ^{11}C methionine, etc. localize in tissues to portray local glucose and protein turnover respectively. When taken up into the cell an emitted positron collides with an electron within 1–2 millimetres of its release and annihilates itself and the interacting electron; this produces two gamma photons which travel in opposite directions, that is at 180° to one another. These two photons can be detected by a ring of detectors situated around the patient and an image can be formed with good resolution.

Positron emission tomography of the thorax has a number of applications for the clinical assessment of patients. In the thorax, the primary use in non-HIV infected individuals has been the identification of malignant versus benign disease and defining the extent of disease using ^{18}F-FDG. These findings have been generated from patients with lung cancer and lymphoma and should have similar appearances in patients with HIV infection. It is likely that ^{18}F-FDG imaging will have a higher sensitivity than gallium scanning in the localization of abnormal lymph nodes although the specificity may be similar. The resolution of the PET imaging should allow more accurate localization of nodes and absolute quantification may allow separation of reactive nodes from malignant nodes. However this remains to be established.

ASSESSMENT OF DRUG DELIVERY

The increasing fascination with delivery of drugs to the respiratory tree demands the increasing involvement of nuclear medicine to measure the deposition of drugs. This will allow rational selection of the most appropriate delivery systems for antibiotics and so the clinical effectiveness of inhaled antibiotics can then be assessed. The use of PET radiopharmaceuticals ^{18}F FDG, ^{11}C

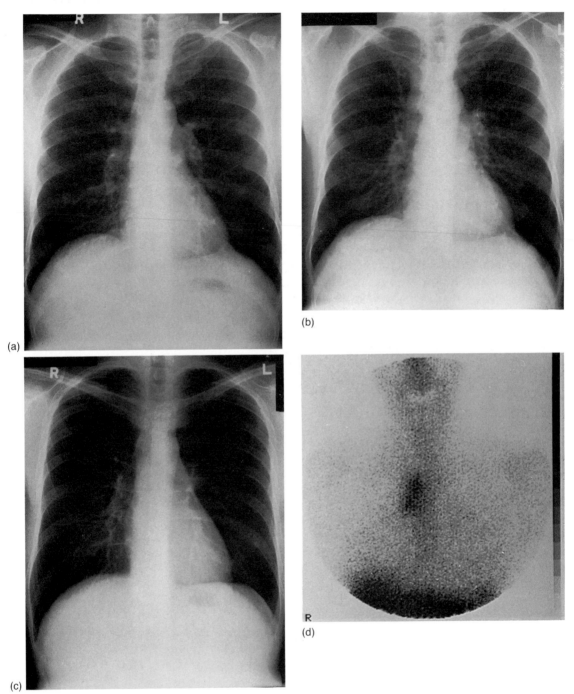

Fig. 5.8 The chest radiograph appearance (a) before; (b) following the gallium and FDG PET scans; (c) after radiotherapy, in a patient presenting with retrosternal chest ache. (d) The gallium accumulation is apparent in the retrosternal region and (e) FDG accumulation in the same region, with no accumulation elsewhere. The chest radiograph was initially normal (a) and later found to be abnormal (b). The diagnosis of a lymphoma was made on biopsy.

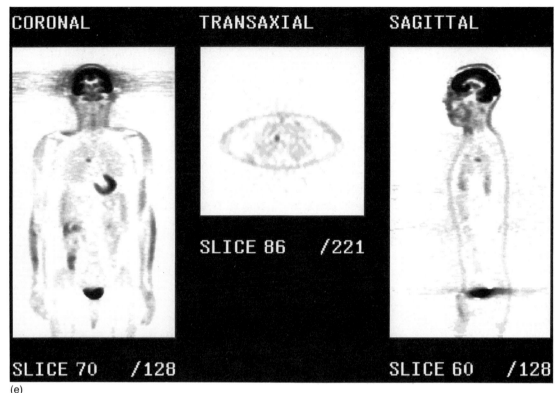

CORONAL　　　TRANSAXIAL　　　SAGITTAL

SLICE 86　　/221

SLICE 70　　/128　　　　　SLICE 60　　/128

(e)

Fig. 5.8 *(cont.)*

methionine may allow the localization of tumors within the lung, mediastinum or soft tissues and by repeat scanning assess the response of tumors to therapy.

Inhaled drug therapy in patients with HIV infection can be divided into the use of drugs (1) as prophylaxis or as treatment for the opportunistic infections, and (2) directed at tumors found in the lung. Radionuclides and the use of the gamma camera or positron emission camera have a role to play in both aspects of monitoring drugs.

The targeting of inhaled therapy to the lung is dependent on the dose of drug delivered to the lung and the specific site required for the therapy, e.g. small or large airways. Radionuclides can be used to directly or indirectly label drugs to assess their distribution within the body or the lung, e.g.

^{18}F fluconazole, ^{123}I iodopentamidine, ^{99m}Tc human serum albumin. Their specific use in the lung is to provide a means of assessing drug delivery using aerosols.

One of the areas in which indirect radionuclide markers have been used is in the assessment of delivery of nebulized pentamidine. Since the introduction of nebulized pentamidine for treatment and prophylaxis via a Respirgard II nebulizer (Montgomery *et al.*, 1987) a variety of nebulizer delivery systems have been tried with varying success. This is not surprising when one considers the variable pulmonary deposition of pentamidine measured using indirect radionuclide markers (O'Doherty *et al.*, 1988, 1990, 1993; Thomas *et al.*, 1991; Smaldone *et al.*, 1991; Ferretti *et al.*, 1994). The increased recurrence of PCP in the upper lobes may also be explained by the lower deposition in the apices compared with the lower lobes, and this deposition may be altered by lying the patient down (O'Doherty *et al.*, 1988). The deposition using indirect labels gives an indication of the amount of drug deposited but not the rate at which it leaves the lung (which can be investigated using a direct label of pentamidine, ^{123}I iodopentamidine (O'Doherty *et al.*, 1993)). Deposition of pentamidine in children is also likely to be different to adults, given the differences in ventilation in children (smaller airways, higher respiratory rate, different airway opening and closing pressures, and airway compliance). Perhaps surprisingly it appears that equivalent or lower doses of the drug are needed in a Respirgard II nebulizier in order to achieve similar lung concentrations of drug to that achieved in adults using the Respirgard II nebulizer (O'Doherty *et al.*, 1993).

Although one can predict that an efficient nebulizer producing a small particle size should produce good peripheral penetration of a drug, this requires *in vivo* confirmation since often the drug in question is an antibiotic (which may not have any measurable immediate effects on the airway) and therefore the quantity of drug delivered should be known in order to assess its effectiveness. A nebulized drug may fail either because the drug is unsuitable or because insufficient drug is deposited in the region of the lung where it is to be effective. The use of radionuclides has a great deal to offer in both evaluation of drug delivery methods and in organ disposition (O'Doherty *et al.*, 1993; Davis *et al.*, 1992).

NUCLEAR MEDICINE, THE AIDS CLINICIAN AND A 'CASH POOR' ENVIRONMENT

The key tests that can be performed depend on access to delivery of gallium and a technetium generator. In a breathless patient with a normal chest radiograph or a nondiagnostic chest radiograph the investigation of choice is ^{99m}Tc DTPA aerosol transfer scan. All units have access to a technetium generator and DTPA is available as kits, therefore the scan is available every day of the week. The test could be performed without a gamma camera by using a scintillation probe linked to a computer (IBM) to generate the curves. This would allow a confident diagnosis of pulmonary abnormality and a high probability of an alveolitis on the day of referral. If patients have a pyrexia of unknown origin (PUO) then gallium is the investigation of choice. In the Western world, this scan might also be performed in HIV-infected patients with continuing weight loss as a screening investigation.

Nuclear medicine procedures are cost effective in patients where there may be no particular localizing features associated with particular symptoms. The procedures can localize abnormalities for more accurate anatomical localization by CT or MRI or more appropriate invasive investigation.

FUTURE

It is clear that with the advent of highly sensitive and specific diagnostic tests such as immunofluorescence and the polymerase chain reaction which promise rapid and early diagnosis of opportunistic infection, that to be of value imaging techniques either have to offer rapid differential diagnoses of high sensitivity or display the extent of disease within the thorax. It is therefore likely in future that imaging procedures that take 24–48 hours to achieve a diagnosis will have limited use.

There are several areas that will expand as HIV-positive patients live longer and so present with different problems. These are:

1. Rapid methods of imaging infection with more novel radiopharmaceuticals. These may include the currently available Infecton^{TM} but will proceed to chemotactic

peptides and Fab fragments (possibly of anti E selectin), hopefully labeled with ^{99m}Tc.

2. The development of suitable imaging for Kaposi's sarcoma to define the total body tumor load. Although thallium has shown limited uptake it is almost certainly not capable of defining the tumor load and new methods are still needed.

3. The use of PET isotopes in the assessment of tumor distribution and response to cytotoxic therapy.

REFERENCES

Baron, A.L., Steinbach, L.D., Leboit, P.E. *et al.* (1990) Osteolytic lesions of bacillary angiomatosis in HIV infection: radiologic differentiation from AIDS-related Kaposi sarcoma. *Radiology*, **177**, 77–81.

Bitran, J., Beckerman, C., Weinstein, R. *et al.* (1987) Patterns of gallium-67 scintigraphy in patients with acquired immunodeficiency syndrome and the AIDS related complex. *J. Nucl. Med.*, **28**, 1103–1106.

Bradburne, R.M., Ettensohn, D.B., Opal, S.M. and McCool, F.D. (1989) Relapse of *Pneumocystis carinii* pneumonia in the upper lobes during aerosol pentamidine prophylaxis. *Thorax*, **44**, 591–3.

Buscombe, J., Lui, D., Ensing, G. *et al.* (1990) ^{99m}Tc human immunoglobulin (HIgG): first results of a new agent for the localisation of infection and inflammation. *Eur. J. Nucl. Med.*, **16**, 649–55.

Buscombe, J., Oyen, W.J.G. Grant *et al.* (1993) Indium-111-labelled polyclonal human immunoglobulin: Identifying focal infection in patients positive for human immunodeficiency virus. *J. Nucl. Med.*, **34**, 1621–25.

Chien, S.-M., Rawji, M., Mintz, S. *et al.* (1992) Changes in hospital admission pattern in patients with human immunodeficiency virus infection in the era of *P. carinii* prohylaxis. *Chest*, **102**, 1035–9.

Cordes, M., Roll, D., Langer, M. *et al.* (1989) Diagnostic value of early gallium-67 scans (4 h p.i.) in patients with AIDS and PCP. *Eur. J. Nucl. Med.*, **15**, 172.

Cregler, L.L., Sosa, I., Ducey, S. and Abbey, S. (1990) Myopericarditis in acquired immunodeficiency syndrome diagnosed by gal-lium scintigraphy. *J. Natl. Med. Assoc.*, **82**, 511–13.

Davis, S.D., Henschke, C.I., Chamides, B.K. and Wescott, J.L. (1987) Intrathoracic Kaposi sarcoma in AIDS patients: radiographic-pathologic correlation. *Radiology*, **163**, 495–500.

Davis, S.S., Hardy, J.G., Newman, S.P. and Wilding, I.R. (1992) Gamma scintigraphy in the evaluation of pharmaceutical dosage forms. *Eur. J. Nucl. Med.*, **19**, 971–86.

Ferretti, P.P., Versari, A., Gafa, S.I. *et al.* (1994) Pulmonary deposition of aerosolised pentamidine using a new nebuliser: efficiency measurements *in vitro* and *in vivo*. *Eur. J. Nucl. Med.*, **21**, 399–406.

Fineman, D.S., Palestro, C.J., Kim, C.K. *et al.* (1989) Detection of abnormalities in febrile AIDS patients with In-111-labelled leucocyte and Ga-67 scintigraphy. *Radiology*, **170**, 677–80.

Fischman, J.A., Strauss, H.W., Fishman, A.J. *et al.* (1991) Imaging of *Pneumocystis carinii* pneumonia with ^{111}In-labelled non-specific polyclonal IgG: an experimental study in rats. *Nuc. Med. Commun.*, **12**, 175–87.

Ganz, W.I., Serafini, A.N., Ganz, S.S. *et al.* (1988) Diagnostic pattern of Ga-67 uptake in lymphocytic interstitial pneumonitis. *J. Nucl. Med.*, **29**, 887–8.

Goldenberg, D.M., Sharkey, R.M., Udem, S. *et al.* (1994) Immunoscintigraphy of *Pneumocystis carinii* pneumonia in AIDS patients. *J. Nucl. Med.*, **35**, 1028–34.

Hunninghake, G.W., Line, B.R., Szapiel, S.V. *et al.* (1981) Activation of inflammatory cells increases the localization of gallium-67 at sites of disease. *Clin. Res.*, **29**, 171A.

Kramer, E.L., Sanger, J.J., Garay, S.M. *et al.* (1987) Gallium-67 scans of the chest in patients with acquired immunodeficiency syndrome. *J. Nucl. Med.*, **28**, 1107–14.

Leach, R., Davidson, C., O'Doherty, M.J. *et al.* (1991) Noninvasive management of fever and breathlessness in HIV positive patients. *Eur. J. Respir. Med.*, **4**, 19–25.

Lee, V.W., Rosen, M.P., Baum, A. *et al.* (1988) AIDS-related Kaposi's sarcoma: Findings on thallium-201 scintigraphy. *AJR*, **151**, 1233–5.

Lee, V.W., Fuller, J.D., O'Brien, M.J. *et al.* (1991) Pulmonary Kaposi sarcoma in patients with AIDS: Scintigraphic diagnosis with sequential thallium and gallium scanning. *Radiology*, **180**, 409–12.

Mason, G.R., Effros, R.M., Uszler, J.M. *et al.*

(1985) Small solute clearance from the lungs of patients with cardiogenic and noncardiogenic pulmonary edema. *Chest*, **88**, 327–34.

Miller, R.F. (1990) Nuclear medicine and AIDS. *Eur. J. Nucl. Med.*, **16**, 103–18.

Monaghan, P., Provan, I., Murray, C. *et al.* (1991) An improved radionuclide technique for the detection of altered pulmonary permeability. *J. Nucl. Med.*, **32**, 1945–9.

Montgomery, A.B., Debs, R.J., Luce, J.M. *et al.* (1987) Aerosolised pentamidine as sole treatment for *Pneumocystis carinii* in patients with the acquired immunodeficiency syndrome. *Lancet*, **ii**, 480–3.

O'Doherty, M.J., Page, C.J., Bradbeer, C.S. *et al.* (1987) Alveolar permeability in HIV patients with *Pneumocystis carinii* pneumonia. *Genitourin. Med.*, **63**, 268–70.

O'Doherty, M.J., Thomas, S., Page, C. *et al.* (1988a) Differences in the relative efficiency of nebulisers for pentamidine administration. *Lancet*, **ii**, 1283–6.

O'Doherty, M.J., Thomas, S.H.L., Page, C.J. *et al.* (1988b) Does inhalation of pentamidine in the supine position increase deposition in the upper part of the lung? *Chest*, **97**, 1343–8.

O'Doherty, M.J., Page, C.J., Bradbeer, C.S. *et al.* (1989) The place of lung 99mTc DTPA aerosol transfer in the investigation of lung infections in HIV positive patients. *Resp. Med.*, **83**, 395–401.

O'Doherty, M.J., Revell, P., Page, C.J. *et al.* (1990a) Donor leucocyte imaging in patients with AIDS. A preliminary communication. *Eur. J. Nucl. Med.*, **17**, 327–33.

O'Doherty, M., Thomas, S., Page, C. *et al.* (1990b) Pulmonary deposition of nebulised pentamidine. The effect of nebuliser type, dose and volume of fill. *Thorax*, **45**, 460–4.

O'Doherty, M.J., Thomas, S.H.L., Gibb, D. *et al.* (1993a) Deposition of aerosolized pentamidine in children. *Thorax*, **48**, 220–6.

O'Doherty, M.J., Thomas, S.H.L., Page, C.J. *et al.* (1993b) Lung deposition of aerosolised pentamidine using a direct radiolabel, 123I iodopentamidine. *Nucl. Med. Commun.*, **14**, 8–11.

O'Doherty, M.J. and Miller, R.F. (1993c) Aerosols for therapy and diagnosis. *Eur. J. Nucl. Med.* **20**, 1201–13.

Ognibene, F.P., Masur, H., Rogers, P. *et al.* (1988) Nonspecific interstitial pneumonitis without evidence of *Pneumocystis carinii* in asymptomatic patients infected with human immunodeficiency virus (HIV). *Ann. Intern. Med.*, **109**, 179–83.

Palestro, C.J. (1994) The current role of gallium imaging in infection. *Seminars Nucl. Med.*, **24**, 128–41.

Pitkin, A.D., Grant, A.D., Foley, N.M. and Miller, R.F. (1993) Changing patterns of respiratory disease in HIV positive patients in a referral centre in the United Kingdom 1986–7 and 1990–1. *Thorax*, **48**, 204–7.

Podzamczer, D., Ricart, I., Bolao, F. *et al.* (1990) Gallium-67 scan for distinguishing follicular hyperplasia from other AIDS-associated disease in lymph nodes. *AIDS*, **4**, 683–5.

Rinderknecht, J., Shapiro, L., Krauthammer, M. *et al.* (1980) Accelerated clearance of small solvents from the lungs in interstitial lung disease. *Am. Rev. Respir. Dis.*, **121**, 105–17.

Rosso, J., Guillon, J.M., Parrot, A. *et al.* (1992) Technetium-99m-DTPA aerosol and gallium-67 scanning in pulmonary complications of human immunodeficiency virus infection. *J. Nucl. Med.*, **33**, 81–7.

Robinson, D.S., Cunningham, D.A., Dave, S. *et al.* (1991) Diagnostic value of lung clearance of 99mTc DTPA compared with other non-invasive investigations in *Pneumocystis carinii* pneumonia in AIDS. *Thorax*, **46**, 722–6.

Rubin, R.H., Fischman, A.J., Needleman, M. *et al.* (1989a) Radiolabelled, nonspecific, polyclonal human immunoglobulin in the detection of focal inflammation by scintigraphy: comparison with gallium-67 citrate and technetium-99m-labelled albumin. *J. Nucl. Med.*, **30**, 385–9.

Rubin, R.H., Fischman, A.J., Callahan, R.J. *et al.* (1989b) 111-In-labelled nonspecific immunoglobulin scanning in the detection of focal infection. *N. Engl. J. Med*, **321**, 935–40.

Schiff, R.G., Kabat, L., Kamain, N. *et al.* (1987) Gallium scanning in lymphoid interstitial pneumonitis in children with AIDS. *J. Nucl. Med.*, **28**, 1915–19.

Smaldone, G.C., Fuhrer, J., Stiegbigel, R.T. and McPeck, M. (1991) Factors determining pulmonary deposition of aerosolised pentamidine in patients with human immunodeficiency virus infection. *Am. Rev. Respir. Dis.*, **143**, 727–37.

Smith, R.L., Berkowitz, K.A. and Lewis, M.L. (1992) Pulmonary disposition of gallium-67 in patients with *Pneumocystis* pneumonia: An analysis using bronchoalveolar lavage. *J. Nucl. Med.*, **33**, 512–15.

Stafianakis, G.N., Jabir, A.M., Beach, R. *et al.*

(1989) Increased gallium-67 pulmonary activity in human immunodeficiency virus (HIV) positive non-AIDS, non-ARC, non-iv drug abusers: correlation with tobacco smoking. *J. Nucl. Med.*, **29**, 829.

Susskind N., H., Weber, D.A., Volkow, D. *et al.* (1991) Increased lung permeability following long-term use of free-base cocaine (crack). *Chest*, **100**, 903–9.

Thomas, S.H.L., O'Doherty, M.J., Page, C.J. *et al.* (1991) Which apparatus for inhaled pentamidine? A comparison of pulmonary deposition via eight nebulisers. *Eur. Respir. J.*, **4**, 616–22.

Tuazon, C.V., Delaney, M.D., Simon, G.L. *et al.* (1985) Utility of gallium-67 scintigraphy and bronchial washings in the diagnosis and treatment of *Pneumocystis carinii* pneumonia in patients with the acquired immunodeficiency syndrome. *Am. Rev. Respir. Dis.*, **132**, 1087–92.

Tumeh, S.S., Rosenthal, D.S., Kaplan, W.D. *et al.* (1987) Lymphoma: evaluation with Ga-67 SPECT. *Radiology*, **164**, 111–14.

Tumeh, S.S., Belville, J.S., Pugatch, R. and McNeil, B. (1992) Ga-67 scintigraphy and computed tomography in the diagnosis of *Pneumocystis carinii* pneumonia in patients with AIDS. A prospective comparison. *Clin. Nucl. Med.*, **17**, 387–94.

Van der Wall, H., Murray, I.P.C., Jones, P.D. *et al.* (1991) Optimising technetium 99m diethylene triamine penta-acetate lung clearance in patients with the acquired immunodeficiency syndrome. *Eur. J. Nucl. Med.*, **18**, 235–40.

Wells, A.U., Hansell, D.M., Harrison, N.K. *et al.* (1993) Clearance of inhaled ^{99m}Tc DTPA predicts the clinical course of fibrosing alveolitis. *Eur. Respir. J.*, **6**, 797–802.

Woolfenden, J.M., Carrasquillo, J.A., Larson, S.M. *et al.* (1987) Acquired immunodeficiency syndrome. Ga-67 citrate imaging. *Radiology*, **162**, 383–7.

Zuckier, L.S., Ongseng, F. and Goldbarb, C.R. (1988) Lymphocytic interstitial pneumonitis: a cause of pulmonary gallium-67 uptake in a child with acquired immunodeficiency syndrome. *J. Nucl. Med.*, **29**, 707–11.

6

MOLECULAR BIOLOGY OF *PNEUMOCYSTIS CARINII* INFECTION

Ann E. Wakefield and Robert F. Miller

PNEUMOCYSTIS CARINII – A MEMBER OF THE FUNGAL KINGDOM

Since *Pneumocystis carinii* was first described, the organism has been variously thought of both as a protozoan and as a fungus based on morphological characteristics and response to therapeutic agents. In the absence of an effective method of *in vitro* culture of the organism (Sloand *et al.*, 1993), molecular techniques have contributed to the understanding of the taxonomy of *P. carinii*. The first genetic locus to be examined was that of the gene encoding the 18S ribosomal RNA from rat-derived *P. carinii* and this was found to show homology to fungal sequences (Edman *et al.*, 1989a; Stringer *et al.*, 1989). Subsequently, a 6.8 kilobase pair fragment of mitochondrial DNA encoding 7 contiguous genes, apocytochrome b, NADH dehydrogenase subunits 1, 2, 3 and 6, cytochrome oxidase subunit II and the small subunit ribosomal RNA, has been analyzed and all the genes showed fungal homology (Pixley *et al.*, 1991). Although *P. carinii* has certain characteristics which are atypical of many fungi, for example, the lack of ergosterol in the plasma membrane (Kaneshiro *et al.*, 1994), and the lack of response to antifungal chemotherapeutic agents, the taxonomic assignment of *P. carinii* to the fungal kingdom has been further

supported by the cloning and sequencing of additional *P. carinii* genes. These include the genes encoding dihydrofolate reductase (DHFR) (Edman *et al.*, 1989b), thymidylate synthase (TS) (Edman *et al.*, 1989c), β-tubulin (Dyer *et al.*, 1992), α-tubulin (Zhang and Stringer, 1993), transcription factor IID (Meade and Stringer, 1991), cation transporting ATPase (Meade and Stringer, 1991, 1995), the AROM protein (Banerji *et al.*, 1993), actin (Fletcher *et al.*, 1994) and translation elongation factor EF3 (Ypma-Wong, Fonzi and Syphera, 1992).

HOST SPECIES SPECIFICITY OF *P. CARINII* INFECTION

The existence of different types of *P. carinii* has been recognized, and early research described differences between the rat- and human-derived organisms, proposing the name *Pneumocystis jiroveci* for the latter (Frenkel, 1976). Immunological data have contributed to the understanding of host specificity of *P. carinii* infection. Antigenic differences between *P. carinii* isolated from different hosts have been observed, by the characterization of proteins and glycoproteins separated by electrophoresis. Most antibodies elicited to *P. carinii* from one host species do not cross-react with antigen

AIDS and Respiratory Medicine. Edited by A. Zumla, M.A. Johnson and R.F. Miller. Published in 1997 by Chapman & Hall, London. ISBN 0 412 60140 0

preparations of *P. carinii* from another host species (Gigliotti *et al.*, 1986, 1988, 1992; Graves *et al.*, 1986a, b; Kovacs *et al.*, 1988; Linke *et al.*, 1989; Bauer *et al.*, 1993). Serological studies in man have detected a high frequency of antibodies to *P. carinii* in the general population and have shown differential responses to specific antigens (Peglow *et al.*, 1990). The frequency and pattern of antibodies to high molecular weight *P. carinii* antigens have been shown to vary in different areas of the world (Smulian *et al.*, 1993).

Functional studies on the transmission of the infection also show differences among isolates of *P. carinii*. Although the parasite is transmissible between animals of the same species by the airborne route under controlled experimental conditions (Hughes, 1987), a number of studies involving cross-infectivity of *P. carinii* isolated from one species into a second host species have indicated that *P. carinii* infection is host-species-specific. Attempts to transmit *P. carinii*, by either intranasal or intrapulmonary inoculation, from dogs to immunosuppressed guinea pigs, from rats to immunosuppressed mice or hamsters, from mice to nude rats and from humans to nude or immunosuppressed rats, have all been unsuccessful (Frenkel, Good and Shultz, 1966; Minielly, Mills and Holley, 1969; Farrow *et al.*, 1972; Furuta and Katsumoto, 1987). Recent experiments, using molecular techniques that could distinguish between ferret- and mouse-derived *P. carinii*, have demonstrated the restricted host range of ferret-derived *P. carinii* when attempting to transmit ferret-derived *P. carinii* to SCID mice by intratracheal inoculation (Gigliotti *et al.*, 1993).

Analysis of genetic diversity amongst *P. carinii* from different host species has been carried out. Chromosome analysis by pulsed field gel electrophoresis has shown that the karyotypes of rat- and human-derived *P. carinii* were of a similar size range but that

the banding patterns were different (Hong *et al.*, 1990). Further studies with rat-, mouse- and ferret-derived *P. carinii* have reported different karyotypes with 14 bands for the rat-derived *P. carinii*, 15 bands for the mouse-derived *P. carinii* and 9 bands for the ferret-derived *P. carinii* (Weinberg and Durant, 1994a). Hybridization of *P. carinii* gene probes to electrophoretically separated chromosomes has also been informative in demonstrating differences in genotype between isolates of *P. carinii* from different host species (Stringer *et al.*, 1993; Weinberg *et al.*, 1994a, b). Sequence analyses of a portion of a mitochondrial genome encoding the large subunit ribosomal RNA (LSU rRNA) (Sinclair *et al.*, 1991), a segment of gene encoding the β-tubulin gene (Edlind *et al.*, 1992) and the nuclear ribosomal RNA operon (Stringer *et al.*, 1993; Liu and Leibowitz, 1993) have shown that *P. carinii* from rats and humans are different. Further sequence data from the mitochondrial LSU rRNA gene of *P. carinii* in thoroughbred foals showed that it is distinct from rat-, mouse-, rabbit-, ferret- and human-derived *P. carinii* (Peters *et al.*, 1994a). Analysis of the gene encoding thymidylate synthase has shown high levels of DNA and amino acid sequence divergence among isolates of rat-, human-, mouse- and rabbit-derived *P. carinii* (Mazars *et al.*, 1995) and also ferret-derived organisms (Keely *et al.*, 1994). Genetic divergence has also been observed among these isolates at a portion of the *arom* locus, involved in aromatic amino acid biosynthesis. The aromatic amino acid biosynthetic pathway is found in bacteria, plants and lower eukaryotes but is absent in mammals. Aromatic amino acid biosynthesis in fungi is dependent on the pre-chorismate pathway; steps 2 to 6 of this pathway are catalysed by a single pentafunctional protein called AROM, which is encoded by a single *arom* gene. The *arom* gene from *P. carinii* has been cloned and characterized and found to have conventional fungal organization (Banerji *et al.*, 1993). The divergence among these isolates ranged from 7% to 22% at the DNA sequence level and 7% to 26% at the amino acid sequence level (Banerji *et al.*, 1995). These cumulative data strongly suggest that *P. carinii* infection is host-species-specific. The results demonstrate that human-derived *P. carinii* is genetically distinct from isolates from other mammalian host species, and suggest that *P. carinii* infection in man is not a zoonosis, acquired from a reservoir of parasites in the infected lungs of an animal host.

GENETIC DIVERSITY AMONG ISOLATES OF *P. CARINII* FROM THE SAME HOST SPECIES

Genetic diversity has also been observed among isolates of *P. carinii* from the same host species. Two distinct types of *P. carinii* have been identified in the infected lungs of rats. These two types were originally distinguished by the difference in migration of chromosomal bands by pulsed field gel electrophoresis (Cushion *et al.*, 1993). These two types (named 'prototype' and 'variant') could also be distinguished by the differential hybridization of chromosomes to a *P. carinii* major surface glycoprotein gene probe, the presence or absence of an intron in the 18S rRNA gene and the DNA sequence of the gene encoding the 18S rRNA. Sequence analysis of a number of other genes has also revealed relatively high levels of genetic divergence between the two types (Keely *et al.*, 1994; Ortiz-Rivera *et al.*, 1995; Sunkin and Stringer, 1995).

Two genetically diverse types of *P. carinii* have also been detected in the infected lungs of ferrets. Preliminary data from analysis of the *arom* locus have demonstrated that the two ferret-derived *P. carinii* sequences showed 15% divergence from each other, and ferret-derived *P. carinii* type A showed 18% divergence and type B showed 16% divergence from the rat-derived *P. carinii* sequences. Similar divergence was found in the

analysis of the deduced amino acids sequence. The two types of *P. carinii* were both isolated from the same infected lung, suggesting that co-infection of ferret lung with two genetically distinct strains of *P. carinii* may occur (Banerji, Lugli and Wakefield, 1994).

In most cases, however, the extent of genetic diversity among isolates of *P. carinii* from the same host species has been found to be lower than that from different host species. Low levels of genetic diversity have been reported among human-derived *P. carinii*. Studies of a portion of the nuclear ribosomal RNA operon from human-derived *P. carinii* from five HIV-infected patients in the USA showed that, although the sequence of this gene was different from that of rat-derived *P. carinii*, each of the human-derived sequences was identical (Liu and Leibowitz, 1993). In another study of 12 patients, the nucleotide sequence of the gene encoding the mitochondrial LSU rRNA of *P. carinii* was compared (Lee *et al.*, 1993). Five of the samples contained sequences which were identical to the original description (Sinclair *et al.*, 1991). In six of the samples, sequences containing between one and three single base polymorphisms were observed. In one patient, the sequence appeared to be a hybrid of human- and rat-derived *P. carinii* sequences (Lee *et al.*, 1993). Samples of human-derived *P. carinii* obtained from various geographical locations – USA, Brazil, Zimbabwe and Britain – have also been examined by sequence analysis of the mitochondrial LSU rRNA. This study revealed striking lack of sequence variation between these isolates, with only a single base polymorphism, seen in the same position as that previously reported. In addition, this study showed a lack of sequence variation between samples obtained from one geographical location (London) over a four-and-a-half year period (Wakefield *et al.*, 1994a). A similar lack of genetic variation was seen when the sequence of the *arom* gene was compared in isolates of human-derived *P. carinii* obtained from the same geographical locations (Banerji *et al.*, 1995). The results from this study also indicated that the infection in some of the individuals may not have been clonal. These data question the hypothesis that the relative prevalence of *P. carinii* pneumonia in humans in different locations is due to strain differences, although analysis at other informative loci, such as those encoding antigenically important epitopes, may reveal differences among these isolates.

A study of samples from 28 HIV-infected patients in France also utilized sequence analysis of the mitochondrial LSU rRNA. Again, only low levels of genetic diversity were observed with single base polymorphisms at the same residues as in the previous studies (Latouche *et al.*, 1994). Sequence variation between isolates of human-derived *P. carinii* has also been examined at the internal transcribed spacer (ITS) regions, which are located between the 18S, 5.8S and 26S rRNA gene sequences in the nuclear rRNA operon (Liu and Leibowitz, 1993). Four different ITS sequence types has been identified in samples of human-derived *P. carinii*. Some of the samples appeared to be infected with two different types (Lu *et al.*, 1994, 1995a). Preliminary data from another study suggest that this locus may provide a useful tool for epidemiological studies (Tsolaki *et al.*, 1996).

DIAGNOSIS OF *P. CARINII* PNEUMONIA USING THE POLYMERASE CHAIN REACTION

The detection of *P. carinii* by DNA amplification using the polymerase chain reaction (PCR) has been developed for the diagnosis of *P. carinii* pneumonia. PCR detection methods have been designed to a number of different loci of the *P. carinii* genome including the gene encoding the mitochondrial LSU rRNA (Wakefield *et al.*, 1990a, b), the 5S

rRNA (Kitada *et al.*, 1991), the 18S rRNA (Lipschik *et al.*, 1992; Borensztein *et al.*, 1992), and thymidylate synthase (Olsson *et al.*, 1993). A number of different types of clinical samples have been used in these studies including invasive samples such as bronchoalveolar lavage, but also non-invasive samples such as induced sputum (Wakefield *et al.*, 1991), and nasopharyngeal samples from pediatric patients where sample collection is more difficult and sample volume usually very small (Richards, Wakefield and Mitchell, 1994). PCR detection of *P. carinii* has also been applied to oropharyngeal samples from HIV-infected patients with respiratory symptoms. When compared to histochemical staining of bronchoalveolar lavage fluid, the sensitivity of detection by PCR in the oropharyngeal samples was 78% (Wakefield *et al.*, 1993).

In an atypical form of human *P. carinii* infection, a granulomatous intrapulmonary response occurs, *P. carinii* cysts are enclosed by a palisade of histiocytes and only very small numbers of *P. carinii*, undetectable by silver staining, are present within the alveoli. Transbronchial biopsies are frequently negative because of the patchy nature of the disease and firm diagnosis may need to be established by open lung biopsy. DNA amplification on samples of bronchoalveolar lavage from these patients has been demonstrated to be positive, although the amount of DNA detected is lower than that seen in patients with typical presentation of disease (Wakefield *et al.*, 1994b).

A number of studies have compared PCR detection of *P. carinii* with conventional silver staining and with detection using immunofluorescence using specific anti-*P. carinii* antibodies. Using the primer pair to the mitochondrial LSU rRNA, PCR detection was demonstrated to be more sensitive than immunofluorescence for the detection of *P. carinii* in samples of bronchoalveolar lavage (Tamburrini *et al.*, 1993a; Leigh *et al.*, 1993a), induced sputum (Leigh *et al.*,

1992; Evans *et al.*, 1995), bronchoalveolar washings, induced sputum and spontaneous sputum (Roux *et al.*, 1994; Cartwright, Nelson and Gill, 1994; Leibovitz *et al.*, 1995). The PCR technique was demonstrated to be especially valuable in the detection of *P. carinii* in non-invasive samples. In a study, again using the primer pair designed to the mitochondrial LSU rRNA gene, PCR was performed on induced sputum samples from 49 patients in France and was found to have a sensitivity and specificity of 100%, compared to 46.5% and 100% respectively with standard histochemical and immunofluorescence staining (Chouaid *et al.*, 1995).

A number of comparative studies have been undertaken to evaluate the efficacy of the different PCR primer pairs, designed to different regions of the *P. carinii* genome, in the detection of *P. carinii* (Lu *et al.*, 1995b). In a study comparing three different primer pairs, those designed to the mitochondrial LSU rRNA were found to exhibit greater sensitivity and specificity than primers to the gene encoding the 5S rRNA or dihydrofolate reductase (DHFR) (DeLuca *et al.*, 1995). The levels of sensitivity of the PCR method of detection have been examined. Levels of sensitivity were increased by subsequent Southern hybridization of the amplification products with an internal probe. Using this method of detection, with primers and probe to the mitochondrial LSU rRNA gene, detection at the level of one to two organisms has been demonstrated (Peters *et al.*, 1992a; DeLuca *et al.*, 1995). Nested PCR, at the same locus using the primer pair pAZ102-X and pAZ102-Y in the second round PCR, has an equivalent sensitivity (Wakefield, unpublished results). Hemi-nested PCR at this locus has also been shown to be effective (Tamburrini *et al.*, 1993; Peters *et al.*, 1994). It has been suggested that the levels of *P. carinii*-specific amplification product in respiratory samples from HIV-infected patients decrease as a response to anti-*P. carinii* therapy (Wakefield *et al.*, 1993, 1994;

Evans *et al.*, 1995). These data are supported by studies on the rat model of the infection, where semi-quantitative PCR has been used to monitor response to treatment (O'Leary *et al.*, 1995).

A number of studies have examined samples of blood and serum for the presence of *P. carinii* DNA, with conflicting results. In a study using primers designed to the gene encoding DHFR, *P. carinii* DNA has been detected in samples of serum from 12 of 14 HIV-infected patients with *P. carinii* pneumonia (Schluger *et al.*, 1992), whereas studies using other *P. carinii*-specific primers have suggested that the detection of *P. carinii* DNA in serum and circulating cells is not a good diagnostic marker of infection (Tamburrini *et al.*, 1993, 1994; Evans *et al.*, 1995). In the rat model of *P. carinii* infection, conflicting results have also been reported. *P. carinii* DNA has been detected in samples of serum, using primers designed to the DHFR gene (Schluger *et al.*, 1992; Sepkowitz *et al.*, 1993). In contrast, in two other studies, using PCR primers designed to the mitochondrial LSU rRNA, no *P. carinii* DNA was detected by PCR in samples of whole blood, although *P. carinii* was detected in the lung lavage and lung homogenate (Evans *et al.*, 1995; O'Leary *et al.*, 1995). The utility of blood or serum as an effective clinical sample for the diagnosis of *P. carinii* pneumonia remains to be established.

ACQUISITION AND PERSISTENCE OF *P. CARINII* INFECTION

It has been widely assumed that *P. carinii* pneumonia in the immunocompromised host results from reactivation of latent infection acquired during childhood. This view has been supported by the presence of high levels of antibody elicited to *P. carinii* in the normal population at an early age (Meuwissen *et al.*, 1977; Pifer *et al.*, 1978; Wakefield *et al.*, 1990c). Reports of nosocomial clusters of *P. carinii* pneumonia among immunocompromised patients, however, challenged this concept of latent infection (Santiago-Delphin *et al.*, 1988; Chave *et al.*, 1991; Jacobs *et al.*, 1991). Moreover, studies using monoclonal antibodies, and the more sensitive technique of DNA amplification, have failed to reveal evidence of *P. carinii* colonization in lung tissue obtained at postmortem or in bronchoalveolar lavage fluid from immunocompetent individuals (Millard and Heryet, 1988; Peters *et al.*, 1992b; Matusiewicz *et al.*, 1994). In addition, experiments with SCID mice failed to demonstrate latent infection at extrapulmonary sites (Cheng, Gigliotti and Harmsen, 1993). Additional data has come from the dexamethasone-induced rat model of *P. carinii* pneumonia, which has been used to determine the period of persistence of *P. carinii* in the lungs after a primary episode of *P. carinii* pneumonia. The organisms were found to be cleared from the lungs of at least 75% of animals within one year of an episode of *P. carinii* pneumonia, implying that the persistence of latent organisms is limited (Vargas *et al.*, 1995).

Animal experiments with the rat model of *P. carinii* pneumonia have demonstrated that *P. carinii* infection is acquired by an airborne route (Hughes, 1987). It is assumed that infection in the human host is similarly acquired. A recent study has shown that DNA sequences identical to *P. carinii* have been detected in samples of the air spora of rural Oxfordshire, and suggests that *P. carinii* may have an environmental phase of its life cycle (Wakefield, 1994, 1996). Seasonal variation in *P. carinii* infection in HIV-positive patients has been reported, with peaks in the late Spring and late Summer/early Autumn which may be related to variations in environmental temperature and humidity, factors that are important for growth and sporulation of fungi (Hoover *et al.*, 1991; Miller, Grant and Foley, 1992; Vanheims, Hirschel and Morabia, 1992). These data lend support to the currently held

view that *P. carinii* infection in the immunocompromised results from *de novo* acquisition of the organism, and not from reactivation of latent infection.

Some studies have suggested, however, that transient carriage of the parasites may occur in the lungs of immunocompetent hosts. *P. carinii* DNA has been detected by the polymerase chain reaction in the lungs of immunocompetent sentinel rats housed near immunosuppressed *P. carinii*-infected rats and disappeared rapidly from the lungs of these sentinel rats when they were isolated from the immunosuppressed infected animals (Sepkowitz *et al.*, 1993). Immunocompetent health care workers in an AIDS unit exposed to patients with *P. carinii* have been shown to have higher serum antibodies to *P. carinii* than health care workers based in a unit for the care of the elderly. These data suggest that asymptomatic carriage may have occurred as a result of environmental exposure (Leigh *et al.*, 1993b).

Recurrent episodes of *P. carinii* pneumonia are a relatively common occurrence in HIV-infected individuals. In a recent study, sequence analysis at the mitochondrial LSU rRNA was undertaken in isolates of *P. carinii* from 10 patients with 2 episodes of *P. carinii*. In 5 of the patients, genetically distinct isolates were associated with each episode (Keely *et al.*, 1995). Samples from HIV-infected individuals undergoing one, two or three episodes of *P. carinii* pneumonia have been examined in another study, by sequence analysis of the ITS regions. Ten different types of *P. carinii* were identified. In four of seven patients with recurrent episodes of pneumonia, the sequence types observed at the second episode were different to those of the first (Tsolaki *et al.*, 1996). These cumulative data suggest that recurrent episodes of *P. carinii* pneumonia result from reinfection from an exogenous source as well as reactivation of a previously acquired infection.

SUMMARY

Application of molecular biological techniques to the study of *P. carinii* support the taxonomic assignment of this organism to the fungal kingdom and demonstrate that different strains of the organism infect different mammalian host species. Co-infection with genetically distinct strains of *P. carinii* may occur within one mammalian host species but in general genetic diversity among isolates of *P. carinii* from a single host species is lower than that between isolates obtained from different host species.

In clinical samples of bronchoalveolar lavage and induced sputum, the polymerase chain reaction using *P. carinii*-specific oligonucleotide primers has been found to be more effective than conventional histochemical or immunofluorescence staining for detection of the organism. Evaluation of the PCR method of detection has demonstrated its efficacy in the diagnosis of *P. carinii* pneumonia, especially on non-invasive samples.

Clinical disease in rats and in humans appears to arise in the majority of cases by *de novo* infection with the organism, acquired by the airborne route, rather than by reactivation of latent organisms. Recurrent episodes of *P. carinii* pneumonia in HIV-infected individuals may result from re-infection from an exogenous source as well as reactivation of a previously acquired infection.

REFERENCES

Banerji, S., Wakefield, A.E., Allen, A.G. *et al.* (1993) The cloning and characterisation of the *arom* gene of *Pneumocystis carinii*. *J. Gen. Microbiol.*, **139**, 2901–14.

Banerji, S., Lugli, E.B. and Wakefield, A.E. (1994) Identification of two genetically distinct strains of *Pneumocystis carinii* in infected ferret lungs. *J. Euk. Microbiol.*, **41**, 73S.

Banerji, S., Lugli, E.B., Miller, R.F. and Wakefield, A.E. (1995) Analysis of genetic diversity at the *arom* locus in isolates of *Pneumocystis carinii*, *J. Euk. Microbiol.*, **42**, 657–9.

Bauer, N.L., Paulsrud, J.R., Bartlett, M.S. *et al.* (1993) *Pneumocystis carinii* organisms obtained from rats, ferrets and mice are antigenically different. *Infect. Immun.*, **61**, 1315–19.

Borensztein, L., Hatin, I., Simonpoli, A.-M. *et al.* (1992) An alternative to DNA extraction for the diagnosis of *Pneumocystis carinii* pneumonia by polymerase chain reaction using a new oligonucleotide probe. *Mol. Cell Probes*, **6**, 361–65.

Cartwright, C.P., Nelson, N.A. and Gill, V.J. (1994) Development and evaluation of a rapid and simple procedure for detection of *Pneumocystis carinii* by PCR. *J. Clin. Microbiol.*, **32**, 1634–38.

Chave, J.-P., David, S., Wauters, J. -P. *et al.* (1991) Transmission of *Pneumocystis carinii* from AIDS patients to other immuno-suppressed patients: a cluster of *Pneumocystis carinii* pneumonia in renal transplant recipients. *AIDS*, **5**, 927–32.

Cheng, W., Gigliotti, F. and Harmsen, A.G. (1993) Latency is not an inevitable outcome of infection with *Pneumocystis carinii*. *Infect. Immun.*, **61**, 5406–5409.

Chouaid, C., Roux, P., Lavard, I. *et al.* (1995) Use of the polymerase chain reaction technique on induced-sputum samples for the diagnosis of *Pneumocystis carinii* pneumonia in HIV-infected patients. *Am. J. Clin. Pathol.*, **104**, 72–72.

Cushion, M.T., Zhang, J., Kaselis, M. *et al.* (1993) Evidence for two genetic variants of *Pneumocystis carinii* co-infecting laboratory rats. *J. Clin. Microbiol.*, **31**, 1217–23.

De Luca, A., Tamburrini, E., Ortona, E. *et al.* (1995) Variable efficiency of three primer pairs for the diagnosis of *Pneumocystis carinii* pneumonia by the polymerase chain reaction. *Mol. Cell. Probes*, **9**, 333–40.

Dyer, M., Volpe, F., Delves, C.J. *et al.* (1992) Cloning and sequence of a β-tubulin cDNA from *Pneumocystis carinii*: possible implications for drug therapy. *Mol. Microbiol.*, **6**, 991–1001.

Edlind, T.D., Bartlett, M.S., Weinberg, G.A. *et al.* (1992) The β-tubulin gene from rat and human isolates of *Pneumocystis carinii*. *Mol. Microbiol.*, **6**, 3365–73.

Edman, J.C., Kovacs, J.A., Masur, H. *et al.* (1989a) Ribosomal RNA sequences show *Pneumocystis carinii* to be a member of the fungi. *Nature*, **334**, 519–22.

Edman, J.C., Edman, U., Cao, M. *et al.* (1989b) Isolation and expression of the *Pneumocystis carinii* dihydrofolate reductase gene. *Proc. Natl*

Acad. Sci, USA **86**, 8625–9.

Edman, U., Edman, J.C., Lundgren, B. and Santi, D.V. (1989c) Isolation and expression of the *Pneumocystis carinii* thymidylate synthase gene. *Proc. of the Natl Acad. Scie.*, USA, **86** 6503–7.

Evans, R., Joss, A.W.L., Pennington, T.H. and Ho-Yen, D.O. (1995) The use of a nested polymerase chain reaction for detecting *Pneumocystis carinii* from lung and blood in rat and human infection. *J. Med. Microbiol.*, **42**, 209–13.

Farrow, B.R.H., Watson, A.D.J., Hartly, W.J. and Huxtable, C.R.R. (1972) *Pneumocystis pneumonia* in the dog. *Comp. Pathol.*, **82**, 447–53.

Fletcher, L.D., McDowell, J.M., Tidwell, R.R. *et al.* (1994) Structure, expression and phylogenetic analysis of the gene encoding actin I in *Pneumocystis carinii. Genetics*, **137**, 743–50.

Frenkel, J.K., Good, J.T. and Shultz, J.A. (1966) Latent pneumocystis infection of rats, relapse and chemotherapy. *Lab. Invest.*, **15**, 1559–77.

Frenkel, J.K. (1976) *Pneumocystis jiroveci* n. sp. from man: morphology, physiology and immunology in relation to pathology. *Natl Cancer Inst. Monogr.*, **43**, 13–30.

Furuta, T. and Katsumoto, U. (1987) Intra and inter species transmission and antigenic differences of *Pneumocystis carinii* derived from rat and mouse. *Jpn Exper. Med.*, **57**, 11–17.

Gigliotti, F., Stokes, D.C., Cheatham, A.B. *et al.* (1986) Development of murine monoclonal antibodies to *Pneumocystis carinii. J. Infect. Dis.*, **154**, 315–22.

Gigliotti, F., Ballou, L.R., Hughes, W.T. and Mosley, B.D. (1988) Purification and initial characterisation of a ferret *Pneumocystis carinii* surface antigen capable of inducing protective anitbody. *J. Infect. Dis.*, **158**, 848–54.

Gigliotti, F. (1992) Host species-specific antigenic variation of a mannosylated surface glycoprotein of *Pneumocystis carinii. J. Infect. Dis.*, **165**, 329–36.

Gigliotti, F., Harmsden, A.G., Haidaris, C.G. and Haidaris, P.J. (1993) *Pneumocystis carinii* is not universally transmissible between mammalian species. *Infect. and Immun.*, **61**, 2886–90.

Graves, D.C., McNabb, S.J.N., Worley, M.A. *et al.* (1986a) Analyses of rat *Pneumocystis carinii* antigens recognised by human and rat antibodies by using Western immunoblotting. *Infect. Immun.*, **54**, 96–103.

Graves, D.C., McNabb, S.J.N., Ivey, M.H. and Worley, M.A. (1986b) Development and charac-

terisation of monoclonal antibodies in *P. carinii. Infect. Immun.*, **51**, 125–33.

Hong, S.T., Steel, P.E., Cushion, M.T. *et al.* (1990) *Pneumocystis carinii* karyotypes. *J. Clin. Microbiol.*, **28**, 1785–95.

Hoover, D.R., Graham, N.M.H., Bacellar, H. *et al.* (1991) Epidemiologic patterns of upper respiratory illness and *Pneumocystis carinii* pneumonia in homosexual men. *Am. Rev. Respir. Dis.*, **144**, 756–9.

Hughes, W.T. (1987) Pneumocystis carinii Pneumonitis. Vol. 1; CRC Press, Florida.

Jacobs, J.L., Libby, D.M., Winters, R.A. *et al.* (1991) A cluster of *Pneumocystis carinii* pneumonia in adults without predisposing illnesses. *N. Engl. J. Med.*, **324**, 246–50.

Kaneshiro, E.S., Ellis, J.E., Jayasimhula, K. and Beach, D.H. (1994) Evidence for the presence of metabolic sterols in *Pneumocystis*: identification and initial characterisation of *Pneumocystis carinii* sterols. *J. Euk. Microbiol.*, **41**, 78–85.

Keely, S., Pai, H.-J., Baughman, R. *et al.* (1994) *Pneumocystis* species inferred from analysis of multiple genes. *J. Euk. Microbiol.*, **41**, 945

Keely, S.P., Stringer, J.R., Baughman, R.P. *et al.* (1995) Genetic variation among *Pneumocystis carinii hominis* isolates in recurrent pneumocystosis. *J. Infect. Dis.*, **172**, 595–8.

Kitada, K., Oka, S., Kimura, S. *et al.* (1991) Detection of *Pneumocystis carinii* sequences by polymerase chain reaction: animal models and clinical application to non-invasive specimens. *J. Clin. Microbiol.*, **29**, 1985–90.

Kovacs, J.A., Halpern, J.L., Suran, J.C. *et al.* (1988) Identification of antigens and antibodies specific for *Pneumocystis carinii. J. Immunol.*, **140**, 2023–3.

Latouche, S., Roux, P., Poirot, J.L. *et al.* (1994) Preliminary results of *Pneumocystis carinii* strain differentiation by using molecular biology. *J. Clin. Microbiol.*, **32**, 3052–3.

Lee, C.-H., Lu, J.-J., Bartlett, M.S. *et al.* (1993) Nucleotide sequence variation in *Pneumocystis carinii* strains that infect humans. *J. Clin. Microbiol.*, **31**, 754–57.

Leibovitz, E., Pollack, H., Moore, T. *et al.* (1995) Comparison of PCR and standard cytological staining for detection of *Pneumocystis carinii* from respiratory specimens from patients with or at high risk of infection by human immunodeficiency virus. *J. Clin. Microbiol.*, **33**, 3004–3007.

Leigh, T.R., Wakefield, A.E., Peters, S.E. *et al.*

(1992) Comparison of DNA amplification and immunofluorescence for detecting *Pneumocystis carinii* in patients receiving immunosuppressive therapy. *Transplantation*, **54**, 468–70.

Leigh, T.R., Gazzard, B.G., Rowbottom, A. and Collins, J.V. (1993a) Quantitative and qualitative comparison of DNA amplification by PCR with immunofluorescence staining for diagnosis of *Pneumocystis carinii* pneumonia. *J. Clin. Pathol.*, **46**, 140–44.

Leigh, T.R., Millet, M.J., Jameson, B. and Collins, J.V. (1993b) Serum titres of *Pneumocystis carinii* antibody in health care workers caring for patients with AIDS. *Thorax*, **48**, 619–21.

Linke, M.J., Cushion, M.T. and Walzer, P.D. (1989) Properties of the major antigens of rat and human *Pneumocystis carinii*. *Infect. Immun.*, **57**, 1547–55.

Lipschik, G.Y., Gill, V.J., Lundgren, J.D., *et al.* (1992) Improved diagnosis of *Pneumocystis carinii* infection by polymerase chain reaction on induced sputum and blood. *Lancet*, **340**, 203–206.

Liu, Y. and Leibowitz, M.J. (1993) Variation and *in vitro* splicing of group I introns in rRNA genes of *Pneumocystis carinii*. *Nucl. Acids Res.*, **21**, 2415–21.

Lu, J.-J., Bartlett, M.S., Shaw, M.M. *et al.* (1994) Typing of *Pneumocystis carinii* strains that infect humans based on nucleotide sequence variations of internal transcribed spacers of rRNA genes *J. Clin. Microbiol.*, **32**, 2904–12.

Lu, J.-J., Bartlett, M.S., Smith, J.W. and Lee, C.-H. (1995a) Typing of *Pneumocystis carinii* strains with type-specific oligonucleotide probes derived from nucleotide sequences of internal transcribed spacers of rRNA genes. *J. Clin. Microbiol.*, **33**, 2973–77.

Lu, J.-J., Chen, C.-H., Bartlett, M.S. *et al.* (1995b) Comparison of six different PCR methods for detection of *Pneumocystis carinii*. *J. Clin. Microbiol.*, **33**, 2785–788.

Matusiewicz, S.P., Ferguson, R.J., Greening, A.P. *et al.* (1994) *Pneumocystis carinii* in bronchoalveolar lavage fluid and bronchial washings. *Br. Med. J.*, **308**, 1206–7.

Mazars, E., Odberg-Ferragut, C., Dei-Cas, E. *et al.* (1995) Polymorphism of the thymidylate synthase gene of *Pneumocystis carinii* from different host species. *J. Euk. Microbiol.*, **42**, 26–32.

Meade, J.C. and Stringer, J.R. (1991) PCR amplification of DNA sequences from the transcription factor IID and cation transport-ing ATPase genes in *Pneumocystis carinii*. *J. Protozool.*, **38**, 66–8.

Meade, J.C. and Stringer, J.R. (1995) Cloning and characterization of an ATPase gene from *Pneumocystis carinii* which closely resembles fungal H^+ ATPases. *J. Euk. Microbiol.*, **42**, 298–307.

Meuwissen, J.H.E.T., Tauber, I., Leevwenberg, A.D.E.M. *et al.* (1977) Parasitologic and serologic observations of infection with *Pneumocystis* in humans. *J. Infect. Dis.*, **136**, 43–49.

Millard, P.R. and Heryet, A.R. (1988) Observations favouring *Pneumocystis carinii* pneumonia as a primary infection: a monoclonal antibody study on paraffin sections. *J. Pathol.*, **154**, 365–70.

Miller, R.F., Grant, A.D. and Foley, N.M. (1992) Seasonal variation in presentation of *Pneumocystis carinii* pneumonia. *Lancet*, **339**, 747–8.

Minielly, J.A., Mills, S.D. and Holley, K.E. (1969) *Pneumocystis carinii* pneumonia. *Canadian Medical Association Journal*, **100**, 846–54.

O'Leary, T.J., Tsai, M.M., Wright, C.F. and Cushion, M.T. (1995) Use of semiquantitative PCR to assess onset and treatment of *Pneumocystis carinii* infection in rat model. *J. Clin. Microbiol.*, **33**, 718–24.

Olsson, M., Elvin, K., Lofdahl, S. and Linder, E. (1993) Detection of *Pneumocystis carinii* DNA in sputum and bronchoalveolar lavage samples by polymerase chain reaction. *J. Clin. Microbiol.*, **31**, 221–26.

Ortiz-Rivera, M., Liu, Y., Felder, R. and Leibowitz, M.J. (1995) Comparison of coding and spacer region sequences of chromosomal rRNA-coding genes of two sequevars of *Pneumocystis carinii*. *J. Euk. Microbiol.*, **42**, 44–49.

Peglow, S.L., Smulian, A.G., Linke, M.J. *et al.* (1990) Serologic responses to *Pneumocystis carinii* antigens in health and disease. *J. Infect. Dis.*, **161** 296–306.

Peters, S.E., Wakefield, A.E., Banerji, S. *et al.* (1992a) Quantification of the detection of *Pneumocystis carinii* by DNA amplification. *Mol. Cell. Probes*, **6**, 115–117. Pneumonia thoroughbred foals: identification of a genetically distinct organism by DNA amplification. *J. Clin. Microbiol*, **32**, 213–16.

Peters, S.E., Wakefield, A.E., Sinclair, K. *et al.* (1992b) A search for latent *Pneumocystis carinii* infection in post-mortem lungs by DNA amplification. *J. Pathol.*, **166**, 195–8.

Peters, S.E., Wakefield, A.E., Whitwell, K.E. and Hopkin, J.M. (1994) *Pneumocystis carinii* pneumonia in thoroughbred foals: identification of a genetically distinct organism by DNA amplification. *J. Clin. Microbiol.*, **32**, 213–16.

Pifer, L.L., Hughes, W.T., Stagno, S. and Woods, D. (1978) *Pneumocystis carinii* infection; evidence for high prevalence in normal and immunosuppressed children. *Pediatrics*, **61**, 35–41.

Pixley, F.J., Wakefield, A.E., Banerji, S. and Hopkin, J.M. (1991) Mitochondrial gene sequences show fungal homology for *Pneumocystis carinii*. *Mol. Microbiol.*, **5**, 1347–51.

Richards, C.G.M., Wakefield, A.E. and Mitchell, C.D. (1994) Detection of *Pneumocystis* DNA in nasopharygneal aspirates of leukaemic infants with pneumonia. *Arch. Dis. Child.*, **71**, 254–55.

Roux, P., Lavrard, I., Poirot, J.L. *et al.* (1994) Usefulness of PCR for detection of *Pneumocystis carinii* DNA. *J. Clin. Microbiol.*, **32**, 2324–26.

Santiago-Delphin, E.A., Mora, E., Gonzalez, Z.A. *et al.* (1988) Factors in an outbreak of *Pneumocystis carinii* in a transplant unit. *Transplant Proc.*, **XXS** 1; 462–65.

Schluger, N., Godwin, T., Sepkowitz, K. *et al.* (1992) Application of DNA amplification to pneumocystosis: presence of serum *Pneumocystis carinii* DNA during human and experimentally induced *Pneumocystis carinii* pneumonia. *J. Exp. Med.*, **176**, 1327–333.

Sepkowitz, K., Schluger, N., Godwin, T. *et al.* (1993) DNA amplification in experimental pneumocystosis: characterisation of serum *Pneumocystis carinii* DNA and potential *P. carinii* carrier states. *J. Infect. Dis.*, **168**, 421–6.

Sinclair, K., Wakefield, A.E., Banerji, S. and Hopkin, J.M. (1991) *Pneumocystis carinii* organisms derived from rat and human hosts are genetically distinct. *Mol. Biochem. Parasitol.*, **45**, 183–4.

Sloand, E., Laughon, B., Armstrong, M. *et al.* (1993) The challenge of *Pneumocystis carinii* culture. *J. Euk. Microbiol.*, **40**, 188–95.

Smulian, A.G., Sullivan, D.W., Linke, M.J. *et al.* (1993) Geographic variation in the humoral response to *Pneumocystis carinii*. *J. Infect. Dis.*, **167**, 1243–7.

Stringer, S.L., Stringer, J.R., Blase, M.A. *et al.* (1989) *Pneumocystis carinii*: sequence from ribosomal RNA implies a close relationship with fungi. *Exp. Parasitol.*, **68**, 450–61.

Stringer, J.R., Stringer, S.L., Zhang, J. *et al.* (1993) Molecular genetic distinction of *Pneumocystis*

from rats and humans. *J. Euk. Microbiol.*, **40**, 733–41.

Sunkin, S.M. and Stringer, J.R. (1995) Transcription factor genes from rat *Pneumocystis carinii*. *J. Euk. Microbiol.*, **42**, 12–20.

Tamburrini, E., Mencarini, P., De Luca, A. *et al.* (1993a) Diagnosis of *Pneumocystis carinii* pneumonia: specificity and sensitivity of polymerase chain reaction in comparison with immunofluorescence in bronchoalveolar lavage specimens. *J. Med. Microbiol.*, **38**, 449–53.

Tamburrini, E., Mencarini, P., De Luca, A. *et al.* (1993b) Simple and rapid two-step polymerase chain reaction for diagnosis of *Pneumocystis carinii* infection. *J. Clin. Microbiol.*, **31**, 2788–89.

Tamburrini, E., Mencarini, P., De Luca, A. *et al.* (1994) Detection of *Pneumocystis* DNA in serum and circulating cells is not a good diagnostic marker for pneumocystosis in HIV patients. *J. Euk. Microbiol.*, **41**, 112S.

Tsolaki, A.G., Miller, R.F., Underwood, A.P. *et al.* (1996) Genetic diversity at the ITS regions of the rRNA operon among isolates of *Pneumocystis carinii* from HIV infected individuals with recurrent pneumonia. *J. Infect. Dis.*, **174**, 141–56.

Wakefield, A.E., Pixley, F.J., Banerji, S. *et al.* (1990a) Amplification of mitochondrial ribosomal RNA sequences from *Pneumocystis carinii* DNA of rat and human origin. *Mol. Biochem. Parasitol.*, **43**, 69–76.

Wakefield, A.E., Pixley, F.J., Banerji, S. *et al.* (1990b) Detection of *Pneumocystis carinii* with DNA amplification. *Lancet*, **336**, 451–3.

Wakefield, A.E., Stewart, T.J., Moxon, E.R. *et al.* (1990c) Infection with *Pneumocystis carinii* is prevalent in healthy Gambian children. *Trans. Roy. Soc. Trop. Med. Hyg.*, **84**, 800–802.

Wakefield, A.E., Guiver, L., Miller, R.F. and Hopkin, J.M. (1991) DNA amplification on induced sputum samples for diagnosis of *Pneumocystis carinii* pneumonia. *Lancet*, **337**, 1378–9.

Wakefield, A.E., Miller, R.F., Guiver, L.A. and Hopkin, J.M. (1993) Oropharyngeal samples for detection of *Pneumocystis carinii* by DNA amplification. *Q. J. Med.*, **86**, 401–6.

Wakefield, A.E., Fritscher, C., Malin, A. *et al.* (1994a) Analysis of genetic diversity in human-derived *Pneumocystis carinii* isolated from four geographical locations. *J. Clin. Microbiol.*, **32**, 2959–61.

Wakefield, A.E., Miller, R.F., Guiver, L.A. and Hopkin, J.M. (1994b) Granulomatous

Pneumocystis carinii pneumonia: DNA amplification studies on bronchoscopic alveolar lavage samples. *J. Clin. Pathol.*, **47**, 664–66.

Wakefield, A.E. (1994) Detection of DNA sequences identical of *Pneumocystis carinii* in samples of ambient air. *J. Euk. Microbiol.*, **41**, 116S.

Wakefield, A.E. (1996) DNA sequences identical to *Pneumocystis carinii* f. sp *carinii* and *Pneumocystis carinii* f. sp. *hominis* in samples of air spores. *J. Clin. Microbiol.*, **34**, 1754–9.

Weinberg, G.A. and Durant, P.J. (1994a) Genetic diversity of *Pneumocystis carinii* derived from infected rats, mice, ferrets and cell cultures. *J. Euk. Microbiol*, **41**, 223–8.

Weinberg, G.A., Dykstra, C.C., Durant, P.J. and Cushion, M.T. (1994b) Chromosomal localization of 20 genes to five distinct pulsed field gel

karyotypic forms of rat *Pneumocystis carinii*. *J. Euk. Microbiol.*, **41**, 117S.

Vanheims, P., Hirschel, B. and Morabia, A. (1992) Seasonal incidence of *Pneumocystis carinii* pneumonia. *Lancet*, **339**, 1182.

Vargas, S.L., Hughes, W.T., Wakefield, A.E. and Oz, S. (1995) Limited persistence and subsequent elimination of *Pneumocystis carinii* from the lungs after *P. carinii* pneumonia. *J. Infect. Dis.*, **172**, 506–510.

Ympa-Wong, M.F., Fonzi, W.A. and Sypherd, P.S. (1992) Fungus-specific translation elongation factor 3 gene present in *Pneumocystis carinii*. *Infect. Immun.*, **60**, 4140–5.

Zhang, J. and Stringer, J.R. (1993) Cloning and characterization of an alpha-tubulin-encoding gene from rat-derived *Pneumocystis carinii*. *Gene*, **123**, 137–41.

7

PROPHYLAXIS AND TREATMENT OF *PNEUMOCYSTIS CARINII* PNEUMONIA

Marc C.I. Lipman and Margaret A. Johnson

Pneumocystis carinii pneumonia (PCP) was the firstly widely reported major opportunistic infection of the AIDS epidemic (Gottblieb *et al.*, 1981). Its importance has never diminished and it has remained one of the commonest AIDS events in the developed world (Hoover *et al.*, 1993). The recognition that it is an early and (with prophylaxis) often avoidable AIDS illness has promoted an increased interest in its presentation and management. The improved survival times that are now seen following an episode of PCP have accounted almost exclusively for the increase in overall AIDS survival (Jacobson *et al.*, 1993). The prophylaxis and treatment of PCP is therefore a vital part of current HIV management. This chapter addresses drug therapy as it applies to clinical practice. It also covers management strategies and ventilatory support; it concludes with a discussion of factors that predict clinical outcome.

PROPHYLAXIS

WHEN TO PROPHYLAX

Prior to HIV infection, PCP prophylaxis was used successfully in transplantation and oncology (Hughes *et al.*, 1977). The progressive nature of HIV-related immunodeficiency means that two forms of prophylaxis are needed: primary (where the individual is perceived to be at great risk of PCP); and secondary (to prevent recurrence following an episode of PCP). With HIV infection, it also follows that prophylaxis must be lifelong. Therefore the therapies used must be safe and (to achieve any form of compliance) 'user friendly'.

In the case of primary prophylaxis, determining the point where the benefits outweigh the risks and disadvantages of drug therapy is also crucial. Data from the Multicenter AIDS Cohort Study (MACS) of homosexual and bisexual men without AIDS revealed that the incidence of PCP in subjects not using prophylaxis rose from 0.5% at 6 months in men with a baseline blood CD4 T lymphocyte count of >200 cells/μl (>0.2 × 10^9/l), to 8.4% in those with CD4 <200 (Phair *et al.*, 1990). Thus a CD4 count of <200 cells/μl (or a CD4 to total lymphocyte ratio of <20%, which yielded similar results in this study) has been recommended as the level at which primary prophylaxis should be offered (US Public Health Service Task Force, 1993).

There are however several other points that arise from the data. First, the median CD4 count at which PCP occurred was less than 100 cells. Therefore if a CD4 count of 200 is used as the cut-off, there will be a number of asymptomatic individuals on a potentially toxic drug who with or without prophylaxis would not develop PCP for quite some time.

AIDS and Respiratory Medicine. Edited by A. Zumla, M.A. Johnson and R.F. Miller. Published in 1997 by Chapman & Hall, London. ISBN 0 412 60140 0

Some patients may therefore choose to wait until their CD4 count has declined below 200 cells before they start prophylaxis. Second, in a multivariate analysis, symptoms or signs of oral thrush or fever were independent predictors of the development of PCP. 60% of subjects with a CD4>200 had either or both of these symptoms prior to PCP (Phair *et al.*, 1990). Third, within the MACS and also the Prospective Study of Pulmonary Complications of HIV Infection (PSPC–a multicenter cohort drawn from all HIV risk groups and including subjects with a previous AIDS diagnosis), a small but appreciable number of individuals developed PCP with CD4 counts higher than 200. In the PSPC this was 16% of all cases (Wallace, personal communication). Nevertheless the importance of advocating a CD4 count <200 to start PCP prophylaxis was shown in the latter study where the cumulative risk at 6 months for an individual not using any prophylaxis was 23 times that of someone starting therapy at this level (Wallace, personal communication).

Once an individual has had an episode of PCP the risk of recurrence is up to 60% at twelve months (Kovacs and Masur, 1988). Whether this reflects their general state of immune dysfunction, local pulmonary damage occurring at the first episode or even clinical reactivation by their first disease-inducing strain of *Pneumocystis* is unclear (Walzer, 1991). However current guidelines advocate lifelong PCP prophylaxis in HIV-infected adults with either prior PCP or CD4 counts <200 cells/μl or constitutional symptoms (documented oral thrush or fever of unknown cause of >37.8C (100°F) persisting >2 weeks) or clinical AIDS (US Public Health Service Task Force, 1993).

THERAPEUTIC OPTIONS

Trimethoprim/sulfamethoxazole

A good prophylactic agent would be safe and without side effects, effica-cious, easily administered and cheap, and also provide cover against a number of different organisms. This ideal has not yet been reached though currently trimethoprim/sulfamethoxazole (co-trimoxazole, TMP/SMX) is the drug of choice. Like many of the early therapies used against PCP, TMP/SMX was adopted in humans after initial success in the steroid-treated rodent model of PCP (Hughes *et al.*, 1974). TMP and SMX target sequential steps in the folate synthesis pathway. TMP selectively inhibits the *Pneumocystis* dihydrofolate reductase enzyme (Allegra *et al.*, 1987a), and SMX inhibits dihydropteroate synthetase. The two drugs act synergistically, and in a fixed dose combination (TMP/SMX ratio of 1:5 or 80 mg: 400 mg per single strength tablet), they have become the most commonly prescribed prophylactic drug on the basis of wide availability, reasonable cost and efficacy. Trimethoprim is not an effective agent when used alone for PCP prophylaxis or treatment.

Fischl's randomized, unblinded study of primary prophylaxis in 60 patients with biopsy-proven Kaposi's sarcoma revealed a striking reduction in PCP incidence in subjects taking TMP/SMX 960 mg twice daily (Fischl, Dickenson and La Voie, 1988). After 2 years' follow up, 16 of 30 subjects on no therapy had developed PCP compared to none on study drug. However adverse reactions occurred in 50% of patients taking TMP/SMX; and in one third of these the drug had to be stopped.

The commonest reactions to TMP/SMX are fever, skin rash (normally of morbilliform type, though occasionally severe and involving the mucous membranes), headache, nausea, gastro-intestinal upset and bone marrow toxicity (predominantly granulocytopenia and thrombocytopenia). Nephritis and biochemical liver dysfunction have also been reported. All of these reactions are much more common when the drug is used at the higher treatment dose for continuous periods (Masur, 1992). Toxicity usually occurs within a few days of starting therapy. Folinic acid supplements do not affect the incidence of hematologic toxicity.

Recent trials have investigated the use of lower doses of TMP/SMX, and now also incorporate other PCP prophylactic regimes. For example the Dutch AIDS Treatment Group's randomized comparison of oral TMP/SMX at either 480 mg or 960 mg per day or aerosolized pentamidine 300 mg per month given via a Respirgard II jet nebulizer (Schneider *et al.*, 1992). Here 213 subjects with a CD4 count <200 and no previous PCP were followed for a mean time of 9 months. Six of 71 (11%) patients in the pentamidine arm developed PCP compared to none of those on TMP/SMX (either dosage, $p=0.002$). However the oral drug was again not particularly well tolerated with a cumulative incidence of adverse events in the first three months of 21% and 26% for lower and higher dose TMP/SMX compared with 0% in the pentamidine group. This was also reflected in the much greater proportion of subjects discontinuing TMP/SMX than pentamidine.

The effect of thrice weekly TMP/SMX 960 mg has been prospectively compared to monthly pentamidine (300 mg via an ultrasonic nebulizer) or dapsone 100 mg per week plus pyrimethamine 25 mg per week (Mallolas *et al.*, 1993). Here a similar low rate of PCP was seen (TMP/SMX, 3% per year of observation, 95% confidence intervals 0–6.3%). Again, adverse reactions and discontinuation of therapy were much more common in the oral therapy arms compared to pentamidine. A potential problem with intermittent therapy is that unless strictly adhered to, the regime may be allowed to lapse to the point that inadequate prophylaxis is being achieved and subsequent breakthrough occurs.

TMP/SMX is also the drug of choice for secondary PCP prophylaxis. This was shown in the ACTG 021 trial which compared oral TMP/SMX 960 mg per day with monthly nebulized pentamidine (300 mg via a Respirgard II) in 310 AIDS patients also taking zidovudine (Hardy *et al.*, 1992). Here, adjusting for initial CD4 count, the risk of recurrence was 3.25 times higher in the pentamidine group. Interestingly, although a greater number of subjects taking TMP/SMX discontinued medication due to toxicity, the drug was much better tolerated overall than expected. A history of adverse effects during treatment dose did not appear to predict drug toxicity when TMP/SMX was used subsequently as secondary prophylaxis.

ACTG 021 also demonstrated another potential advantage of TMP/SMX in that the drug conferred some degree of protection against clinically significant bacterial infections (Hardy *et al.*, 1992). This 'cross prophylaxis' has also been seen in a significant reduction in the incidence of cerebral toxoplasmosis in a retrospective study of patients taking 960 mg TMP/SMX twice daily two times per week compared to nebulized pentamidine (Carr *et al.*, 1992). Thus, provided an individual can tolerate it, TMP/SMX at a dose of 480–960 mg per day or 960 mg thrice weekly should be recommended as first-line PCP prophylaxis. In our center we use a starting dose of 960 mg once daily, and adjust this according to patient tolerance as necessary (Table 7.1).

Pentamidine

As described in the previous section, pentamidine isethionate has been the other drug predominantly used for PCP prophylaxis. Its poor oral absorption means that it must be given parenterally, though when used in nebulized form the lack of consequent systemic side effects is a great advantage over TMP/SMX. Pentamidine has a long intrapulmonary half life (Waldman, Pearce and Martin, 1973) and therefore can be given as intermittent therapy. When used as primary prophylaxis at 300 mg/month given via a

Respirgard II nebulizer, the cumulative yearly incidence of PCP was 9% compared to 27% with placebo (Hirschel *et al.*, 1991).

The San Francisco Community Prophylaxis Trial demonstrated that 4-weekly 300 mg nebulized pentamidine was superior to either 150 mg or 30 mg nebulized pentamidine fortnightly given via a Respirgard II jet nebulizer (Leoung *et al.*, 1990). This effect was most striking in those patients using the drug for secondary PCP prophylaxis. The study also showed that pulmonary symptoms of cough (36% of study participants) and wheeze (11%) were common with pentamidine inhalation (Leoung *et al.*, 1990) and it is now routine practice to give a bronchodilator (e.g. a β_{-2} agonist) before inhaling the drug.

A placebo-controlled study of inhaled pentamidine as secondary prophylaxis using the ultrasonic Fisoneb showed that the relapse rate at 6 months fell from 50% on placebo to 9% with pentamidine. The aerosol delivery characteristics of the Fisoneb meant that after 5 loading doses of 60 mg within a fortnight, 60 mg every 2 weeks could be used as the prophylactic dose (Montaner *et al.*, 1991).

Pentamidine has largely been replaced by TMP/SMX due to the latter's enhanced protective effect against PCP. There are however other issues that pertain to pentamidine's use. First, when administered as an aerosol, the particle size must be such that alveolar deposition is maximal. This requires either particular jet nebulizers (e.g. Respirgard II) or the more expensive ultrasonic nebulizers. Added to the cost of the equipment is the high price of the drug itself: in the United Kingdom in 1994 on a monthly basis this made pentamidine prophylaxis approximately nine times more expensive than TMP/SMX (Miller, 1994). Second, there is a potential risk that the process of nebulization (and any associated coughing) may increase the transmission of respiratory diseases such as tuberculosis to either other patients or members of staff. Cer-

tainly health care workers supervising pentamidine administration have been reported to develop acute circumoral paresthesiae and bronchospasm (Miller, 1994). Third, the clinical presentation of PCP (and therefore its early detection) may be altered. For example the use of nebulized pentamidine predisposes to 'atypical' radiographic upper zone shadowing (Fahy *et al.*, 1992) and possibly pneumothorax (Sepkowitz *et al.*, 1991). There is less evidence to confirm, however, the early reports that PCP diagnosis using induced sputum or bronchoalveolar lavage is compromised in pentamidine users (Fahy *et al.*, 1992). Fourth, pentamidine's selective pulmonary deposition may not protect against extrapulmonary pneumocystis, though this condition is rare.

There is an increasing trend in profoundly immunosuppressed HIV-infected individuals (i.e. CD4 count <50 cells/μl) who cannot tolerate TMP/SMX to prescribe more frequent pentamidine nebulizers, e.g. 300 mg per fortnight. Whether this policy results in less breakthrough is currently unclear (Golden *et al.*, 1993) (Table 7.1). Another option is to combine fortnightly or even more frequent nebulizers with drugs such as dapsone 100 mg per day in patients with multiple recurrences of PCP.

Other drugs

Several other drugs active against *Pneumocystis* have been proposed as prophylactic agents. These include the folate synthesis inhibitor **dapsone**, often paired with **pyrimethamine**. Although this combination acts at the same metabolic steps as TMP/SMX, when used as primary prophylaxis at a dosage of dapsone 50 mg per day and pyrimethamine 50 mg per week it was no more effective than inhaled pentamidine 300 mg per month (at 18 months, 5.5% of subjects had developed PCP); and less well tolerated (Girard *et al.*, 1993). However, in a large, direct comparison of dapsone 50 mg twice per day, TMP/SMX

Table 7.1 Recommended *Pneumocystis carinii* pneumonia prophylaxis

	Drug	*Dose*	*Comments*
First line	Trimethoprim/ sulfamethoxazole	960 mg OD	May be equally effective at 480 mg/day or 960 mg × 3/week
			Possible protection against cerebral toxoplasmosis and bacterial infections
Second line	Pentamidine	300 mg/month via jet nebulizer	Dosage frequency should be increased if CD4 <50, or if 2° prophylaxis
		60 mg/fortnight via ultrasonic nebulizer	
Third line	Dapsone	100 mg OD	Additional pyrimethamine 25–50 mg/week may give protection against cerebral toxoplasmosis
Fourth line	Intravenous/intramuscular pentamidine	4 mg/kg single infusion every 2–4 weeks	Potential severe local and systemic side effects

960 mg twice per day and nebulized pentamidine 300 mg per month as primary prophylaxis in subjects taking zidovudine 500 mg per day, by intention to treat analysis, the 3 regimes were of equivalent efficacy (Bozzette *et al.*, 1995). In this study 40–50% of patients switched at least once from either oral therapy due to adverse events, compared with 12% in the pentamidine arm. By 'on treatment analysis', TMP/SMX was the superior prophylaxis provided it could be tolerated.

Dapsone 100 mg per day may be useful prophylaxis in patients intolerant or failing on TMP/SMX and pentamidine (Table 7.1). However, in a small retrospective study of thrice weekly dapsone 100 mg in just such a population, 39% discontinued study drug due to adverse reactions (Jorde, Horowitz and Wormser, 1993). Pyrimethamine appears to add little to dapsone's effect against PCP (Falloon *et al.*, 1994) but is important when considering 'cross prophylaxis' against reactivation of cerebral toxoplasmosis (Girard *et al.*, 1993). Dapsone is contraindicated in patients with glucose-6-phosphate dehydrogenase (G-6-PD) deficiency because of the risk of hemolysis.

Current fourth-line options include monthly **intravenous** (Ena *et al.*, 1994) or **intramuscular pentamidine**. In one report, when the latter regime was used at 300 mg per month, as both primary and secondary prophylaxis, there was little reported PCP breakthrough and minimal toxicity (Cheung *et al.*, 1993). Other drugs that are effective in treating PCP also have been tried as prophylaxis. These include **atovaquone**, **clindamycin** plus **primaquine** and **trimethoprim** plus **dapsone**. Evidence for their effect is anecdotal (Kay and Dubois, 1990) and trials of these agents as PCP treatments suggest that one might expect them to be no better than TMP/SMX in terms of efficacy or in some cases toxicity. The combination of **sulfadoxine** and **pyrimethamine** (Fansidar) appears to be much less effective than other regimes (Gottlieb *et al.*, 1984).

It is important to remember that **antiretroviral therapy** reduces the risk of progression to PCP and therefore offers some degree of protection against the development of pneumonitis (Fischl, Dickenson and La Voie, 1990). Many subjects currently in trials of prophylactic agents will also be taking antiretrovirals. The interactions between these different drugs may be of some importance.

TREATMENT

EMPIRICAL THERAPY

As a rule of thumb, treatment should never be deferred in an HIV-positive individual with suspected PCP. The question whether microbiological/cytological diagnosis is necessary is perhaps more controversial (Tu, Biem and Detsky, 1993). Patients with PCP on appropriate therapy typically take 4–8 days to show signs of clinical improvement, and up to 2 weeks before radiographic change occurs. Therefore diagnostic confirmation provides reassurance that the patient is on the correct treatment during this early, potentially stormy, period.

Trimethoprim/sulfamethoxazole

TMP/SMX is the current drug of choice for all episodes of PCP. Used in the fixed combination of TMP 20 mg/kg/day and SMX 100 mg/kg/day, in 3–4 divided doses, it can

be given as either oral or intravenous therapy. Most clinicians advocate a 21-day treatment course to insure maximal eradication of the *Pneumocystis* cysts and trophozoites. Given intravenously each dose should be diluted 1:25 in 5% dextrose in water or normal saline and infused over 1–1.5 hours. The standard oral dose is 1920 mg 3 or 4 times per day depending on the patient's weight.

In a randomized treatment trial comparing intravenous TMP/SMX with once daily intravenous pentamidine (4 mg/kg/day) the 2 drugs were found to have equally good efficacy (approximately 70% overall survival) and equally high toxicity (approximately 30%) (Klein *et al.*, 1992). TMP/SMX's toxicity can be greatly reduced if dosage adjustments are performed to maintain serum TMP between 5–8μg/ml (equivalent to 100–150 μg/ml of SMX) with no loss of efficacy (Sattler *et al.*, 1988). In practice this can be achieved by using a reduced dosage (15 mg/kg/day TMP and 75 mg/kg/day SMX) if toxicity occurs (Sattler *et al.*, 1988).

The oral formulation is well absorbed and can be used either as initial (outpatient) therapy in patients with mild to moderate PCP (Table 7.2) or as a switch from intravenous drug when there are signs of clinical improvement. During treatment, patients should have twice weekly monitoring of blood count, renal and hepatic function.

Table 7.2 grades the severity of *P. carinii* pneumonia. PAO_2–PaO_2 (alveolar to arterial oxygen tension gradient) indicates the overall efficiency of the lungs in oxygenation. It can be derived from blood gas analysis since

$$PAO_2 = PIO_2 - \frac{PaCO_2}{R}$$

where PIO_2 = inspired oxygen tension at sea level = 20 kPa (150 mmHg). $PaCO_2$ = partial pressure of carbon dioxide; R = the gas exchange ratio, usually 0.8–1. It should be noted that *Pneumocystis* pneumonia physically reduces the amount of lung available for

Table 7.2 Grading of severity of *Pneumocystis carinii* pneumonia. (Modified from Miller, R.F., 1994. Reproduced from *Drug and Therapeutics Bulletin*, **32**, 12–15, with permission)

	Mild	Moderate	Severe
Symptoms and signs	Breathless on exertion +/- cough and fever	Breathless on minimal exertion, occasionally at rest; cough and fever	Breathless at rest; cough and fever
Blood gas tensions (room air, at rest)	$PaO_2 > 11$ kPa (>83 mmHg)	PaO_2 8.1–11 kPa (61–83 mmHg)	$PaO_2 < 8$ kPa (<60 mmHg)
Arterial oxygen saturations	$SaO_2 > 94\%$ at rest; with exercise >90%	SaO_2 90–94% at rest; with exercise <90%	$SaO_2 < 90\%$ at rest
Alveolar-arterial oxygen gradient	PAO_2–$PaO_2 < 4.7$ kPa (<35 mmHg)	PAO_2–PaO_2 4.7–6 kPa (35–45 mmHg)	PAO_2–$PaO_2 > 6$ kPa (>45 mmHg)
Chest radiograph	Normal or minor perihilar shadowing	Diffuse interstitial shadowing	Extensive interstitial shadowing and alveolar shadowing

PaO_2 = partial pressure of oxygen
SaO_2 = arterial oxygen saturation, measured by non-invasive pulse oximetry
PAO_2–PaO_2 = alveolar to arterial oxygen tension gradient.

alveolar ventilation. This produces a rise in the alveolar–arterial gradient, the magnitude of which reflects the amount of acute lung damage. In health, PAO_2–PaO_2 is <2.5 kPa (<20 mmHg).

Adverse reactions to high dose TMP/SMX are similar to those found using prophylactic doses (Jung and Paauw, 1994). If rash or fever develops, symptomatic relief can be given and PCP treatment can then often be continued. A large number of patients (especially if taking concurrent zidovudine) may develop leukopenia, thrombocytopenia or anemia. In one study these constituted 35% of major toxicities and 28% of all adverse events (Medina *et al.*, 1990). Folinic acid (leukovorin) has been used to reduce this. A recent report suggested that folinic acid (dosage 7.5 mg per day of its L-isomer) did not prevent hematological toxicity; it also increased therapeutic failure and mortality (Safrin, Lee and Sande, 1994). It was postu-lated that this effect arose from folinic acid antagonizing TMP/SMX's blockage of the *Pneumocystis* folate pathway (Safrin, Lee and Sande, 1994).

A patient who is intolerant of TMP/SMX during treatment has no greater risk of hy-persensitivity on rechallenge (Hardy *et al.*, 1992). Desensitization programs have been used with some success in patients starting TMP/SMX prophylaxis (Jung and Paauw, 1994).

Pentamidine

The inconvenience of administering pen-tamidine parenterally has severely limited its use as a first-line drug. It is as effective as TMP/SMX in severe PCP (Klein *et al.*, 1992); dosage reduction can also reduce the fre-quency and severity of adverse events (Sattler *et al.*, 1988). These include hypotension (now rarely clinically important with slow rates of infusion), nephrotoxicity, arrhythmias, leukopenia, pancreatitis and hyper- or hypoglycemia. Biochemical renal impairment (usually an isolated rise in serum creatinine) is seen in almost two-thirds of patients on 4 mg/kg/day. It can be managed often by dose reduction (2–3 mg/kg/day) with no apparent loss of efficacy (Sattler *et al.*, 1988) or with less frequent dosing (with a glomerular filtration rate of >10 ml/min, the drug should be given every 48 hours after 7 days of conventional therapy) (Miller, 1994). Pentamidine's toxic effect tends to occur early in therapy; though dysglycemias may be seen once the drug has been stopped. Nephrotoxicity appears to predict the risk of subsequent blood sugar abnormalities (Kovacs and Masur, 1988).

Currently, intravenous pentamidine is administered as 4 mg/kg once daily for 21 days. It is given in 250 ml of 5% dextrose in water over 1.5–2 hours (Miller, 1994). During therapy blood pressure, blood count, glucose, calcium and electrolytes should be closely monitored.

The use of intramuscular or nebulized pentamidine for PCP treatment is now rare. This relates to the high frequency of painful sterile abscesses produced by regular intramuscular injection; and the high relapse rate associated with nebulized treatment (Masur, 1992).

Other specific PCP treatments

PCP can be graded as mild, moderate or severe depending on a combination of symptoms and signs, blood gas oxygen tensions or oxygen saturations or estimated alveolar-arterial oxygen tension gradients, and chest radiographic appearances (Table 7.2). Whilst TMP/SMX and pentamidine are considered the best therapies for severe PCP, other drugs may be useful when either the patient is failing or intolerant of these; or if the episode of PCP is mild.

The combination of oral **dapsone** 100 mg/day and **trimethoprim** 20 mg/kg/day had similar efficacy (90% response rate) to oral TMP/SMX when used in mild to moderate PCP (Medina *et al.*, 1990). Its toxicity profile was similar to TMP/SMX though overall it was better tolerated. Methemoglobinemia was seen in 3% of dapsone treated patients, though the clinical implications of this are uncertain. Dapsone and trimethoprim are therefore a useful oral combination in patients with mild to moderate PCP unable to tolerate TMP/SMX. This has received further support from the recently reported ACTG 108 trial which compared oral TMP/SMX 1920 mg thrice daily with dapsone 100 mg per day plus TMP 300 mg thrice daily and oral clindamycin 600 mg thrice daily plus primaquine base 30 mg per day in this patient population (Hardy *et al.*, 1994). No difference was seen between the three arms in either time to treatment failure, treatment failure (all <10%) or dose-limiting toxicity (24–36%).

Clindamycin plus **primaquine** was first used in intravenous form, though recent trials have demonstrated its efficacy as an oral preparation (Black *et al.*, 1994; Hardy *et al.*, 1994). Adverse effects tend to be mild, though in the ACTG 044 trial skin rash was seen in 62% of 60 subjects, whilst methemoglobinemia occurred in 40%. Diarrhea was noted in 11% of subjects (Black *et al.*, 1994). The association of clindamycin with the development of pseudomembranous colitis means that careful evaluation needs to be performed in all patients with diarrhea on this drug. Like dapsone, primaquine is contraindicated in patients with G-6-PD deficiency.

Combination clindamycin and primaquine were originally used as 'salvage therapy' in patients failing on TMP/SMX and pentamidine (Noskin *et al.*, 1992). Of 28 patient episodes, 24 (86%) responded to a combined intravenous and oral schedule, and survived at least 30 days from the end of treatment. Although these are impressive results, this illustrates the difficulty of determining whether it is a slow response to the initial therapy given, any adjunctive treatments used (e.g. corticosteroids) or the test drug itself that is responsible for the effects seen in trials of salvage therapy.

Atovaquone (BW 566C80) has also been investigated as a PCP treatment. Although its precise mechanism of action against *Pneumocystis* is unknown, it appears to demonstrate true microbicidal activity in the steroid-treated rat model of acute PCP. In a double-blind comparison of 322 patients with mild to moderate PCP randomized to receive either oral atovaquone 750 mg three times per day or oral TMP/SMX 1920 mg thrice daily, the test drug was found to be much less effective though produced fewer treatment limiting side effects (7% – the commonest being rash, nausea and diarrhea, compared to 20% with TMP/SMX) (Hughes *et al.*, 1993). Of subjects, 20% on atovaquone and 7% on TMP/SMX did not respond to therapy; and within 4 weeks of completing treatment there were 11 deaths in the atovaquone group, compared to only 1 with TMP/SMX ($p=0.003$).

In its current formulation, atovaquone is variably absorbed. This is important, as in Hughes' study, therapeutic outcome was closely related to the plasma concentration of the drug (Hughes *et al.*, 1993). Therefore as a suspension with increased bioavailability, atovaquone may be an effective oral alternative to current therapies with few side effects. When using the tablet form now available, it is recommended that it be taken with a fatty meal to enhance its absorption.

Trimetrexate (TMTX) is a dihydrofolate reductase inhibitor that *in vitro* is 1500 times more potent than trimethoprim (Allegra *et al.*, 1987a). As *Pneumocystis* lacks the folate membrane transport system necessary to take up classical folate structures, **folinic acid** (leukovorin) must be co-administered

with TMTX to protect the host cell from drug toxicity. A recent double-blind study compared intravenous TMTX 45 mg/m² once daily plus leukovorin 20 mg/m² six hourly with intravenous TMP/SMX 120 mg/kg/day in 215 patients with moderate to severe PCP. TMTX and leukovorin was less effective than TMP/SMX (failure rate at day 21 was 38% compared to 20% respectively; $p=0.008$); and there was a significant difference in survival which also favored TMP/SMX (Sattler *et al.*, 1994). Serious and treatment limiting adverse events, including hematological toxicity, were less in the TMTX group. The side-effect profiles were similar in the two study arms. TMTX plus leukovorin may be useful therefore in moderate to severe PCP where first-line therapy has failed. This trial did not confirm reports of a high relapse rate following TMTX treatment that has been seen in other studies (Masur, 1992).

Its role as 'salvage therapy' has been documented by Allegra *et al.* (1987b) where at a lower dose than used in the above trial (TMTX 30 mg/m² plus leukovorin as above), a 69% response and survival rate were seen. Combining TMTX with a sulfa drug such as dapsone may be the best hope yet for moderate to severe PCP.

The polyamine synthesis inhibitor **Eflornithine** (difluoromethyl ornithine, DFMO) has been studied in small numbers of patients as salvage therapy. In a retrospective review of 31 patients, a 68% response rate was seen when intravenous DFMO was given at 400 mg/kg daily for 14 days. Bone marrow suppression occurred in 48% of cases though only 5 patients needed to stop therapy. Phlebitis at the infusion site was noted in 52% of cases (Smith *et al.*, 1990).

ADJUNCTIVE THERAPY

Corticosteroids

The use of either oral or intravenous corticosteroids started within 72 hours of the initiation of specific PCP treatment has been shown to reduce the risk of death by one half in patients with moderate or severe PCP (Bozzette *et al.*, 1990; National Institutes of Health, 1990). The mechanism of this effect is unclear, but it may be that steroids act to damp down the pulmonary inflammatory response associated with dying *Pneumocystis*. The beneficial effects seen in the more hypoxic patients would then reflect the fact that these people have the greatest degree of pulmonary compromise due to PCP, and thus have the most to lose from a host response which further reduces arterial oxygenation. It follows from this that steroids must be given early in treatment, and may be less useful in milder forms of disease. Teasing out the effectiveness of steroids in this latter group is made even harder by the efficacy of current PCP treatments in such patients.

In practice, steroids are recommended in patients who are hypoxic with a PaO_2 <9.3 kPa (<70 mmHg) or an alveolar-arterial oxygen gradient >4.7 kPa (>35 mmHg). Table 7.2 gives the method of calculation. If using non-invasive pulse oximetry to monitor the patient, then in most people this is equivalent to arterial O_2 saturations of <92% at rest.

Different steroid regimes have been employed (NIH, 1990). The most commonly used is oral prednisolone 40 mg twice daily for 5 days, followed by 40 mg once daily for 5 days and then 20 mg once daily on days 11–21. With intravenous administration, shorter courses of high doses of either methylprednisolone or hydrocortisone have been successfully used (Miller, 1994). The potential concern of reactivation of mycobacterial, fungal and viral diseases does not appear to be much of a problem with these steroid regimes. In one study, local herpetic infection and oral thrush (as well as steroid-induced hyperglycemia) were seen more frequently following corticosteroids (Bozzette *et al.*, 1990).

Ventilatory support

The last few years have seen a greater flexibility in the clinical approach to PCP-associated respiratory failure. This has mirrored improvements in the early recognition of disease, the management of patients failing on first-line therapy (including the use of adjunctive steroids), patient selection for mechanical ventilation, and post-ventilation survival (Lipman and Johnson, 1992).

The use of non-invasive ventilatory support techniques such as continuous positive airway pressure (CPAP) via a tight-fitting face or nose mask can buy time for the specific PCP therapies to take effect (Miller and Semple, 1991). The mechanism by which CPAP works is unclear, but it probably acts as a 'pneumatic splint' throughout the airway, thus improving oxygenation. In general it is well tolerated and often its use is associated with an important reduction in the patient's sensation of breathlessness. CPAP circuits can be especially useful when a patient deteriorates following a bronchoscopy. Provided pneumothoraces have been excluded, CPAP will often tide the patient over this self-limiting episode. It should be noted that barotrauma itself is a rare complication of CPAP, as are also gastric aspiration and mask pressure necrosis.

If a patient continues to deteriorate despite maximal specific and adjunctive therapies, then formal mechanical ventilation may be necessary. In general terms most authorities advocate ventilation for first-episode PCP and severe post-bronchoscopy deterioration. Whenever a patient is ventilated it is important to try and set clear goals so that an individual will not remain mechanically supported with an ever-decreasing chance of recovery. Decisions regarding ventilation should be made on an individual basis, and if at all possible take into account the wishes of the patient and their next of kin (Lipman and Johnson, 1992).

MANAGEMENT STRATEGIES IN THE TREATMENT OF PCP

THERAPEUTIC OPTIONS IN PCP

There is an increasing trend towards the outpatient management of PCP. This requires that the patient is able to cope at home, understands the need for regular review and that the (initially mild to moderate) PCP is responding to treatment. Oral TMP/SMX 1920 mg three or four times/day depending on weight is currently the favored combination. It is effective in at least 90% of such patients (Medina *et al.*, 1990). If, despite symptomatic relief, this were not tolerated, then intravenous TMP/SMX, oral TMP plus dapsone, or clindamycin plus primaquine, could be given. In its current formulation, oral atovaquone would be a third-line option.

Moderate to severe PCP (Table 7.2) should always be managed in a hospital setting with initially either intravenous TMP/SMX or intravenous pentamidine together with adjunctive steroid therapy. If a patient fails on one of these, then if possible they should be switched to the other drug with at least 48 hours' overlap to allow for adequate tissue levels of the new drug. Patients who need to switch drugs have a greatly increased mortality (Wharton *et al.*, 1986) though this may reflect the severity of the underlying disease in these patients rather than the drug change itself.

There appears to be no advantage in combining TMP/SMX with pentamidine. Patients failing on these drugs with moderate or severe PCP should be offered intravenous trimetrexate and leukovorin or clindamycin and primaquine. Eflornithine is also an option.

Patient compliance should always be considered in someone developing PCP whilst on prophylaxis. If this were adequate, and this is genuine prophylactic failure, then there is a tendency to assume that the *Pneumocystis* is drug resistant and to initiate therapy with another drug. There is little hard evidence to support this view (US Public Health Service Task Force, 1993).

DETERIORATION ON TREATMENT

Patients on treatment may deteriorate either rapidly or over several days or weeks. When there is an acute decline, precipitating causes such as pneumothorax (especially after any respiratory procedure), acute pulmonary edema (secondary to fluid overload and perhaps hypoalbuminemia), or a drug-induced event (e.g. hypotension, arrhythmias or hypoglycemia with pentamidine infusions) should be considered. Deterioration over a few hours may be due to a preceding bronchoscopic procedure. A marked decline within the first 24–48 hours of admission is quite common. It is this patient population which appear to gain most from adjunctive steroids and CPAP.

A more gradual deterioration, or a failure to improve, may reflect PCP that is not responding, a copathogen that has been missed, drug-associated anemia or, again, fluid overload. Here therapeutic options include diuresis, further diagnostic investigation (e.g. repeat bronchoscopy or open lung biopsy), adding in treatments against suspected copathogens or switching PCP therapy. It should be noted that with both TMP/SMX and pentamidine, improvements in oxygenation often do not occur for several days. Of the two, a faster response is seen with TMP/SMX (Sattler *et al.*, 1988). The initial drug therapy may therefore influence the time that treatment is changed.

SURVIVAL AND PREDICTORS OF OUTCOME

Overall survival following an episode of PCP has dramatically improved since the early 1980s. Within the MACS cohort, men diagnosed with PCP in 1990–91 had one-tenth the risk of dying of those who developed PCP in

1984–85. Median survival following PCP rose significantly over the same period from 12.8 months to 26.3 months (Jacobson *et al.*, 1993). This finding appears to reflect widespread use of effective PCP prophylaxis, early recognition of disease and perhaps the beneficial effect of corticosteroids.

The severity of the pneumonia is an important predictor of outcome. Thus grading the episode by symptoms and signs, degree of hypoxemia and extent of radiographic shadowing has clinical relevance (Table 7.2). Biochemical tests that imply a poor outcome include low serum albumin at time of admission and persistently elevated serum lactate dehydrogenase despite therapy. A marked pulmonary inflammatory response characterized by a bronchoalveolar lavage neutrophilia or edema on transbronchial biopsy is also a poor prognostic sign. A combination of these different features can be used to create a score predictive of an individual's chance of survival (Speich *et al.*, 1992). A recent retrospective study in 576 patients demonstrated that this can also be achieved using more readily available clinical data obtained at admission (alveolar-arterial oxygen gradients, total lymphocyte count and body mass index) (Bennett *et al.*, 1994). It should be noted that the effect of steroid co-administration was not investigated in this study.

Once a patient has reached the point of requiring ventilation, there appear to be few useful predictors of outcome (Lipman and Johnson, 1992). However, post-ventilation survival has also risen over time from at best 14% prior to 1985 to about 50% on most units experienced in the management of HIV (Lipman and Johnson, 1992). This final point is of some importance, as knowledge of what can be reasonably achieved using current drug therapies has enabled health care workers to provide a standard of medical care which seeks to enhance both the length and the quality of their patients' lives.

REFERENCES

Allegra, C.J., Kovacs, J.A., Drake, J.C. *et al.* (1987a) Activity of antifolates against *Pneumocystis carinii* dihydrofolate reductase and identification of a potent new agent. *J. Exp. Med.*, **165**, 926–31.

Allegra, C.J., Chabner, B.A., Tuazon, C.U. *et al.* (1987b) Trimetrexate for the treatment of *Pneumocystis carinii* pneumonia in patients with the acquired immunodeficiency syndrome. *N. Engl. J. Med.*, **317**, 978–85.

Bennett, C.L., Weinstein, R.A., Shapiro, M.F. *et al.* (1994) A rapid preadmission method for predicting inpatient course of disease for patients with HIV-related *Pneumocystis carinii* pneumonia. *Am. J. Respir. Crit. Care Med.*, **150**, 1503–7.

Black, J.R., Feinberg, J., Murphy R.L., *et al.* (1994) Clindamycin and primaquine therapy for mild-to-moderate episodes of *Pneumocystis carinii* pneumonia in patients with AIDS: AIDS clinical trial group 044. *Clin. Infect. Dis.*, **18**, 905–13.

Bozzette, S.A., Sattler, F.R., Chiu, J. *et al.* (1990) A controlled trial of early adjunctive treatment with corticosteroids for *Pneumocystis carinii* pneumonia in the acquired immunodeficiency syndrome. *N. Engl. J. Med.*, **323**, 1451–57.

Bozzette, S.A., Finkelstein, D.M., Spector, S.A. *et al.* (1995) A randomized trial of three antipneumocystis agents in patients with advanced human immunodeficiency virus infection. NIAID AIDS Clinical Trials Group. *N. Engl. J. Med.*, **332**, 693–99.

Carr, A., Tindall, B., Brew, B.J. *et al.* (1992) Low-dose trimethoprim-sulfamethoxazole prophylaxis for toxoplasmic encephalitis in patients with AIDS. *Ann. Intern. Med.*, **117**, 106–11.

Cheung, T.W., Matta, R., Neibart, E. *et al.* (1993) Intramuscular pentamidine for the prevention of *Pneumocystis carinii* pneumonia in patients infected with human immunodeficiency virus. *Clin. Infect. Dis.*, **16**, 22–25.

Ena, J., Amador, C., Pasqua, F. *et al.* (1994) Once-a-month administration of intravenous pentamidine to patients infected with human immunodeficiency virus as prophylaxis for *Pneumocystis carinii* pneumonia. *Clin. Infect. Dis.*, **18**, 901–4.

Fahy, J.V., Chin, D P., Schnapp, L.M. *et al.* (1992) Effect of aerosolized pentamidine prophylaxis on the clinical severity and diagnosis of

Pneumocystis carinii pneumonia. *Am. Rev. Respir. Dis.*, **146**, 844–48.

Falloon, J., Lavelle, J., Ogata-Arakaki, D. *et al.* (1994) Pharmacokinetics and safety of weekly dapsone and dapsone plus pyrimethamine for prevention of Pneumocystis pneumonia. *Antimicrob. Agents Chemother.*, **38**, 1580–87.

Fischl, M.A., Dickinson, G.M. and La Voie, L. (1988) Safety and efficacy of sulfamethoxazole and trimethoprim chemoprophylaxis for *Pneumocystis carinii* pneumonia in AIDS. *JAMA*, **259**, 1185–89.

Fischl, M.A., Richman, D.D., Hansen, N. *et al.* (1990) The safety and efficacy of zidovudine (AZT) in the treatment of subjects with mildly symptomatic human immunodeficiency type 1 (HIV) infection. *Ann. Intern. Med.*, **112**, 727–37.

Girard, P.M., Landman, R., Gaudebout, C. *et al.* (1993) Dapsone-pyrimethamine compared with aerosolized pentamidine as primary prophylaxis against *Pneumocystis carinii* pneumonia and toxoplasmosis in HIV infection. *N. Engl. J. Med.*, **328**, 1514–20.

Golden, J.A., Katz, M.H., Chernoff, D.N. *et al.* (1993) A randomized trial of once-monthly or twice-monthly high-dose aerosolised pentamidine prophylaxis. *Chest*, **104**, 743–50.

Gottlieb, M.S., Schanker, H., Fan, P. *et al.* (1981) Pneumocystis pneumonia – Los Angeles. *MMWR* **30**, 250–52.

Gottlieb, M.S., Knight, S., Mitsuyasu, R. *et al.* (1984) Prophylaxis of *Pneumocystis carinii* infection in AIDS with pyrimethamine-sulfadoxine. *Lancet*, **ii**, 398–99.

Hardy, W.D., Feinberg, J., Finkelstein, D.M. *et al.* (1992) A controlled trial of trimethoprim-sulfamethoxazole or aerosolized pentamidine for secondary prophylaxis against *Pneumocystis carinii* pneumonia in patients with the acquired immunodeficiency syndrome. *N. Engl. J. Med.*, **327**, 1842–48.

Hardy, W.D., Bozzette, S., Safrin, S. *et al.* (1994) Results from recent therapeutic trials for opportunistic infections from the United States. *AIDS*, **8**, S4, 15s.

Hirschel, B., Lazzarin, A., Chopard, P. *et al.* (1991) A controlled study of inhaled pentamidine for primary prevention of *Pneumocystis carinii* pneumonia. *N. Engl. J. Med.*, **324**, 1079–83.

Hoover, D.R., Saah, A.J., Bacellar, H. *et al.* (1993) Clinical manifestations of AIDS in the era of pneumocystis prophylaxis. *N. Engl. J. Med.*, **329**, 1922–26.

Hughes, W.T., McNabb, P.C., Makres, T.D. and Feldman, S. (1974) Efficacy of trimethoprim and sulfamethoxazole in the prevention and treatment of *Pneumocystis carinii* pneumonitis. *Antimicrob. Agents Chemother.*, **5**, 289–93.

Hughes, W.T., Kuhn, S., Chaudhary, S. *et al.* (1977) Successful chemoprophylaxis for *Pneumocystis carinii* pneumonitis. *N. Engl. J. Med.*, **297**, 1419–26.

Hughes, W., Leoung, G., Kramer, F. *et al.* (1993) Comparison of atovaquone (566C80) with trimethoprim-sulfamethoxazole to treat *Pneumocystis carinii* pneumonia in patients with AIDS. *N. Engl. J. Med.*, **328**, 1521–27.

Jacobson, L.P., Kirby, A.J., Polk, S. *et al.* (1993) Changes in survival after acquired immunodeficiency syndrome (AIDS): 1984–1991. *Am. J. Epidemiol.*, **138**, 952–64.

Jorde, U.P., Horowitz, H.W. and Wormser, G.P. (1993) Utility of dapsone for prophylaxis of *Pneumocystis carinii* pneumonia in trimethoprim-sulfamethoxazole-intolerant, HIV-infected individuals. *AIDS*, **7**, 355–59.

Jung, A.C. and Paauw, D.S. (1994) Management of adverse reactions to trimethoprim-sulfamethoxazole in human immunodeficiency virus-infected patients. *Arch. Intern. Med.*, **154**, 2402–6.

Kay, R. and Dubois, R.E. (1990) Clindamycin/primaquine therapy and secondary prophylaxis against *Pneumocystis carinii* pneumonia in patients with AIDS. *S. Med. J.*, **83**, 403–4.

Klein, N.C., Duncanson, F.P., Lenox, T.H. *et al.* (1992) Trimethoprim-sulfamethoxazole versus pentamidine for *Pneumocystis carinii* pneumonia in AIDS patients: results of a large prospective randomised treatment trial. *AIDS*, **6**, 301–5.

Kovacs, J.A., and Masur, H. (1988) *Pneumocystis carinii* pneumonia: therapy and prophylaxis. *J. Infect. Dis.*, **158**, 254–59.

Leoung, G.S., Feigal, D.W. Jr., Montgomery, A.B. *et al.* (1990) Aerosolized pentamidine for prophylaxis against *Pneumocystis carinii* pneumonia – the San Francisco Community Prophylaxis Trial. *N. Engl. J. Med.*, **323**, 769–75.

Lipman, M.C.I. and Johnson, M.A. (1992) Resuscitation in HIV. *Genitourin. Med.*, **68**, 151–53.

Mallolas, J., Zamora, L., Gatell, J.M. *et al.* (1993) Primary prophylaxis for *Pneumocystis carinii* pneumonia: a randomized trial comparing cotrimoxazole, aerosolized pentamidine and dapsone plus pyrimethamine. *AIDS*, **7**, 59–64.

Masur, H. (1992) Prevention and treatment of Pneumocystis pneumonia. *N. Engl. J. Med.*, **327**, 1853–60.

Medina, I., Mills, J., Leoung, G. *et al.* (1990) Oral therapy for *Pneumocystis carinii* pneumonia in the acquired immunodeficiency syndrome: a controlled trial of trimethoprim-sulfamethoxazole versus trimethoprim-dapsone. *N. Engl. J. Med.*, **323**, 776–82.

Miller, R.F. and Semple, S.J.G. (1991) Continuous positive airway pressure ventilation for respiratory failure associated with *Pneumocystis carinii* pneumonia. *Respir. Med.*, **85**, 135–38.

Miller, R.F. (1994) Prevention and treatment of *Pneumocystis carinii* pneumonia in patients infected with HIV. *Drug Ther. Bull.*, **32**, 12–15.

Montaner, J.S.G., Lawson, L.M., Gervais, A. *et al.* (1991) Aerosol pentamidine for secondary prophylaxis of AIDS-related *Pneumocystis carinii* pneumonia. *Ann. Intern. Med.*, **114**, 948–53.

National Institutes of Health–University of California Expert Panel for Corticosteroids as Adjunctive Therapy for Pneumocystis Pneumonia. (1990) Consensus statement on the use of corticosteroids as adjunctive therapy for Pneumocystis pneumonia in the acquired immunodeficiency syndrome. *N. Engl. J. Med.*, **323**, 1500–4.

Noskin, G.A., Murphy, R.L., Black, J.R. and Phair, J.P. (1992) Salvage therapy with clindamycin/primaquine for *Pneumocystis carinii* pneumonia. *Clin. Infect. Dis.*, **14**, 183–88.

Phair, J.P., Munoz, A., Detels, R. *et al.* (1990) The risk of *Pneumocystis carinii* pneumonia among men infected with human immunodeficiency virus type 1. *N. Engl. J. Med.*, **322**, 160–65.

Safrin, S., Lee, B.L. and Sande, M.A. (1994) Adjunctive folinic acid with trimethoprim-sulfamethoxazole for *Pneumocystis carinii* pneumonia in AIDS patients is associated with an increased risk of therapeutic failure and death. *J. Infect. Dis.*, **170**, 912–17.

Sattler, F.R., Cowan, R., Nielsen, D. and Ruskin, J. (1988) Trimethoprim-sulfamethoxazole compared with pentamidine for treatment of *Pneumocystis carinii* pneumonia in the acquired immunodeficiency syndrome. *Ann. Intern. Med.*, **109**, 280–87.

Sattler, F.R., Frame, P., Davis, R. *et al.* (1994) Trimetrexate with leucovorin versus trimethoprim-sulfamethoxazole for moderate to severe episodes of *Pneumocystis carinii* pneumonia in patients with AIDS. *J. Infect. Dis.*, **170**, 165–72.

Schneider, M.M.E., Hoepelman, A.I.M., Eeftinck-Schattenkerk, J.K.M. *et al.* (1992) A controlled trial of aerosolized pentamidine or trimethoprim-sulfamethoxazole as primary prophylaxis against *Pneumocystis carinii* pneumonia in patients with human immunodeficiency virus infection. *N. Engl. J. Med.*, **327**, 1836–41.

Sepkowitz, K.A., Telzak, E.E., Gold, J.M.W. *et al.* (1991) Pneumothorax in AIDS. *Ann. Intern. Med.*, **114**, 455–59.

Smith, D., Davies, S., Nelson, M. *et al.* (1990) *Pneumocystis carinii* pneumonia treated with eflornithine in AIDS patients resistant to conventional therapy. *AIDS*, **4**, 1019–21.

Speich, R., Opravil, M., Weber R. *et al.* (1992) Prospective evaluation of a prognostic score for *Pneumocystis carinii* pneumonia in HIV-infected patients. *Chest*, **102**, 1045–48.

Tu, J.V., Biem, H.J. and Detsky, A.S. (1993) Bronchoscopy versus empirical therapy in HIV-infected patients with presumptive *Pneumocystis carinii* pneumonia. A decision analysis. *Am. Rev. Respir. Dis.*, **148**, 370–77.

US Public Health Service Task Force on Antipneumocystis Prophylaxis in Patients Infected with Human Immunodeficiency Virus Infection (1993) Recommendations for prophylaxis against *Pneumocystis carinii* pneumonia for persons infected with human immunodeficiency virus. *AIDS*, **6**, 46–55.

Waldman, R.H., Pearce, D.E. and Martin, R.A. (1973) Pentamidine isethionate levels in lungs, livers, and kidneys of rats after aerosol or intramuscular administration. *Am. Rev. Respir. Dis.*, **108**, 1004–6.

Walzer, P.D. (1991) Immunopathogenesis of *Pneumocystis carinii* infection. *J. Lab. Clin. Med.*, **118**, 206–16.

Wharton, J.M., Coleman, D.L., Wofsy, C.B., *et al.* (1986) Trimethoprim-sulfamethoxazole or pentamidine for *Pneumocystis carinii* pneumonia in the acquired immunodeficiency syndrome: a prospective randomised trial. *Ann. Intern. Med.*, **105**, 37–44.

Mario C. Raviglione and Paul P. Nunn

INTRODUCTION

Tuberculosis competes with the measles virus and *Streptococcus pneumoniae* for the dubious distinction of causing the highest number of deaths each year from a single infectious agent. The World Health Organization (WHO) has recently estimated that nearly 90 million new cases and 30 million deaths may occur in the decade 1990–1999 (Dolin, Raviglione and Kochi, 1994). Tuberculosis kills more adults each year than any other communicable disease (WHO, 1992). Tuberculosis alone accounted for 3.4% of all disability adjusted life years (DALYs) lost globally in 1990, and as much as 4.7% of all the DALYs lost in Sub-Saharan Africa (World Bank, 1993).

Even so, in spite of the burden it places on society, few diseases of public health significance are as neglected as tuberculosis. Governments of developing countries have consistently ignored it. In those few which did recognize the problem, lack of resources hampered attempts to develop adequate tuberculosis control programmes. As a result, tuberculosis never declined: it was just forgotten on the agenda of public health problems. In some industrialized countries, on the other hand, control programs were dismantled under the impression that the disease was no longer a problem. In part as a result, we face today a resurgence of tuberculosis: after decades of decline, tuber-culosis cases began to increase in some countries around the mid-1980s. This increase, which will be discussed below, prompted the recognition of the problem at an international level and new efforts to revitalize control activities.

In this chapter, we will concentrate on the impact of HIV on the epidemiology of tuberculosis in a worldwide context.

BASIC EPIDEMIOLOGY OF TUBERCULOSIS

TUBERCULOSIS TRANSMISSION AND INFECTION

Tuberculosis is caused by three related organisms, *Mycobacterium tuberculosis*, *Mycobacterium africanum*, and *Mycobacterium bovis*, of which by far the most frequent organism involved in human disease is *M. tuberculosis*. *M. africanum* is rarely found outside Africa, and *M. bovis* is usually transmitted via the digestive tract through contaminated milk from cows suffering from bovine tuberculosis.

By far the most common route of infection for man is person-to-person spread via the respiratory route. Tubercle bacilli are expelled into the environment in water droplets by a person suffering from pulmonary or laryngeal tuberculosis during coughing, sneezing, singing or even just speaking. They are then inhaled by the susceptible host, in whose

AIDS and Respiratory Medicine. Edited by A. Zumla, M.A. Johnson and R.F. Miller. Published in 1997 by Chapman & Hall, London. ISBN 0 412 60140 0

lungs the bacilli elicit non-specific acute responses, and are ingested by macrophages. If non-specific immunity proves inadequate, the bacilli spread to regional lymph nodes and, occasionally, beyond, to distant sites. As cell-mediated immunity to *M. tuberculosis* develops, bacilli are usually confined intracellularly within granulomatous lesions where they can persist for years. At this stage, infection can be demonstrated by local induration to intradermal injection of tuberculin.

The risk of infection depends largely on the degree of exposure to an infectious case which is determined by the density of infected droplet nuclei in the air inhaled by a contact, and by the length of time the contact has to breathe such air (Geuns, van Meijer and Styblo, 1975; Styblo, 1991). Contacts exposed to a sputum smear-positive case, or to a case with radiological cavitation, are thus most likely to become infected, since these types of case excrete the most bacilli. The intimacy of contact is also a risk factor: those sharing the same bed are at greater risk than those sharing only a living room, or a work space. The frequency, or force, with which an index case coughs may also influence the chances of contacts becoming infected. Thus the risk factors for infection are largely extrinsic to the individual contact.

There is suggestive evidence from two outbreaks of tuberculosis in AIDS-care settings that HIV renders patients more susceptible to infection, but this has yet to be conclusively proven (Di Perri *et al.*, 1989; Daley *et al.*, 1992).

BREAKDOWN AND DISEASE

Following infection by *M. tuberculosis*, it has been estimated that disease will develop in only 5% to 10% of HIV-negative individuals during their lifetimes, with variations in different locations (Sutherland, 1976). The shorter the interval following infection, the greater the likelihood of disease. In newborns and small children especially, disease can develop rapidly within weeks or months following infection, either at the primary site or in metastatic foci. Serious forms of tuberculosis, such as miliary tuberculosis and tuberculous meningitis, may develop. These forms of tuberculosis also occur in adolescents and adults, but less frequently. In the majority of cases, however, tuberculosis develops later in life as a result of reactivation of an initially dormant infection. Less often, but especially where the risk of infection with tubercle bacilli is high, disease can also arise as a result of exogenous reinfection (Styblo, 1991).

Adolescents, young adults, and especially women of child-bearing age are most likely to experience breakdown of a latent infection, and there is some evidence that those aged over 60 are also at greater risk. This latter phenomenon should not be confused with the increase in incidence rates of tuberculosis that occurs with age in most developing countries, which is largely due to the fact that, having lived longer, elderly people are more likely to be infected than those younger. It is now well established that the most potent risk factor for tuberculosis disease is tuberculosis-infected individuals is HIV (Rieder *et al.*, 1989; Selwyn *et al.*, 1989).

Race or ethnicity has often been considered to give rise to vulnerability to tuberculosis. This is probably due to two factors: first, the introduction of tuberculosis among populations with no previous experience of the disease – and therefore no acquired resistance – has led to very high rates of disease, and of mortality. Examples are the African troops brought to Europe to fight in the trenches in the First World War, who had disease rates several times greater than those of their French-born comrades (Stead, 1992). Mortality rates among native Americans during the eighteenth and early nineteenth centuries were much higher than those of the immigrant groups (Grigg, 1958). Secondly, disease rates are higher among certain disadvantaged ethnic groups, particularly immigrants (Rieder *et al.*, 1994). This is probably mostly related to their socio-economic conditions, which in turn reflects the chances of becoming infected and of subsequent breakdown. No specific genetic susceptibility factor has yet been identified in humans and shown to vary by ethnicity.

Several other factors are known to enhance the probability of developing disease, once infected. These include silicosis, immunosuppressive treatment, malnutrition, diabetes, chronic renal failure, gastrectomy and jejunoileal bypass (Rieder *et al.*, 1989), but since these are comparatively rare, they have little impact on the epidemiology of tuberculosis. In sum, the risk factors for disease following infection are largely intrinsic to the individual.

It follows from the above that probably the most important determinant of infection and disease in a community is the prevalence of sputum smear-positive cases, i.e. cases which excrete large numbers of bacilli and are therefore infectious (Geuns, van Meijer and Styblo, 1975; Styblo, 1991), while HIV is the factor most able to upset the balance between man and the tubercle bacillus and cause major upward shifts in tuberculosis disease incidence. On the other hand, sputum smear-negative cases are much weaker transmitters of tubercle bacilli (Geuns, van Meijer and Styblo, 1975), and extrapulmonary cases, unless draining tuberculous pus, are not infectious at all.

THE IMPACT OF HIV INFECTION ON TUBERCULOSIS EPIDEMIOLOGY

The extent of overlap between the population infected with HIV and that infected with tuberculosis determines the number of perons co-infected and therefore at increased risk of developing active tuberculosis. The overlap also determines in what populations the interaction will have the greatest impact. In industrialized countries the large majority of the tuberculosis-infected populations is elderly and at minimal risk of HIV infection. However, among certain population groups, such as the inhabitants of inner-city slum areas with high unemployment, communities consisting of individuals born in high prevalence areas, or those with high rates of substance abuse, the proportion of tuberculosis-infected young adults is more like that found in developing countries (Altarac *et al.*, 1993). In the developing world, infection with *M. tuberculosis* is common at young ages, and about half of the total adult population is infected (Sudre, ten Dam and Kochi, 1992).

Worldwide, in 1990, WHO estimated the number of persons latently infected with tubercle bacilli, but without disease, to be about 1.7 billion, i.e. one-third of the human population (Sudre, ten Dam and Kochi, 1992). Approximately one billion of them live in Asia, where the impact of HIV on the tuberculosis situation is likely to have catastrophic consequences for the often poorly organized and already overburdened tuberculosis programmes. In the developing countries of Sub-Saharan Africa and Latin America about 171 and 117 million people, respectively are estimated to be infected with tuberculosis (Sudre, ten Dam and Kochi, 1992).

The size of the HIV-associated tuberculosis epidemic can be predicted using WHO's global estimates of HIV infection (WHO, 1995a) and the prevalence of tuberculosis infection in the age group at high risk of HIV infection (15–49 years). Assuming that the risk of being infected with *M. tuberculosis* and that of being infected with HIV are independent (which is clearly not the case), by mid-1995 nearly 6 million persons were living with the dual infection (Figure 8.1). If their annual risk of developing tuberculosis is

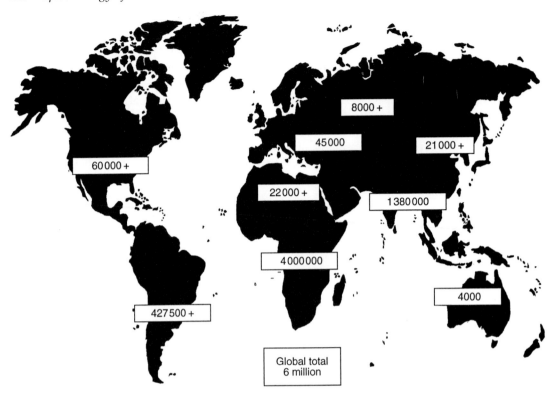

Fig. 8.1 Estimated global distribution of adults (15-49 years) infected with HIV and tuberculosis, mid-1995.

between 5% and 15% (Selwyn *et al.*, 1989, 1992; Allen *et al.*, 1992; Guelar *et al.*, 1993; Antonucci *et al.*, 1995), more than half a million cases of HIV-attributable tuberculosis could have occurred in this age group of the population that year; the greatest majority occurring in developing countries. By the year 2000, when the total number of co-infected persons may be higher than 8 million (WHO, 1993), the number of HIV-attributable tuberculosis cases in the same age group is likely to approach one million. Including cases estimated to occur in the pediatric and older adult populations and assuming more realistically that the risks of being infected with *M. tuberculosis* and HIV are not independent, an even higher number of cases of tuberculosis will be attributable to HIV by the year 2000. These figures are close to those

estimated by different methods and these are outlined below.

TUBERCULOSIS MORBIDITY

TUBERCULOSIS CASE NOTIFICATIONS AND INCIDENCE

In countries with efficient tuberculosis control programs, case notifications would closely approximate to the true incidence of tuberculosis, which, in turn, would provide an accurate measure of the burden of disease caused by tuberculosis. In practice, however, the incidence of tuberculosis is difficult to obtain. Case notifications only represent a fraction of the true incident cases, particularly in areas like Sub-Saharan Africa where only a minority of the population has

Table 8.1 Average tuberculosis notification rates by WHO Region (World Health Organization, 1992)

WHO region	1984–1986		1989–1991		1984–86 and 1989–91	
	Cases	*Rate*	*Cases*	*Rate*	*Cases*	*Rate*
African	264,037	66.8	365,465	79.6	38.4	19.0
American	227,277	34.2	207,790	32.7	−8.6	−4.5
Eastern Mediterranean	212,872	64.9	281,182	74.7	32.1	15.1
European	307,617	37.4	242,643	29.6	−21.1	−20.8
South-East Asia	1,338,896	115.5	1,874,950	146.2	39.9	26.6
Western Pacific	600,185	42.6	826,507	54.5	37.7	27.9
Global	2,951,884	61.8	3,798,538	74.6	28.7	20.8

access to health care services. Alternatives are therefore necessary for estimating the size of the disease burden due to tuberculosis and also for estimating the proportion of the incident cases that are actually identified and treated in a country. This is normally achieved by measuring the annual risk of infection (see page 125).

An alternative approach might be to measure incidence directly as is done in community-based surveys of childhood acute respiratory infections. However, while surveys could provide a reasonable estimate of incidence, even in the worst affected developing countries, incidence is rarely above 2 to 3 cases per 1000 population. Tuberculosis is therefore a relatively rare disease, in comparison, say, to measles, and precise measurement of incidence would require a very large sample size. Screening 10 000 people by sputum microscopy or miniature radiography would only detect some 20 or 30 cases, with wide confidence intervals, and is prohibitively expensive. It is thus rarely done, even as a research exercise.

Notwithstanding the limitations of the data, WHO recently published tuberculosis notifications worldwide (WHO, 1994a, b) which were provided by its member states and other sources. Table 8.1 compares the average tuberculosis case notifications and

rates (per 100 000 population) during the period 1984–1986 to those of the period 1989–1991, with the percentage change between the two periods. Overall, 3.8 million cases of tuberculosis were reported annually around 1990: 49% in the South-East Asian Region, 22% in the Western Pacific Region, 10% in the African Region, 8% in the Eastern Mediterranean Region, 6% in the European Region and 5% in the American Region (Figure 8.2). The notification rates (per 100 000 population) increased by 20.8% between the two periods. This increase was shared by four WHO regions: the African, the Eastern Mediterranean, the South-East Asian and the Western Pacific. In the American and European regions the average number of cases around 1990 was lower than the average number of cases around 1985. Thus, in developing countries worldwide, tuberculosis case notifications are on the increase (Figure 8.3).

However, as mentioned above, data on tuberculosis case notifications do not necessarily represent the incidence of tuberculosis. Rather, they reflect the efficiency of case-finding and reporting activities of the national tuberculosis control programs. In many instances, the performance of these programs is poor, and the reported data are only minimal estimates. In addition, case definitions vary

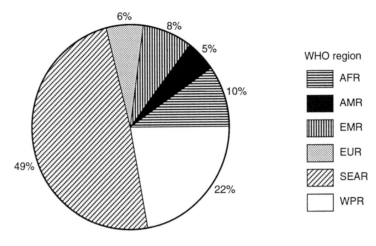

Average total: 3798538 cases

AFR: Sub-Saharan Africa; AMR: Americas; EMR: Eastern Mediterranean;
EUR: Europe; SEAR: South-East Asia; WPR: Western Pacific.

Fig. 8.2 Distribution of notified tuberculosis cases in the world. Average for 1989-1991, by WHO Region (World Health Organization, 1994a, b).

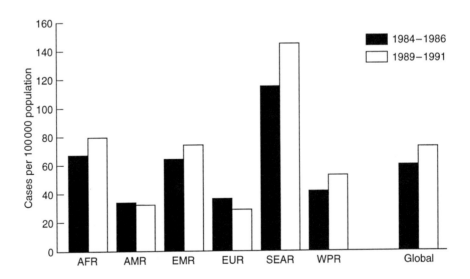

AFR: Sub-Saharan Africa; AMR: Americas; EMR: Eastern Mediterranean;
EUR: Europe; SEAR: South-East Asia; WPR: Western Pacific.

Fig. 8.3 Case rates (per 100 000) of tuberculosis by WHO region. Averages for 1984-1986 and 1989-1991 (World Health Organization, 1994a, b).

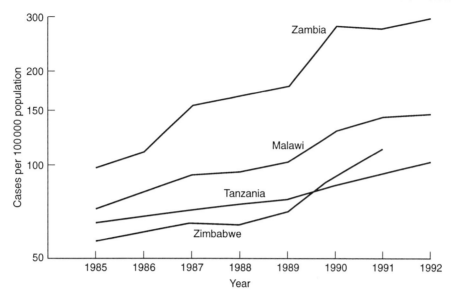

Fig. 8.4 Tuberculosis notification rates (per 100 000) in selected African countries during the period 1985-92.

among countries. Thus, the data shown include all cases, both new and those being re-treated (WHO, 1994a). In spite of these limitations, in countries with well organized and well supported control programs, case notifications may be a reasonable proxy of the incidence of tuberculosis, and, provided that the circumstances of the control program remain more or less stable, may provide useful data on the trend of incidence. In addition, notifications are useful for obtaining rates by age, sex and risk group.

IMPACT OF HIV ON TUBERCULOSIS CASE NOTIFICATIONS

Tuberculosis notifications have increased markedly in those countries known to have a high prevalence of HIV infection. A comparison between the average of the period 1984–1986 and that of 1989–1991 shows the following percentage increases: 67% in Burundi; 205% in the Central African Republic; 73% in Malawi; 133% in Rwanda; 37% in Tanzania; 141% in Zambia; and 48%

in Zimbabwe (WHO, 1994a). A large part of this increase can be attributed to the HIV epidemic. Figure 8.4 shows the trend in tuberculosis notification rates in a few African countries. Less dramatic, yet important increases have been seen in other regions of the world. In Chiang Mai and Chiang Rai, Northern Thailand, where HIV has made rapid inroads, a 5%–7% increase in tuberculosis registrations has been reported during 1990–1992 (Bamrungtrakul, Akarasewi and Viriyakittja, 1993).

In the USA, after 30 years of decline, there was an increase in the number of tuberculosis cases reported annually between 1986 and 1992 (Centers for Disease Control, 1993a), although 1993 saw a reduction for the first time in 8 years (Centers for Disease Control, 1994). In New York City the increase began in 1979. In Central Harlem, New York, notifications increased over 130% in the period 1979–1989 (Brudney and Dobkin, 1991). The increase in the United States has been attributed to HIV and the foreign-born. The latter accounted for 60% of the total increase from 1986 through to 1992, and particularly those increases occurring in Asians, Hispanics, the female population and persons other than those aged 25–44 (Cantwell *et al.*, 1994). HIV was probably responsible for about 50% of the excess cases (a few would have been both foreign-born and attributable to HIV) and had the greatest impact on morbidity among whites, blacks, males and persons aged 25–44 years (Cantwell *et al.*, 1994). Also contributing to the increase were cutbacks in funding for public health programs and worsening socio-economic conditions in inner city areas (Brudney and Dobkin, 1991).

The situation in Western, Central and Eastern Europe is rather different. Although increased case notifications have also been observed in many countries, the HIV epidemic seems to be less important. In Western Europe the main factor producing an increase in tuberculosis case notification is immigration of persons from high prevalence areas (Raviglione *et al.*, 1993a, b). Indeed, in countries such as The Netherlands and Switzerland, the numbers of cases in foreign-born persons now exceeds the numbers occurring in the native-born population. Nevertheless, HIV is having some epidemiological impact on tuberculosis in Europe: increases in case notifications in the southern European countries, such as Spain, are thought to be largely due to the occurrence of HIV among the drug-using population (Raviglione *et al.*, 1993a). In Central and Eastern Europe, increasing trends are probably related to a variety of factors, such as the economic recession, malnutrition, poor living conditions existing in some countries, and war in others (Raviglione *et al.*, 1994).

INCIDENCE OF TUBERCULOSIS AMONG HIV-INFECTED PERSONS

Cohort studies have shown that the risk of developing active tuberculosis among HIV-

infected persons also infected with *Mycobacterium tuberculosis* is much higher than among tuberculous-infected but HIV-seronegative persons.

While the *lifetime* risk of tuberculosis in persons with tuberculosis infection alone is estimated to be only 5–10% (Sutherland, 1976), the *annual* risk of developing active tuberculosis in a person co-infected with HIV and *M. tuberculosis* ranges from 5% to 15% (Selwyn *et al.*, 1989, 1992; Allen *et al.*, 1992; Guelar *et al.*, 1993; Antonucci *et al.*, 1995), with an estimated lifetime risk above 30%. It is these figures which have brought about a reconsideration of the role of preventive therapy in tuberculosis-infected individuals.

However, HIV infection gives rise to a significant number of falsely negative tuberculin skin tests (Okwera *et al.*, 1990), and if preventive therapy is contemplated in the dually infected, it is clearly important to establish the risk of tuberculosis not only in tuberculin skin-test positive individuals, but also in those with negative tests. Three studies from Italy, Spain and the United States have shown that anergic (i.e. skin tests negative to most antigens used) HIV-infected persons also have an increased risk of developing active tuberculosis, which presumably reflects the prevalence of tuberculosis infection in the communities concerned (Selwyn *et al.*, 1992; Guelar *et al.*, 1993; Antonucci *et al.*, 1995).

A recent study in Italy has evaluated the risk of tuberculosis based on the tuberculin skin-test status and on the level of CD4$^+$ T lymphocytes. Among HIV-infected tuberculin-positive persons the incidence of tuberculosis was 5.4 per 100 person-years, as opposed to 3 per 100 person-years in anergic HIV-infected persons, and 0.45 per 100 person-years in non-anergic tuberculin-negative persons (Antonucci *et al.*, 1995). Among tuberculin-positive persons the incidence of tuberculosis was inversely proportional to the level of CD4$^+$ cells, suggesting, as one might expect, that the likelihood of developing tuberculosis increases as the degree of immunosuppression worsens. The lower rate among those who were anergic, compared to the tuberculin positive group, probably reflects the fact that many were not actually infected with *M. tuberculosis*.

THE ANNUAL RISK OF INFECTION WITH *M. TUBERCULOSIS*

BASIC CONCEPTS

Infection is a necessary condition for the development of disease, and given some knowledge of the breakdown rate, the measurement of infection can provide an estimate of the disease burden of tuberculosis. In addition, infection is relatively easy to measure in a tuberculin survey, while incidence is much less so for the reasons stated above. Furthermore, Styblo and colleagues in the 1960s developed a method for using data from tuberculin surveys to derive the probability for an uninfected person to become infected with *M. tuberculosis* (Styblo, van Meijer and Sutherland, 1969). This, measured in a period of one year, is called the annual risk of tuberculosis infection (ARTI) and expresses the rate of transmission of *M. tuberculosis* within the community.

Tuberculin surveys measure the prevalence of cell-mediated immune reactions to specially prepared, standardized tuberculin, such as RT-23 (Statens Seruminstitut, Copenhagen, Denmark) or PPD-S (Centers for Disease Control, Atlanta, USA), in previously sensitized individuals. Ideally, infection rates are obtained at different times using the same technique and testing a representative sample with the same age range. In this way the risk of infection can be calculated and thus the level and trend of the ARTI can be estimated (Styblo, van Meijer and Sutherland, 1969; ten Dam, 1985). However, an estimate of the ARTI can also be derived from a single survey. Since BCG also gives rise to tuberculin reactions,

normally only BCG-unvaccinated subjects are selected. Increasingly, though, there are limitations to tuberculin surveys. BCG coverage rates are now very high in most countries, and it can be reasonably assumed that those who are BCG-negative are likely to be different in other ways from those who have been vaccinated. Thus, confining the surveys to such individuals very likely introduces bias. False-negative tuberculin tests are also common in high HIV prevalence areas.

Intuitively one would expect a connection between the numbers of infectious cases in a community and the numbers of individuals being infected. Styblo (1985) examined the relationship between the ARTI and the incidence of smear-positive pulmonary tuberculosis using various data from developing countries and from The Netherlands before chemotherapy was widely available. Assuming that the prevalence of smear-positive tuberculosis was twice the incidence in communities without widespread availability of chemotherapy, a linear relationship between ARTI and incidence of smear-positive tuberculosis was found. In countries with a moderate to high incidence of tuberculosis, a 1% ARTI corresponds to an incidence of 50 to 60 new infectious (sputum smear-positive) cases of tuberculosis per 100 000 population (Styblo, 1985). In those countries examined, the ratio of sputum smear-positive cases to sputum-negative and extrapulmonary cases remains roughly constant, at around 0.8. The total number of cases of all kinds can thus be estimated (Murray, Styblo and Rouillon, 1990).

This linear relationship, however, may not hold at low levels of ARTI, when the proportion of cases resulting from endogenous reactivation, which are related to past rather than current levels of ARTI, will increase, and the probability that a positive tuberculin test truly indicates infection with *M. tuberculosis* falls. In particular, if the ARTI is rapidly declining, for each ARTI level, many more cases than predicted by this model will occur, as incidence will begin to fall only at a later stage when the cohorts of infected persons will have been replaced by cohorts of uninfected ones. The availability of effective treatment may also upset the relationship since infectious cases will presumably have rather less time to infect their contacts. In addition, in areas with high prevalence of HIV infection, the relationship may be further affected, as disease develops much more rapidly and frequently following infection in HIV-infected patients (Di Perri *et al.*, 1989; Daley *et al.*, 1992).

In spite of the limitations of tuberculin surveys, however, no better method for estimation of the disease burden due to tuberculosis in countries with less than complete case notification has yet been identified. Results of tuberculin skin-test surveys performed in developing countries between the 1950s and 1987 were reviewed (Cauthen, Pio and ten Dam, 1988). The highest estimates for ARTI were in Sub-Saharan Africa and in South and East Asia (1% to 2.5%). In North Africa and the Middle East, the ARTI was probably between 0.5% and 1.5%, similar to that in Central and South America and the Caribbean. In industrialized countries and in some of the former socialist countries, the ARTI is much lower than that estimated for developing countries. In The Netherlands, for instance, the ARTI was estimated to be less than 0.01% in 1990 (Broekmans, 1993), and in the Czech Republic it was 0.046% in the late 1980s (Trnka, Dankova and Svandova, 1993).

How many people worldwide are therefore infected with *M. tuberculosis*? WHO estimates that about one third of the world's population (1.7 billion people in 1990, probably close to 2 billion in 1995) is infected with *M. tuberculosis*, the great majority of which reside in developing countries (Sudre *et al.*, 1992). In industrialized countries, 80% of infected individuals are aged 50 years or more, as opposed to 23% in developing countries (Sudre, ten Dam and Kochi, 1992). Natural mortality will therefore result in a rapid disappearance from the industrialized countries of cohorts of infected individuals as long as current control methods are maintained, and there are no fundamental shifts in the relationship between *M. tuberculosis* and its human host. On the other hand, many decades will be necessary to achieve the elimination of tuberculosis from the developing world, even if current control methods are greatly improved.

THE IMPACT OF HIV ON THE ANNUAL RISK OF INFECTION

The most significant effect of HIV is to increase the incidence of tuberculosis and also to increase the absolute numbers of cases. The annual risk of infection will therefore likely increase in high HIV prevalence areas, all other factors being equal. This increase may be offset, to some extent, by the fact that a greater proportion of cases of HIV-associated tuberculosis is extrapulmonary or sputum-smear negative, and therefore less infectious (Elliott *et al.*, 1993a). In addition, since the infectiousness of tuberculosis is a function of duration as well as of intensity of exposure, the impact of HIV on the ARTI for tuberculosis may be further attenuated since the survival of such patients is considerably shorter than HIV-negative cases of tuberculosis. This scenario may be analogous to the situation in The Netherlands during the Second World War when tuberculosis notifications greatly increased, but the estimated ARTI for the same period continued to fall (Styblo, van Meijer and Sutherland, 1969). In that instance it was hypothesized that the poor nutrition levels of the population led to a marked increase in early tuberculosis mortality. This increased mortality balanced the increased incidence resulting in no effect on transmission. It remains to be seen whether the same will occur in high HIV prevalence areas.

Recent work on the molecular epidemiology of tuberculosis in New York and San Francisco has questioned a fundamental tenet of tuberculosis epidemiology, which is that about 90% of cases of pulmonary tuberculosis arise from reactivation of latent disease. The extension of this argument is that reinfection is uncommon. By use of RFLP analysis it was shown in the two studies that over a third of the cases of active tuberculosis appear to be due to recent infection. However, HIV and/or AIDS diagnosis was clearly a risk factor for such recent transmission, and, indeed, it remains unclear to what extent this phenomenon occurs in populations in which HIV infection is uncommon (Small *et al.*, 1994; Alland *et al.*, 1994).

TUBERCULOSIS MORTALITY

With the introduction of effective chemotherapy, mortality from tuberculosis has become a less useful indicator of the magnitude of the tuberculosis problem, but instead has become a more useful indicator of the quality of local tuberculosis control measures, at least in areas without HIV (Styblo and Sutherland, 1974; WHO, 1991). Without chemotherapy, tuberculosis is often fatal, as was shown in a number of studies before chemotherapy became available (Drolet, 1938; Lindhart, 1939; Berg, 1939; Galtung Hansen, 1955; Olakowski, 1973). Without treatment, about 50% to 60% of tuberculosis patients will die within a 5-year period. Fatality is highest among smear-positive patients, ranging from 53% to 66% within five years from diagnosis (Rutledge and Crouch, 1919; Lindhart, 1939; Olakowski, 1973).

Even in the chemotherapy era, tuberculosis mortality may be relatively high. In a study in England and Wales among 1222 cases notified in 1983–1985, the case fatality rate was 12.9% (Cullinan and Meredith, 1991). Factors associated with death were age and radiographic extent of the disease. How-ever, co-infection with HIV seems to be an even stronger factor determining mortality, and in one study in a low-income country, deaths were about 4 times more common among HIV-infected patients than uninfected patients (Nunn *et al.*, 1992). Not all deaths, however, were due to tuberculosis. Further follow-up of this same cohort suggested that the relative risk of dying from tuberculosis was about 3 times greater for HIV-infected patients with tuberculosis than for HIV-uninfected patients, while the relative risk for death from causes other than tuberculosis was over 13 (Nunn, unpublished data). In the industrialized world, in contrast, mortality due to tuberculosis does not appear to be increased among HIV-infected patients compared to HIV-uninfected patients (Small *et al.*, 1991). This difference may well be due to the more effective nature of the regimens used in industrialized countries, and in particular, the use of rifampicin throughout treatment, whereas, in the African studies, rifampicin was rarely included in the continuation phase of therapy. In addition, care for other opportunistic infections and AIDS/HIV related complications would not have been as readily available in Africa.

While in the industrialized world, diagnosis is usually rapid, treatment available, and tuberculosis mortality low (Raviglione *et al.*, 1993a), most developing countries do not report data on tuberculosis mortality. Therefore, as in the case of incidence, global figures must be estimated.

ESTIMATES AND PROJECTIONS OF THE GLOBAL TUBERCULOSIS BURDEN

ESTIMATES OF TUBERCULOSIS INCIDENCE AND MORTALITY

For reasons already mentioned, incidence of tuberculosis cannot be obtained from reported data and therefore has to be estimated. Various approaches have been used since the early 1980s. Using notification data, Bulla (1981) estimated that worldwide in 1976–1977 there were 2.8 million new cases of tuberculosis (68.4 cases per 100 000 population) and 380 000 deaths (9.2 per 100 000 population). Since they were based on notifications, these figures clearly underestimate the true picture. Styblo and Rouillon (1981) attempted to improve the accuracy by including data derived from ARTI estimates and concluded that in 1977 about 3.7 million cases of sputum smear-positive tuberculosis and another 4 million cases of smear-negative pulmonary disease and extrapulmonary tuberculosis occurred, with a total estimate of 7.7 million cases.

Further work by Murray, Styblo and Rouillon (1990) used the relationship established by Styblo (1985) between the ARTI and the incidence of sputum smear-positive tuberculosis. The various regional ARTI in developing countries were derived mainly from survey data reviewed by Cauthen and colleagues (Cauthen, Pio and ten Dam, 1988). The incidence of sputum smear-positive tuberculosis in the developing world in 1990 was estimated to be 77 per 100 000 population, corresponding to 3.2 million cases. Including sputum smear-negative and extrapulmonary cases it was estimated that a total of 7.1 million cases of tuberculosis had occurred in developing countries in 1990, of whom 2.5 million were estimated to have died (Murray, Styblo and Rouillon, 1990). Sudre, ten Dam and Kochi (1992) also included industrialized countries and estimated that the global number of cases of tuberculosis in 1990 was around 8 million with nearly 3 million deaths.

More recently, WHO and the World Bank have estimated incidence by country (World Bank, 1993; WHO, 1994a) utilizing available information on the ARTI for developing countries, and notification data for low prevalence industrialized countries (Figure 8.5). Dolin *et al.* (Dolin, Raviglione and Kochi, 1993, 1994) used a different region-based approach, in which, for low prevalence countries, estimates were based on reported case notifications (Cheah, 1992; Statistics Canada, 1993; Raviglione *et al.*, 1993a, 1994; Centers for Disease Control, 1993b). For other areas, the incidence of the most populated countries with an established surveillance system within each region was estimated from the notification data and information on case coverage, and applied to populations in subregions to calculate regional totals. Mortality was derived using published case-fatality rates for industrialized countries (Raviglione *et al.*, 1993b), and estimating from available data overall rates for Eastern Europe (Raviglione *et al.*, 1994) and Latin America. For all other developing countries, it was assumed that all cases reported are treated and 5% of treated cases are not reported. Finally, case-fatality rates of 55% for untreated cases and 15% for treated cases were used (Dolin, Raviglione and Kochi, 1993, 1994). From Tables 8.2 and 8.3 it can be seen that tuberculosis has a devastating effect in the developing world, where 95% of the 7.5 million world's tuberculosis cases occurred in 1990. Of these cases 80% are in their productive years (15–59 years of age). About 1.3 million cases and 450 000 deaths from tuberculosis in developing countries occur in children under the age of 15 years (WHO, 1989). Overall, 98% of 2.5 million tuberculosis deaths in 1990 occurred in the developing world. Tuberculosis is estimated to cause over 25% of avoidable adult deaths in the developing world (Murray, Styblo and Rouillon, 1990).

In 1990, over 315 000 cases and 100 000 deaths from tuberculosis worldwide were thought to be attributable to HIV infection, i.e. 4.2% of all cases and 4.6% of all tuberculosis deaths (Dolin, Raviglione and Kochi, 1994). However, for the year 2000, these estimates are, respectively, 1.4 million (13.8%) and 500 000 (4.2%).

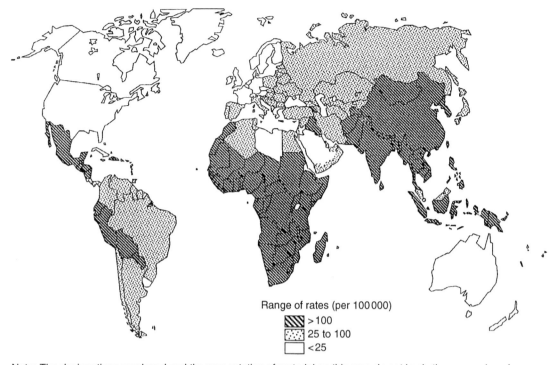

Fig. 8.5 Estimated incidence rates, 1990 (World Health Organization, 1994a).

FUTURE BURDEN OF TUBERCULOSIS INCIDENCE AND MORTALITY

Forecasting future incidence and mortality is difficult in the absence of reliable data and can be based only on figures available at the time of modelling. Therefore, any projection exercise must be viewed critically.

Several factors are important in determining the future epidemiology of tuberculosis. First, the world's population is increasing. Second, children born in past decades in regions with high population growth rates are now reaching the ages where the incidence of tuberculosis is highest. Even if the age-specific rates of new cases remain unchanged, the changing size of the population age groups will now begin to cause a large increase in the number of new tuberculosis cases, and also deaths if adequate control programs are not available.

Third, excessive population density, famine, war, and natural disasters are resulting in ever larger groups of displaced and malnourished people in crowded living conditions. These persons are clearly at high risk of tuberculosis.

Fourth, age-specific tuberculosis incidence rates are expected to rise in those areas of the world where HIV infection is highly prevalent. It is hard to imagine how the HIV pandemic can avoid having a major negative impact on the tuberculosis situation, particularly in the decades which will follow the year 2000.

The most recent estimates on the future

Table 8.2 Estimated tuberculosis incidence and HIV-attributable tuberculosis cases in 1990, 1995 and 2000 (Dolin et al., 1994)

Region	1990			1995			2000		
	Total TB cases	Rate[a]	HIV-attributed TB cases	Total TB cases	Rate[a]	HIV-attributed TB cases	Total TB cases	Rate[a]	HIV-attributed TB cases
South-East Asia	3,106,000	237	66,000	3,499,000	241	251,000	3,952,000	247	571,000
Western Pacific[b]	1,839,000	136	19,000	2,045,000	140	31,000	2,255,000	144	68,000
Africa	992,000	191	194,000	1,467,000	242	380,000	2,079,000	293	604,000
Eastern Mediterranean	641,000	165	9,000	745,000	168	16,000	870,000	168	38,000
Americas[c]	569,000	127	20,000	606,000	123	45,000	645,000	120	97,000
Eastern Europe[d]	194,000	47	1,000	202,000	47	2,000	210,000	48	6,000
Industrialized countries[e]	196,000	23	6,000	204,000	23	13,000	211,000	24	26,000
Total	7,537,000	143	315,000 (4.2%)	8,768,000	152	738,000 (8.4%)	10,222,000	163	1,410,000 (13.8%)
Increase since 1990	143			16.3%			35.6%		

[a]Crude incidence rate per 100,000 population.
[b]Includes all countries of the Western Pacific Region of WHO, except Japan, Australia and New Zealand.
[c]Includes all countries of the American Region of WHO, except USA and Canada.
[d]Eastern European and independent states of the former USSR.
[e]Western European, USA, Canada, Japan, Australia and New Zealand.

Table 8.3 Estimated total tuberculosis deaths and HIV-attributable tuberculosis deaths in 1990, 1995 and 2000. Estimates assume regional treatment coverage rates remain at their 1990 level (Dolin *et al.*, 1994)

Region	1990 deaths		1995 deaths		2000 deaths	
	Total	HIV-attributed	Total	HIV-attributed	Total	HIV-attributed
South-East Asia	1,087,000	23,000	1,225,000	88,000	1,383,000	200,000
Western Pacific[a]	644,000	7,000	716,000	11,000	789,000	24,000
Africa	393,000	77,000	581,000	150,000	823,000	239,000
Eastern Mediterranean	249,000	4,000	290,000	6,000	338,000	15,000
Americas[b]	114,000	4,000	121,000	9,000	129,000	19,000
Eastern Europe[c]	29,000	<200	30,000	<600	32,000	<900
Industrialized countries[d]	14,000	<500	14,000	1,000	15,000	2,000
All regions	2,530,000	116,000 (4.6%)	2,977,000	266,000 (8.9%)	3,509,000	500,000 (14.2%)
Increase since 1990			17.7%		38.7%	

[a]Includes all countries of the Western Pacific Region of WHO, except Japan, Australia and New Zealand.
[b]Includes all countries of the American Region of WHO except USA and Canada.
[c]Eastern Europe and independent states of former USSR.
[d]Western Europe, USA, Canada, Japan, Australia and New Zealand.

burden of tuberculosis suggest that worldwide tuberculosis cases will increase from 7.5 million in 1990 to 10.2 million by the year 2000, and that tuberculosis deaths will increase from 2.5 million in 1990 to 3.5 million in the same period (Dolin, Raviglione and Kochi, 1994) (Tables 8.2 and 8.3). If the effectiveness and availability of tuberculosis control do not improve substantially, over 30 million tuberculosis deaths and nearly 90 million new cases are expected to occur in the last decade of this century (Dolin, Raviglione and Kochi, 1994). Nearly 3 million tuberculosis deaths and 8 million cases will occur due to HIV infection (Figures 8.6 and 8.7).

EVIDENCE OF THE HIV–TUBERCULOSIS INTERACTION

On a more local scale a great deal of data has already been obtained which sheds light on the impact, present and future, of HIV on the epidemiology of tuberculosis. First, in countries where both tuberculosis and HIV infections are common, the HIV seroprevalence among tuberculosis patients is severalfold higher than that found among the general population (Narain, Raviglione and Kochi, 1992). In many Eastern and Southern African countries the HIV seroprevalence among tuberculosis cases is very high (Table 8.4). In Uganda during the period 1990–1992, the relative risk for HIV infection among patients with tuberculosis in four sentinel hospitals compared to women attending antenatal clinics at the same hospitals was 5.9 (95% CI 5.1–6.9) (Aisu *et al.*, 1992). In Tanzania, where the HIV seroprevalence was 29% in 1991–1992 among patients with tuberculosis, the odds ratio for HIV infection was 5.4 for patients with sputum smear-positive tuberculosis, using blood donors as controls (Chum *et al.*, 1992).

In Latin America, surveys showed an HIV seroprevalence among tuberculosis cases be-

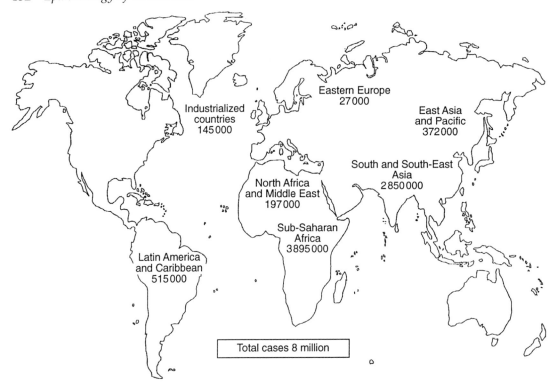

Industrialized
countries
145 000

Eastern Europe
27 000

East Asia
and Pacific
372 000

South and South-East
Asia
2 850 000

North Africa
and Middle East
197 000

Sub-Saharan
Africa
3 895 000

Latin America
and Caribbean
515 000

Total cases 8 million

Fig. 8.6 HIV-attributable cases of tuberculosis estimated to occur in the world during the period 1990–1999.

tween 5% and 39% in recent years (Table 8.4). In South-East Asia, HIV seroprevalence is rapidly increasing. Among tuberculosis cases diagnosed in Chiang Mai, Northern Thailand, it increased from 5% in 1989 to 40% in 1994 (Payanandana *et al.*, 1995) and in one hospital in Bombay, India, from 2.3% in 1988–1989 to 8.9% in 1992–1993 (Mohanty, Sundarani and Pasi, 1993).

HIV infection is not confined to adults with diagnosed tuberculosis. In Lusaka, Zambia, as many as 37% of hospitalized children with a diagnosis of tuberculosis were HIV-infected in 1990–1991, as opposed to 11% of non-tuberculosis controls (Chintu *et al.*, 1993), although a number of these cases may not, in fact, have had tuberculosis. In 1992, this percentage increased to 56% (Luo *et al.*, 1994). In Côte d'Ivoire, the seroprevalence to both

HIV-1 and HIV-2 combined was 11.8% in children in 1989–1990 (Sassan-Morokro *et al.*, 1994), while in the Dominican Republic, 6.6% of children with tuberculosis were HIV-seropositive (Espinal *et al.*, 1993).

In industrialized countries, HIV seroprevalence among tuberculosis cases varies greatly. In 28 clinics of 17 cities of the USA it was 12.5% in 1992; however, it ranged between 0 and 66% (Onorato *et al.*, 1993). In Western Europe, the HIV seroprevalence was 2% in Portugal and 24% in Barcelona, Spain (Raviglione *et al.*, 1993b; Caylà *et al.*, 1993). In 1991 in France, the minimum level of HIV seroprevalence was 6%, with a peak of 16.4% in Paris (Schwoebel and Jougla, 1993). Only limited and non-representative data are available from Central and Eastern Europe: in Poland the seroprevalence was 3.5% in

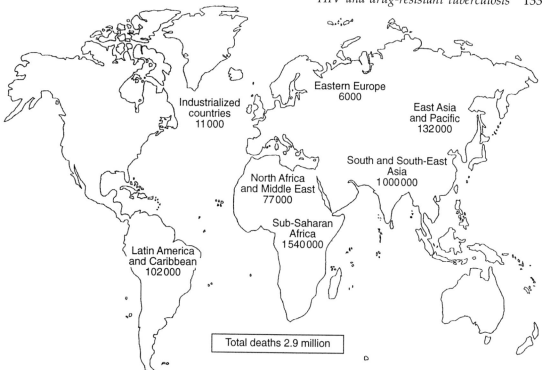

Fig. 8.7 HIV-attributable tuberculosis deaths estimated to occur in the world during the period 1990-1999 (WHO Tuberculosis Programme).

1991 and in Romania 1.6% in 1991–1992 (Raviglione *et al.*, 1994). In New South Wales, Australia, only 1.4% of tuberculosis cases were HIV-infected in 1992 (Anonymous, 1993).

It is also important to determine the extent of the HIV/AIDS-related morbidity and mortality due to tuberculosis. In most developing countries tuberculosis is clearly the most important opportunistic infection observed among HIV-infected patients because it is common, transmissible to both HIV-infected and -uninfected persons, and is a life-threatening disease, but it is relatively easily treated, and can be prevented. In Africa, for instance, as many as 54% of patients with AIDS or HIV infection have tuberculosis (McLeod *et al.*, 1989; Mbaga *et al.*, 1990; Lucas *et al.*, 1993), and in South-East Asia as many as 68% had tuberculosis in

some studies (Kaur *et al.*, 1992); Tansuphaswasdikul, 1993). The frequency of tuberculosis among HIV-infected patients is summarized in Table 8.5. A recent study in Zambia suggested that 42% of all HIV-related expenditures in a district hospital were due to HIV-associated tuberculosis (Foster, personal communication).

HIV AND DRUG-RESISTANT TUBERCULOSIS

There is much anecdotal, but little published evidence that drug resistance is becoming a more important barrier to effective national tuberculosis programs. The available information suggests there may be high levels of drug resistance, particularly in Asia and parts of Africa (Van der Werf, 1989; Kim and Hong, 1992; Chandrasekaran, Jagota and

Table 8.4 HIV seroprevalence among patients with tuberculosis in selected countries. Studies in adults are shown, followed by studies in children

Selected country (reference)	Year	Total no. of TB cases	HIV$^{(+)}$ (%)
Studies in adults			
Lusaka, Zambia (Elliott *et al.*, 1993)	1989	249	73
Kampala, Uganda (Eriki *et al.*, 1991)	1988/89	59	66
Four sites, Uganda (Aisu *et al.*, 1992)	1990/92	1770	44
Tanzania (Chum *et al.*, 1992)	1991/92	3369	29
Abidjan, Côte d'Ivoire (De Cock *et al.*, 1991)	1989/90	2043	40
Cité Soleil, Haiti (Clermont *et al.*, 1990)	1989/90	143	39
Rio de Janeiro, RJ, Brazil (Kritski *et al.*, 1993)	1989	136	5.2
Campinas, SP, Brazil (Kritski *et al.*, 1994)	1990/1991	140	6.4
Salvador, BA, Brazil (Kritski *et al.*, 1994)	1990/1991	90	7.8
Buenos Aires, Argentina (Pilheu *et al.*, 1993)	1992/1993	117	21.3
Thailand (Payanandana *et al.*, 1995)	1994	n.s.	10 (1.4–39.7)
Chiang Mai, Thailand (Payanandana *et al.*, 1995)	1994	n.s.	39.7
Bombay, India (Mohanty *et al.*, 1993)	1992/1993	684	8.9
Manipur State, India (Ibopishak, 1993)	1992/1993	148	11.5
USA (Onorato *et al.*, 1993)	1992	n.s.	12.5(0–66)
Barcelona, Spain (Caylà *et al.*, 1993)	1992	1081	24.3
France (Schwoebel and Jougla, 1993)	1991	4181	6
New South Wales, Australia (Anonymous, 1993)	1992	424	1.4
Studies in children			
Lusaka, Zambia (Chintu *et al.*, 1993)	1990/1991	237	37
Lusaka, Zambia (Luo *et al.*, 1994)	1991/1992	120	55.8
Abidjan, Côte d'Ivoire (Sassan-Morokro *et al.*, 1994)	1989/1990	289	11.8
Santo Domingo, Dominican Republic (Espinal *et al.*, 1993)	1991/1992	120	6.6

Table 8.5 Frequency of tuberculosis among HIV-infected or AIDS patients

Country/region	Source	%
Africa (McLeod *et al.*, 1989; Mbaga *et al.*, 1990; Lucas *et al.*, 1993)	clinical/autopsy	20–54
South-East Asia: India (Kaur *et al.*, 1993); Thailand (Tansuphaswadikul, 1993)	clinical	52–68
Latin America: Brazil (Dalcolmo and Kritski, 1993; Sanches *et al.*, 1990); Mexico (Jessurum *et al.*, 1990)	autopsy/surveillance	24–28
Caribbean: Haiti (Pape *et al.*, 1985)	clinical	23
Europe: Italy (Girardi *et al.*, 1994); England and Wales (Watson *et al.*, 1993)	surveillance	5–11
Europe: Spain (Iribarran *et al.*, 1989; Barber *et al.*, 1992)	clinical	36–37
United States (Cauthen *et al.*, 1990)	surveillance	4

Chaudhuri, 1992; Braun *et al.*, 1992; Kochi, Vareldzis and Styblo, 1993; Frieden *et al.*, 1993). Unfortunately, adequate surveillance of drug resistance has been performed in only a few countries and does not allow any definite conclusion. Most of the published work has suffered from one or more of three major deficiencies, rendering interpretation difficult, if not impossible. The first of these is selection bias. Most surveys on drug resistance have been centered on major hospitals and other institutions to which patients with problems, including drug resistance, are more likely to be referred. Second, many papers fail to distinguish clearly between those patients who had received previous treatment and those who had not. Third, non-standard or unclear laboratory methods are described, resulting in unclear definitions of what was meant by resistance. Thus, there is an urgent need to establish surveillance of drug resistance at country level to obtain data which are standardized and comparable within and between countries. In addition, the impact of the HIV epidemic on the level of antituberculosis drug resistance is unknown.

While the many reports of multidrug resistant tuberculosis (MDR-TB) from the United States have noted the association with HIV, there is no intrinsic reason why HIV should give rise to resistant tuberculosis. Rather, the social conditions to which HIV is linked are the more likely risk factors, such as substance abuse and concomitant poor adherence. However, because of the extraordinarily high risk of active tuberculosis within a short period of time among co-infected persons (Di Perri *et al.*, 1989; Daley *et al.*, 1992), HIV infection can 'telescope' an epidemic of drug resistant tuberculosis, permitting its manifestations to be seen in months rather than years. Evidence for this comes from the findings of recent studies based on fingerprinting techniques (restriction fragment length polymorphism, or RFLP) which suggest that recent

transmission accounts for two-thirds of all drug-resistant tuberculosis in one American city, and that HIV/AIDS is a major risk factor for recent transmission (Alland *et al.*, 1994). It is this mechanism which lies at the root of the current association of HIV and MDR-TB in the USA.

In contrast, a number of studies in the USA (Shafer *et al.*, 1991; Chawla *et al.*, 1992), Haiti (Long *et al.*, 1991) and Africa (Githui *et al.*, 1992; Braun *et al.*, 1992), have measured resistance in more representative groups of patients and have not found an excess of resistance in the HIV-positive groups (Nunn and Felten, 1994).

The epidemiological impact of resistance on tuberculosis control, and the degree to which it is influenced by HIV, will depend on the number, cost and efficacy of the drugs available to treat tuberculosis. There are, in current use in the developing world, six drugs for the treatment of tuberculosis: isoniazid, rifampicin, pyrazinamide, ethambutol, streptomycin and thiacetazone. The first three are the most essential. HIV, however, has rendered the use of streptomycin inadvisable, because of the risk of parenteral transmission of HIV with a drug that has to be given by injection in situations where sterilization of needles and syringes cannot be guaranteed. This risk has not, so far, been supported by observation. More important, HIV gives rise to severe, occasionally fatal, cutaneous hypersensitivity reactions in patients treated with thiacetazone (Nunn *et al.*, 1991). The armamentarium available for treating tuberculosis in developing countries is thus somewhat reduced. Furthermore, if thiacetazone is replaced by ethambutol, there is the risk that ethambutol resistance will become more common, and thus create the conditions for rifampicin resistance. It is resistance to rifampicin that carries the greatest risk of poor outcome. This 'domino theory' of drug resistance is presented in more detail in a recent review (Nunn and Felten, 1994).

RESEARCH PRIORITIES ON TUBERCULOSIS EPIDEMIOLOGY

Research on HIV-associated tuberculosis has been fundamental to understand the relationship between the two diseases. However, several research issues still need to be addressed in order to insure control of tuberculosis in the face of HIV (WHO 1995b).

Many data already exist on the impact of HIV on the incidence of tuberculosis, but this probably needs to be re-examined in each region as the HIV epidemic expands. The reasons for this are that health service planners need to know the likely impact of HIV in advance. This impact will depend on the level of infection with *M. tuberculosis* in the country or region concerned, as well as the breakdown rate caused by HIV. In most countries, data on tuberculosis infection levels are too old to be of much contemporary use. Furthermore, it is theoretically possible that the impact will vary with geographically specific strains of either HIV or *M. tuberculosis*. Lastly, such studies can be a major element in the advocacy efforts that will be required in many countries in order to obtain the resources necessary to contain the 3–10 fold increase in tuberculosis notifications that could occur.

Further work is required to determine the most effective and efficient way of treating patients with tuberculosis who also have HIV. The amount of work per patient contributed by each health care worker needs to be minimized in the light of projected HIV-induced increases in incidence, and this is likely to require development and evaluation of new management strategies for tuberculosis.

The basic assumption underlying tuberculosis control policy should be re-examined in the light of HIV. For example, one of the major tenets of modern tuberculosis control is passive case finding. That is, it has been considered more efficient to wait until patients present with their symptoms, rather than actively searching in the community for patients with tuberculosis. This approach makes a number of assumptions. First, that patients with tuberculosis have symptoms. Second, that when symptoms occur, patients attend the health services. Third, that patients have confidence in those services. Little is known of the degree to which HIV may modify people's perception of their symptoms: a person attending a local healer with low-grade fever due to HIV may not think of attending the local health center when he or she gets a cough as well. The extreme overcrowding of clinics and hospitals in some developing countries must act, at least to some extent, as a disincentive to attend. In addition, the stigma now being attached in some societies to AIDS, and the widespread recognition that tuberculosis is often a feature of AIDS, may well act as a further disincentive. Lastly, the effect on the public of the severe skin reactions that can occur in HIV-infected tuberculosis patients treated with thiacetazone is not yet known.

Other epidemiologic studies are needed. These include those (1) to monitor tuberculosis drug resistance in patients with HIV infection; (2) to determine more accurately the causes of morbidity and mortality in HIV positive patients with tuberculosis; (3) to assess the epidemiological impact of the increased recurrence rate of tuberculosis among HIV positive patients; and (4) to obtain further data from larger studies on the impact of HIV on tuberculosis transmission and particularly on the annual risk of tuberculosis infection.

CONCLUSIONS

The impact of HIV represents a frame-shift in the epidemiology of tuberculosis. The equilibrium between man and the tubercle bacillus has already been disturbed in a major way in some countries, and we have not even seen yet the full impact of HIV in Asia, whence two-thirds of the world's tuberculosis at present arises. Our current knowledge, however, is sufficient to show us the desperate necessity of insuring that national tuberculosis control programs in countries at risk of HIV are rapidly made as efficient as possible. The work of Karel Styblo and his colleagues showed that the epidemiological cycle of tuberculosis could be effectively broken by good tuberculosis control. Epidemiological work should now focus on establishing that the same can be done even in the baleful presence of HIV.

REFERENCES

Aisu, T., Raviglione, M.C., Narain, J.P. *et al.* (1992) Monitoring HIV-associated tuberculosis in Uganda. Abstract 43D. *Proceedings of the World Congress on Tuberculosis*, Bethesda, Maryland, USA, 16–19 November 1992.

Alland, D., Kalkut, G.E., Moss, A.R. *et al.* (1993) Transmission of tuberculosis in New York City. An analysis by DNA fingerprinting and conventional epidemiologic methods. *New England Joournal of Medicine*, **330**, 1710–16.

Allen, S., Batungwanayo, J., Kerlikowske, K. *et al.* (1992) Two-year incidence of tuberculosis in cohorts of HIV-infected and uninfected urban Rwandan women. *American Review of Respiratory Diseases*, **146**, 1439–44.

Altarac, D., Raucher, B., Back, S. and Nichols, S.E. (1993) A reevaluation of PPD testing in a high risk cohort. Abstract 1357. *Proceedings of the 33rd Interscience Conference on Antimicrobial Agents and Chemotherapy*, New Orleans, LA, USA, 17–20 October 1993.

Anonymous (1993) Tuberculosis and Mycobacteria-atypical. *New South Wales Public Health Bulletin*, Suppl. 4, No. S-5:32.

Antonucci, G., Girardi, E., Raviglione, H.C., Ippolito, G. *et al.* (1995) Risk factors for tuberculosis in HIV-infected persons. A prospective cohort study. *Journal of the American Medical Association*, **274**, 143–8.

Bamrungtrakul, T., Akarasewi, P. and Viriyakit-tja, D. (1993) Trends of HIV-1 coinfection among tuberculosis patients, Thailand, 1989–1992. Abstract n. S-2(3). *Proceedings of the 17th Eastern Regional Conference on Tuberculosis and Respiratory Diseases of the IUATLD, Eastern Region*, Bangkok, Thailand, 1–4 November 1993.

Barber, J., Ocana, I., Ruiz, I. *et al.* (1992) Tuberculosis and AIDS. Abstract No. P39. *Proceedings of the III European Conference on Clinical Aspects and Treatment of HIV Infection*, Paris, France, 12–13 March 1992.

Berg, G. (1939) The prognosis of open pulmonary tuberculosis. A clinical-statistical analysis. *Acta Tuberculosea Scandinavica*, suppl. IV, vii–viii, 1–207.

Braun, M.M., Kilburn, J.O., Smithwick, R.W. *et al.* (1992) HIV infection and primary resistance to antituberculosis drugs in Abidjan, Côte d'Ivoire. *AIDS*, **6**, 1327–30.

Broekmans, J.F. (1993) Evaluation of applied strategies in low-prevalence countries, in *Tuberculosis. A Comprehensive International Approach* (eds L.B. Reichman and E.S. Hershfield), Marcel Dekker, New York.

Brudney, K. and Dobkin, J. (1991) Resurgent tuberculosis in New York City. Human immunodeficiency virus, homelessness, and the decline of tuberculosis control programs. *American Review of Respiratory Diseases*, **144**, 745–9.

Bulla, A. (1981) Worldwide review of officially reported tuberculosis morbidity and mortality (1967-1971-1977). *Bulletin of the International Union Against Tuberculosis*, **56**, 111–17.

Cantwell, M.F., Snider, D.E. Jr, Cauthen, G.M. and Onorato, I.M. (1994) Epidemiology of tuberculosis in the United States, 1985 through 1992. *Journal of the American Medical Association*, **272**, 535–9.

Cauthen, G.M., Pio, A. and ten Dam, H.G. (1988) Annual risk of tuberculous infection. Geneva, World Health Organization, 1988 (unpublished document WHO/TB/88.154; available on request from the Tuberculosis Programme, World Health Organization, 1211 Geneva 27, Switzerland).

Cauthen, G.M., Bloch, A.B., Snider, D.E. Jr. (1990) Reported AIDS patients with tuberculosis in the United States. Abstract n.Th.C.725. *Proceedings of the VI International Conference on AIDS*, San Francisco, California USA, 20–24 June 1990.

Caylà, J.A., Galdos-Tangüis, H., Jansà, J.M. *et al.* (1993) La tuberculosi a Barcelona. Informe 1992. *Programa de Prevencio i Control de la Tuberculosi a Barcelona*. Servei d'Epidemiologia, Institut Municipal de la Salut, Barcelona 1993.

Centers for Disease Control (1993a) Tuberculosis morbidity – United States, 1992. *Morbidity and Mortality Weekly Report*, **42**, 696–704.

Centers for Disease Control and Prevention (1993b) *Tuberculosis Statistics in the United States, 1991.* Atlanta, GA.

Centers for Disease Control (1994) Expanded tuberculosis surveillance and tuberculosis morbidity – United States, 1993. *Morbidity and Mortality Weekly Report,* **43**, 361–6.

Chandrasekaran, S., Jagota, P. and Chaudhuri, K. (1992) Initial drug resistance to antituberculosis drugs in urban and rural district tuberculosis programme. *Indian Journal of Tuberculosis,* **39**, 171–5.

Chawla, P., Klapper, P., Kamholz, S. *et al.* (1992) Drug-resistant tuberculosis in an urban population including patients at risk for human immunodeficiency virus infection. *American Review of Respiratory Diseases,* **146**, 280–4.

Cheah, D. (1992) Tuberculosis notification rates, Australia, 1991. *Communicable Diseases Intelligence,* **16**, 398–400.

Chintu, C., Bhat, G., Luo, L. *et al.* (1993) Seroprevalence of human immunodeficiency virus type 1 infection in Zambian children with tuberculosis. *Pediatric Infectious Disease Journal,* **12**, 499–504.

Chum, H.L., Graf, P., O'Brien, R.J. *et al.* (1992) The impact of HIV infection on tuberculosis in Tanzania. Abstract 41B. *Proceedings of the World Congress on Tuberculosis,* Bethesda, Maryland, USA, 16–19 November 1992.

Clermont, H.C., Chaisson, R.E., Davis, H.A. *et al.* (1990) HIV-1 infection in adult tuberculosis patients in Cité Soleil, Haiti. Abstract. Th.B.490. *Proceedings of the VI International Conference on AIDS,* San Francisco, California, USA, 20–24 June 1990.

Cullinan, P. and Meredith, S.K. (1991) Deaths in adults with notified pulmonary tuberculosis 1983-5. *Thorax,* **46**, 347–50.

Dalcolmo, M.P. and Kritski, A.L. (1993) Tuberculosis y co-infección por VIH. *Revista Argentina del Torax,* **54**, 29–34.

Daley, C.L., Small, P.M., Schecter, G.F. *et al.* (1992) An outbreak of tuberculosis with accelerated progression among persons infected with the human immunodeficiency virus. An analysis using restriction-fragment-length polymorphism. *New England Journal of Medicine,* **326**, 231–5.

De Cock, K.M., Gnaore, E., Adjorlolo, G. *et al.* (1991) Risk of tuberculosis in patients with HIV-I and HIV-II infections in Abidjan, Ivory Coast. *British Medical Journal,* **302**, 496–9.

Di Perri, G., Cruciani, M., Danzi, M.C. *et al.* (1989) Nosocomial epidemic of active tuberculosis among HIV-infected patients. *Lancet,* **2**, 1502–504.

Dolin, P.J., Raviglione, M.C. and Kochi, A. (1993) Estimates of future global tuberculosis morbidity and mortality. *Morbidity and Mortality Weekly Report,* **42**, 961–4.

Dolin, P.J., Raviglione, M.R. and Kochi, A. (1994) Global tuberculosis incidence and mortality during 1990–2000. *Bulletin of the World Health Organization,* **72**, 213–20.

Drolet, G.J. (1938) Present trend of case fatality rates in tuberculosis. *American Review of Tuberculosis,* **37**, 125–51.

Elliott, A.M., Hayes, R.J., Halwiindi, B. *et al.* (1993a) The impact of HIV on infectiousness of pulmonary tuberculosis: a community study in Zambia. *AIDS,* **7**, 981–7.

Elliott, A.M., Halwiindi, B., Hayes, R.J. *et al.* (1993b) The impact of human immunodeficiency virus on presentation and diagnosis of tuberculosis in a cohort study in Zambia. *Journal of Tropical Medicine and Hygiene,* **96**, 1–11.

Eriki, P.P., Okwera, A., Aisu, T. *et al.* (1991) The influence of human immunodeficiency virus infection on tuberculosis in Kampala, Uganda. *American Review of Respiratory Disease,* **43**, 185–7.

Espinal, M., Reingold, A., Gonzales, G. *et al.* (1993) HIV infection and TB-treatment response in children with tuberculosis. Abstract PO-C19-3060. *Proceedings of the IX International Conference on AIDS,* Berlin, Germany, 6–11 June, 1993.

Frieden, D.R., Sterling, T., Pablos-Mendez, A. *et al.* (1993) The emergence of drug-resistant tuberculosis in New York City. *New England Journal of Medicine,* **328**, 521–6.

Galtung Hansen, O. (1955) Tuberculosis mortality and morbidity and tuberculin sensitivity in Norway. World Health Organization, Copenhagen (unpublished document WHO EURO 84/15; available on request from the Tuberculosis Programme, World Health Organization, 1211 Geneva 27, Switzerland).

Geuns, H.A., van Meijer, J., Styblo, K. (1975) Results of contact examination in Rotterdam, 1967–1969. *Bulletin of the International Union Against Tuberculosis,* **50**, 107–21.

Girardi, E., Antonucci, G., Armignacco, O. *et al.* (1994) Tuberculosis and AIDS: a retrospective, longitudinal, multicenter study on Italian AIDS patients. *Journal of Infection,* **28**, 261–9.

Githui, W., Nunn, P.P., Juma, E. *et al.* (1992) Cohort study of HIV-positive and HIV-negative tuberculosis, Nairobi, Kenya: comparison of bacteriological results. *Tubercle and Lung Disease*, **73**, 203–9.

Grigg, E.R.N. (1958) The arcana of tuberculosis. With a brief epidemiologic history of the disease in the USA. *American Review of Tuberculosis and Pulmonary Diseases*, **78**, 151–72, 426–53, and 583–603.

Guelar, A., Gatell, J.M., Verdejo, J. *et al.* (1993) A prospective study of the risk of tuberculosis among HIV-infected patients. *AIDS*, **7**, 1345–9.

Ibopishak Singh, I. (1993) HIV infection amongst tuberculosis patients at tuberculosis hospital, Chingeirong, Manipur. Abstract n.OP 48. *Proceedings of the 17th Eastern Regional Conference on Tuberculosis and Respiratory Diseases of the IUATLD*, Eastern Region, Bangkok, Thailand, 1–4 November 1993.

Iribarran, J.A., Arrizabalaga, J., Garde, C. *et al.* (1989) Tuberculosis in AIDS patients. Abstract Th.B.P.65:426. *Proceedings of the V International Conference on AIDS*, Montreal, Canada, 4–9 June 1989.

Jessurum, J., Angeles-Angeles, A. and Gasman, N. (1990) Comparative demographic and autopsy findings in acquired immunodeficiency syndrome in two Mexican popullations. *Journal of Acquired Immunodeficiency Syndrome*, **3**, 579–83.

Kaur, A., Babu, P.G., Jacob, M. *et al.* (1992) Clinical and laboratory profile of AIDS in India. *Journal of Acquired Immunodeficiency Syndrome*, **5**, 883–9.

Kim, S.J. and Hong, Y.P. (1992) Drug resistance of *Mycobacterium tuberculosis* in Korea. *Tubercle and Lung Disease*, **73**, 219–24.

Kochi, A., Vareldzis, B. and Styblo, K. (1993) Multi-drug resistant tuberculosis and its control. *Research Microbiology*, **144**, 104–10.

Kritski, A.L., Werneck-Barroso, E., Armandas Vieira, M. *et al.* (1993) HIV infection in 567 active pulmonary tuberculosis patients in Brazil. *Journal of Acquired Immunodeficiency Syndrome*, **6**, 1008–12.

Kritski, A.L., Dalcolmo, M.P., Fiuza de Melo, *et al.* (1994) Association between tuberculosis and HIV in Brazil. *Bulletin of the Pan American Health Organization*, **28**: (in press).

Lindhart, M. (1939) The statistics of pulmonary tuberculosis in Denmark, 1925-34. A statistical investigation on the occurrence of pulmonary tuberculosis in the period 1925-34. Worked out on the basis of the Danish National Health Service File of notified cases and of deaths. Ejnar Munksgaard, Copenhagen.

Long, R., Scalcini, M., Manfreda, J. *et al.* (1991) Impact of human immunodeficiency virus type 1 on tuberculosis in rural Haiti. *American Review of Respiratory Diseases*, **143**, 69–73.

Lucas, S.B., Nounnou, A., Peacock, C. *et al.* (1993) The mortality and pathology of HIV infection in a West African city. *AIDS*, **7**, 1569–79.

Luo, C., Chintu, C., Bhat, G. *et al.* (1994) Human immunodeficiency virus type-1 infection in Zambian children with tuberculosis: changing seroprevalence and evaluation of a thiacetazone-free regimen. *Tubercle and Lung Disease*, **75**, 110–15.

Mbaga, J.M., Pallangyo, K.J., Bakari, M. and Aris, E.A. (1990) Survival time of patients with acquired immunodeficiency syndrome: experience with 274 patients in Dar-Es-Salaam. *East African Medical Journal*, **67**, 95–9.

McLeod, D.T., Neill, P., Robertson, W. *et al.* (1989) Pulmonary diseases in patients infected with the human immunodeficiency virus in Zimbabwe, Central Africa. *Transactions of the Royal Society of Tropical Medicine and Hygiene*, **83**, 691–7.

Mohanty, K.C., Sundarani, R.M. and Pasi, R.B. (1993) Changing trend of HIV infection in tuberculosis and pulmonary diseases patients, since 1988, at Bombay. Abstract n.OP 49. *Proceedings of the 17th Eastern Regional Conference on Tuberculosis and Respiratory Diseases of the IUATLD*, Eastern Region, Bangkok, Thailand, 1–4 November 1993.

Murray, C.J.L., Styblo, K and Rouillon, A. (1990) Tuberculosis in developing countries: burden, intervention and cost. *Bulletin of the International Union Against Tuberculosis and Lung Disease*, **65**, 6–24.

Narain, J.P., Raviglione, M.C. and Kochi, A. (1992) HIV-associated tuberculosis in developing countries: epidemiology and strategies for prevention. *Tubercle and Lung Disease*, **73**, 311–21.

Nunn, P., Kibuga, D., Gathua, S. *et al.* (1991) Cutaneous hypersensitivity reactions due to thiacetazone in HIV-1 seropositive patients treated for tuberculosis. *Lancet*, **337**, 627–30.

Nunn, P., Brindle, R., Carpenter, L. *et al.* (1992) Cohort study of human immunodeficiency virus infection in patients with tuberculosis in

Nairobi, Kenya. Analysis of early (6-month) mortality. *American Review of Respiratory Diseases*, **146**, 849–54.

Nunn, P. and Felten, M. (1994) Surveillance of resistance to antituberculosis drugs in developing countries. *Tubercle and Lung Disease*, **75**, 163–7.

Okwera, A., Eriki, P.P., Guay, L.A. *et al.* (1990) Tuberculin reactions in apparently healthy HIV-seropositive and HIV-seronegative women – Uganda. *Morbidity and Mortality Weekly Report*, **39**, 638–9 and 645–6.

Olakowski, T. (1973) Assignment report on a tuberculosis longitudinal survey, National Tuberculosis Institute, Bangalore WHO Project: India 0103. World Health Organization, Geneva, Regional Office for South East Asia (unpublished document WHO SEA/TB/129; available on request from the Tuberculosis Programme, World Health Organization, 1211 Geneva 27, Switzerland).

Onorato, I., McCombs, S., Morgan, M. and McCray, E. (1993) HIV infection in patients attending tuberculosis clinics, United States, 1988–1992. Abstract n. 1363. Proceedings of the 33rd Interscience Conference on Antimicrobial Agents and Chemotherapy, New Orleans, Louisiana, USA, 17–20 October 1993.

Pape, J.W., Liautaud, B., Thomas, F. *et al.* (1985) The acquired immunodeficiency syndrome in Haiti. *Annals of Internal Medicine*, **103**, 674–8.

Payanandana, V., Klòdphuang, B., Talkitkul, N. and Tornee, S. (1995) Information in preparation for an External Review of the National Tuberculosis Programme, Thailand, 1995, Bangkok: Tuberculosis Division, Department of Communicable Disease Control, Ministry of Public Health.

Pilheu, J.A., Yunis, A.S., De Salvo, M.C. *et al.* (1993) Infeccion por VIH en pacientes tuberculosos. *Revista Argentina del Torax*, **54**, 7–11.

Raviglione, M.C., Sudre, P., Rieder, H.L. *et al.* (1993a) Secular trends of tuberculosis in Western Europe. *Bulletin of the World Health Organization*, **71**, 297–306.

Raviglione, M.C., Sudre, P., Esteves, K. *et al.* (1993b) Tuberculosis – Western Europe, 1974–1991. *Morbidity and Mortality Weekly Report*, **42**, 628–31.

Raviglione, M.C., Rieder, H.L., Styblo, B. *et al.* (1994) Tuberculosis trends in Eastern Europe and the former USSR. *Tubercle and Lung Disease*, **75**, 400–16.

Rieder, H.L., Cauthen, G.M., Comstock, G.W. and Snider, D.E. Jr. (1989) Epidemiology of tuberculosis in the United States. *Epidemiological Reviews*, **11**, 79–98.

Rieder, H.L., Zellweger, J.-P., Raviglione, M.C. *et al.* (1994) Tuberculosis control in Europe and international migration. *European Respiratory Journal*, **7**.

Rutledge, C.J.A. and Crouch, J.B. (1919) The ultimate results in 1,694 cases of tuberculosis treated at the Modern Woodmen of America Sanitorium. *American Review of Tuberculosis*, **2**, 755–63.

Sanches, K., Almeida, E., Pinto, M. *et al.* (1990) AIDS and tuberculosis in the state of Rio de Janeiro, Brazil. Abstract n.Th.C.731. Proceedings of the VI International Conference on AIDS, San Francisco, California, USA, 20–24 June 1990.

Sassan-Morokro, M., De Cock, K.M., Ackah, A. *et al.* (1994) Tuberculosis and HIV infection in children in Abidjan, Côte d'Ivoire. *Transactions of the Royal Society of Tropical Medicine and Hygiene*, **88**, 178–81.

Schwoebel, V. and Jougla, E. (1993) Tuberculose et infection VIH en France. *Revue Epidémiologique et de Santé Publique*, **41**, 505–8.

Selwyn, P.A., Hartel, D., Lewis, V.A. *et al.* (1989) A prospective study of the risk of tuberculosis among intravenous drug users with human immunodeficiency virus infection. *New England Journal of Medicine*, **320**, 545–50.

Selwyn, P.A., Sckell, B.M., Alcabes, P. *et al.* (1992) High risk of active tuberculosis in HIV-infected drug users with cutaneous anergy. *Journal of the American Medical Association*, **268**, 504–9.

Shafer, R.W., Chirgwin, K.D., Glatt, E.A. *et al.* (1991) HIV prevalence, immunosuppression, and drug resistance in patients with tuberculosis in an area endemic for AIDS. *AIDS*, **5**, 399–405.

Small, P.M., Schecter, G.F., Goodman, P.C. *et al.* (1991) Treatment of tuberculosis in patients with advanced human immunodeficiency virus infection. *New England Journal of Medicine*, **324**, 289–94.

Small, P.M., Hopewell, P.C., Singh, S.P. *et al.* (1994) The epidemiology of tuberculosis in San Francisco. A population-based study using conventional and molecular methods. *New England Journal of Medicine*, **330**, 1703–9.

Stead, W.W. (1992) Genetics and resistance to tuberculosis. Could resistance be enhanced by genetic engineering? *Annals of Internal Medicine,* **116**, 937–41.

Statistics Canada, Canadian Centre for Health Information (1993) *Tuberculosis Statistics 1991.* Catalogue 82.220, Ottawa.

Styblo, K., van Meijer, J. and Sutherland, I. (1969) The transmission of tubercle bacilli, its trend in human population. Tuberculosis Surveillance Research Unit, Report No. 1. *Bulletin of the International Union Against Tuberculosis,* **42**, 5–104.

Styblo, K. and Sutherland, J. (1974) Epidemiological indices for planning, surveillance and evaluation of tuberculosis programmes. *Bulletin of the International Union Against Tuberculosis and Lung Disease,* **49**, 66–73.

Styblo, K. and Rouillon, A. (1981) Estimated global incidence of smear-positive pulmonary tuberculosis. Unreliability of officially reported figures on tuberculosis. *Bulletin of the International Union Against Tuberculosis,* **56**, 118–26.

Styblo, K. (1985) The relationship between the risk of tuberculosis infection and the risk of developing infectious tuberculosis. *Bulletin of the International Union Against Tuberculosis,* **60**, 117–19.

Styblo, B. (1991) *Epidemiology of Tuberculosis.* Royal Netherlands Tuberculosis Association, The Hague, The Netherlands.

Sudre, P., ten Dam, G. and Kochi, A. (1992) Tuberculosis: a global overview of the situation today. *Bulletin of the World Health Organization,* **70**, 149–59.

Sutherland, I. (1976) Recent studies in the epidemiology of tuberculosis, based on the risk of being infected with the tubercle bacilli. *Advances in Tuberculosis Research,* **19**, 1–63.

Tansuphaswasdikul, S. (1993) Thai experiences on the diagnostic approaches and management of pulmonary complications in HIV infection. Abstract n. *Proceedings of the 17th Eastern Regional Conference on Tuberculosis and Respiratory Diseases of the IUATLD,* Eastern Region, Bangkok, Thailand, 1–4 November 1993.

Ten Dam, H.G. (1985) Surveillance of tuberculosis by means of tuberculin surveys. Geneva, World Health Organization (unpublished document WHO/TB/85.145; available on request from the Tuberculosis Programme, World Health Organization, 1211 Geneva 27, Switzerland).

Trnka, L., Dankova, D. and Svandova, E. (1993) Six years' experience with the discontinuation of BCG vaccination. +. Risk of tuberculosis infection and disease. *Tubercle and Lung Disease,* **74**, 167–72.

Van der Werf, T.S. (1989) High initial drug resistance in pulmonary tuberculosis in Ghana. *Tubercle,* **70**, 249–55.

Watson, J.M., Meredith, S.K., Whitmore-Overton, E. *et al.* (1993) Tuberculosis and HIV: estimates of the overlap in England and Wales. *Thorax,* **48**, 199–203.

World Bank (1993) *World Development Report 1993. Investing in Health.* Oxford University Press, New York.

World Health Organization (1989) *Childhood Tuberculosis and BCG Vaccine.* EPI Update Supplement, Geneva.

World Health Organization. Tuberculosis Unit (1991) *Tuberculosis Surveillance and Monitoring.* Report of a WHO Workshop. Geneva, 20–22 March 1991. Geneva. (unpublished document WHO/TUB/91.163; available on request from the Tuberculosis Programme, World Health Organization, 1211 Geneva 27, Switzerland).

World Heath Organization. Division of Epidemiological Surveillance and Health Situation and Trend Assessment (1992) *Global Health Situation and Projections. Estimates.* WHO/HST/92.1, Geneva.

World Health Organization. Global Programme on AIDS (1993) *The HIV/AIDS Pandemic: 1993 Overview,* Doc. no. WHO/GPA/CNP/EVA/93.1 (WHO, Geneva, Switzerland, 1993).

World Health Organization. Tuberculosis Programme (1994a) *Tuberculosis notification update. December 1993.* Geneva (unpublished document WHO/TB/93.175; available on request from the Tuberculosis Programme, World Health Organization, 1211 Geneva 27, Switzerland).

World Health Organization (1994b) Tuberculosis. *Weekly Epidemiological Record,* **69**, 77–80.

World Health Organization, Global Programme on AIDS (1995a) The current global situation of the HIV/AIDS pandemic. *Weekly Epidemiological Record,* **70**, 192–6.

World Health Organization (1995b) *Tuberculosis and HIV research: working towards solutions.* WHO/TB/95, 193.

CLINICAL ASPECTS OF ADULT TUBERCULOSIS IN HIV-INFECTED PATIENTS

9

Adam S. Malin and Kevin M. De Cock

THE THREE CLINICAL FACES OF TUBERCULOSIS

Prior to the development of chemotherapy, tuberculosis frequently progressed, unabated, to cause severe cavitary lung disease. Persons with tuberculosis expectorated large numbers of bacilli from pulmonary foci and these highly infectious secretions could then directly infect the mucosa of the respiratory and gastrointestinal tracts. Thus, common features included indolent ulcers of the tongue and mouth, frequent involvement of the larynx and middle ear, and severe gastrointestinal disease (Marshall, 1993).

With the advent of effective antituberculous drugs and a system for pasteurizing milk, the incidence of both gastrointestinal and laryngeal disease fell. In this post-chemotherapy era, disease occurred more usually in the very young or elderly and otherwise debilitated, such as those with uremia, malignancy, diabetes or alcoholism. The very young tended to present with miliary or meningeal disease; the older group with features of either chronic organ involvement, particularly pulmonary disease, or, less commonly, widespread dissemination.

Today, a third clinical face is recognized, that of the 'new tuberculosis' (Snider and Roper, 1992), a manifestly different clinical entity from its predecessors. This new syndrome results from the emergence of HIV infection as the strongest risk factor for developing tuberculosis that has been recognized. This chapter will discuss the influence of HIV on tuberculous disease, drawing comparisons where appropriate with the clinical features of tuberculosis not associated with HIV.

THE NEW TUBERCULOSIS

HIV infection has profoundly influenced the epidemiology and clinical expression of tuberculosis. The effects of HIV include:

1. an increased susceptibility to reactivation of latent tuberculous infection;
2. rapid progression following primary infection;
3. an increased risk of recurrent disease following certain therapeutic regimens;
4. documented instances of reinfection after treatment;
5. increased case rates in many developing countries and in some communities in industrialized countries;

AIDS and Respiratory Medicine. Edited by A. Zumla, M.A. Johnson and R.F. Miller. Published in 1997 by Chapman & Hall, London. ISBN 0 412 60140 0

6. a change in the clinical picture;
7. a change in the descriptive characteristics of persons affected; and
8. a marked increase in mortality despite treatment.

Of all the risk factors for the development of tuberculosis, HIV is by far the most potent, the relative risk for developing tuberculosis being 6–100 in HIV-infected persons when compared with HIV-negative individuals (Nunn *et al.*, 1994). The greatest increases in case rates are occurring in populations in developing countries and in selected groups in affluent countries that have high rates of co-infection with *Mycobacterium tuberculosis* and HIV.

Tuberculosis often precedes other opportunistic infections in HIV-infected persons by about two years (Barnes *et al.*, 1991). Another facet of the interaction between HIV infection and tuberculosis is the effect of tuberculosis on the natural history of HIV disease itself. Although this is not firmly established, there is some evidence that tuberculosis may enhance the progression of HIV disease (Forte *et al.*, 1992; Pape *et al.*, 1993; Toossi *et al.*, 1993; Whalen *et al.*, 1995). Thus, efforts to improve treatment of tuberculosis and prevent its spread play an important role in the therapeutic approach to HIV/AIDS.

REACTIVATION, PRIMARY INFECTION, RECURRENCE, OR REINFECTION?

Early studies (Selwyn *et al.*, 1989) showing the increased risk for tuberculosis in HIV-infected persons suggested that the majority of cases resulted from reactivation of latent tuberculous infection in the face of waning immunity. More recent studies (Small *et al.*, 1994; Alland *et al.*, 1994) using restriction fragment length polymorphism (RFLP) indicate that 30–40% of tuberculosis cases in New York City and San Francisco may represent recently acquired infections. HIV-infected persons were especially likely to belong to a cluster of infection presumed recently acquired.

HIV-infected persons who acquire tuberculosis are particularly prone to rapidly progressive primary disease (Centers for Disease Control, 1991, 1992; Daley *et al.*, 1992; Edlin *et al.*, 1992; Pearson *et al.*, 1992; Snider and Roper, 1992), which may develop within a few weeks of exposure. An investigation of a drug-resistant outbreak in a New York State prison demonstrated that HIV infection was not associated with becoming infected *per se* (disease cases plus asymptomatic skin test convertors), but once infected, the HIV-positive inmates were significantly more likely to develop disease than HIV-negative inmates ($p < 0.001$) (Valway *et al.*, 1994). The same feature has also been noted among residents of a housing facility for HIV-infected individuals (Daley *et al.*, 1992).

Prior tuberculosis does not necessarily protect a person with advanced HIV disease from reinfection; exogenous reinfection has been well described, involving both drug sensitive and resistant strains. It may be impossible clinically to distinguish between reinfection following treatment and relapse.

THE ALTERED SPECTRUM OF TUBERCULOSIS IN PATIENTS CO-INFECTED WITH HIV

Data describing clinical features of co-infected individuals come from cross-sectional and cohort studies.

Clinical differences in HIV-infected persons include:

1. a higher proportion of extrapulmonary tuberculosis (Barnes, Le and Davidson, 1993; Berenguer *et al.*, 1992; Colebunders *et al.*, 1989; De Cock *et al.*, 1991; Elliott *et al.*, 1990; Gilks *et al.*, 1990; Houston *et al.*, 1994; Kelly, Burnham and Radford, 1990);
2. a higher proportion with tuberculosis at

more than one site (Houston *et al.*, 1994; Shafer *et al.*, 1991);

3. a lower rate of tuberculin skin test positivity (Barnes *et al.*, 1991; Houston *et al.*, 1994; Shafer *et al.*, 1991);

4. more frequent atypical chest radiographs (Elliott *et al.*, 1990; Houston *et al.*, 1994);

5. a lower frequency of sputum smear positivity;

6. a higher rate of adverse drug effects (Nunn, Porter and Winstanley, 1993);

7. a higher death rate (Chaisson and Slutkin, 1989; De Cock *et al.*, 1992; Elliott, 1995).

The important clinical features are discussed below.

Pulmonary tuberculosis

The clinical manifestations of pulmonary disease can be categorized as chronic pulmonary, atypical pneumonic, and mass lesions. Typical chronic pulmonary tuberculosis occurs as a manifestation of recrudescent disease in the lung in an individual with a relatively intact immune system. There are several sites of predilection including the posterior segment of the upper lobe and the apical segment of the lower lobe. Cavitation and fibrosis in the upper zones are a hallmark of this type of disease. However, rupture of an upper zone focus can lead to bronchial spread and involve the lower lobes. Regional lymphadenopathy is usually absent.

Atypical pneumonic features usually progress directly from primary infection, and intrathoracic adenopathy is often present. However, in individuals with marked immune deficiency such features may also occur as a consequence of recrudescence. Pulmonary tuberculomas, as in other parts of the body, present as mass lesions and are often mistaken for malignancy.

Symptomatology is varied. Early primary infection may be asymptomatic or associated with constitutional symptoms such as fever, cough, weight loss, anorexia, chills and sweats. Thus, the presentation can easily be mistaken for symptoms of HIV disease. Severe cough with marked sputum production is usually a feature of fairly advanced cavitary disease. In most cases, sputum production is mucopurulent in type, a common finding in symptomatic HIV infection alone. Hemoptysis is a feature of prolonged disease and arises as a consequence of caseous sloughing, endobronchial erosion, pulmonary artery erosion (Rasmussen's aneurysm) or aspergillous superinfection of a cavity. Chest pain suggests parietal pleural involvement with or without an effusion. Painless serofibrinous pleurisy may occur at an early stage, but the patient may not present until other symptoms intervene.

Over two-thirds of HIV-infected tuberculosis patients will have pulmonary involvement (Barnes, Le and Davidson, 1993). The symptoms and signs are often indistinguishable from other causes of HIV-related respiratory diseases. Differences occur between early and late HIV infection and for the sake of clarity, one can classify these into two separate, albeit artificial, categories: (1) those with relatively higher CD4 T-lymphocyte counts who tend to present with a more typical clinical picture of chronic pulmonary tuberculosis; a predilection for involvement of the upper lobes; cavitary disease; uncommon extrapulmonary involvement; higher rates of sputum positivity and tuberculin skin test positivity; and (2) those who are more immunocompromised and tend to present with patchy reticular or alveolar shadowing; no predilection for the upper lobes; much more common extrapulmonary involvement; and lower rates of sputum positivity and tuberculin skin test positivity (Barnes, Le and Davidson, 1993; Colebunders *et al.*, 1989). Indeed, sputum positivity rates tend to parallel those seen in HIV-uninfected reactivation tuberculosis (similar to early HIV disease) and HIV-uninfected primary/miliary tuberculosis (similar to late HIV disease).

Extrapulmonary tuberculosis

Spread giving rise to extrapulmonary disease can be mucosal, where highly infectious respiratory secretions are expectorated and bathe the mucosa of the gastrointestinal and respiratory tracts. Alternatively, spread may occur through blood and lymphatics from an established primary or chronic focus. Mucosal spread usually arises in those patients with high bacillary loads, typically in long-standing, untreated cavitary disease. Gastrointestinal and laryngeal disease is uncommon in HIV-infected persons, in whom extrapulmonary disease arising from lymphohematogenous spread is the rule.

The relative frequency of pulmonary and extrapulmonary disease depends on the degree of immune deficiency in the patients studied. In the US, over 70% of tuberculosis patients with advanced HIV-disease have extrapulmonary tuberculosis, as compared with 24–45% of those with less severe immune deficiency (Chaisson *et al.*, 1987). The extrapulmonary sites most commonly involved include lymph nodes, blood, pleura, meninges and pericardium. In Africa, studies in Zambia (Elliott *et al.*, 1990), Zaire (Colebunders *et al.*, 1989), Zimbabwe (Houston *et al.*, 1994), Kenya (Gilks *et al.*, 1990), and Côte d'Ivoire (De Cock *et al.*, 1991) have shown similarly increased rates of extrapulmonary disease. The extent of mycobacterial dissemination is often unsuspected, as shown by autopsy data from West Africa (Lucas *et al.*, 1993). The frequency of extrapulmonary disease will depend not only on the patient population, but also on the vigor with which extrapulmonary disease is searched for (Githui *et al.*, 1992; Kamanfu *et al.*, 1993). Thus, in a recent prospective analysis of 300 consecutive acute respiratory admissions to a hospital in Bujumbura, Burundi, 18 of 39 (46%) HIV-negative tuberculosis patients had extrapulmonary disease compared with 33 of 109 (30%) HIV-positive patients (Kamanfu *et al.*, 1993).

However, the study was not designed to investigate disease in other sites and in all other studies extrapulmonary disease is more frequent in the HIV-infected.

Miliary TB

Although this name is derived from the resemblance of lesions on the chest radiograph to millet seeds, the term has come to be used for all forms of disseminated tuberculosis. The final nature of miliary tuberculosis reflects the balance between mycobacterial spread by lymphatics and blood, and cell-mediated immunity attempting to control the infection. When cell-mediated immunity is essentially absent, as in advanced HIV disease, there is marked tissue necrosis with gross bacillary replication and lack of a granulomatous response (Kielhofner and Hamill, 1991; Lucas *et al.*, 1993).

Prior to the HIV epidemic, children frequently suffered progressive post-primary disease with mycobacterial spread occurring via the lymphatics and blood prior to the development of effective cell-mediated immunity. During the blood-borne phase, there is seeding of foci throughout the body. In the presence of an intact immune system, the foci will lay dormant and may only later progress to chronic organ tuberculosis.

When cell-mediated immunity is more effective, spread tends to be milder and results typically from a chronic active focus, leading to diffuse liver involvement (Kielhofner and Hamill, 1991) and the appearance of choroidal tubercles (Sherman and Nozik, 1992). This disease may be low-grade, protracted and even episodic. Bacillemia will abate in these patients with moderate cell-mediated immunity, and this is accompanied by the development of tuberculin skin-test positivity.

Patients who fail to mount an adequate immune response will succumb to progressive disease. Presentation in these patients is very non-specific and includes malaise, weakness, weight loss, fever, night sweats and, occasionally, rigors. The illness may also be complicated by pleural, peritoneal and meningeal disease (see below). Multiorgan disease occurs with heavy mycobacterial load. This presentation is typical of advanced HIV disease but also occurs, for example, in the elderly (immunosenesence), and in patients with malignancy, uremia, diabetes and alcoholism. A very common presenting feature is non-specific weight loss or 'slim', as described in Sub-Saharan Africa (Lucas *et al.*, 1993). Fever may be absent and thus, importantly, apyrexia does not exclude infection.

In HIV infection, miliary tuberculosis accounts for one of the most frequent forms of extrapulmonary TB. *Mycobacterium tuberculosis* has frequently been isolated from blood of patients in both the US (Barnes *et al.*, 1991; Kramer *et al.*, 1990) and in Africa (Gilks *et al.*, 1990; Vugia *et al.*, 1993). Positive culture rates in the US vary between 26–42%. In one study, a high temperature, miliary shadowing on a chest radiograph or abnormal liver tests were all associated with positive blood culture (Shafer *et al.*, 1989). Failure to diagnose extrapulmonary disease may depend on the extent of diagnostic evaluation. In another study, blood was the only extrapulmonary source in 19% of cases (Kramer *et al.*, 1990). Autopsies of HIV-infected persons dying in Abidjan, Côte d'Ivoire, indicated the extent of undiagnosed disseminated disease prior to death. In 80 cadavers diagnosed with tuberculosis as prime cause of death, all but 10 (88%) showed widely disseminated disease (Lucas *et al.*, 1993).

Lymphadenitis

Tuberculous lymphadenopathy is strongly associated with HIV infection (Barnes, Le and Davidson, 1993; Berenguer *et al.*, 1992; Stein and Libertin, 1990). The differential diag-

nosis includes persistent generalized lymphadenopathy (PGL), Kaposi's sarcoma, atypical mycobacteriosis, and lymphoma. The presence of rapidly enlarging nodes, tenderness or marked asymmetry suggests possible tuberculosis and is against a diagnosis of PGL. *Mycobacterium avium*-complex (MAC) infection of lymph nodes rarely causes tenderness (Modilevsky, Sattler and Barnes, 1989). The presence of intrathoracic disease usually suggests TB, KS, or, less commonly, lymphoma, and is not a feature of PGL (Barnes, Le and Davidson, 1993). Whenever the diagnosis is in doubt, further investigation is required and should include needle aspiration of lymph node biopsy.

Serofibrinous pleurisy with effusion

Prior to the HIV epidemic, pleural tuberculosis was seen early in post-primary disease when, in the absence of treatment, about 65% of patients would go on to develop chronic organ tuberculosis within five years (Roper and Waring, 1955). Pleural tuberculosis could also occur as a complication of chronic tuberculous disease of different organs. The entity of *tuberculous polyserositis* was recognized, referring to patients with co-existent bilateral pleural, peritoneal and pericardial disease. However, most cases are unilateral without involvement of lung parenchyma.

Today, pleural tuberculosis is commonly associated with HIV infection, as noted in several studies in Africa (Elliott *et al.*, 1990; Houston *et al.*, 1994; Kelly, Burnham and Radford, 1990; Pozniak *et al.*, 1994) and the US (Barnes, Le and Davidson, 1993). For example, in Zambia, 84% of all patients with pleural tuberculosis were HIV-positive, compared with 49% of those with pulmonary tuberculosis (odds ratio 3.5, corrected for age and sex, $p<0.001$) (Elliott *et al.*, 1990). Pleural tuberculosis in HIV-infected persons tended to affect a younger age group (Elliott *et al.*, 1990; Kelly, Burnham and Radford, 1990) and to respond well to treatment (Kelly, Burnham and Radford, 1990).

Tuberculous pericarditis

Pericardial disease has been thought to occur as a result of rupture of an adjacent lymph node into the pericardium or from hematogenous spread. At one end of the clinical spectrum, the onset of disease may be subtle without systemic features, cardiovascular symptoms appearing at a late stage. Alternatively, there may be an abrupt systemic illness with fever and pericardial-type pain or cardiac tamponade. Data from a retrospective study in Zimbabwe assessed 61 consecutive patients presenting with tuberculous pericardial effusions. Positive associations were found with HIV infection (odds ratio (OR) 2.5) and, for those infected with HIV, disease at more than one site (OR 6.1).

Tuberculous meningitis and other CNS syndromes

When associated with primary disease, typically in children, meningeal involvement usually occurs several weeks after symptoms of miliary disease, and may be due to rupture of a subependymal tubercle. The clinical picture is somewhat different in those with recrudescent disease. Spread is hematogenous, but arises from chronic tuberculosis of one or other organ.

About 75% of non-HIV infected patients with tuberculous meningitis will have evidence of organ disease outside of the meninges (Kennedy and Fallon, 1979), the other 25% having no clinically apparent extrameningeal disease. In the latter, presumably there is a hidden focus with spread arising from another site such as a lymph node, the genitourinary tract or an osseous site. Presentation is often insidious, with only a mild headache or a vague change in mentation. Fever is usually only low grade and may be absent. Less commonly, there may be abrupt onset of a typical illness mimicking bacterial meningitis. This can be further confused by the presence of a predominant neutrophilia on microscopy of spinal fluid; in one series this was as demonstrated in as many as 31% of HIV-infected persons (Berenguer *et al.*, 1992).

In HIV-infected patients, meningitis is more common than in HIV-seronegative tuberculosis patients (Berenguer *et al.*, 1992; Dube, Holtom and Larsen, 1992). A retrospective study from Madrid assessed the records of over 2000 patients, 21% of whom were HIV-positive. *M. tuberculosis* was isolated from cerebrospinal fluid of 10% of those infected with HIV as compared with only 2% of HIV non-infected tuberculosis patients ($p<0.001$). Lymph node enlargement was more common in those with HIV infection, although clinical features were otherwise indistinguishable (Berenguer *et al.*, 1992). Similar to previous studies prior to the HIV epidemic, extrameningeal tuberculosis was apparent in 65% of cases. An illness lasting more than two weeks prior to presentation and a CD4 T cell count below 200 cells/μl were both associated with a poor outcome.

Tuberculoma and tuberculous abscess formation are uncommon in HIV-infected persons (Bishburg *et al.*, 1986; Dube, Holtom and Larsen, 1992). Most reported cases have been in persons from developing countries where the incidence of disseminated disease is relatively high. A series of ten HIV-positive patients was reported from New Jersey, nine of them intravenous drug users. The authors emphasize that the clustering seen in this particular risk group is probably a consequence of their exposure to both HIV and tuberculosis infections (Bishburg *et al.*, 1986).

A study by Dube and colleagues, which compared 15 tuberculous meningitis patients with HIV infection and 16 without, showed that intracerebral mass lesions were more common in the HIV-infected (60% versus 14%, $p<0.01$) (Dube, Holtom and Larsen, 1992). It is recognized that such mass lesions may present with meningitis, diffuse or focal neurological features, or fits. However, contrary to expectation, this series did not show a correlation between the presence of a mass and a focal neurological deficit, altered level of consciousness, or mortality.

Cerebrospinal fluid may be normal and the diagnosis only indicated by the presence of ring enhancing lesions or lesions of low attenuation on the CT scan. When facilities are available and there is a high index of suspicion, a biopsy may permit early intervention for this potentially treatable condition. Rarely similar lesions also occur in the spine and present with features typical of pressure at this site (Mantzoros, Brown and Dembry, 1993). A wide variety of other neurological syndromes have been described. These are rare and include hemiballismus, decerebrate rigidity and cerebellar syndrome.

Liver disease

Inapparent liver involvement is common in all types of tuberculosis regardless of HIV status. For example, prior to chemotherapy, post-mortem liver histology has demonstrated diffuse, micronodular hepatic involvement in 50–80% of samples from persons with end-stage pulmonary disease (Keilhofner and Hamill, 1991). Prospective evaluation of liver histology in unselected persons with pulmonary tuberculosis showed 75% involvement prior to starting treatment. Disease is usually diffuse but may be focal and mimic metastases or pyogenic abscesses. Occasionally extrahepatic tuberculosis is absent.

The presence of MAC in the liver is common, whilst tuberculous liver involvement in those co-infected with HIV does not appear strikingly more frequent than in those without HIV (Kielhofner and Hamill, 1991). In industrialized countries, MAC disease of the liver is more frequent than hepatic tuberculosis. AIDS patients in general often have raised serum levels of alkaline phosphatase that are difficult to explain, and granulomatous involvement of liver in such patients is uncommon.

Tuberculosis at more than one site

Several studies have established that HIV-infected patients are more likely to present with tuberculosis at more than one site (Elliott *et al.*, 1990; Houston *et al.*, 1994; Pozniak *et al.*, 1994; Stein and Libertin, 1990), making it imperative to sample widely for diagnosis. Common associations include pulmonary plus another extrapulmonary site (Barnes *et al.*, 1991) and pericardial and pleural involvement (Pozniak *et al.*, 1994).

Kramer and colleagues emphasize the importance of taking samples from extrapulmonary sites in those sputum-negative patients with a chest radiograph suggestive of tuberculosis. For example, acid-fast smear examination of stools in HIV-infected patients was positive in 42% of cases, and stool culture in 58%. Similarly, 38% of blood cultures were positive for *M. tuberculosis* (Stein and Libertin, 1990). Another hospital-based study reported a rate of positive urine culture in 77% and blood culture in 56% of patients (Shafer *et al.* 1991).

It should be noted that evidence of *M. tuberculosis* in the stool *per se* does not necessarily indicate extrapulmonary disease, as this may result from swallowed secretions. Other useful but more difficult sites to sample include bone marrow, liver, and lymph node, biopsies from these sites yielding positive results in 50–90% of cases (Shafer *et al.*, 1991). A simple, less-invasive procedure, lymph node fine-needle aspiration, produced a surprisingly high yield, with a sensitivity rate of 87% in patients with confirmed tuberculosis (Pithie and Chicksen, 1992). This study was performed in southern Africa where most mycobacterial disease is due to *M. tuberculosis*. In affluent countries, smear-positivity would not help to distinguish tuberculosis from MAC.

Delay in diagnosis of TB

Late stage HIV-infection is associated with atypical presentations of tuberculosis. For persons with pulmonary tuberculosis, the clinical features are often indistinguishable from other forms of HIV-related respiratory disease. For those with extrapulmonary tuberculosis, multibacillary, disseminated disease is common (Lucas and Nelson, 1994). Given the high prevalence of tuberculosis throughout the world, a high index of suspicion is required in any HIV-infected person with respiratory symptoms, unexplained fever, or weight loss. The extent of investigation will depend on the likelihood of tuberculosis in a given setting and the availability of tests. However, as a minimum, three sputum samples should be examined in undiagnosed cases of pulmonary involvement.

CONCLUSION

There is a major resurgence of tuberculosis throughout the world, which in some areas is largely attributable to HIV infection (WHO, 1995). Increased transmission of tuberculosis is a potential health risk to all, irrespective of HIV status. Multidrug-resistant tuberculosis has emerged in several large cities in the US, has been intimately associated with HIV disease, and has the potential for occurring in resource-poor countries with high rates of HIV infection and weak tuberculosis control programmes. It is essential that we have a clear clinical picture of this protean disease in order to use resources responsibly and to manage patients as effectively as possible.

REFERENCES

Alland, D., Kalkut, G.E., Moss, A.R. *et al.* (1994) Transmission of tuberculosis in New York City. An analysis by DNA fingerprinting and conventional epidemiologic methods [see comments]. *N. Engl. J. Med.*, **330**, 1710–16.

Centers for Disease Control. (1991) Nosocomial transmission of multidrug-resistant tuberculosis among HIV-infected persons – Florida and New York, 1988–1991. *MMWR. Morb. Mortal. Wkly. Rep.*, **40**, 585–91.

Centers for Disease Control. (1992) Transmission of multidrug-resistant tuberculosis among immunocompromised persons in a correctional system – New York, 1991. *MMWR. Morb. Mortal. Wkly. Rep.*, **41**, 507–9.

Barnes, P.F., Bloch, A.B., Davidson, P.T. *et al.* (1991) Tuberculosis in patients with human immunodeficiency virus infection [see comments]. [Review]. *N. Engl. J. Med.*, **324**, 1644–50.

Barnes, P.F., Le, H.Q. and Davidson, P.T. (1993) Tuberculosis in patients with HIV infection. [Review]. *Med. Clin. N. Am.*, **77**, 1369–90.

Berenguer, J., Moreno, S., Laguna, F. *et al.* (1992) Tuberculous meningitis in patients infected with the human immunodeficiency virus [see comments]. *N. Engl. J. Med.*, **326**, 668–72.

Bishburg, E., Sunderam, G., Reichman, L.B. *et al.* (1986) Central nervous system tuberculosis with the acquired immunodeficiency syndrome and its related complex. *Ann. Intern. Med.*, **105**, 210–13.

Chaisson, R.E., Schecter, G.F., Theuer, C.P. *et al.* (1987) Tuberculosis in patients with the acquired immunodeficiency syndrome. Clinical features, response to therapy, and survival. *Am. Rev. Respir. Dis.*, **136**, 570–4.

Chaisson, R.E. and Slutkin, G. (1989) Tuberculosis and human immunodeficiency virus infection. *J. Infect. Dis.*, **159**, 96–100.

Colebunders, R.L., Ryder, R.W., Nzilambi, N. *et al.* (1989) HIV infection in patients with tuberculosis in Kinshasa, Zaire. *Am. Rev. Respir. Dis.*, **139**, 1082–5.

Daley, C.L., Small, P.M., Schecter, G.F. *et al.* (1992) An outbreak of tuberculosis with accelerated progression among persons infected with the human immunodeficiency virus. An analysis using restriction-fragment-length polymorphisms. *N. Engl. J. Med.*, **326**, 231–5.

De Cock, K.M., Gnaore, E., Adjorlolo, G. *et al.* (1991) Risk of tuberculosis in patients with HIV-I and HIV-II infections in Abidjan, Ivory Coast. *Br. Med. J.*, **302**, 496–9.

De Cock, K.M., Soro, B., Coulibaly, I.M. *et al.* (1992) Tuberculosis and HIV infection in sub-Saharan Africa. *JAMA*, **268**, 1581–7.

Dube, M.P., Holtom, P.D. and Larsen, R.A. (1992) Tuberculous meningitis in patients with and without human immunodeficiency virus infection. *Am. J. Med.*, **93**, 520–14.

Edlin, B.R., Tokars, J.L., Grieco, M.H. *et al.* (1992) An outbreak of multidrug-resistant tuberculosis among hospitalized patients with the acquired immunodeficiency syndrome [see comments]. *N. Engl. J. Med.*, **326**, 1514–21.

Elliott, A.M., Luo, N., Tembo, G. *et al.* (1990) Impact of HIV on tuberculosis in Zambia: a cross sectional study [see comments]. *Br. Med. J.*, **301**, 412–15.

Elliott, A.M., Halwiindi, B., Hayes, R.J. *et al.* (1995) The impact of human immunodeficiency virus on mortality of patients treated for tuberculosis in a cohort study in Zambia. *Trans. R. Soc. Trop. Med. Hyg.*, **89**, 78–82.

Forte, M., Maartens, G., Rahelu, M. *et al.* (1992) Cytolytic T-cell activity against mycobacterial antigents in HIV. *AIDS*, **6**, 407–11.

Gilks, C.F., Brindle, R.J., Otiena, L.S. *et al.* (1990) Extrapulmonary and disseminated tuberculosis in HIV-1 seropositive patients presenting to the acute medical services in Nairobi. *AIDS*, **4**, 981–5.

Githui, W., Nunn, P., Juma, E. *et al.* (1992) Cohort study of HIV-positive and HIV-negative tuberculosis, Nairobi, Kenya: comparison of bacteriological results. *Tuber. Lung Dis.*, **73**, 203–9.

Houston, S., Ray, S., Mahari, M. *et al.* (1994) The association of tuberculosis and HIV infection in Harare, Zimbabwe. *Tuber. Lung. Dis.*, **75**, 220–6.

Kamanfu, G., Mlika Cabanne, N., Girard, P.M. *et al.* (1993) Pulmonary complications of human immunodeficiency virus infection in Bujumbura, Burundi. *Am. Rev. Respir. Dis.*, **147**, 658–63.

Kelly, P., Burnham, G. and Radford, C. (1990) HIV seropositivity and tuberculosis in a rural Malawi hospital. *Trans. R. Soc. Trop. Med. Hyg.*, **84**, 725–7.

Kennedy, D.H. and Fallon, R.J. (1979) Tuberculous meningitis. *JAMA*, **241**, 264–8.

Kielhofner, M.A. and Hamill, R.J. (1991) Focal hepatic tuberculosis in a patient with acquired immunodeficiency syndrome. [Review]. *S. Med. J.*, **84**, 401–4.

Kramer, F., Modilevsky, T., Waliany, A.R. *et al.* (1990) Delayed diagnosis of tuberculosis in patients with human immunodeficiency virus infection [see comments]. *Am. J. Med.*, **89**, 451–6.

Lucas, S.B., Hounnou, A., Peacock, C. *et al.* (1993) The mortality and pathology of HIV infection in a west African city [see comments]. *AIDS*, **7**, 1569–79.

Lucas, S. and Nelson, A.M. (1994) Pathogenesis of tuberculosis in human immunodeficiency virus-infected people, in *Tuberculosis. Pathogenesis, Protection and Control.* (ed. B.R. Bloom). American Society for Microbiology, Washington DC, pp. 503–13.

Mantzoros, C.S., Brown, P.D., and Dembry, L. (1993) Extraosseous epidural tuberculoma: case report and review. [Review]. *Clin. Infect. Dis.*, **17**, 1032–6.

Marshall, J.B. (1993) Tuberculosis of the gastrointestinal tract and peritoneum. [Review.] *Am. J. Gastroent.*, **88**, 989–99.

Modilevsky, T., Sattler, F.R. and Barnes, P.F. (1989) Mycobacterial disease in patients with human immunodeficiency virus infection. *Arch. Intern. Med.*, **149**, 2201–5.

Nunn, P.P., Porter, J. and Winstanley, P. (1993) Thiacetazone – avoid like poison or use with care? *Trans. R. Soc. Trop. Med. Hyg.*, **87**, 578–82.

Nunn, P.P., Elliott, A.M. and McAdam, K.P.W.J. (1994) Impact of human immunodeficiency virus on tuberculosis in developing countries. *Thorax*, **49**, 511–18.

Pape, J.W., Jean, S.S., Ho, J.L. *et al.* (1993) Effect of isoniazid prophylaxis on incidence of active tuberculosis and progresssion of HIV infection. *Lancet*, **342**, 268–72.

Pearson, M.L., Jereb, J.A., Frieden, T.R. *et al.* (1992) Nosocomial transmission of multidrug-resistant *Mycobacterium tuberculosis*. A risk to patients and health care workers [see comments]. *Ann. Intern. Med.*, **117**, 191–6.

Pithie, A.D. and Chicksen, B. (1992) Fine-needle extrathoracic lymph-node aspiration in HIV-associated sputum-negative tuberculosis [see comments]. *Lancet*, **340**, 1504–5.

Pozniak, A.L., Weinberg, J., Mahari, M. *et al.* (1994) Tuberculous pericardial effusion associated with HIV infection: a sign of disseminated disease. *Tuber. Lung Dis.*, **75**, 297–300.

Roper, W.H. and Waring, J.J. (1955) Primary serofibrinous pleural effusion in military personnel. *Am. Rev. Tuberc.*, **71**, 616–34.

Selwyn, P.A., Hartel, D., Wasserman, W. *et al.* (1989) Impact of the AIDS epidemic on morbidity and mortality among intravenous drug users in a New York City methadone maintenance program. *Am. J. Public Health*, **79**, 1358–62.

Shafer, R.W., Goldberg, R., Sierra, M. *et al.* (1989) Frequency of *Mycobacterium tuberculosis* bacteremia in patients with tuberculosis in an area endemic for AIDS. *Am. Rev. Respir. Dis.*, **140**, 1611–13.

Shafer, R.W., Kim, D.S., Weiss, J.P. *et al.* (1991) Extrapulmonary tuberculosis in patients with human immunodeficiency virus infection. *Medicine Baltimore*, **70**, 384–97.

Sherman, M.D. and Nozik, R.A. (1992) Other infections of the choroid and retina. Toxoplasmosis, histoplasmosis, Lyme disease, syphilis, tuberculosis, and ocular toxocariasis. [Review.] *Infect. Dis. Clin. N. Am.*, **6**, 893–908.

Small, P.M., Hopewell, P.C., Singh, S.P. *et al.* (1994) The epidemiology of tuberculosis in San Francisco. A population-based study using conventional and molecular methods [see comments]. *N. Engl. J. Med.*, **330**, 1703–9.

Snider, Jr, D.E. and Roper, W.L. (1992) The new tuberculosis [editorial; comment]. *N. Engl. J. Med.*, **326**, 703–5.

Stein, D.S. and Libertin, C.R. (1990) Disseminated intravascular coagulation in association with cavitary tuberculosis. [Review]. *S. Med. J.*, **83**, 60–3.

Toossi, Z., Sierra Madero, J.G., Blinkhorn, R.A. *et al.* (1993) Enhanced susceptibility of blood monocytes from patients with pulmonary tuberculosis to productive infection with human immunodeficiency virus type 1. *J. Exp. Med.*, **177**, 1511–16.

Valway, S.E., Richards, S.B., Kovacovich, J. *et al.* (1994) Outbreak of multi-drug-resistant tuberculosis in a New York State prison, 1991. *Am. J. Epidemiol.*, **140**, 113–22.

Vugia, D.J., Kiehlbauch, J.A., Yeboue, K. *et al.* (1993) Pathogens and predictors of fatal septicemia associated with human immunodeficiency virus infection in Ivory Coast, west Africa. *J. Infect. Dis.*, **168**, 564–70.

Whalen, C., Horsburgh, C.R., Hom, D. *et al.* (1995) Accelerated course of human immunodeficiency virus infection after tuberculosis. *Am. J. Respir. Crit. Care Med.*, **151**, 129–35.

World Health Organization (1995) Tuberculosis and HIV research: working towards solution. WHO/TB/95,193.

PEDIATRIC TUBERCULOSIS AND THE HIV EPIDEMIC

10

Chifumbe Chintu and Alimuddin Zumla

INTRODUCTION

The human immunodeficiency virus (HIV) is one of the major risk factors for the development of tuberculosis (TB) (WHO, 1992a; Raviglione, Narain and Kochi, 1992; Raviglione, Snider and Kochi, 1995). The HIV pandemic and its close association with the resurgence of TB are a cause of grave concern and both have been declared global emergencies by the World Health Organization. TB is one of the most common infectious complications in adult patients infected with HIV in developing countries where HIV seroprevalence rates have been shown to be 4 to 7 times greater than in the general population (Gilks *et al.*, 1990; Elliott *et al.*, 1990; Eriki *et al.*, 1991; Muganga, Nkuadiolandu and Mashako, 1991; Batungwanayo *et al.*, 1993). However, research into the effects of HIV on childhood tuberculosis has lagged behind partly due to the limited influence which it has on the immediate epidemiology of the disease within the community (IUALTD, 1991). Furthermore, there are limitations to designing studies of TB in children. Excellent reviews on childhood TB (Jacobs and Starke, 1993a; Wong and Oppenheimer, 1994; Coovadia, 1994; Donald, 1994) have brought to light the problems associated with assessing the magnitude of the TB problem

in children. The diagnosis of pediatric tuberculosis is conventionally based on a combination of clinical and laboratory criteria (Stegen, Jones and Kaplan, 1969). Sputum and gastric fluid yield of mycobacteria on Ziehl-Neelsen staining is low and often it cannot be obtained from children for examination. Lack of appropriate radiology and laboratory facilities in developing countries add to underdiagnosis and misdiagnosis. Even in countries where advanced diagnostic facilities are available diagnosis can only be culture confirmed in about 40% cases (Starke and Taylor Watts, 1989). Despite these limitations, important data on childhood TB in light of the HIV epidemic are now emerging both from developed countries (Moss *et al.*, 1992; Khouri *et al.*, 1992; Bakshi *et al.*, 1993; Drucker *et al.*, 1994; Gutman *et al.*, 1994) and developing countries (Cathebras *et al.*, 1988; Muganga, Nkuadiolandu and Mashako, 1991; Bhat *et al.*, 1992; Chintu *et al.*, 1993a, b; Sassan-Morokro *et al.*, 1994; Luo *et al.*, 1995). This chapter highlights the changing epidemiological and clinical features of childhood TB in developing countries in light of the HIV epidemic.

EPIDEMIOLOGICAL FEATURES

According to recent estimates, approximately 90 million new cases of TB will occur world-

AIDS and Respiratory Medicine. Edited by A. Zumla, M.A. Johnson and R.F. Miller. Published in 1997 by Chapman & Hall, London. ISBN 0 412 60140 0

wide during the decade 1990 to 2000 (Dolin, Raviglione and Kochi, 1994). In January 1992 the World Health Organization (WHO) estimated that between 9 and 11 million adults and one million children, mostly in developing countries, had been infected with HIV and that in early 1992 approximately 4 million people were infected with both HIV and TB with the great majority (3.12 million) in Sub-Saharan Africa (WHO, 1992a; Raviglione, Snider and Kochi, 1995). Data from Sub-Saharan Africa show that a serious TB epidemic linked to HIV infection is also currently in progress in children (Cathebras *et al.*, 1988; Muganga, Nkuadiolandu and Mashako, 1991; Bhat *et al.*, 1992; Chintu *et al.*, 1993a; Luo *et al.*, 1994; Sassan-Morokro *et al.*, 1994). From a global perspective, comprehensive data on the importance of tuberculosis in HIV-infected children remain scarce.

In contrast to the picture in the USA and Europe, over 80% of HIV infections in Africa are attributable to heterosexual transmission, mother to child transmission and 'other risk factors' account for the remaining 20% (WHO, 1992a). Women acquire HIV as often as men in Africa and the number of children affected by HIV disease is increasing dramatically. HIV-seropositivity rates in pregnant women are estimated to be between 20 to 30% in certain Central Africa countries (WHO, 1995) and significant numbers are thought to transmit the infection to their children. Newborns are particularly vulnerable to TB if the mother has active disease. In a cohort of infants born to HIV-infected mothers in Lusaka followed up for 3 years, 12% of the children developed TB (Hira *et al.*, 1989). In those infants who were HIV-seropositive, TB manifested clinically in more than 25% of cases within the first 2 years of life. A study from Kinshasa, Zaire, showed that TB occurred in 28% of 60 HIV-seropositive infants in the first year of life (Muganga, Nkuadiolandu and Mashako, 1991).

In a 3-year follow up study of 16 HIV-seropositive children aged between 5

and 12 years in Kigali, Rwanda, TB was diagnosed in 4 out of 16 HIV-seropositive children (LePage *et al.*, 1991) while a study from the Central African Republic in 1988 reported 4 out of 37 children with TB were HIV-seropositive (Cathebras *et al.*, 1988). The overall prevalence of HIV-1 in 289 children with TB in Abidjan, Ivory Coast, was 11.8% (Sassan-Morokro *et al.*, 1994). Recent studies from Zambia illustrate that the close association between TB and HIV infection seen in adults also holds true for children (Bhat *et al.*, 1992; Chintu *et al.*, 1993a, b; Luo *et al.*, 1994). The risk of TB in Zambian children was found to be nearly six times greater in HIV-seropositive children relative to HIV-seronegative ones. The HIV seroprevalence rates in children with TB presenting to the University Teaching Hospital in Lusaka, Zambia, have risen at an alarming rate with studies documenting rates of 24% in 1989, 37% in 1990 (Chintu *et al.*, 1993b), 56% in 1991 (Luo *et al.*, 1994a), and 68.9% in 1992 (Luo *et al.*, 1994b). Data from the same studies show that all pediatric age groups are affected by dual infection with TB and HIV. These data reveal a serious TB epidemic closely linked with HIV in children in developing countries.

DIAGNOSIS OF PEDIATRIC TUBERCULOSIS

One of the bugbears of pediatric TB research and clinical practice has been the difficulty with which an accurate diagnosis of TB with or without bacteriological confirmation can be made and the diagnosis of TB in children remains difficult even in the best centers (Glassroth, 1993; Starke, 1993b; Donald, 1994). The diagnosis of pediatric TB continues largely to be a clinical one and this is particularly so in infants and small children in whom the disease is often non-specific and sputum induction or gastric lavage is difficult. Several diagnostic criteria have been devised by pediatricians and combinations of symptoms and signs with diagnostic scoring

Table 10.1   Clinical features of 237 children with tuberculosis in Lusaka, Zambia

Clinical presentation	HIV+ve	HIV−ve	(HIV+ve % of total)
Pneumonia	78	126	32.9
Miliary (disseminated)	3	6	1.3
Pleural effusion	0	5	0
Lymphadenopathy	3	8	1.3
Pericardial effusion	2	2	0.8
Abdominal	0	2	0
Bone	1	0	0.4
Meningitis	1	0	0.4
Total	88	149	37

(Adapted from Chintu *et al.*, 1993a, *Paediatric Infectious Diseases*, with permission.)

appear to be useful (Stegen, Jones and Kaplan, 1969; Cundall, 1986; IUALTD, 1991; Starke, 1993; Donald, 1994). The lack of a definitive diagnostic tool for pediatric tuberculosis is a limiting factor for ascertaining the actual size of the TB problem in children. Current techniques for the diagnosis of TB are resource intensive, slow and not ideally sensitive or specific (Starke, 1993b; Glassroth, 1993; Donald, 1994). The need for more rapid, reliable, sensitive and specific diagnostic tests and improvement of the clinical criteria for the diagnosis of TB remain a high research priority.

CLINICAL FEATURES OF TB IN HIV-INFECTED CHILDREN

A changing pattern of clinical disease is seen in HIV-seropositive adults with TB (Chaisson *et al.*, 1987, 1989; Colebunders *et al.*, 1989; Elliott *et al.*, 1990; Gilks *et al.*, 1990; Barnes *et al.*, 1991; Sudre, ten Dam and Kochi, 1992; Huebner and Castro, 1995; Castro, 1995). These studies have indicated that adult patients with TB co-infected with HIV frequently present with atypical clinical presentations. They often do not produce sputum, and when they do, mycobacteria are often absent from sputum smears on micro-

scopy. Sputum cultures are often negative; the chest X-ray appearances can be atypical and extrapulmonary manifestations appear more common. Studies of clinical presentations of TB in HIV-seropositive children are now emerging. A 10-year retrospective study of 345 HIV-seropositive children in Miami, Florida, USA (Khouri *et al.*, 1992) showed 9 cases of TB. These HIV-seropositive children were shown to have dominant extrapulmonary features. A study of Zambian children with TB co-infected with HIV (Chintu *et al.*, 1993a) indicated that the clinical picture of TB in HIV-infected children does not appear to differ significantly from HIV-seronegative cases, although miliary TB and lymphadenopathy appear to occur more commonly in the HIV-seropositive group (Table 10.1). The predominant clinical presentation of TB in both HIV-seropositive and HIV-seronegative Zambian children is that of pulmonary TB (Figures 10.1–3) and that of lymphadenopathy. Pericardial effusion (Figures 10.4a and 10.4b), meningitis, ascites and bone involvement are less common presentations.

Tuberculosis is a predominant cause of pleural effusions in adult patients and is strongly associated with HIV-1 infection (Batungwanayo *et al.*, 1993). In contrast to this, the results of the Zambian pediatric

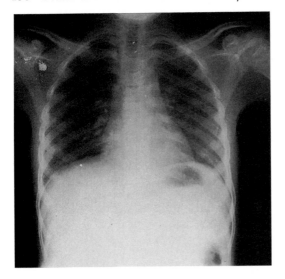

Fig. 10.1 Chest X-ray of an HIV-seropositive child showing interstitial infiltrates and hilar involvement.

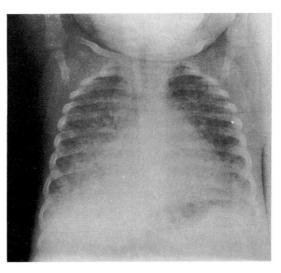

Fig. 10.3 Chest X-ray of a 10-month-old HIV-seropositive child with extensive miliary mottling.

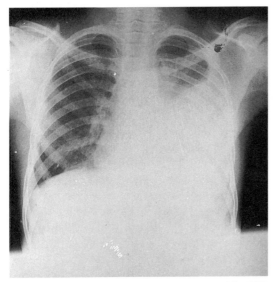

Fig. 10.2 Chest X-ray of an 11-year-old HIV-seropositive child with left-sided tuberculous pleural effusion.

studies show that pleural effusions are not an important feature of TB in HIV-infected children (Chintu *et al.*, 1993a; Luo *et al.*, 1994a).

PATIENT COMPLIANCE AND FOLLOW-UP

Factors responsible in part for the breakdown of TB control programs and the emergence of drug resistance include patients' non-compliance of anti-TB treatment and that of non-attendance at follow-up clinics. In a study of Zambian children with TB, Luo *et al.* (1994) recorded over 50% of children were lost to follow-up within 3 months of initiation of therapy. Prolonged compliance is difficult to achieve even in the more organized health systems in the USA and Europe (Starke, 1993b). Compliance is further hindered by the effects of HIV on the health of children's parents and also by the growing problem of the disintegration of the extended family support system caused by the HIV pandemic. An active search for clinic non-attenders to minimize loss to follow-up should be carried out. Furthermore, education of parents/guardians, provision of better access to health facilities and directly observed therapy may improve management outcome. Non-attendance has several complicated facets to it and operational research

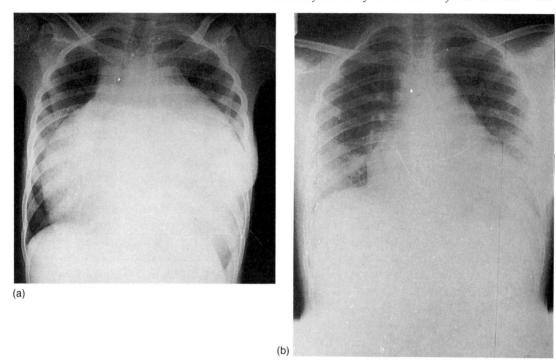

(a)

(b)

Fig. 10.4 (a) Chest X-ray of a 14-year-old HIV-seropositive child with massive pericardial effusion. (b) Same child after four months of anti-TB treatment with rifampicin, isoniazid and pyrazinamide (with prednisolone).

studies should identify the reasons and possible solutions for them. Patient compliance with antituberculous therapy in children will continue to pose one of the most important stumbling blocks for control programs and for clinical studies assessing effective anti-TB treatment and chemoprophylaxis regimens.

ANTI-TB TREATMENT

Recent reviews have dealt with the treatment of TB (Commentary, 1995) and this is discussed in detail elsewhere in this book. Optimal treatment for TB in children infected with HIV has not been established. Data on the efficacy of treatment regimens in children co-infected with TB and HIV are only just emerging and current opinion is that HIV-seropositive children with drug-susceptible TB should receive the same regimen as

HIV-infected adults with TB (two months of isoniazid, rifampicin, pyrazinamide followed by isoniazid and rifampicin for a further four months). In areas of high endemicity, treatment should be continued for a minimum period of 9 months and for at least 6 months after culture conversion as evidenced by 3 negative cultures, or a clinical response is noted. Because it is difficult to monitor toxicity from ethambutol, this agent is less used in children.

In general, children tend to tolerate anti-TB therapy better than adults. While historically most clinical trials of TB chemotherapy have been carried out in adults, literature on short-course chemotherapy in children is accumulating. In the treatment of pulmonary TB and TB lymphadenitis, the use of 3-drug regimens for 6 months (isoniazid, rifampicin, plus pyrazinamide or streptomycin for the first 2 months and rifampicin and isoniazid for the remaining 4 months) is thought to be just as effective as a 9 to 12 month regimen in the treatment of pulmonary TB and TB lymphadenitis (Starke, 1992a, 1993; Biddulph, 1990; Kumar, 1990). While initial response to therapy in both HIV-seropositive and HIV-seronegative children appears encouraging, long-term follow-up studies in developing countries show that HIV-seropositive children with TB appear to have a higher mortality rate (Chintu *et al.*, 1993a, b; Luo *et al.*, 1994). The reasons for a higher mortality rate among HIV-infected children remain to be ascertained. Possible reasons are: an inadequate immune response, drug resistance, or other concomitant HIV-associated complications such as diarrhea, malnutrition and failure to thrive. Corticosteroids (prednisolone or dexamethasone) appear to be useful adjuncts to anti-TB chemotherapy and are beneficial in the management of TB in children when the host inflammatory reaction contributes significantly to tissue damage as occurs in TB meningitis, miliary TB, large pleural effusions and massive pericardial effusions (Figures 10.4a and 10.4b). Data on the usefulness of continuation of lifelong therapy with isoniazid in children co-infected with HIV and TB after completion of anti-TB therapy are not available.

POTENTIAL DANGERS OF ANTI-TB TREATMENT

Cutaneous hypersensitivity reactions attributed to thioacetazone during antituberculous therapy of African adults infected with HIV-1 have been well documented (Nunn *et al.*, 1991). A study of children in Zambia (Chintu *et al.*, 1993b) monitored adverse drug reactions during anti-tuberculous treatment over an 18-month period (1 April 1990 to 31 October 1991) of 237 children with a clinical diagnosis of tuberculosis (125 males and 112 females;

88/237 being HIV-1 seropositive). 22 out of the 237 (9.3%) children with tuberculosis developed hypersensitivity skin reactions during the course of therapy. Adverse skin reactions were seen more frequently amongst HIV-seropositive than HIV-seronegative children. These represented 17 out of 88 HIV-infected children (19.3%) and 3 out of 149 HIV-seronegative children (2.0%). These skin reactions occurred after a period of treatment ranging between 2 to 4 weeks among 14 children on therapy with isoniazid, streptomycin, thioacetazone regimen and 8 children on isoniazid, streptomycin, thioacetazone and rifampicin regimen. Out of the 22 children, 12 developed the Stevens–Johnson syndrome (SJS). All 12 of these children with SJS were HIV-seropositive. The mortality amongst these children who developed the SJS was 91% (11 out of 12 died within three days of onset of the reaction). No further reactions were observed in those 11 children who recovered from the cutaneous hypersensitivity reactions after thioacetazone was discontinued over a period of 6 months of further anti-tuberculous therapy. The results of this study were in part responsible for the recommendations put forward by the WHO to avoid the use of thioacetazone in the treatment of tuberculosis in children infected with HIV (WHO, 1992b). The underlying pathophysiological mechanisms responsible for the development of the Stevens–Johnson syndrome are not clear. Importantly, there appears no adequate explanation as to why only certain HIV-positive individuals should react so adversely to thioacetazone. Identification of clinical or immunological characteristics (of patients who have experienced adverse reactions to thioacetazone) that differentiate them from other HIV-infected patients may be of importance. This analysis could help resource-poor countries to identify at-risk groups and tailor treatment regimens which contain thioacetazone for their HIV-infected individuals.

STRATEGIES FOR PREVENTION OF TB IN HIV-INFECTED CHILDREN

The main strategies currently being practiced in the control of TB in children are to improve the cure rate of adult and pediatric TB, and the widescale BCG vaccination of children. The principles of these strategies still hold true even in the face of the HIV pandemic. Case finding and diagnosing adult and pediatric cases of TB quickly and rendering them non-infectious by adequate treatment could remove a substantial portion of sources of infection. The recent increased burden of HIV-associated TB in children requires interventions to limit its occurrence in HIV-positive individuals.

While preventive therapy for TB in HIV-infected adults has been extensively investigated (O'Brien and Perriens, 1995; De Cock, Grant and Porter, 1995), controlled clinical trials to assess the effects of chemoprophylaxis with anti-TB drugs for the prevention of drug susceptible TB infection without disease in HIV-seropositive children are lacking. The high prevalence rates of TB and HIV in children, the problems encountered with patient compliance and the high cost of administering effective chemoprophylaxis, make chemoprophylaxis in HIV-positive children a low priority in developing countries.

ROLE OF BCG

Routine immunization with BCG at birth is used in most developing countries without the knowledge of HIV status of the children (Bregere, 1988; Quinn, 1989; Weltran and Rose, 1993). The role of BCG vaccination in preventing tuberculosis when given to HIV-infected children remains unknown. Although there have been reports of adverse reactions to BCG such as lymphadenitis, abscess and fistula formation and disseminated disease among HIV-infected individuals receiving BCG, most cases resolved without major complications. Prospective follow-up of a group of infants who were immunized with BCG after birth showed that the frequency of BCG-related lymphadenitis in HIV-infected children did not differ significantly from the group of HIV-uninfected children (Lallemant-Le *et al.*, 1991; O'Brien *et al.*, 1995a, b). It is generally accepted that BCG vaccine is relatively safe in asymptomatic HIV-infected children. Current WHO recommendations for countries where TB is common are that BCG should be administered to infants as early as possible even in cases where the mother is known to be infected with HIV (Tarantola and Mann, 1987; Von Reyn, Clements and Manu, 1987; Quinn, 1989). However, BCG should be withheld from known, symptomatic HIV-infected children.

CONCLUSIONS

TB in HIV-infected children is becoming a major cause of morbidity and mortality in developing countries. Despite the availability of curative therapy, the incidence of TB in children and adults is increasing at an alarming rate and is posing a grave threat to TB control programs in developing countries. This increase is closely linked to the HIV epidemic. Improved methods for the diagnosis of TB in children are required. Several prospective studies to define basic clinical, microbiological and epidemiological features of the resurgence of childhood TB in light of the HIV epidemic are urgently required.

ACKNOWLEDGMENTS

Dr A. Zumla acknowledges support from the Camden and Islington Community Health Services NHS Trust, London, United Kingdom.

REFERENCES

Bakshi, S.S., Alvarez, D. Hilfer, C.L. *et al.* (1993) Tuberculosis in human immunodeficiency virus-infected children. A family infection. *Am. J. Dis. Child.*, **147**, 3, 320–4.

Barnes, P.F., Bloch, A.B., Davidson, P.T. and Snider, D.E. Jr. (1991) Tuberculosis in patients with human immunodeficiency virus infection. *N. Engl. J. Med.*, :1644–9.

Bass, J.B. Jr., Farer, L.S., Hopewell, P.C. *et al.* (1994) Treatment of tuberculosis and tuberculosis infection in adults and children. American Thoracic Society and The Centers for Disease Control and Prevention. *Am. J. Respir. Crit. Care Med.*, **149**;5, 1359–74.

Batungwanayo, J., Taelman, H., Allen, S. *et al.* (1993) Pleural effusion, tuberculosis and HIV-1 infection in Kigali, Rwanda. *AIDS*, **7**, 73–39.

Beyers, N., Gie, R.P., Schaaf, H.S. *et al.* (1994) Delay in the diagnosis, notification and initiation of treatment and compliance in children with tuberculosis. *Tuber. Lung Dis.*, **75**, 4, 260–65.

Bhat, G.J., Diwan, V.K., Chintu, C. *et al.* (1992) HIV, BCG and TB in children: a case control study in Lusaka, Zambia. *J. Trop. Paediatr.*, **VI**, 1–VI:10.

Biddulph, J. (1990) Short course chemotherapy for childhood TB. *Paediatr. Infect. Dis. J.*, **9**, 794–801.

Bregere, P. (1988) BCG vaccination and AIDS. *Bull. Int. Un. TB Lung Dis.*, **63**, 4, 40–1.

Castro, K.G. (1995) Tuberculosis as an opportunistic disease in persons infected with human immunodeficiency virus. *Clin. Infect. Dis*, **21**, suppl. 1, S66–S77.

Cathebras, P., Vohito, J.A., Yete, M.L. *et al.* (1988) Tuberculosis et infection par le virus de l'immunodeficience humaine en Republique Centrafricaine. *Med. Trop.*, **48**, 401–7.

Chaisson, R.E., Shecter, G.F., Theuer, C.P. *et al.* (1987) Tuberculosis in patients with the acquired immunodeficiency syndrome. Clinical features, response to therapy, and survival. *Am. Rev. Respir. Dis.*, **136**, 570–4.

Chaisson, R.E. and Slutkin, G. (1989) Tuberculosis and human immunodeficiency virus infection. *J. Infect. Dis.*, **159**, 1:96–100.

Chintu, C., Bhatt, G., Luo, C. *et al.* (1993a) Seroprevalence of HIV-1 in Zambian children with tuberculosis. *Paediatr. Infect. Dis. J.*, **12**, 499–504.

Chintu, C., Luo, C., Bhat, G. *et al.* (1993b) Cutaneous hypersensitivity reactions to thioacetazone in the treatment of tuberculosis in Zambian children infected with HIV-1. *Arch. Dis. Child.*, **68**, 665–8.

Chintu, C. and Zumla, A. (1995) Childhood

tuberculosis and infection with the human immunodeficiency virus. *J. Roy. Coll. Phys.*, **29**, 2,92–4.

Colebunders, R.L., Ryder, R.W., Nzilambi, N. *et al.* (1989) HIV infection in patients with tuberculosis in Kinshasha, Zaire. *Am. Rev. Respir. Dis.*, **139**, 1082–5.

Commentary (1995) American Thoracic Society: Treatment of tuberculosis infection in adults and children. *Clin. Infect. Dis.*, **21**, 9–27.

Coovadia, H. M. (1994) Tuberculosis in Children, chapter 5 in *A Century of Tuberculosis – A South African Perspective*, (eds H.M. Coovadia and S.R. Benatar), Oxford University Press, Cape Town, pp. 91–110.

Cundall, D.B. (1986) The diagnosis of pulmonary tuberculosis in malnourished Kenyan children. *Ann. Trop. Paed.*, **6**, 249–55.

De Cock, K.M., Grant, A. and Porter, J.H. (1995) Preventive therapy for TB in HIV-infected persons: international recommendations, research and practice. *Lancet*, **345**, 833–6.

Dolin, P.J., Raviglione, M.C. and Kochi, A. (1994) Global tuberculosis incidence and mortality during 1990–2000. *Bull. WHO*, **72**, 213–20.

Donald, P.R. (1994) Diagnostic considerations in management and epidemiology, chapter 15 in *A Century of Tuberculosis – a South African Perspective*, (eds H.M Coovadia and S.R. Benatar), Oxford University Press, Cape Town, pp. 243–57.

Drucker, E., Alcabes, P., Bosworth, W. *et al.* (1994) Childbood tuberculosis in Bronx, New York. *Lancet*, **343**, 1482–5.

Elliott, A.M., Luo, N.P., Tembo, G. *et al.* (1990) Impact of HIV on tuberculosis in Zambia: a cross sectional study. *Br. Med. J.* **301**, 412–15.

Elliott, A.M., Hayes, R.J., Halwindi, B. *et al.* (1993) The impact of HIV on infectiousness of pulmonary tuberculosis: a community study in Zambia. *AIDS*, **7**, 7, 981–7.

Eriki, P.P., Okwera, A., Aisu, T. *et al.* (1991) The influence of human immunodeficiency virus infection in Kampala, Uganda. *Am. Rev. Respir. Dis.*, **143**, 185–7.

Gilks, C.F., Brindle, R.J., Otieno, L.S. *et al.* (1990) Extrapulmonary and disseminated tuberculosis in HIV-1 seropositive patients presenting to the acute medical services in Nairobi. *AIDS*, **4**, 981–5.

Girling, D.J. (1982) Adverse effects of antituberculosis drugs. *Drugs*, **23**, 56.

Glassroth, J. (1993) Diagnosis of tuberculosis. Chapter 8, in *Tuberculosis*, Marcel-Dekker, New

York, pp. 149–65.

Gutman, L.T., Moye, J., Zimmer, B. and Tian, C. (1994) Tuberculosis in human immunodeficiency virus – exposed or infected United States children. *Pediatr. Infect. Dis. J.*, **13**, 11, 963–8.

Hira, S.K., Mwale, C., Kamanga, J. *et al.* (1989) Perinatal transmission of HIV in Zambia. *Br. Med. J.* **299**, 1250–2.

Huebner, R.E. and Castro, K.G. (1995) The changing face of tuberculosis. *Ann. Rev. Med.*, **46**, 47–55.

IUALTD (1991) Tuberculosis in children. Guidelines for diagnosis, prevention and treatment. A statement of the scientific committee of the IUALTD. *Bull. Int. Union Tuber. Lung. Dis.*, **66**, 61–7.

Jacobs, R.F. and Starke, J.R. (1993) Tuberculosis in children. *Med. Clin. N. Am.*, **77**, 6, 1335–13351.

Jones, D.S., Malecki, J.M., Bigler, W.J. *et al.* (1992) Pediatric tuberculosis and human immunodeficiency virus infection in Palm Beach County, Florida. *Am. J. Dis. Child.*, **146**, 10, 1166–70.

Khouri, Y.F., Mastrucci, M.T., Hutto, C. *et al.* (1987) *Mycobacterium tuberculosis* in children with the human immunodeficiency virus infection and routine childhood immunisations. *Lancet*, **2**, 669–72.

Khouri, Y.F., Mastrucci, M.T., Mitchell, C.D. *et al.* (1992) *Mycobacterium tuberculosis* in children with the human immunodeficiency virus infection. *Pediatr. Infect. Dis. J*, **11**, 11, 950–5.

Kumar, K.L., Dhand, R., Singhi, P.D. and Rao K.L.N. (1990) A randomized trial of intermittent short course chemotherapy for childhood tuberculosis. *Pediatr. Infect. Dis. J.*, **9**, 802–6.

Lallemant-Le, C.S., Lallament, M., Cheynier, D. *et al.* (1991) BCG immunization in infants born to HIV-1 seropositive mothers. *AIDS*, **5** 195–9.

LePage, P., Van de Perre, C., Van Vliet, G. *et al.* (1991) Clinical and endocrinologic manifestations in perinatally acquired human immunodeficiency virus type-1 infected children aged 5 years or older. *Am. J. Dis. Child.*, **145**, 11, 1248–51.

Luo, C., Chintu, C., Bhatt, G. *et al.* (1994) HIV-infection in Zambian children with tuberculosis: changing seroprevalence and evaluation of a thiacetazone-free regimen. *Tuber. Lung Dis.*, **75**, 11–115.

Luo, C., Chintu, C., Bhatt, G. *et al.* (1996) Impact of HIV on common paediatric illnesses in Zambia. *J. Trop. Paediatr.*, **41**, 1–5.

Moss, W.J., Dedyo, T., Suarez, M. *et al.* (1992) Tuberculosis in children infected with human immunodeficiency virus: a report of five cases. *Paediatr. Infect. Dis. J.*, **11**, 114–20.

Muganga, N., Nkuadiolandu, A. and Mashako, L.M. (1991) Clinical manifestations of AIDS in children in Kinshasha. *Paediatrie*, **46**, 12, 825–9.

Nunn, P., Kibuga, D., Gathua, S. *et al.* (1991) Cutaneous hypersensitivity reactions due to thiacetazone in HIV-1 seropositive patients treated for tuberculosis. *Lancet*, **339**, 627–30.

O'Brien, R.J. and Perriens, J.H. (1995a) Preventive therapy for tuberculosis in HIV infection: the promise and the reality. *AIDS*, **9**, 665–73.

O'Brien, K.L., Ruff, A.J., Louis, MA. *et al.* (1995b) Bacillus Calmette-Guérin complications in children born to HIV-1 infected women with a review of literature. *Pediatrics*, **95**, 414–18.

Quinn, T.C. (1989) Interactions of the human immunodeficiency virus and tuberculosis and the implication for BCG vaccination. *Rev. Infect. Dis.*, **11**, S379–S384.

Raviglione, M.C., Narain, J.P. and Kochi, A. (1992) HIV-associated tuberculosis in developing countries: clinical features, diagnosis and treatment. *Bull WHO*, **70**, 4, 515–26.

Raviglione, M.C., Snider, D.E. and Kochi, A. (1995) Global epidemiology of tuberculosis. Morbidity and mortality of a worldwide epidemic. *JAMA*, **273**, 3, 220–6.

Report, 1992 Severe hypersensitivity reactions among HIV-seropositive patients with tuberculosis treated with thiacetazone. *WHO Wkly. Epidem. Rec*, 1/2, 1–3.

Sassan–Morokro, M., De Cock, K.M. Ackah, A. *et al.* (1994) Tuberculosis and HIV infection in children in Abidjan, Côte d'Ivoire. *Trans. Roy. Soc. Trop. Med. Hyg.*, **88**, 2, 178–81.

Starke, J.R. (1992) Tuberculosis in children with acquired immunodeficiency syndrome. *Paediatr. Infect. Dis. J.*, **11**, 8, 683–4.

Starke, J.R. (1993a) Tuberculosis in children. Chapter 16 in *Tuberculosis*, Marcel-Dekker, New York, pp. 329–67.

Starke, J.R. (1993b) Childhood tuberculosis. A diagnostic dilemma. *Chest*, **104**, 2, 393–404.

Starke, J.R. and Taylor-Watts, R.T. (1989) Tuberculosis in the paediatric population in Houston, Texas. *Pediatrics*, **84**, 28–35.

Stegen, G., Jones, K. and Kaplan, P. (1969) Criteria for guidance in the diagnosis of tuberculosis.

Pediatrics, **43**, 2, 260–3.

Sudre, P., ten Dam, H.G. and Kochi, A. (1992) Tuberculosis: a global overview of the situation today. *Bull. WHO*, **70**, 149–59.

Tarantola, D. and Mann, J.M. (1987) Acquired immunodeficiency syndrome (AIDS) expanded programmes on immunisation. Special Programme on AIDS. Geneva, WHO, 1987.

Tomlinson, D.R., Moss, F., McCarty, M. *et al.* (1992) Tuberculosis in HIV seropositive individuals – a retrospective analysis. *Int. J. STD. AIDS*, **3**, 1, 38–45.

Von Reyn, C.F., Clements, C.J. and Manu, J.M. (1987) Human immunodeficiency virus and routine childhood immunisations. *Lancet*, **2**, 669–72.

Weltran, A.C. and Rose, D.N. (1993) The safety of Bacille Calmette-Guérin vaccination in HIV infection and AIDS. *AIDS*, **7**, 149–57.

WHO (1992a) Global Programme on AIDS. Current and future dimensions of HIV/AIDS pandemic. A capsule summary. Document WHO/GPA/RES/SF/92.1.

WHO (1992b) Severe hypersensitivity reactions to thiacetazone among HIV-seropositive patients with tuberculosis treated with thiacetazone. *Wkly Epidemiol. Rec.* **67**, 1–3.

WHO (1995) Tuberculosis and HIV research: working towards solutions. II. Impact of HIV on tuberculosis control. WHO/TB/95. **183**, 6–8.

Wirima, J.J. and Harries, A.D. (1991) Stevens–Johnson syndrome during anti-tuberculosis chemotherapy in HIV-seropositive patients: report on six cases. *East Afr. Med. J.*, **68**, 1, 64–6.

Wong, G.W.K. and Oppenheimer, S.J. (1994) Childhood tuberculosis. Chapter 11 in *Clinical Tuberculosis*, (ed. P.D.O. Davies), Chapman & Hall, London, pp. 211–23.

Peter Godfrey-Faussett

Preceding chapters of this book have made it clear that the pattern of tuberculosis has changed, both clinically and epidemiologically. These changes have created new challenges for the diagnosis of tuberculosis and these will be the focus of the present chapter.

INDEX OF SUSPICION

The risk of developing tuberculosis in those already infected with HIV depends on the prevalence of latent infection with *Mycobacterium tuberculosis* and the risk of new infection with the bacillus. An appreciation of these two factors allows one to develop an index of suspicion for the disease. Throughout the developing world, the high risk of infection with *Mycobacterium tuberculosis* has led to the majority of adults being infected and in these societies tuberculosis is being seen as one of the commonest secondary diseases associated with HIV (Gilks *et al.*, 1990; Lucas *et al.*, 1993). In contrast, there is little disease due to *Mycobacterium avium* and this has allowed sputum microscopy to retain its specificity as a diagnostic tool.

Unlike some other organisms discussed in previous chapters, *Mycobacterium tuberculosis* is a virulent pathogen and is therefore able to cause disease in patients with minimal immunosuppression who are infected with HIV. These patients present with features indistinguishable from those seen before the HIV era. As immunosuppression deepens, measured either by the number of CD4-positive lymphocytes or by more clinical markers of immunosuppression, tuberculosis becomes an increasingly disseminated disease and provokes a less brisk immune response. As a result, cavitation becomes rarer, lesions are less confined to the apices and extrapulmonary disease becomes commoner (Jones *et al.*, 1993; Mukadi *et al.*, 1993). A consequence of these changes is that a smaller proportion of patients have positive sputum smears on direct microscopy.

Another consequence of immunosuppression is an increased susceptibility to disease following recent infection, or re-infection (Daley *et al.*, 1992). This may also explain the increase in numbers of cases with disease reminiscent of primary infection with pleural effusions, hilar lymphadenopathy and miliary spread.

THE CLINICAL CHALLENGE

It should be clear from the above that the challenge in the developing world is to document mycobacterial infection in the face

AIDS and Respiratory Medicine. Edited by A. Zumla, M.A. Johnson and R.F. Miller. Published in 1997 by Chapman & Hall, London. ISBN 0 412 60140 0

of reduced numbers of bacilli found in the sputum and the increase in the number of cases of extrapulmonary disease. On the other hand, mycobacterial disease in those infected with HIV in the industrialized world is more frequently due to *Mycobacterium avium*, particularly in those with advanced immunosuppression.

There is therefore a real need to distinguish between different acid-fast bacilli and to use traditional methods involving cultivation may take weeks. The risk of infection with *Mycobacterium tuberculosis* is also less generalized which leads to higher notification rates of HIV-related tuberculosis among those countries in which the pool of people infected with *Mycobacterium tuberculosis* overlaps with those infected with HIV (Guelar *et al.*, 1994).

One of the effects of these changes in clinical and epidemiological features has been to delay the diagnosis. In patients with culture-confirmed tuberculosis in two American inner city hospitals, 20% either died or were discharged before the diagnosis was made (Mathur *et al.*, 1994). In contrast, in countries in Africa where HIV and tuberculosis are common and diagnostic facilities sparse, many patients are being treated on the basis of a presumed diagnosis and overdiagnosis may be as common as delay. For instance, in Malawi, while the number of smear positive cases has doubled since 1985, the number of smear negative cases has quadrupled (Nunn, 1994).

EFFECTS OF HIV ON TRADITIONAL DIAGNOSTIC TECHNIQUES

Radiological diagnosis of tuberculosis has never been ideal. The difficulty in achieving reproducibility and consensus over interpretation was demonstrated long before HIV appeared on the scene (Springett, Wasler and Nyboe, 1967; Khan *et al.*, 1977). HIV has however made the situation still more difficult, with proven disease occurring in the mid and lower zones more commonly than before (Pitchenik *et al.*, 1984; Pitchenik and Robinson, 1985) often with lymphadenopathy (Pastores *et al.*, 1993) and non-specific infiltrates. Even a normal chest radiograph does not exclude active disease (Pedrobotet *et al.*, 1992).

Careful studies of the numbers of bacilli excreted from pulmonary lesions and the response to therapy show that HIV-infected patients have about one log less organisms in the sputum (Brindle *et al.*, 1993) which accords with clinical studies that show a higher proportion of smear-negative, culture-positive disease among HIV-seropositive subjects (Elliott *et al.*, 1990; Githui *et al.*, 1992).

The importance of nosocomial spread of tuberculosis is now widely appreciated and should lead to a higher index of suspicion in those patients who have been hospitalized (Diperri *et al.*, 1989; Coronado *et al.*, 1993; Kent *et al.*, 1994). Specialized units for the care of those infected with HIV will inevitably cluster together patients with active tuberculosis and those most susceptible to infection. In the developing world, the same situation may well apply in general medical facilities where a high proportion of inpatients may be HIV-seropositive and those with undiagnosed tuberculosis may be sharing overcrowded ward space. Early specific diagnosis would allow a rationalization of isolation facilities and early institution of chemotherapy which should prevent ongoing transmission.

Pediatric tuberculosis has always been a difficult diagnosis, with bacteriological confirmation only possible in the minority of cases (Cundall, 1986; Starke and Taylor-Watts, 1989). Although HIV has led to an upsurge in notifications of pediatric disease (Chintu *et al.*, 1993; Drucker *et al.*, 1994) that mirrors the changes in the adult population, the distinction between other respiratory conditions or the effects of the retroviral infection itself is a major challenge. Autopsy studies of adults with HIV infection in West Africa confirm tuberculosis to be a major pathogen (Lucas *et al.*, 1996) but, surprisingly, tuberculosis was seen very rarely in the pediatric age group with bacterial pathogens and *Pneumocystis carinii* predominating (Lucas *et al.*, 1996).

Clinicians faced with a patient who may have tuberculosis will therefore need to take into account the new epidemiology and clinical features of tuberculosis when taking their history and examining their patient. It is hoped that the advances in molecular technologies will soon lead to investigations to confirm or refute the diagnosis.

APPROACHES TO CONFIRM A DIAGNOSIS

Inevitably, new methods of diagnosis will become most available in the parts of the world with least tuberculosis. The emphasis here will be on benefits for the individual patient and resource allocation will be a relatively minor concern. In the parts of the world where tuberculosis is still killing millions and control programs are swamped by the rising tide of HIV-related disease, the role of any new techniques will have to be compared very critically to sputum microscopy which is already capable of detecting those cases most at risk of continuing to spread the epidemic. Nonetheless, the clinical officer in these situations is still faced with many symptomatic people with negative sputum smears, for whom he must decide how best to care (Lherminez, 1993).

The new diagnostic strategies can be broadly divided into those that aim to demonstrate the response of the host to the tubercle bacilli and those that try to detect the bacillus, or some component of it, directly.

HOST RESPONSE TO *MYCOBACTERIUM TUBERCULOSIS*

Tests designed to detect the reaction of the human host to the tubercle bacilli may be based on the immune response, either cellular or humoral, or on less specific markers of the body's defensive mechanisms. Because antibody and cell-mediated responses may be long lasting, the parameters of a given test must be carefully evaluated to allow interpretation. Some tests may be markers of infection with *Mycobacterium tuberculosis*, others of active disease and others of previously treated infection. Furthermore, HIV itself has a profound effect on cellular immune responses and also alters humoral responses so that tests need to be revalidated to determine their role in HIV-related disease.

The tuberculin test, also known as the Mantoux test, is read as the size of induration produced in the skin of the forearm, following the delayed hypersensitivity reaction to an intradermal injection of purified protein derivative of *Mycobacterium tuberculosis*. It has long been the most widely accepted test of whether somebody has been infected with *Mycobacterium tuberculosis* and as such can be used to assess the risk of developing active disease. In regions where tuberculosis is endemic, much of the adult population has been infected with *Mycobacterium tuberculosis* and will have a positive reaction to the tuberculin test. However, the generalized cutaneous anergy seen with advancing immunosuppression, leads to many false negative reactions in the HIV-positive population (Graham *et al.*, 1992; Duncan *et al.*, 1995). Those who are neither anergic nor tuberculin-test positive are the least likely to develop active tuberculosis, while in both the anergic and the tuberculin-positive population the incidence is much greater (Selwyn *et al.*, 1989, 1992). Other cell-mediated tests have also been used to diagnose specific conditions (Choy *et al.*, 1994) and there has been some success in the veterinary field in measuring the gamma-interferon produced by stimulating whole blood with mycobacteria-specific proteins (Rothel *et al.*, 1990), a test that could be adapted for human use.

The idea of detecting specific antibodies against *Mycobacterium tuberculosis* to diagnose exposure, active disease or past history, is attractive and has been actively explored for almost a century. Although impressive results have been obtained with a variety of different targets and formats, none of the tests has entered widespread usage. The reality under which a test will finally be used is often overlooked by enthusiastic researchers. Since tuberculosis is not a common disease, the majority of patients investigated will not have it. The specificity of a test must therefore be extremely high if it is to be useful and the specificity can only be estimated accurately if large numbers of negative control samples are assayed. These negative controls must be taken from patients who might reasonably be investigated for tuberculosis but are in fact known not to have the illness. For a particular population it may be possible to define a cut-off to give a high enough specificity and retain a useful sensitivity (Wilkins and Ivanyi, 1990) or a likelihood ratio can be calculated (Verbon *et al.*, 1993) but until such tests are evaluated prospectively on larger and different populations, they will remain on the research laboratory bench. Ironically, the regions of the world with the highest prevalence of disease, in which new tests would be expected to have the best positive predictive value, are also those in which the diagnosis of smear-negative disease has been less of a priority while so much smear-positive disease remains inadequately treated. Once again, tests that have shown promise in some populations have not been shown to be useful in those infected with HIV (van der Werf *et al.*, 1992) and specific IgG responses appear to be extinguished particularly early (Saltini *et al.*, 1993).

There has also been a considerable amount written about non-specific markers of activation of cells that are important in the control of tuberculous infection. The most widely used test is the level of adenosine deaminase levels, an enzyme involved in purine catabolism, which can be assayed either in serum, or more usefully at the site of disease (Sanchez Hernandez *et al.*, 1991; Chiang *et al.*, 1994). The specificity of the assay will depend on the prevalence of other diseases that provoke a similar immune response (Petterson, Klochars and Weber, 1984). Other markers of macrophage activation such as neopterin may also be useful markers of disease but tend to be higher anyway in patients already infected with HIV (Chiang *et al.*, 1994; Hosp *et al.*, 1994) and so serve little diagnostic role.

DIRECT SEARCH FOR THE TUBERCLE BACILLUS

The poor specificity of indirect tests and the alteration in host responses that follows HIV infection make searching directly for the tubercle bacilli, or its constituents, an attractive option. As mentioned above, the lack of atypical mycobacteria in clinical specimens in developing countries means that sputum microscopy retains a high degree of specificity. Sensitivity however has fallen with the arrival of HIV. One study showed that while 79% of seronegative patients with positive cultures for *Mycobacterium tuberculosis* had positive microscopy also, the corresponding figure for HIV seronegative patients was 66% (Long *et al.*, 1991).

Culture of *Mycobacterium tuberculosis* remains the standard against which other tests must be compared for specificity. In addition to allowing for direct biochemical identification of the organism, it provides material for drug susceptibility testing. It will be some time before confidence in other tests, be they for detection of *Mycobacterium tuberculosis* or for drug susceptibility testing, is sufficient to allow culture to pass into history. However, the slow generation time of *Mycobacterium tuberculosis* does mean that results for traditional culture are not available for weeks rather than days. Radiospirometric culture techniques are a major step forward and are now becoming widely used. Growth is detected rapidly and the species of mycobacteria can then be ascertained, either by traditional means or by molecular tests (Telenti *et al.*, 1994). Furthermore, the technique adapts easily to include drug sensitivity results in a few extra days. The disadvantage of these techniques is the cost and the need to work with radioactive reagents. It is also worth pointing out that the problems of contamination that beset some of the molecular techniques (discussed below) also occur in the routine microbiological setting. Even laboratories used to handling mycobacteria can be demonstrated to be the sources of cross contamination (Small *et al.*, 1993; Das *et al.*, 1993) and 'outbreaks' of tuberculosis have also been attributed to contamination between radiospirometric machines (Small *et al.*, 1993).

The paucibacillary and extrapulmonary nature of HIV-related tuberculosis has led to increasingly invasive searches for specimens that can then be examined by traditional or novel techniques. In Africa, where atypical mycobacteria cause little disease, aspiration of lymph nodes with a wider needle than that used for cytology leads to a satisfying number of cases in whom microscopy shows caseation or acid-fast bacilli, thus avoiding the need for surgical biopsy and histology (Bem *et al.*, 1993). In the industrialized world, induced sputum (Klein and Motyl, 1993; Fishman *et al.*, 1994) or specimens obtained through a fiberoptic bronchoscope improve the yield (de Gracia *et al.*, 1988). These procedures will often be indicated already to exclude other pathologies, so the relatively small numbers of extra cases found beyond those found by microscopy of expectorated sputum should be seen as a bonus.

Blood may be cultured directly onto appropriate media, and has more success in seropositive patients than those without concurrent HIV infection (Shafer *et al.*, 1989).

Bone marrow examination may also increase the yield in patients with disseminated disease (Nichols *et al.*, 1991), as will needle biopsy of abnormal looking intrathoracic or abdominal nodes, under the control of bronchoscopic, ultrasonic, fluoroscopic or computed tomographic control.

ANTIGENS AND STRUCTURAL COMPONENTS

Immunoassays to detect mycobacterial antigens directly in clinical specimens have had some success, particularly with tuberculous meningitis (Radhakrishnan and Mathai, 1991), but tend to work less well on inhomogeneous samples such as sputum or respiratory secretions (Araj *et al.*, 1988). Culturing the specimen for a short time first may improve the accuracy (Raja *et al.*, 1988).

It is also possible to detect other specific bacillary constituents. Gas chromatography and mass spectrometry is cumbersome and expensive but can be modified to use flame ionization detection to pick up tuberculostearic acid, a structural component of mycobacterial cell walls (Herz *et al.*, 1994).

APPROACHES THROUGH MOLECULAR GENETICS

Although mycobacteria raise technical and safety issues when brought into laboratories that are more used to nonpathogenic *Escherichia coli* with less waxy cell walls, the recent advances that have been made in mycobacterial molecular genetics have led to better understanding of pathogenesis and epidemiology as well as to possibilities for diagnosis and avenues to explore for vaccine development (McFadden, 1990; Arruda *et al.*, 1993).

In the diagnostic field, detection of nucleic acids either directly by hybridization to a labeled probe or following amplification of specific sequences of DNA or RNA raises the exciting possibility of sensitive specific diagnosis that would provide an answer within hours rather than days or weeks.

As particular genes are cloned and sequenced, it becomes possible to select target sequences that, while present in every strain of *Mycobacterium tuberculosis*, are not found in any other species so far examined. Such sequences have been used as probes to try to detect small amounts of tuberculous DNA in clinical material (Pao *et al.*, 1988) or (as mentioned above) in early cultures. Sadly, the rheology of sputum and the resistance of the mycobacterial cell wall to standard procedures for extracting nucleic acids have led to a disappointingly poor sensitivity and the only commercial probe to be released was withdrawn when it was realized that it was little better than microscopy, despite considerably more effort and expense.

The description of the polymerase chain reaction using a thermostable DNA polymerase (Saiki *et al.*, 1988) has led to a flurry of activity to produce diagnostic tests for tuberculosis. In principle the exquisite sensitivity of PCR combined with the inherent specificity of the target DNA sequence makes it an attractive option. The first paper using PCR as a diagnostic test for tuberculosis appeared in 1989 (Brisson-Noel *et al.*, 1989) and since then there have been over 60 similar publications, attesting to the perceived importance of new diagnostic tools but also highlighting the difficulties experienced in taking the technique from the research bench into the routine lab. Nor is PCR the only amplification technique being developed with commercial backers. Ligase Chain Reaction (Winndeen, Batt and Wiedmann, 1993), Transcription Mediated Amplification (Gen-probe 'Amplified *Mycobacterium tuberculosis* Direct' assay (Jonas *et al.*, 1993; Miller, Hernandez and Cleary, 1994)) and Strand Displacement Amplification (Walker *et al.*, 1992; Spargo *et al.*, 1993), are all capable of exponential amplification of nucleic acids from a specific target, either by cycling the temperature (PCR, LCR) or by the dynamics of specific enzymes at a constant temperature (TMA, SDA). The limiting steps are likely to be similar for all these techniques, namely how to prevent contamination of reactions with the products of previous assays and how best to extract the mycobacterial nucleic acid from clinical material in a form that is easily amplified.

False positive results will usually be caused by contamination occurring at some stage from the collection of the sample to the analysis of the amplified product. That contamination occurs in routine settings has been known for a long time (Aber *et al.*, 1980) and reconfirmed by molecular techniques (Small *et al.*, 1993). However, all the amplification techniques are particularly susceptible to 'carryover' problems, where infinitesimal amounts of previous reactions are allowed to get into the reactions being prepared, by contaminating reagents, pipettes, laboratory staff's clothing or skin or through aerosols produced by opening the lids from microcentrifuge tubes.

The scale of the problem was demonstrated in a comparison of seven different laboratories, all of whom had already developed PCR-based assays with a view to diagnosing tuberculosis (Noordhoek *et al.*, 1994). In four of these labs, specificity was less than 80% and in the remaining labs the sensitivity was rather disappointing with only 60% of the samples with 5000 *Mycobacterium bovis* cells per ml being detected.

Measures to prevent contamination include strict physical separation of amplified product from the area where reactions are being set up, with dedicated equipment and no access to staff coming from the 'contaminated area' (Kwok and Higuchi, 1989). A three-room system adds additional security by preventing any DNA from entering the lab in which stock solutions are prepared and opened (Wilson *et al.*, 1993). Incorporating deoxy-uracil triphosphate into the reaction mixture, in the place of deoxy-thymidine means that amplified product can be rendered unamplifiable by uracil-N-glycosylase at the start of each reaction, leaving genuine target DNA unaffected (Longo *et al.*, 1990). Despite these precautions some false positives will continue to occur, so that all samples should be processed in duplicate and only considered positive if both duplicates contain product.

PCR works best with ultrapure reagents and solutions of predetermined concentrations. It is therefore not surprising that DNA extracted from complex body fluids, such as sputum, should sometimes be contaminated with substances that inhibit the polymerase. Although false negative results are a less common problem than false positives, the addition of target DNA that has been genetically engineered to produce a product of a different size when amplified by the same PCR, allows them to be quantified (Andersen *et al.*, 1993; Kox *et al.*, 1994).

'Nested' PCR involves amplifying DNA directly from a clinical sample and then taking a small aliquot of the resulting products and re-amplifying them using primers internal to the first set on the same target (Pierre *et al.*, 1991). The advantages are that any inhibiting substances that were extracted along with the DNA from the original sample and that may reduce the efficiency of the polymerase, will be diluted during the second reaction. The overall amplification will be increased, leading to greater sensitivity (although theoretically, single copies of the target sequence should be detectable with a single PCR). The product from the first reaction will only re-amplify if it is indeed the correct product of the same sequence as the original target, which reduces the need for a secondary hybridization or method to insure specificity. Furthermore, the product from the second reaction will not be amplified by the first reaction, so that carry-over contamination may be able to

be reduced, particularly if the number of cycles for the second reaction (which determines the degree of amplification) is not too many. However, these advantages are usually overshadowed by the fact that the reaction tube has to be opened half way through the assay and material transferred to a new set of tubes. This increases the likelihood of tube-to-tube contamination and cannot be performed within the strict segregation of amplified product from reaction tubes described above.

Despite a few small studies that found positive PCRs in patients with asymptomatic tuberculous infection, or previous fully treated disease (Walker *et al.*, 1992; Schluger *et al.*, 1994), a consensus is now emerging from the thousands of specimens that have been tested (Eisenach *et al.*, 1991; Clarridge *et al.*, 1993; Noordhoek *et al.*, 1994; Kox *et al.*, 1994). It seems that PCR can indeed detect DNA from *Mycobacterium tuberculosis* within a day from clinical samples. The sensitivity of most assays is similar to that of culture and the specificity is also very high if appropriate care and controls are used. Defining the sensitivity and specificity obviously depends on which patients are considered to have tuberculosis and which are not and there is still a great need for prospectively designed studies that include close follow-up of patients for at least six months after specimens are submitted. PCR also remains positive for longer than either microscopy or culture once a patient starts treatment (Levee *et al.*, 1994) although more studies are needed to quantify this more accurately.

The newer amplification techniques, particularly TMA, will reach similar consensus more rapidly as the trials will be larger and better designed and with the experience of PCR to look to. The challenges for the large commercial companies that are now taking these tests into the marketplace will be to develop closed lysis systems that do not require repeated opening of reaction vessels and also methods to detect the amplified product that do not require the tube to be opened again. Such systems are already practical and will overcome the most significant problem with amplification based diagnostics, that of contamination. However, it must be borne in mind that, so far, no test has proved to be much more sensitive than culture and that the use of BACTEC (Becton Dickenson) radiospirometric culture with probes, commercially available from Gen-probe, may give a culture result in only a week. Furthermore, the hope that nucleic acids would be detectable after amplification from the blood of those with extrapulmonary and blood-culture negative tuberculosis, or in children with culture negative disease, remains a dream at present, although a blood-based PCR assay has now been described for patients with pulmonary disease (Condos *et al.*, 1996).

OTHER MOLECULAR APPLICATIONS

DNA fingerprinting

Molecular technologies have also proved useful in uncovering new aspects of the epidemiology of tuberculosis. The description of a repetitive mobile element within the genome of *Mycobacterium tuberculosis* has allowed much clearer distinctions to be drawn between different isolates (Hermans *et al.*, 1990) and other genetic markers can confirm and extend these distinctions (Ross *et al.*, 1992; Van Soolingen *et al.*, 1993). This has allowed transmission to be documented both in the community (Yang *et al.*, 1995) and in nosocomial settings (Daley *et al.*, 1992). Most interesting have been prospective studies in communities in Switzerland (Genewein *et al.*, 1993) and the US (Small *et al.*, 1994; Alland *et al.*, 1994) which have demonstrated that a considerable number of new tuberculosis cases are due to recent transmission and that the routes of transmission are frequently missed by routine contact tracing. Combining the polymorphism of

these mobile elements with PCR allows a more rapid technique for determining whether isolates are part of a cluster of transmission and in principle can be applied directly to clinical samples without the need for a cultured isolate (Haas *et al.*, 1993).

DRUG RESISTANCE

Although particular DNA fingerprints do not predict resistance to anti-tuberculosis drugs (Godfrey-Faussett, 1993), DNA fingerprinting has been used successfully to follow outbreaks of drug resistant tuberculosis (Shafer *et al.*, 1995). The molecular mechanisms of resistance to the major anti-tuberculosis drugs are rapidly being elucidated (Zhang *et al.*, 1992; Telenti *et al.*, 1993; Banerjee *et al.*, 1994; Honore and Cole, 1994). This has led to the possibility of rapid diagnosis of drug resistance, either through single stranded conformational polymorphism analysis (Telenti *et al.*, 1993a) or by direct sequencing of the region of the gene containing the majority of the relevant mutations (Telenti *et al.*, 1993b). These techniques are most suited for detection of rifampicin resistance, since the great majority of isolates have mutations in a short region of the rpoB gene that encodes for the beta-subunit of RNA polymerase. Such tests will need to be streamlined further before they are practical either for surveillance or routine diagnosis but it is likely that they will soon be available in larger centers for individual clinical decisions.

CONCLUSIONS

The diagnosis of tuberculosis remains a challenge and nowhere more so than in the context of HIV-infected patients. Although molecular tools are now showing some promise and may lead to more rapid confirmation of the diagnosis, it remains unclear whether they will greatly enhance the sensitivity of existing culture methods.

Some patients will continue to suffer from tuberculosis and to spread the disease in their communities through the negligence of their physician, whose index of suspicion was too low. However, even when the diagnosis is considered, there will be a significant number of patients with pulmonary tuberculosis in whom a confirmed diagnosis will not be made and with extrapulmonary or pediatric disease the number of undiagnosed patients will be larger. The proportion of patients remaining undiagnosed will depend upon the facilities available – most patients with HIV-related tuberculosis live in areas where sputum culture is not available, let alone more invasive procedures. There will therefore always remain a place for the 'therapeutic trial' but it must be used with caution. Not only must response to therapy be adequately and objectively documented but also the initiation of a trial of therapy must not be allowed to prevent a continuing search for other causes. Neither rifampicin nor streptomycin are specific in their action against *Mycobacterium tuberculosis* so that if they are included in the therapeutic trial, improvement may result from treatment of other organisms. On the other hand, unless good supervision is available, it may be dangerous to introduce a regimen specifically for therapeutic trials as some patients may be overlooked and left on inadequate treatment with consequent risk of recurrence and the development of drug resistance.

ACKNOWLEDGMENTS

PG-F is funded by the Beit Memorial Medical Fellowship. I am grateful to Rachel Baggaley and Marian Bruce for her comments on this manuscript.

REFERENCES

Aber, V.R., Allen, B.W., Mitchison, D.A. *et al.* (1980) Quality control in tuberculosis bacteriology. 1. Laboratory studies on isolated positive cultures and the efficiency of direct smear examination. *Tubercle*, **61**, 123–33.

Alland, D., Kalkut, G.E., Moss, A.R. *et al.* (1994) Transmission of tuberculosis in New York City – An analysis by DNA fingerprinting and conventional epidemiologic methods. *N. Engl. J. Med.*, **330**, 1710–16.

Andersen, A.B., Thybo, S., Godfrey-Faussett, P. and Stoker, N.G. (1993) Polymerase chain reaction for detection of *Mycobacterium tuberculosis* in sputum. *Eur. J. Clin. Microbiol. Infect. Dis.*, **12**, 922–7.

Araj, G.F., Fahmawi, B.H., Chugh, T.D. and Abusalim, M. (1993) Improved detection of mycobacterial antigens in clinical specimens by combined enzyme-linked immunosorbent assays. *Diagn. Microbiol. Infect. Dis.*, **17**, 119–27.

Arruda, A., Bomfim, G., Knights, R. *et al.* (1993) Cloning of an *M. tuberculosis* DNA fragment associated with entry and survival inside cells. *Science*, **261**, 1454–7.

Banerjee, A., Dubnau, E., Quemard, A. *et al.* (1994) inhA, a gene encoding a target for isoniazid and ethionamide in *Mycobacterium tuberculosis*. *Science*, **263**, 227–30.

Bem, C., Patil, P.S., Elliott, A.M. *et al.* (1993) The value of wide-needle aspiration in the diagnosis of tuberculous lymphadenitis in Africa. *AIDS*, **7**, 1221–5.

Brindle, R.J., Nunn, P.P., Githui, W. *et al.* (1993) Quantitative bacillary response to treatment in HIV-associated pulmonary tuberculosis. *Am. Rev. Respir. Dis.*, **147**, 958–61.

Brisson-Noel, A., Gicquel, B., Lecossier, D. *et al.* (1989) Rapid diagnosis of tuberculosis by amplification of mycobacterial DNA in clinical samples. *Lancet*, **ii**, 1069–71.

Chiang, C.S., Chiang, C.D., Lin, J.W. *et al.* (1994) Neopterin, soluble interleukin-2 receptor and adenosine deaminase levels in pleural effusions. *Respiration*, **61**, 150–4.

Chintu, C., Bhat, G., Luo, C. *et al.* (1993) Seroprevalence of HIV type 1 infection in Zambian children with TB. *Pediatr. Infect. Dis.*, **12**, 499–504.

Choy, E.H.S., Chiecobianchi, F., Panayi, G.S. and Kingsley, G.H. (1994) Synovial fluid lymphocyte proliferation to tuberculin protein product derivative – a novel way of diagnosing tuberculous arthritis. *Clin. Exp. Rheumatol.*, **12**, 187–90.

Clarridge, J.E., Shawar, R.M., Shinnick, T.M. and Plikaytis, B.B. (1993) Large-scale use of polymerase chain reaction for detection of *Mycobacterium-tuberculosis* in a routine mycobacteriology laboratory. *J. Clin. Microbiol.*, **31**, 2049–56.

Condos, R., McClune, A., Rom, W.N. and Schluger, N.W. (1996) Peripheral-blood-based PCR assay to identify patients with active pulmonary tuberculosis. *Lancet*, **347**, 1082–5.

Coronado, V.G., Becksague, C.M., Hutton, M.D. *et al.* (1993) Transmission of multidrug-resistant *Mycobacterium-tuberculosis* among persons with human immunodeficiency virus infection in an urban hospital – epidemiologic and restriction fragment length polymorphism analysis. *J. Infect. Dis.*, **168**, 1052–5.

Cundall, D.B. (1986) The diagnosis of pulmonary tuberculosis in malnourished Kenyan children. *Ann. Trop. Paediatr.*, **6**, 249–55.

Daley, C.L., Small, P.M., Schecter, G.F. *et al.* (1992) An outbreak of tuberculosis with accelerated progression among persons infected with human immunodeficiency virus. *N. Engl. J. Med.*, **326**, 231–5.

Das, S., Chan, S.L., Allen, B.W. *et al.* (1993) Application of DNA fingerprinting with IS986 to sequential mycobacterial isolates obtained from pulmonary tuberculosis patients in Hong Kong before, during and after short-course chemotherapy. *Tuber. Lung Dis.*, **74**, 47–51.

de Gracia, J., Curull, V., Vidal, R. and Morell, F. (1988) Diagnostic value of bronchoalveolar lavage in suspected pulmonary tuberculosis. *Chest*, **93**, 329–32.

Diperri, G., Danzi, M., DeChecchi, G. *et al.* (1989) Nosocomial epidemic of active tuberculosis among HIV-infected patients. *Lancet*, **ii**, 1502–4.

Drucker, E., Alcabes, P., Bosworth, W. and Sckell, B. (1994) Childhood tuberculosis in the Bronx, New York. *Lancet*, **343**, 1482–5.

Duncan, L.E., Elliott, A., Hayes, R.J. *et al.* (1995) Tuberculin sensitivity and HIV-1 status of patients attending a sexually transmitted diseases clinic in Lusaka, Zambia: a cross-sectional study. *Trans. Roy. Soc. Trop. Med. Hyg.*, **89**, 37–40.

Eisenach, K.D., Sifford, M.D., Cave, M.D. *et al.* (1991) Detection of *Mycobacterium-tuberculosis* in sputum samples using a polymerase chain reaction. *Am. Rev. Respir. Dis.*, **144**, 1160–3.

Elliott, A.M., Luo, N., Tembo, G. *et al.* (1990) Impact of HIV on tuberculosis in Zambia: a cross sectional study. *Br. Med. J.*, **301**, 412–15.

Fishman, J.A., Roth, R.S., Zanzot, E. *et al.*

(1994) Use of induced sputum specimens for microbiologic diagnosis of infections due to organisms other than *Pneumocystis carinii*. *J. Clin. Microbiol.*, **32**, 131–4.

Genewein, A., Telenti, A., Bernasconi, C. *et al.* (1993) Molecular approach to identifying route of transmission of tuberculosis in the community. *Lancet*, **342**, 841–4.

Gilks, C.F., Brindle, R.J., Otieno, L.S. *et al.* (1990) Extrapulmonary and disseminated tuberculosis in HIV-1 seropositive patients presenting to the acute medical services in Nairobi. *AIDS*, **4**, 981–5.

Githui, W.A., Nunn, P.P., Juma, E. *et al.* (1992) Cohort study of HIV infection in tuberculosis patients, Nairobi, Kenya: comparison of bacteriological results. *Tuber. Lung Dis.*, **73**, 203–9.

Godfrey-Faussett, P., Mortimer, P., Jenkins, P.A. and Stoker, N.G. (1992) Evidence of transmission of tuberculosis by DNA fingerprinting. *Br. Med. J.*, **305**, 221–3.

Godfrey-Faussett, P., Stoker, N.G., Scott, J.A.G. *et al.* (1993) DNA fingerprints from *Mycobacterium tuberculosis* do not change during the development of rifampicin resistance. *Tuber. Lung Dis.*, **74**, 240–3.

Graham, N.M.H., Nelson, K.E., Solomon, L. *et al.* (1992) Prevalence of tuberculin positivity and skin test anergy in HIV-1-seropositive and HIV-1-seronegative intravenous drug users. *JAMA*, **267**, 369–73.

Guelar, A., Gatell, J.M., Verdejo, J. *et al.* (1993) A prospective study of the risk of tuberculosis among HIV-infected patients. *AIDS*, **7**, 1345–9.

Haas, W.H., Butler, W.R., Woodley, C.L. and Crawford, J.T. (1993) Mixed-linker polymerase chain reaction – a new method for rapid fingerprinting of isolates of the *Mycobacterium tuberculosis* complex. *J. Clin. Microbiol.*, **31**, 1293–8.

Hermans, P.W.M., van Sollingen, D., Dale, J.W. *et al.* (1990) Insertion element IS986 from *Mycobacterium tuberculosis*: a useful tool for diagnosis and epidemiology of tuberculosis. *J. Clin. Microbiol.*, **28**, 2051–8.

Herz, A., Leichsenring, M., Felten, M. *et al.* (1994) The diagnosis of pulmonary tuberculosis by gas chromatographic detection of tuberculostearic acid using flame ionisation detectors. *Eur. J. Clin. Invest.*, **24**, 114–8.

Honore, N. and Cole, S.T. (1994) Streptomycin resistance in Mycobacteria. *Antimicrob. Agents Chemother.*, **38**, 238–42.

Hosp, M., Elliott, A., Raynes, J. *et al.* (1994)

Neopterin beta-2-microglobulin and acute phase proteins in Zambian patients with tuberculosis. *Pteridines*, **4**, 99–100.

Jonas, V., Alden, M.J., Curry, J.I. *et al.* (1993) Detection and identification of *Mycobacterium tuberculosis* directly from sputum sediments by amplification of rRNA. *J. Clin. Microbiol.*, **31**, 2410–6.

Jones, B.E., Young, S.M.M., Antoniskis, D. *et al.* (1993) Relationship of the manifestations of tuberculosis to CD4 cell counts in patients with human immunodeficiency virus infection. *Am. Rev. Respir. Dis.*, **148**, 1292–7.

Kent, R.J., Uttley, A.H.C., Stoker, N.G. *et al.* (1994) Evidence for nosocomial transmission of tuberculosis in an HIV care centre in the United Kingdom. *Br. Med. J.*, **309**, 639–40.

Khan, M.A., Kovnat, D.M., Bachus, B. *et al.* (1977) Clinical and roentgenographic spectrum of pulmonary tuberculosis in adults. *Am. J. Med.*, **62**, 31–8.

Klein, R.S. and Motyl, M. (1993) Frequency of pulmonary tuberculosis in patients undergoing sputum induction for diagnosis of suspected *Pneumocystis-carinii* pneumonia. *AIDS*, **7**, 1351–5.

Kox, L.F.F., Rhienthong, D., Miranda, A.M. *et al.* (1994) More reliable PCR for detection of *Mycobacterium tuberculosis* in clinical samples. *J. Clin. Microbiol.*, **32**, 672–8.

Kwok, S. and Higuchi, R. (1989) Avoiding false positives with PCR. *Nature*, **339**, 237–8.

Levee, G., Glaziou, P., Gicquel, B. and Chanteau, S. (1994) Follow-up of tuberculosis patients undergoing standard anti-tuberculosis chemotherapy by using a polymerase chain reaction. *Res. Microbiol.*, **145**, 5–8.

Lherminez, R.H. (1993) Urgent need for a new approach to the diagnosis of tuberculosis in developing countries in the decade of AIDS. *Trop. Geogr. Med.*, **45**, 145–9.

Long, R., Scalcini, M., Manfreda, J. *et al.* (1991) The impact of HIV on the usefulness of sputum smears for the diagnosis of tuberculosis. *Am. J. Public Health*, **81**, 1326–8.

Longo, M.C., Berninger, M.S. and Hartley, J.L. (1990) The use of uracil DNA glycosylase to control carry-over contamination in polymerase chain reactions. *Gene*, **93**, 125–8.

Lucas, S.B., Hounnou, A., Peacock, C. *et al.* (1993) The mortality and pathology of HIV infection in a West African City. *AIDS*, **7**, 1569–79.

Lucas, S.B., Peacock, C.S., Hounnou, A. *et al.* (1996) Diseases in children with and without HIV in Abidjan, Côte d'Ivoire: an autopsy study. *Br. Med. J.*, **312**, 335–8.

Mathur, P., Sacks, L., Auten, G. *et al.* (1994) Delayed diagnosis of pulmonary tuberculosis in city hospitals. *Arch. Intern Med.*, **154**, 306–10.

McFadden, J. (ed.) (1990) *Molecular Biology of the Mycobacteria*. Academic Press, London.

Miller, N., Hernandez, S.G. and Cleary, T.J. (1994) Evaluation of Gen-Probe amplified *Mycobacterium tuberculosis* direct test and PCR for direct detection of *Mycobacterium tuberculosis* in clinical specimens. *J. Clin. Microbiol.*, **32**, 393–7.

Mukadi, Y., Perriens, J.H., Stlouis, M.E. *et al.* (1993) Spectrum of immunodeficiency in HIV-1-infected patients with pulmonary tuberculosis in Zaire. *Lancet*, **342**, 143–6.

Nichols, L., Florentine, B., Lewis, W. *et al.* (1991) Bone marrow examination for the diagnosis of mycobacterial and fungal infections in the acquired immunodeficiency syndrome. *Arch. Pathol. Lab. Med.*, **115**, 1125–32.

Noordhoek, G.T., Kolk, A.H.J., Bjune, G. *et al.* (1994) Sensitivity and specificity of PCR for detection of *Mycobacterium tuberculosis* – a blind comparison study among seven laboratories. *J. Clin. Microbiol.*, **32**, 277–84.

Nunn, P. (1990) Impact of HIV – Discussion, in *Tuberculosis: Back to the Future.* (eds J.D.H. Porter and K.P.W.J. McAdam) John Wiley, Chichester, pp. 49–52.

Pao, C.C., Lin. S.S., Wu, S.Y. *et al.* (1988) The detection of mycobacterial DNA sequences in uncultured clinical specimens with cloned *Mycobacterium tuberculosis* DNA as probes. *Tubercle*, **69**, 27–36.

Pastores, S.M., Naidich, D.P., Aranda, C.P. *et al.* (1993) Intrathoracic adenopathy associated with pulmonary tuberculosis in patients with human immunodeficiency virus infection. *Chest*, **103**, 1433–7.

Pearson, M.L., Jereb, J.A., Frieden, T.R. *et al.* (1992) Nosocomial transmission of multidrug-resistant *Mycobacterium tuberculosis*: a risk to patients and health care workers. *Ann. Intern. Med.*, **117**, 191–6.

Pedrobotet, J., Gutierrez, J., Miralles, R. *et al.* (1992) Pulmonary tuberculosis in HIV-infected patients with normal chest radiographs. *AIDS*, **6**, 91–3.

Petterson, T., Klockars, M. and Weber, T. (1984) Pleural fluid adenosine deaminase in rheumatoid arthritis and systemic lupus erythematosus. *Chest*, **86**, 273.

Pierre, C., Lecossier, D., Boussougant, Y. *et al.* (1991) Use of reamplification protocol improves sensitivity of detection of mycobacterium TB in clinical samples by amplification of DNA. *J. Clin. Microbiol.*, **29**, No. 4, 712–17.

Pitchenik, A.E., Cole, C., Russell, B.W. *et al.* (1984) Tuberculosis, atypical mycobacteriosis, and AIDS among Haitian and non-Haitian patients in South Florida. *Ann. Intern. Med.*, **101**, 641–5.

Pitchenik, A.E. and Robinson, H.A. (1985) The radiographic appearance of tuberculosis in patients with the acquired immunodeficiency syndrome. *Am. Rev. Respir. Dis.*, **131**, 393–6.

Radhakrishnan, V.V. and Mathai, A. (1991) A dot-immunobinding assay for the laboratory diagnosis of tuberculous meningitis and its comparison with enzyme-linked immunosorbent assay. *J. Appli. Bacteriol.*, **71**, 428–33.

Raja, A., Machicao, A.R., Morrissey, A.B. *et al.* (1988) Specific detection of *Mycobacterium tuberculosis* in radiometric cultures by using an immunoassay for antigen 5. *J. Infect. Dis.*, **158**, 428–33.

Ross, B.C., Raios, K., Jackson, K. and Dwyer, B. (1992) Molecular cloning of a highly repeated DNA element from *Mycobacterium-tuberculosis* and its use as an epidemiological tool. *J. Clin. Microbiol.*, **30**, 942–6.

Rothel, J.S., Jones, S.L., Corner, L.A. *et al.* (1990) A sandwich enzyme immunoassay for bovine interferon-gamma and its use for the detection of tuberculosis in cattle. *Aust. Vet. J*, **67**, 134–7.

Saiki, R.K., Gelfand, D.H., Stoffel, S. *et al.* (1988) Primer-directed enzymatic amplification of DNA with a thermostable DNA polymerase. *Science*, **239**, 487–91.

Saltini, C., Amicosante, M., Girardi, E. *et al.* (1993) Early abnormalities of the antibody response against *Mycobacterium-tuberculosis* in human immunodeficiency virus infection. *J. Infect. Dis.*, **168**, 1409–14.

Sanchez Hernandez, I.M., Pantoja, C. Ussetti, P. *et al.* (1991) Pleural fluid adenosine deaminase and lysozyme levels in the diagnosis of tuberculosis. *Chest*, **100**, 1479–80.

Schluger, N.W., Kinney, D., Harkin, T.J. and Rom, W.N. (1994) Clinical utility of the polymerase chain reaction in the diagnosis of infections due to *Mycobacterium tuberculosis*. *Chest*, **105**, 1116–21.

Selwyn, P.A., Hartel, D., Lewis, V.A. *et al.* (1989) A prospective study of the risk of tuberculosis among intravenous drug users with human immunodeficiency virus infection. *N. Engl. J. Med.*, **320**, 545–50.

Selwyn, P.A., Sckell, B.M., Alcabes, P. *et al.* (1992) High risk of active tuberculosis in HIV-infected drug users with cutaneous anergy. *JAMA*, **268**, 504–8.

Shafer, R.W., Goldberg, R., Sierra, M. and Glatt, A.E. (1989) Frequency of *Mycobacterium tuberculosis* bacteremia in patients with tuberculosis in an area endemic for AIDS. *Am. Rev. Respir. Dis.*, **140**, 1611–3.

Shafer, R.W., Small, P.M., Larkin, C. *et al.* (1995) Temporal trends and transmission patterns during the emergence of multidrug resistant tuberculosis in New York City; a molecular epidiomologic assessment. *J. Infect. Dis.*, **171**, 170–6.

Small, P.M., McClenny, N.B., Singh, S.P. *et al.* (1993) Molecular strain typing of *Mycobacterium tuberculosis* to confirm cross-contamination in the mycobacteriology laboratory and modification of procedures to minimise occurrence of false-positive cultures. *J. Clin. Microbiol.*, **31**, 1677–82.

Small, P.M., Hopewell, P.C., Singh, S.P. *et al.* (1994) The epidemiology of tuberculosis in San Francisco – A population-based study using conventional and molecular methods. *N. Engl. J. Med.*, **330**, 1703–9.

Spargo, C.A., Haaland, P.D., Jurgensen, S.R. *et al.* (1993) Chemiluminescent detection of strand displacement amplified DNA from species comprising the *Mycobacterium tuberculosis* complex. *Mol. Cell Probe.*, **7**, 395–404.

Springett, V.H., Waaler, H.Th. and Nyboe, J. (1967) Results of the study on X-ray readings of the ad hoc committee for the study of classification and terminology in tuberculosis. *Bull. Int. Union Tuber. Lung Dis.*, **17**, 107–31.

Starke, J.R., Taylor-Watts, K.T. (1989) Tuberculosis in the pediatric population of Houston, Texas. *Pediatrics*, **84**, 28–35.

van Soolingen, D., Dehaas, P.E.W., Hermans, P.W.M. *et al.* (1993) Comparison of various repetitive DNA elements as genetic markers for strain differentiation and epidemiology of *Mycobacterium tuberculosis*. *J. Clin. Microbiol.*, **31**, 1987–95.

Telenti, M., Dequiros, J.F.B., Alvarez, M. *et al.* (1994) The diagnostic usefulness of DNA probe for *Mycobacterium tuberculosis* complex (Gen-

Probe(R)) in BACTEC cultures versus other diagnostic methods. *Infection*, **22**, 18–23.

Telenti, A., Imboden, P., Marchesi, F. *et al*. (1993a) Detection of rifampicin-resistance mutations in *Mycobacterium tuberculosis*. *Lancet*, **341**, 647–50.

Telenti, A., Imbodem P., Marchesi, F. *et al*. (1993b) Automated detection of rifampicin-resistant *Mycobacterium tuberculosis* by polymerase chain reaction and single-strand conformation polymorphism analysis. *Antimicrob. Agents Chemother.*, **37**, 2054–8.

van der Werf, T.S., Das, P.K., Van Soolingen, D. *et al*. (1992) Sero-diagnosis of tuberculosis with A60 antigen enzyme-linked immunosorbent assay: failure in HIV-infected individuals in Ghana. *Med. Microbiol. Immunol.*, **181**, 71–6.

Verbon, A., Weverling, G.J., Kuijper, S. *et al*. (1993) Evaluation of different tests for the serodiagnosis of tuberculosis and the use of likelihood ratios in serology. *Am. Rev. Respir. Dis.*, **148**, 378–84.

Walker, G.T., Little, M.C., Nadeau, J.G. and Shank, D.D. (1992a) Isothermal in vitro amplification of DNA by a restriction enzyme/DNA polymerase system. *Proc. Natl. Acad. Sci. USA*, **89**, 392–6.

Walker, D.A., Taylor, I.K., Mitchell, D.M. and Shaw, R.J. (1992b) Comparison of polymerase chain reaction amplification of two mycobacterial DNA sequences, IS6110 and the 65 kDa antigen gene, in the diagnosis of tuberculosis. *Thorax*, **47**, 690.

Wilkins, E.G.L. and Ivanyi, J. (1990) Potential value of serology for diagnosis of extrapulmonary tuberculosis. *Lancet*, **336**, 641–4.

Wilson, S.M., McNerney, R., Nye, P.M. *et al*. (1993) Progress towards a simplified polymerase chain reaction and its application to the diagnosis of tuberculosis. *J. Clin. Microbiol.*, **31**, 776–82.

Winndeen, E.S., Batt, C.A. and Wiedmann, M. (1993) Non-radioactive detection of *Mycobacterium-tuberculosis* LCR products in a microtitre plate format. *Mol. Cell Probe*, **7**, 179–86.

Yang, Z.H., Mtoni, I., Chonde, M. *et al*. (1995) DNA finger-printing and phenotyping of *Mycobacterium tuberculosis* isolates from HIV-seropositive and HIV-seronegative patients in Tanzania. *J. Clin. Microbiol.*, **33**, 1064–9.

Zhang, Y., Heym, B., Allen, B. *et al*. (1992) The catalase-peroxidase gene and isoniazid resistance of *Mycobacterium* TB. *Nature*, **358**, 591–3.

MANAGEMENT OF MYCOBACTERIAL INFECTIONS IN AIDS

Geoff M. Scott and Janet H. Darbyshire

INTRODUCTION

The treatment of tuberculosis in association with HIV is essentially not different from that of patients without HIV infection and follows well-established principles. The choice of chemotherapy regimen may be limited by cost or toxicity or be influenced by the likelihood of multiple drug resistance. Because patients with HIV are likely to be immunosuppressed and to become more so with time, there is some debate about whether one or more drugs should be continued after completing a course of treatment. As patients with HIV are more likely to relapse or acquire new infection, preventive therapy for life may be desirable. In areas of high prevalence of HIV and tuberculosis (as in Sub-Saharan Africa), tuberculosis remains the major cause of death in AIDS (Kassim *et al.*, 1995). Strategies for chemoprophylaxis in these high risk groups must be considered.

The treatment of disseminated *Mycobacterium avium-intracellulare* complex (MAC) infection has become an important clinical issue only since the HIV epidemic. Because the disease used to be rare, successful treatment regimens were not established by clinical trials before AIDS. MAC is constitutively resistant to many first-line anti-tuberculosis drugs but regimens including newer drugs have now been shown to have modest activity in terms of reduction of symptoms and clearance of bacteremia. However, whereas tuberculosis tends to occur at an early stage of immunosuppression in HIV infection, significant MAC infection is associated with severe immunosuppression. The life expectancy of individuals with these different mycobacterial infections is therefore different and influences the approach to treatment and the expectation of cure.

The transmission of mycobacteria from HIV-infected to other individuals has become an important public health issue and guidelines for the prevention of such transmission have recently been published and will be reviewed.

EVALUATION OF PATIENTS WITH MYCOBACTERIAL INFECTION FOR TREATMENT

In many circumstances, the definitive diagnosis is delayed. The diagnosis depends on local patterns of infection. A positive blood culture or a positive fecal smear for AFBs in a Caucasian patient with a very low CD4 cell

AIDS and Respiratory Medicine. Edited by A. Zumla, M.A. Johnson and R.F. Miller. Published in 1997 by Chapman & Hall, London. ISBN 0 412 60140 0

Table 12.1 Rate of isolation of *Mycobacterium* spp. according to specimen type and smear positivity – cumulative percentage culture positive by week after setting up culture (UCLH)

Week	M. tuberculosis All specimens, smear −	+	++	All	MAC Specimen Blood or bone marrow	Respiratory[b]	Other[c]
1	0	0	4	3	ND[a]	0	0
2	5	21	57	26	15	3	18
3	52	63	90	67	49	14	72
4	68	84	98	81	64	47	87
5	83	89	98	89	88	72	95
6	87	100	100	93	95	81	97
7	95			98	95	94	97
8	95			98	97	100	100
>8	97			98[d]	100		

[a]ND, blood cultures not examined in week 1.
[b]resp = BAL, sputum and induced sputum.
[c]other includes stool, rectal biopsy, lymph nodes and pleural fluid.
[d]some specimens from patients known to have tuberculosis were negative on culture at 12 weeks.
MAC = *Mycobacterium avium-intracellulare* complex

count (e.g. <100/μl) in the UK is very likely (though not exclusively) to indicate MAC infection; a patient in Africa with sputum smear-positive disease is much more likely to be suffering from tuberculosis. The treatment regimen for each disease is not wholly satisfactory for the other and it may occasionally be necessary to cover both possibilities when choosing the initial regimen. The treatment can then be modified as the results of culture and identification tests become available. In general, in technically advanced countries, for patients with low CD4 counts it is wise to use regimens suitable for MAC infection but which are also effective against tuberculosis. Most patients with mycobacteremia have MAC infection, although *M. tuberculosis* may also occur (Saltzman *et al.*, 1986).

Many cases of tuberculosis are sputum smear-negative but culture-positive. It is possible for skilled microbiology laboratory staff to provisionally identify a mycobacterial species from the appearances of early growth on Lowenstein–Jensen egg agar although this method is not totally reliable. The expected intervals between the receipt of a specimen and positive culture according to the smear result in University College London Hospitals (UCLH) are indicated in Table 12.1. The nature of the specimens yielding positive information differs between species. Blood and bone marrow cultures, exclusively from AIDS patients, represent 55% of specimens yielding MAC. Of the respiratory specimens, only 11% are smear-positive, as are 18% of feces or rectal biopsies. Therefore in only about 7% of cases will direct smear give any intimation that an AIDS patient has MAC infection. 50% of all cultures are visible between weeks three and four after setting up the culture.

In this institution, so few patients with AIDS have tuberculosis that the comparisons have been made with cultures from all patients. If a specimen is smear-positive and particularly if it is strongly positive, then more than 50% of specimens will be culture-positive for *M. tuberculosis* between weeks two and three. These data, preferably derived from the physician's own institution, will indicate how likely it is that a patient does *not* have mycobacterial disease as time after collecting the specimens passes. Sometimes it will not be possible to make a bacteriological diagnosis at all and the clinician will have to make a difficult decision on the clinical evidence available.

TUBERCULOSIS

TREATMENT

The type of tuberculosis varies with the stage of immunosuppression in an AIDS patient and many patients have peripheral $CD4^+$ counts in the normal range and have classical focal and even cavitatory pulmonary disease. Those with severe immunosuppression due to HIV are likely to have disseminated multibacillary tuberculosis. The theoretical basis for the use of combinations of drugs with different actions against active disease with high numbers of replicating organisms has been summarized by Grosset (1990).

The currently recommended regimens of chemotherapy have been developed from a series of well-controlled trials in large numbers of subjects with pulmonary tuberculosis, mainly sputum smear-positive, which were conducted before the advent of AIDS. The most widely recommended is a six-month regimen of isoniazid plus rifampicin with an initial two months of pyrazinamide, together with ethambutol (or streptomycin) if initial resistance to one agent is suspected or thought to be likely (Committee on Treatment, 1988; Ormerod, 1990; Centers for Disease Control, 1989; Joint Tuberculosis Committee, 1994). However, the strategy of adding a fourth drug to the initial regime has not formally been demonstrated to be of value in the context of preventing the development of secondary resistance. Personal choice of the physician often determines the actual regimen used

(Small *et al.*, 1991; van Deutekom, 1990) and physician compliance with guidelines has always been poor, contributing in part to the emergence of resistant strains.

In developing countries, for reasons of cost, the initial two-month phase may be followed by isoniazid plus thiacetazone for six months. If rifampicin and pyrazinamide are not available, thiacetazone plus isoniazid should be given for at least 12 months with streptomycin for at least the first month. National tuberculosis programmes in E. Africa using short-course chemotherapy have been moderately successful, achieving cure rates in the region of 75% (Rouillon and Enarson, 1991) or better (Murray *et al.*, 1991).

There have been no controlled trials in HIV-infected individuals of sufficient size to detect differences in efficacy between regimens in these individuals. Small clinical studies suggest that regimens based on rifampicin and isoniazid, particularly if adequately supervised, are as effective in AIDS as in immunocompetent individuals (Small *et al.*, 1991), but the mortality in a group with HIV, at least in Africa, is likely to be much higher than in those without and this is borne out in observational studies (Grosset, 1992; Githui *et al.*, 1992; Ackah *et al.*, 1995; Perriëns *et al.*, 1995). However, regimens based on thiacetazone and isoniazid are less efficacious, due, at least in part, to increased toxicity particularly to thiacetazone (Nunn *et al.*, 1991; Githui *et al.*, 1992; Hawken *et al.*, 1993; World Health Organization, 1992) which may be life threatening and therefore limit its use. This has serious implications for countries with high incidences of both HIV and tuberculosis where isoniazid and thiacetazone are the only affordable anti-tuberculosis drugs.

Okwera and colleagues (Okwera *et al.*, 1994) have done a controlled study to evaluate thiacetazone toxicity. The regimens were, however, completely different: isoniazid (H), rifampicin (R) and pyrazinamide (Z) versus streptomycin (S), thiacetazone (T) and isoniazid. The rates of adverse drug reactions and particularly skin rashes were significantly higher to STH compared with HRZ, which also had more impressive sterilizing activity at two months of treatment. Harries and co-workers (Harries *et al.*, 1995) have recently compared a standard regimen in Malawi with one excluding thiacetazone: a two-month intensive regimen with streptomycin, rifampicin, isoniazid and pyrazinamide, followed by six months of either isoniazid and ethambutol compared with isoniazid and thiacetazone. The outcomes were similar and showed that considerable savings could be made by restricting rifampicin to the early supervised phase in hospital.

Whereas Elliott and Foster (1996) take a view that the serious side-effects of thiacetazone outweigh its advantage as a cheap component of antituberculosis regimens, and that its use should now be completely discontinued, others (Rieder and Enarson, 1996; van Gorkom and Kibuga, 1996) have argued that many countries cannot afford to do without the drug altogether. Economically, it has been suggested that ethambutol should replace thiacetazone as the companion to isoniazid in the continuation phase (essentially to prevent the emergence of resistance) when the HIV prevalence in tuberculosis exceeds 90% (van Gorkom and Kibuga, 1996).

The frequencies of adverse reactions to thiacetazone vary from country to country in different studies and approached 30% in Singapore before the AIDS epidemic. Furthermore, life-threatening adverse events occasionally occur with any anti-mycobacterial regimen (Aquinas *et al.*, 1972; Girling, 1987; Mitchell *et al.*, 1995) and most patients do not have significant side effects. It is of considerable interest that patients with AIDS have an increasing likelihood of side-effects to many drugs, and in particular, folate antagonists such as co-trimoxazole.

Intermittent regimens which can be more easily supervised are of particular value in difficult patient groups (e.g. injection drug users) who are likely to be at increased risk of both tuberculosis and HIV. Encouraging results of directly observed therapy have recently been reported from both the USA and South Africa (Alwood *et al.*, 1994; Wilkinson, 1994).

It has been recommended that antituberculosis treatment should be continued for longer in patients with HIV infection than those without but there is little evidence to support this (Small *et al.*, 1991). Clearly, if conversion to sputum culture negativity has been prolonged despite adequate chemotherapy, it would be wise to continue treatment, preferably supervised, but each case should be judged on its merits. In such cases, doubts about compliance and absorption of drugs should be raised.

There is some evidence that tuberculosis may recur as the immunosuppression due to HIV progresses (Hawken *et al.*, 1993) and prolonged preventive therapy after completion of a successful eradicative regime, for example with isoniazid alone, may be justified (Perriëns *et al.*, 1991, 1995; Hawken *et al.*, 1993). In the more recent study, Perriëns used isoniazid with rifampicin twice weekly (supervised once a week) for post-treatment chemoprophylaxis in Zaire and showed a modest reduction in the risk of relapse but no effect on mortality.

DRUG RESISTANCE

Outbreaks of multidrug resistant (MDR) tuberculosis in HIV-infected individuals have been reported in the USA (Centers for Disease Control, 1991; Menzies *et al.*, 1995). It has been considered that these are likely to have arisen because of inadequate regimens of chemotherapy or poor compliance with therapy, but it is possible that HIV-infected individuals may be more likely to develop resistant strains of *M. tuberculosis* than those without. Some of the problems have without doubt arisen because of the gradual withdrawal of specialist services for managing tuberculosis which followed the fall in the prevalence of the disease in developed countries (Iseman, 1994). Vareldzis and co-workers (1994) have also drawn attention to the gradual increase in drug resistance in isolates from developing countries, suggesting that the increasing use of more effective drugs including rifampicin in National Control Programs may be as potent an influence on the emergence of resistance as the prevalence of HIV infection. However, this is not always borne out in individual countries where careful intensive tuberculosis control is being practiced (Glynn *et al.*, 1995).

Selection of drug-resistant mutants occurs rapidly if a single antituberculosis drug is taken when there is a large dividing pool of organisms, that is at the time of diagnosis of active tuberculosis. The mechanisms of antimicrobial resistance are as found in isolates from patients without AIDS (Heym *et al.*, 1994). The rate of resistance to individual antibiotics in a rapidly dividing population varies between 10^{-4} and 10^{-9}. Theoretically, lack of compliance with medication will only influence this if patients take some but not all of their prescribed drugs or if some but not others are absorbed. Otherwise, the outcome of failure to comply (by taking all the drugs but intermittently) should result in a failure to achieve successful killing of the organisms and therefore failure of cure. The few patients (without HIV) who relapse after short-course chemotherapy regimens tend to do so with fully sensitive organisms. Thus, even if lack of compliance may be more common in some groups of HIV-infected individuals, this should not in itself select for MDR strains.

MDR is likely to occur by the sequential emergence of resistance in an individual patient (the 'domino' effect) (Grange, 1990). For example, isoniazid preventive therapy

given in error to someone who has active disease will rapidly select for isoniazid resistance. Subsequent treatment with isoniazid plus rifampicin will then select for rifampicin resistance. At best it will be some months before the discovery of the isoniazid resistance because of the natural delay in culture and sensitivity tests. The addition of a third drug at this stage will then select for further resistance because, effectively, monotherapy with rifampicin has been given. The eventual outcome is the selection of a strain with multiple drug resistance (MDR) which can then be transmitted to others. There is good evidence that such transmission has occurred within health care settings between HIV-infected individuals and to health care workers (Centers for Disease Control, 1991; Menzies *et al.*, 1995). Resistance can appear to newer antibiotics within a very short time of their introduction (Sullivan *et al.*, 1995).

Occasionally, failure of what seems to be an optimal regime is seen (Sunderam *et al.*, 1987). Although failure of compliance must account for most of these cases, a recent report showed that MDR strains are likely to have arisen because of poor differential absorption of anti-tuberculosis drugs in AIDS patients (Patel, Belmonte and Crowe, 1995). One patient had ileo-cecal tuberculosis but there are other infections of the bowel common in AIDS which could account for this observation.

The selection of antibiotics for the empirical therapy of tuberculosis must take into account the known patterns of antibiotic resistance in the population. At present, in the UK, in most patients it is sufficient to start treatment with three drugs (rifampicin, isoniazid and pyrazinamide) (Ormerod, 1990, 1992; Joint Tuberculosis Committee, 1994). However, in a population or individual with an organism at increased risk of resistance, it is recommended that therapy should be started with four (including ethambutol) or even five (including ethambutol and streptomycin) antituberculosis drugs, until the results of initial sensitivity tests are known. If MDR tuberculosis is suspected on the basis of a contact history with MDR or prior history of inadequately treated disease, it may be preferable to delay starting treatment until results of sensitivity tests of the current isolate are available. In such a patient, if therapy is required, it should be started with at least four drugs to which the organism is likely to be sensitive based on the history of prior treatment and the treatment supervised. The rapid results for sensitivity tests obtained using the BACTEC radiometric antibiotic sensitivity system may be valuable in these circumstances (Siddiqi *et al.*, 1984), as conventional sensitivity testing results may take as long as 12 weeks from starting to process sputum. Physicians in charge of tuberculosis treatment must have clear protocols to follow to prevent the emergence of resistance. In the case of established MDR tuberculosis, second-line drugs have to be used, with their attendant toxicity. These second-line drugs have been re-reviewed by Bass *et al.*, members of an *ad hoc* committee of the American Thoracic Society (1995). Newer drugs (macrolides, rifamycins and fluoroquinolones), mainly now used to treat MAC infection, also have an important role to play in the management of resistant tuberculosis infection (Mitchison, Ellard and Grosset, 1988).

Goble and co-workers (1993) and Iseman (1993) have written of their experiences in managing large numbers of patients with tubercle resistant to a median of six drugs (including rifampicin and isoniazid). Previous use of a drug for more than a month predicted reduced sensitivity to that agent. Such patients required prolonged hospitalization, unusual combinations of drugs and only 65% of a group of 171 patients had a favorable response in terms of sputum clearance in the short term, despite the use of regimens appropriate to the sensitivity of isolates. There was a high rate of serious side-effects. The most important lesson is

that to use second-line drugs without isoniazid or rifampicin is to return to a time when responses were not as consistent as we would now expect and a few patients appeared not to respond to treatment at all.

If there is doubt about compliance, as there may be in patients with HIV and tuberculosis, particularly drug abusers and others with a chaotic lifestyle, fully supervised (directly observed) daily or intermittent therapy (DOT) will be more successful than a daily self-administered regimen, and is widely recommended (Alwood *et al.*, 1994; Weis *et al.*, 1994). This can be simply arranged by keeping patients in hospital for the critical first two months of treatment. Some patients will avoid treatment even in hospital. In outpatients, however, DOT is a novelty and is difficult and expensive to organize. Issues of trust between physician and patient are raised simply by the suggestion of supervised therapy which may have an adverse effect on management.

If regimens without isoniazid or a rifamycin or both have to be used, either because the isolate is resistant or because of adverse reactions, the length of the treatment course must be prolonged. Guidelines suggest that rifampicin and ethambutol alone should be given for a year in people without HIV but for 18 months (or for at least 6 months after sputum culture conversion) in those with HIV. Prolonged use of ethambutol, or its use in renal failure, require monitoring for ocular toxicity.

PREVENTIVE THERAPY

Preventive therapy has been recommended for HIV-infected individuals with strongly positive tuberculin tests, particularly if there has been no history of BCG immunization (Advisory Committee, 1990; International Union, 1994b; Joint Tuberculosis Committee, 1994). However, such guidance depends on the prevalence of tuberculosis in the population. In many parts of the world, tuberculin tests are positive in a high proportion of the population but may be negative in individuals with severe immunosuppression. In populations of low tuberculosis endemicity (e.g. middle class, white, non-Hispanic males in the USA), a strongly positive tuberculin test may indicate exposure to tuberculosis which may reactivate due to HIV-induced immunosuppression. This is particularly so where BCG immunization is not routinely given.

Initially, there was a suggestion among skin-test positive intravenous drug users in New York that isoniazid could prevent overt tuberculosis (Selwyn *et al.*, 1989). Similar observations were made in Spain (Moreno *et al.*, 1993). Standard regimens of chemoprophylaxis of isoniazid alone for 6 to 12 months have been shown to reduce the risk of tuberculosis in studies in Haiti (Pape *et al.*, 1993) and Zambia (Wadhawan *et al.*, 1992) over a follow-up period of 2 to 6 years. INAH alone reduced the relapse rate from 10% to 2% but most of this advantage was in the first two years. It is very important to exclude active disease before starting monotherapy to prevent the emergence of resistance, and this may be extremely difficult in developing countries (Porter and McAdam, 1992). For this reason, preventive regimens in which rifampicin and/or pyrazinamide are added to isoniazid for a limited period are being evaluated.

Even if preventive therapy works at least in the short-term, the logistics and costs of effective programs must be considered in the light of the prevalence of tuberculosis in the community, the ability to diagnose disease early, the success of treatment of established disease, the relative importance of reinfection rather than reactivation, the likelihood of compliance and drug toxicity (DeCock, Grant and Porter, 1995: O'Brien and Perriëns, 1995). In this equation the suggestions that prevention of tuberculosis may delay the progression of HIV disease (Pape *et al.*, 1993) and that

untreated tuberculosis accelerates the course of HIV disease must be taken into consideration.

MYCOBACTERIUM AVIUM-INTRACELLULARE INFECTION

TREATMENT

A basic principle of treatment of all mycobacterial diseases is that the use of at least two drugs to which the organism is sensitive will prevent the emergence of resistant strains. In addition, in tuberculosis, the use of additional drugs in the initial intensive phase has led to effective treatment of shorter duration. Before AIDS, disseminated MAC was such a rare disease (Holland *et al.*, 1994) that there was no consensus about how it should be treated (Banks, 1989). The *in vitro* measurement of drug sensitivity to MAC is less reliable than to *M. tuberculosis* and does not necessarily predict *in vivo* activity. For this institution, the percentage of strains given as fully sensitive to various relevant antibiotics are: clarithromycin 92%; ciprofloxacin 73%; ethambutol 29%; isoniazid 5%; rifabutin 4%; rifampicin, streptomycin, pyrazinamide, amikacin and clofazimine each <1%. Killing of intracellular organisms is perhaps more important than the agar incorporation methods usually used (Yajko *et al.*, 1989), although in AIDS many of the mycobacteria are extracellular. Despite their apparent lack of *in vitro* activity, clinically useful antibiotics against MAC include aminoglycosides (particularly amikacin), ethambutol, some rifamycins, fluoroquinolones, macrolides and clofazimine (Young, 1988). Of the fluoroquinolones, sparfloxacin is more active against MAC *in vitro* than ofloxacin which in turn is more active than ciprofloxacin (Grosset, 1992).

Newer additions to these drugs include the macrolides such as clarithromycin (Peters and Clissold, 1992). This drug is more active against MAC than azithromycin and erythromycin (Gornyski, Gutman and Allen, 1989), is active against MAC in beige mice (Klemens, DeStefano and Cynamon, 1992) and works intracellularly (Perronne *et al.*, 1990; Yajko *et al.*, 1992). It is also more active against MAC than against *M. tuberculosis*. It is better absorbed than erythromycin; like other macrolides, it is concentrated intracellularly but is predominantly excreted in the urine after hepatic metabolism. Side-effects mainly relating to the gastrointestinal tract are fewer than with erythromycin but, as with all antibiotics, still affect about 20% of subjects. Three percent of subjects may discontinue the drug because of side-effects at low dosage (Bahal and Nahata, 1992) but inevitably, the risk of side-effects increases with dose. In the first controlled study in AIDS, one half of the subjects discontinued treatment at a dose of 2 g twice a day. In a large treatment study, the highest dose was associated with most rapid clearance of bacteremia but also with accelerated mortality in the group – presumably because so many discontinued (Chaisson *et al.*, 1994).

Rifapentine (Dickinson and Mitchison, 1987a; Parenti, 1989) has a longer half-life than rifampicin and is more active against *M. tuberculosis* but it has not found a particular role in the management of mycobacterioses in AIDS. On the other hand, rifabutin is a semi-synthetic derivative of rifamycin S with better pharmacokinetics and activity than rifampicin against MAC (Dickinson and Mitchison, 1987b; Gangadharam *et al.*, 1987; O'Brien, Lyle and Snider, 1987; Heifets and Iseman, 1985). Though poorly soluble in water, the drug is rapidly absorbed from the gastrointestinal tract and this absorption is not affected by food. Peak levels in serum of 0.5 mg/L are achieved by 4 h after a single dose of 300 mg and the terminal half life is 16 h. The drug achieves high concentrations in urine and bile and, more importantly, is concentrated in tissues such as lung to levels five or ten times those of serum. Rifabutin

appears to be somewhat more active than rifampicin against MAC *in vitro*. MICs for sensitive *M. tuberculosis* strains are <0.01 mg/l rifabutin but for MAC range from 0.015–2.0 mg/L. The drug has comparable toxicity to rifampicin, but toxicity of the drug alone is almost impossible to assess because it is always given in combination. Toxicity may be greater in those with disseminated rather than local mycobacterial disease but there are several confounding factors to account for this observation.

Rifabutin, like other rifamycins, enhances the hepatic clearance of drugs like zidovudine. Rare side-effects of rifabutin include thrombocytopenia and uveitis (Shafran *et al.*, 1994). The co-administration of fluconazole increases rifabutin serum levels, hence its activity (Narang *et al.*, 1994) and toxicity (Fuller, Stanfield and Craven, 1994).

Several regimens based on combinations of a rifamycin, ethambutol and clofazimine have been tried in small series of patients with MAC in AIDS with limited success (Dautzenberg *et al.*, 1991b; Hoy *et al.*, 1990; Kemper *et al.*, 1992). Combination therapy results in blood culture-negativity for MAC in about 20% of patients for regimens containing ciprofloxacin, ethambutol, rifampicin with amikacin or clofazimine (Chiu *et al.*, 1990; Kemper *et al.*, 1992; de Lalla, Maserati and Scarpellini, 1992). Another multidrug regimen as originally proposed by Agins and co-workers (1989) and by Hoy and co-workers (1990), with rifabutin, clofazimine, ethambutol and isoniazid may be tried, and may well be successful in clearing mycobacteremia with relief of symptoms for a substantial period. The greatest improvement in the activity of a regimen seems to be achieved by using rifabutin instead of rifampicin although this has not been formally proved. Nevertheless, it is surprising how slowly bacteria are killed by combinations of highly active drugs in the presence of advanced AIDS.

A balance must be struck between the aim of killing MAC without selecting resistance, which is probably best achieved by using a combination of four or even five antibiotics (Hoy *et al.*, 1990) and their toxicity and cost, and the quality of life of the patient with advanced disease who is often already on treatment for other conditions. Nevertheless, MAC is, even more so than tuberculosis, a disseminated infection and although it occurs at a late stage of HIV infection, treatment may lead to improvement of unpleasant symptoms such as fever and diarrhea. Perhaps it is just as acceptable to use simple combinations such as a rifamycin with ethambutol (Heifets, Iseman and Lindholm-Levy, 1988).

Monotherapy with clarithromycin was shown to reduce bacteremia and was well tolerated, but inevitably drug resistance emerged (Dautzenberg *et al.*, 1991a; Chaisson *et al.*, 1994). Treatment with clarithromycin alone may reduce bacteremia if the strains are 'sensitive' *in vitro* (MIC ≤2 mg/l) but not if they are 'resistant' (MIC ≥32 mg/l). However, the *in vitro* measurement of sensitivity is not particularly accurate (Heifets and Iseman, 1985; Heifets *et al.*, 1988, 1992; Dautzenberg *et al.*, 1991a). Clofazimine does not protect against the emergence of resistance to clarithromycin (DeWit *et al.*, 1993).

Other smaller uncontrolled studies with azithromycin (Young *et al.*, 1991), ethambutol, clofazimine or rifampicin (Kemper *et al.*, 1992) have been reported (reviewed in Masur *et al.*, 1993). Clofazimine, rifampicin or sparfloxacin used alone each failed to suppress MAC bacteremia.

The only randomized controlled trial published to date comparing multidrug regimens has demonstrated the superiority of the combination of rifabutin plus clarithromycin plus ethambutol over rifampicin plus ethambutol plus clofazimine plus ciprofloxacin in patients with AIDS and AMC bacteremia (Shafran *et al.*, 1996). Benefit was seen in both bacteriological response and survival. Among

187 patients with a positive baseline culture in the central laboratory, 69% of the three-drug group and only 29% ($p < 0.001$) of the four-drug group became culture-negative and response was also more rapid in the three-drug group. The median survival was 8.6 months in the three-drug and 5.2 months in the four-drug group ($p = 0.001$). The development of uveitis in 24 of the first 63 patients randomized to the three-drug regimen (Shafran *et al.*, 1994) led to a halving of the dose of rifabutin. Even though the 300 mg dose was less effective than the 600 mg dose in clearing bacteremia, in this combination it was still more effective than the four-drug regimen. Uveitis was much less common with the reduced dose of rifabutin and the only other significant difference in adverse events between the groups was an alteration in taste, which occurred in 9 patients in the three-drug and 1 in the four-drug groups ($p = 0.02$).

The interaction between rifabutin and clarithromycin has important implications for the dosages of both drugs when used together. The considerable increase in plasma levels of both rifabutin and its active metabolite (DATRI 001 study group, 1994a) may account for the increased risk of uveitis when it is given with clarithromycin. The reduction by about half of the clarithromycin levels when given with rifabutin (DATRI 001 Study group, 1994b; Wallace *et al.*, 1995) may mean that a dose of 1000 mg twice a day (as in the trial) may achieve levels similar to those of the recommended dose of 500 mg twice a day without. This is important as an ongoing trial of combination therapy in MAC bacteremia has recently been modified because an interim analysis has shown better survival in the group taking 500 mg twice daily than in that taking 1000 mg twice a day (Cohn *et al.*, 1996). May and coworkers (1996) have shown the superiority, in terms of bacteriological relapse by 6 months, of the three-drug regimen of clarithromycin plus ethambutol plus rifabutin over a two-drug regimen of clarithromycin plus clofazimine in a study of 134 patients. However, there was no significant difference in the proportions who died.

In most clinical studies, the activity of an antibiotic or a combination has been judged by reduction in counts of MAC in blood after short-duration therapy but also by resolution of fever and prevention of weight loss. There is little expectation of cure. In interpreting studies where the endpoint is MAC bacteremia, it is important to appreciate that the presence of antibiotic in the blood may compromise isolation of the organism, suggesting increased efficacy. Some patients appear to have transient MAC bacteremia which is of doubtful clinical significance. In many patients, symptoms recur even though monotherapy is continued, suggesting that clinical (and perhaps microbiological) resistance can develop in as short a time as one month after starting monotherapy.

PREVENTIVE THERAPY

There have been two large placebo-controlled trials of rifabutin prophylaxis which included a total of 1146 HIV patients with peripheral CD4 lymphocyte counts less than $200/\mu l$ (Nightingale *et al.*, 1993, discussed in Masur, 1993). In this trial 566 patients received rifabutin for a mean of 218 days. The development of MAC bacteremia was reduced by about one half in the rifabutin group; the relative risk for MAC bacteremia in the combined study population for the rifabutin compared to the placebo group was 0.45 (95% CI 0.32 to 0.63; $p<0.001$). No survival benefit was demonstrated in these trials but morbidity was significantly reduced. Resistant strains were not selected by rifabutin prophylaxis. Toxicity leading to cessation of treatment, comprising neutropenia, rash, nausea and hepatitis, occurred in 16% of rifabutin and 8% of placebo patients. Rash and discolored

urine occurred as often in placebo as in treated patients.

A randomized controlled trial of clarithromycin at a dose of 500 mg twice daily versus placebo in 667 HIV-infected individuals with $CD4^+$ counts of $<100/\mu l$ followed for a mean of 427 days in the clarithromycin and 402 days in the placebo group showed a reduction in the risk of MAC bacteremia from 16 to 6% (Pierce *et al.*, 1996). Eleven of 19 isolates tested in the treated group became resistant to clarithromycin. There was also a significant reduction in mortality from 41 to 32% (relative reduction 25%; $p = 0.026$) in the clarithromycin group but a significant increase in gastrointestinal side-effects in the treated group.

A second trial compared three different prophylaxis regimens in 693 patients with CD4 counts below $100/\mu l$: once-weekly azithromycin or daily rifabutin or both (Havlir *et al.*, 1996). The proportions with disseminated MAC infection at 1 year in the three groups were 7.6, 15.3 and 2.8% respectively, representing a relative reduction in the risk of disseminated MAC infection (after adjusting for baseline CD4 counts which were higher in the combination group) of 72% ($p<0.001$) for combination therapy compared to rifabutin alone and 47% ($p = 0.03$) compared to azithromycin alone. The relative reduction for azithromycin compared to rifabutin was 47% ($p = 0.008$). Two of 18 isolates of MAC from patients receiving azithromycin alone, but none of the five from patients receiving both drugs, were resistant to both azithromycin and clarithromycin. None of the 21 isolates from the patients receiving rifabutin alone or the five from those receiving both drugs were resistant to rifabutin. There were no significant differences in survival between the groups but there were differences in the incidence of adverse events. In particular, gastrointestinal symptoms were significantly more common in the two-drug group and in the azithromycin group compared to the rifabutin group. Overall, dose-limiting adverse events were more common in the two-drug group.

Although there is now evidence of the benefits of prophylaxis for disseminated MAC infection in terms of the prevention of MAC bacteremia but also improved survival, there still remains a number of issues about the optimum regimen and when it should be started. A panel of the Public Health Service and the Infectious Disease Society of America has recommended a level of 75 CD4 cells in patients who have had opportunistic diseases but others may wait for longer (Kaplan *et al.*, 1995; Ostroff *et al.*, 1995; Horsburgh, 1996). A further issue concerns the interactions of the drugs used for prophylaxis with the many other drugs taken by individuals with advanced HIV infection. Fluconazole affects the serum levels of both clarithromycin and rifabutin and the interaction with the HIV-protease inhibitors may be even more important (Horsburgh, 1996). The balance between prophylaxis and therapy for an infection depends on many factors and is particularly complex in MAC infection in individuals with HIV infection. The indiscriminate, routine use of preventive therapy against MAC with any of the newer antimicrobials in HIV-infected individuals would be a very expensive strategy.

TREATMENT GUIDELINES FOR MYCOBACTERIAL INFECTIONS IN HIV INFECTION

Guidelines on the management of tuberculosis and other mycobacterial infections in association with HIV have been published, both for technically advanced and developing countries (Ormerod, 1990, 1992; Centers for Disease Control, 1989; Advisory Committee for the Elimination of Tuberculosis, 1989, 1990; IUATLD, 1988; WHO and IUATLD, 1994). However, as in this article, very little of the advice is based on the results of controlled studies in AIDS patients.

PREVENTING THE TRANSMISSION OF MYCOBACTERIAL DISEASE

Because of the outbreaks of nosocomial infection of tuberculosis in HIV infected individuals (Report, 1991), guidelines for the control of tuberculosis in health care settings have also been published (IUATLD and WHO, 1994a; Centers for Disease Control, 1990, 1994).

CROSS INFECTION WITH MAC

MAC is a common infection in patients with advanced AIDS. It is presumed that patients become colonized after exposure to environmental mycobacteria in the water supply (von Reyn *et al.*, 1994; Singh and Yu, 1994) and that natural inhibition of the infection is lost with progression of immunosuppression. However, MAC is relatively unusual in the water supply compared with other atypical mycobacterial species (Peters *et al.*, 1995). There is a suspicion that the organism can be transmitted from one patient to another, and this would be particularly likely if a patient with MAC had diarrhea from whatever cause, the stools being heavily contaminated with bacilli. However, it is not clear what contribution cross infection may make to the likelihood of acquiring MAC. Molecular biology techniques are being applied to establish the relatedness of strains from patients and the water supply in units (von Reyn *et al.*, 1994). All patients with diarrhea (whatever the cause) should be nursed in source isolation.

CROSS INFECTION WITH *M. TUBERCULOSIS*

M. tuberculosis is transmitted most effectively by the aerosol route but the number of infectious particles generated by smear-positive individuals is relatively small and prolonged exposure is usually required to effect transmission (Riley, 1982). Because they are highly susceptible to tuberculosis, the most effective indicators of the transmission of tuberculosis in hospitals and other institutions are the immunosuppressed; children (George *et al.*, 1985); patients with AIDS (Chaisson *et al.*, 1987; Daley *et al.*, 1992; Festenstein and Grange, 1991); and the elderly (Stead *et al.*, 1985). These papers draw attention to the risk of patients *acquiring* rather than reactivating tuberculosis in later life, an observation which clearly anticipated the problems which are now seen in AIDS (Godfrey-Faussett *et al.*, 1994). Occasionally, large outbreaks occur in hospitals, particularly when the disease is not suspected and a large aerosol is generated (Hutton *et al.*, 1990).

Patients with tuberculosis in HIV often have non-pulmonary disease so are theoretically less likely to transmit the disease than those with classical cavitatory disease and this is borne out by some observational evidence. Family contacts of HIV-positive individuals with tuberculosis in Zaire are less likely to have evidence of infection than those of HIV-negative individuals (Elliott *et al.*, 1993). This should not make the carer complacent: transmission was just as likely if the index case was smear-positive and the rate of tuberculosis in the contacts was the same. In Kenya, HIV positivity in the index case had little effect on the overall likelihood of contacts having tuberculosis (Nunn *et al.*, 1994).

There has been clear evidence of transmission of tuberculosis from HIV-infected patients to others, even from a patient who was sputum smear-negative but culture-positive (Di Perri *et al.*, 1989). Despite the fact that healthy adults are relatively unlikely to develop tuberculosis, carers of HIV-infected individuals have caught tuberculosis from their patients and in some instances this has proved to be with MDR strains (Pearson *et al.*, 1992).

Several sets of guidelines have been published to reduce the risk of spread of tuberculosis from one patient to another or to a carer (Centers for Disease Control, 1990;

IUATLD, 1994a; WHO and IUATLD, 1994).

The most recent guidelines from the TB Infection-Control Guidelines Work Group (Centers for Disease Control, 1994), take a rigorous and stringent approach to the problem. In the UK, a simple strategy of source isolation of tuberculous patients for the first two weeks of therapy is widely accepted (Joint Tuberculosis Committee, 1994). The recent recommendations from the USA suggest that a risk assessment is carried out for each clinical area where there may be patients with tuberculosis with the aim of identifying and reducing the perceived risks to other patients and Health Care Workers. An appropriate control program can then be implemented. Most hospitals have very satisfactory and appropriate programs enshrined in Infection Control Policies. The detection of nosocomial transmission (Edlin *et al.*, 1992; Kent *et al.*, 1994), however, stresses the need to determine ways in which the risks can be reduced. Wenger and co-workers successfully applied stringent precautions according to these guidelines, in the face of a major continuing outbreak of nosocomial MDR tuberculosis in Miami (Wenger *et al.*, 1995).

Features of a patient which enhance the risk of transmission include smear-positivity and cavitatory disease of the lungs or infection of the larynx. Other important factors are the natural delay in diagnosis of tuberculosis and the rapid progression of disease in immunocompromised individuals. Many patients infected with HIV have CXR appearances which are not typical of tuberculosis, some 20% having normal CXRs, others having lobar shadowing or diffuse shadowing like *Pneumocystis carinii* pneumonia (see Chapter 4). Delayed diagnosis leads to delays in implementing treatment and source isolation which are the critical steps to reduce infectivity. Procedures which enhance transmission in health care settings include bronchoscopy (the organism being aerosolized or transmitted directly on an inadequately decontaminated endoscope), endotracheal intubation and suction, irrigation of an abscess and autopsy. Induction of sputum or administration of aerosolized pentamidine may also be important.

The tenets of reducing the risk of transmission involve identification of infectious cases and treatment and source isolation of those cases. Control of environment and protection of health care workers are also important.

Identification of infectious cases

Because there is usually a protracted delay between the onset and detection of disease, doctors caring for those at high risk of tuberculosis (e.g. HIV-infected individuals or immigrants) must have a high degree of suspicion when there are respiratory symptoms or lymphadenopathy. Diagnosis is straightforward if a patient has a classical cavitatory lesion on chest X-ray but this is unusual in advanced HIV disease where the disease is more likely to be disseminated. Diffuse chest X-ray changes will at first be ascribed to *Pneumocystis carinii* pneumonia and the confirmatory diagnosic procedures (bronchoscopy or induced sputum) may be risky.

All bronchoalveolar lavage, sputum and induced sputum specimens from HIV-infected patients must be examined for mycobacteria. Cultures will take a matter of weeks (Table 12.1 above). Acid-fast bacilli seen in profusion in feces or isolated from blood cannot be assumed to be MAC. We have seen several patients with tuberculosis presenting in this way. Furthermore in a patient with multibacillary disease, although the colonial appearance of the isolate on primary culture was that of MAC, the strain turned out to be MDR *M. tuberculosis*. Hopefully, rapid identification techniques based on DNA sequencing should soon be available but these will not become universally available and delays in diagnosis must continue to occur. If fingerprinting of strains is possible (Saunders, 1995), then this should be done routinely on all strains for a unit in order to identify episodes of cross-infection which have occurred.

Treatment

Providing an organism is sensitive, and that the treatment is taken and absorbed, it is perceived that the risk of transmission is so reduced after two weeks of treatment that source isolation is no longer necessary. The sputum is not necessarily free of viable bacilli by this time but there is usually a several log-fold reduction in numbers. It may be wise to extend the period of source isolation in those with open cavitatory multibacillary smear-positive disease and also in AIDS when MDR is suspected (IUATLD, 1994a).

The US recommendations that patients should remain in source isolation until the patient is improving clinically and has had three consecutive negative sputum smears may be somewhat over-restrictive. However, if MDR strains are likely, then arguably patients should remain in source isolation throughout their hospitalization.

Whatever the status of infectivity, it is safer for patients and staff for those with tuberculosis to be at home with appropriate contact tracing for close contacts. On discharge from hospital, continuing therapy is of such importance that directly observed therapy should be arranged when indicated. Treatment should be modified on results of culture and sensitivity.

The question of malabsorption of anti-tuberculosis therapy in AIDS has arisen so recently that there are no guidelines as to appropriate investigation or action. Spot urine tests for rifampicin and isoniazid are very easy to perform and if negative indicate that the patient is either not taking or is not absorbing therapy. A positive urine test does not, however, indicate that sufficient of either drug has been absorbed to guarantee cure.

Source isolation of infectious cases

Patients with open tuberculosis in hospital should be nursed in a separate room or area either individually or in cohort with other tuberculous patients. The wearing of masks **by patients** visiting other parts of the hospital to reduce the dissemination of aerosols has been recommended. However, this is ineffective in the case of surgical masks as they may hold up large particles (which are not a significant risk) and do not prevent the dissemination of aerosols. It is not appropriate to ask patients to wear HEPA filtered masks. The risks of transmission by transient contact is very low (Riley, 1982).

Family and close contacts of an index case should be traced and investigated according to local procedures, with due regard to previous BCG immunization and the possibility of partners also having HIV infection (Nunn *et al.*, 1994).

Occupational health guidance of health care workers infected with HIV should indicate the risks of working with patients who are a significant risk of infection to susceptible individuals.

Engineering or environmental control

Optimally, isolation rooms should be ventilated in such a way that there is negative pressure in the room in relation to the local ward environment. If no mechanical ventilation is available, the window should be open to dilute aerosols. Exhausted air should be filtered, particularly if the exhaust duct is positioned near to air intakes for air conditioning. Alternatively, the air inside a room can be recirculated through a high efficiency particulate air (HEPA) filter. Ultraviolet irradiation may be used as a disinfectant in air conditioning systems, in an isolation room or more generally in other areas where there may be tuberculous patients: there is no evidence as to efficacy. Continued maintenance is important because radiation from

tubes falls quite rapidly with time and they become much less active when covered with dust.

Protection of health care workers

Surgical masks are relatively inefficient in protecting against the inhalation of 1–5μM particles, compared to respirators fitted with HEPA filters (Weber *et al.*, 1993). This has led to the recommendation in the US that health care workers should wear a HEPA filter respirator when entering a room where tuberculous patients are isolated. However, this recommendation has caused much controversy (Wilcox, 1995) and there are very cogent reasons for not wearing such masks. The first is that there is no guarantee of their efficiency in preventing the inhalation of tubercle bearing aerosols. The second is that the mask creates a physical and psychological barrier between staff and patients, many of whom already feel ostracized by being in isolation. Thirdly, patients with tuberculosis are not usually identified from the time they become infectious. Finally, the masks have to be fitted individually and are not efficient for those with beards. Calculations suggest that they would be very expensive for the benefit conferred (Nettleman *et al.*, 1994; Adal *et al.*, 1994).

Use of BCG?

Weltman and Rose (1993) have reviewed the literature on complications of BCG immunization in HIV. There is no place for the immunization of skin-test negative patients with HIV using BCG. It is unlikely to be effective and *Mycobacterium bovis* BCG may disseminate in immunosuppressed individuals. Mass immunization campaigns with BCG have revealed a small increase in complications with HIV (Bregère, 1988; Quinn, 1989) but others have found that the local complication rates (lymphadenitis and fistula) are similar between

HIV infected and uninfected children (ten Dam, 1990). Cases of systemic BCGosis immunized in error should be treated with conventional chemotherapy (e.g. rifampicin, isonazid and ethambutol) and usually respond very well. The organism is not sensitive to pyrazinamide.

There is a strong case for immunization of healthy health-care workers in whom there is no good evidence of previous immunization or natural infection with mycobacteria. The practice of pre-employment screening of all staff using tuberculin skin testing is widely used in some countries. In areas where BCG is not routinely given at birth or in early teenage, then most of the adult population will be tuberculin skin-test negative. A balance has then to be struck between the value of skin-test conversion as a marker for infection of a health-care worker exposed to tuberculosis and the potential protective effect of BCG against disease.

In summary, a comprehensive approach to the reduction of transmission of tuberculosis in health care facilities must be adopted. This involves improved identification of cases, adequate treatment, appropriate facilities to prevent the transmission of aerosols and protection of health-care workers.

REFERENCES

Ackah, A.N., Coulibaly, D., Digbeu, H. *et al.* (1995) Response to treatment, mortality, and CD4 lymphocyte counts in HIV-infected persons with tuberculosis in Abidjan, Côte d'Ivoire. *Lancet*, **345** 607–10.

Adal, K.A., Anglim, A.M., Palumbo, C.L. *et al.* (1994) The use of high-efficiency particulate air-filter respirators to protect hospital workers from tuberculosis. *New England Journal of Medicine*, **331**, 169–73.

Advisory Committee for Elimination of Tuberculosis (ACET), Centers for Disease Control (1989) Tuberculosis and Human Immunodeficiency virus infection. *Morbidity and Mortality Weekly Reports*, **38**, 236–50.

Advisory Committee for the Elimination of Tuberculosis, Centers for Disease Control (1990) Screening for tuberculosis and tuberculous infection in high risk populations and the use of preventive therapy for tuberculosis in the US. *Morbidity and Mortality Weekly Reports*, **39**, RR8: 1–12.

Agins, B.D., Berman, D.S., Spicehandler, D. *et al.* (1989) Effect of combined therapy with ansamycin, clofazimine, ethambutol and isoniazid for *Mycobacterium avium* infection in patients with AIDS. *Journal of Infectious Diseases*, **159**, 784–7.

Alwood, K., Keruly, J., Moore-Rice, K. *et al.* (1994) Effectiveness of supervised intermittent therapy for tuberculosis on HIV-infected patients. *AIDS*, **8**, 1103–8.

Aquinas, Sr. M., Allan, W.G.L., Horsfall, P.A.L. *et al.* (1972) Adverse reactions to daily and intermittent rifampicin regimens for pulmonary tuberculosis in Hong Kong. *British Medical Journal*, **i**, 765–71.

Bahal, N. and Nahata, M. (1992) The new macrolide antibiotics: azithromycin, clarithromycin, dirithromycin and roxithromycin. *Annals of Pharmacotherapeutics*, **26**, 46–55.

Banks, J. (1989) Treatment of pulmonary disease caused by opportunist mycobacteria. *Thorax*, **44**, 449–54.

Bass, J.B., Farer, L.S., Hopewell, P.C. *et al.* (1995) Treatment of tuberculosis and tuberculosis infection in adults and children. *Clinical Infectious Diseases*, **21**, 9–27.

Bregère, P. (1988) BCG vaccination and AIDS. *Bulletin of the International Union against Tuberculosis*, **63**, 40–1.

Centers for Disease Control (1989) Tuberculosis and human immunodeficiency virus infections: recommendations of the Advisory Committee for the Elimination of Tuberculosis (ACET). *Morbidity and Mortality Weekly Reports*, **38**, 236–8, 243–50.

Centers for Disease Control (1991) Nosocomial transmission of multi-drug resistant tuberculosis amongst HIV-infected persons – Florida and New York 1988-1991. *Morbidity and Mortality Weekly Reports*, **40**, 585–91.

Centers for Disease Control (1994) Guidelines for preventing the transmission of *Mycobacterium tuberculosis* in health-care facilities. *Morbidity and Mortality Weekly Reports*, **40**, 585–91.

Chaisson, R.E., Schecter, G.F., Theuer, C.P. *et al.* (1987) Tuberculosis in patients with the acquired immunodeficiency syndrome. *American Review of Respiratory Disease*, **136**, 570–4.

Chaisson, R.E., Benson, C.A., Dube, M.P. *et al.* (1994) Clarithromycin therapy for bacteremic *Mycobacterium avium* complex disease. *Annals of Internal Medicine*, **121**, 905–11.

Chiu, J., Nussbaum, J., Bozette, S. *et al.* (1990) Treatment of disseminated *Mycobacterium avium* complex infection in AIDS with amikacin, ethambutol, rifampin and ciprofloxacin. *Annals of Internal Medicine*, **113**, 358–61.

Cohn, D.L., Fisher, E., Franchino, B. *et al.* (1996) Comparison of two doses of clarithromycin in a randomised trial of four 3-drug regimens for treatment of disseminated *Mycobacterium avium* complex disease in AIDS: excess mortality associated with high-dose clarithromycin. 11th International Conference on AIDS, Vancouver, July 1996, abstract LB B 6025.

Committee on Treatment of the International Union Against Tuberculosis and Lung Disease (1988) Antituberculosis regimens of chemotherapy. Recommendations. *Bulletin of the International Union Against Tuberculosis and Lung Disease*, **63**, 60–4.

Daley, C.L., Small, P.M., Schecter, G.F. *et al.* (1992) An outbreak of tuberculosis with accelerated progression among persons infected with the human immunodeficiency virus. *New England Journal of Medicine*, **326**, 231–41.

DATRI 001 Study Group (1994a) Clarithromycin (CL) plus rifabutin (RFB) for MAC prophylaxis: evidence for drug interaction. First National Conference on Human Retroviruses and Related Infections, December 1993, Washington DC.

DATRI 001 Study Group (1994b) Co-administration of clarithromycin (CL) alters the concentration–time profile of rifabutin (RFB). 34th Interscience Conference on Antimicrobial Agents and Chemotherapy, October 1994, Orlando Florida. Abstract A2, p. 3.

Dautzenberg, B., Truffot, C., Legris, S. *et al.* (1991a) Activity of clarithromycin against *Mycobacterium avium* infection in patients with the acquired immune deficiency syndrome: a controlled clinical trial. *American Review of Respiratory Disease*, **144**, 564–9.

Dautzenberg, B., Truffot, Ch., Mignon, A. *et al.* (1991b) Rifabutin in combination with clofazimine, isoniazid and ethambutol in the treatment of AIDS patients with infections due to opportunist mycobacteria. *Tubercle*, **72**, 168–75.

De Cock, K.M., Grant, A. and Porter, J.D.H. (1995) Preventive therapy for tuberculosis in HIV-infected persons: international recommendations, research, and practice. *Lancet*, **345**, 833–6.

de Lalla, F., Maserati, R. and Scarpellini, P. (1992) Clarithromycin-ciprofloxacin-amikacin for therapy of *Mycobacterium avium* bacteraemia in patients with AIDS. *Antimicrobial Agents and Chemotherapy*, **36**, 1567–9.

De Wit, S., D'Abbraccio, M., De Mol, P. and Clumeck, N. (1993) Acquired resistance to clarithromycin as combined therapy in *Mycobacterium avium intracellulare* infection. *Lancet*, **341**, 53–4.

Di Perri, G., Cruciani, M., Danzi, M.C. *et al.* (1989) Nosocomial epidemic of active tuberculosis among HIV-infected patients. *Lancet*, **ii**, 1502–4.

Dickinson, J.M. and Mitchison, D.A. (1987a) In vitro properties of rifapentine (MDL473) relevant to its use in intermittent chemotherapy of tuberculosis. *Tubercle*, **68**, 113–8.

Dickinson, J.M. and Mitchison, D.A. (1987b) In vitro activity of new rifamycins against rifampicin-resistant *M. tuberculosis* and MAIS-complex mycobacteria. *Tubercle*, **68**, 177–82.

Edlin, B.R., Tokars, J.I., Grieco, M.H. *et al.* (1992) An outbreak of multidrug-resistant tuberculosis among hospitalized patients with the acquired immunodeficiency syndrome. *New England Journal of Medicine*, **326**, 1514–21.

Elliott, A.M., Hayes, R.J., Halwiindi, B. *et al.* (1993) The impact of HIV on infectiousness of pulmonary tuberculosis: a community study in Zambia. *AIDS*, **7**, 981–7.

Elliott, A.M. and Foster S.D. (1996) Thiacetazone: time to call a halt? *Tubercle and Lung Disease*, **77**, 27–9.

Festenstein, F. and Grange, J.M. (1991) Tuberculosis and the acquired immune deficiency syndrome. *Journal of Applied Bacteriology*, **71**, 19–30.

Fuller, J.D., Stanfield, L.E.D. and Craven, D.E. (1994) Rifabutin prophylaxis and uveitis. *New England Journal of Medicine*, **330**, 1315–6.

Gangadharam, P.R.J., Perumal, V.K., Jairam, B.T. *et al.* (1987) Activity of rifabutin alone or in combination with clofazimine or ethambutol or both against acute and chronic experimental *Mycobacterium intracellulare* infections. *American Review of Respiratory Disease*, **136**, 329–33.

George, R.H., Gully, P.R., Gill, O.N. *et al.* (1985) An outbreak of tuberculosis in a children's hospital. *Journal of Hospital Infection*, **8**, 129–42.

Girling, D.J. (1978) The hepatic toxicity of anti-tuberculosis regimens containing isoniazid, rifampicin and pyrtazinamide. *Tubercle*, **59**, 13–32.

Githui, W., Nunn, P., Juma, E. *et al.* (1992) Cohort study of HIV-positive and HIV-negative tuberculosis, Nairobi, Kenya: comparison of bacteriological results. *Tubercle and Lung Disease*, **73**, 203–9.

Glynn, J.R., Jenkins, P.A., Fine, P.E.M. *et al.* (1995) Patterns of initial and acquired antituberculosis drug resistance in Karonga District, Malawi, *Lancet*, **345**, 907–10.

Goble, M., Iseman, M.D., Madsen, L.A. *et al.* (1993) Treatment of 171 patients with pulmonary tuberculosis resistant to isoniazid and rifampin. *New England Journal of Medicine*, **328**, 527–32.

Godfrey-Faussett, P., Githui, W., Batchelor, B. *et al.* (1994) Recurrence of tuberculosis in an endemic area may be due to relapse or reinfection. *Tubercle and Lung Disease*, **75**, 199–202.

Goldberger, M. and Masur, H. (1994) Clarithromycin therapy for *Mycobacterium avium* complex disease in patients with AIDS: potential and problems. *Annals of Internal Medicine*, **121**, 974–5.

Gornyski, E., Gutman, S. and Allen, (1989) Comparative antimicrobial activities of difloxacin, temafloxacin, enoxacin, pefloxacin, reference fluoroquinolones and a new macrolide clarithromycin. *Antimicrobial Agents and Chemotherapy*, **33**, 591–2.

Grange, J.M. (1990) Drug resistance and tuberculosis elimination. *Bulletin of the International Union against Tuberculosis and Lung Disease*, **65** (2–3), 57–9.

Grosset, J.H. (1990) Present and new drug regimens in chemotherapy and chemoprophylaxis of tuberculosis. *Bulletin of the International Union against Tuberculosis and Lung Disease*, **65**, 86–91.

Grosset, J.H. (1992) Treatment of tuberculosis in HIV infection. *Tubercle and Lung Disease*, **73**, 378–83.

Harries, A.D., Menwe, L. N'O., Maher, D. *et al.* (1995) Regimen containing short-term rifampicin for pulmonary tuberculosis in HIV-infection. *Lancet*, **345**, 264–5.

Havlir, D.V., Dube, M.P., Sattler, F.R. *et al.* (1996) Prophylaxis against disseminated *Mycobacterium avium* complex with weekly azithromycin, daily rifabutin, or both. *New England Journal of Medicine*, **335**, 392–8

Hawken, M., Nunn, P., Gathua, S. *et al.* (1993) Increased recurrence of tuberculosis in HIV-1 infected patients in Kenya. *Lancet*, **342**, 332–7.

Heifets, L.B. and Iseman, M.D. (1985) Determination of *in vitro* susceptibility of mycobacteria to Ansamycin. *American Review of Respiratory Disease*, **132**, 710–1.

Heifets, L.B., Iseman, M.D. and Lindholm-Levy, P.J. (1988) Combinations of rifampin or rifabutine plus ethambutol against *Mycobacterium avium* complex. *American Review of Respiratory Disease*, **137**, 711–15.

Heifets, L.B., Lindholm-Levy, P.J. and Iseman, M.D. (1988) Rifabutine: minimal inhibitory and bactericidal concentrations for *mycobacterium* tuberculosis. *American Review of Respiratory Disease*, **137**, 719–21.

Heifets, L.B., Lindholm-Levy, P.J. and Comstock, R.D. (1992) Clarithromycin minimal inhibitory and bactericidal concentrations against *Mycobacterium avium*. *American Review of Respiratory Disease*, **145**, 856–8.

Heym, B., Honoré, N., Truffot-Pernot, C. *et al.* (1994) Implications of multidrug resistance for the future of short course chemotherapy of tuberculosis. *Lancet*, **344**, 293–8.

Holland, S.M., Eisenstein, E.M., Kuhns, D.B. *et al.* (1994) Treatment of refractory disseminated nontuberculous mycobacterial infection with interferon gamma. *New England Journal of Medicine*, **330**, 1348–55.

Horsburgh, C.R. (1996) Advances in the prevention and treatment of *Mycobacterium avium* disease. *New England Journal of Medicine*, **355**, 428–30

Hoy, J., Mijch, A., Sandland, M. *et al.* (1990) Quadruple-drug therapy for *Mycobacterium avium-intracellulare* bacteraemia in AIDS patients *Journal of Infectious Diseases*, **161**, 801–5.

Hutton, M., Stead, W.W., Cauthen, G. *et al.* (1990) Nosocomial transmission of tuberculosis associated with a draining abscess. *Journal of Infectious Diseases*, **161**, 286–95.

International Union against Tuberculosis and Lung Disease (1988) Antituberculosis regimens of chemotherapy. *Bulletin of the International Union against Tuberculosis and Lung Diseases*, **63**, 60–4.

International Union against Tuberculosis and Lung Disease (IUATLD) and Tuberculosis Programme of the WHO (1994a) Control of tuberculosis in health care settings. *Tubercle and Lung Disease*, **75**, 94–5.

International Union against Tuberculosis and Lung Disease (IUATLD) and the Global Programme on AIDS and the Tuberculosis Programme of the World Health Organisation (WHO) (1994b) TB preventive therapy in HIV-infected individuals. *Tubercle and Lung Disease*, **75**, 96–8.

Iseman, M.D. (1993) Treatment of multidrug-resistant tuberculosis. *New England Journal of Medicine*, **329**, 784–91.

Iseman, M.D. (1994) Evolution of drug-resistant tuberculosis: a tale of two species. *Proceedings of the National Academy of Sciences USA*, **91**, 2428–9.

Joint Tuberculosis Committee of the British Thoracic Society (1994) Control and prevention of tuberculosis in the UK: code of practice. *Thorax*, **49**, 1193–1200.

Kaplan, J.E., Masur, H., Holmes, K.K. *et al.* (1995) USPHS/IDSA guidelines for the prevention of opportunistic infections in persons infected with human immunodeficiency virus: an overview. *Clinical Infectious Diseases*, **21** (suppl 1), S12–31.

Kassim, S., Sassan-Morokro, M., Ackah, A. *et al.* (1995) Two-year follow-up of persons with HIV-1 and HIV-2-associated pulmonary tuberculosis treated with short course chemotherapy in West Africa. *AIDS*, **9**, 1185–91.

Kemper, C.A., Meng, T.C., Nussbaum, J. *et al.* (1992) Treatment of *Mycobacterium avium* complex bacteremia in AIDS with a four-drug oral regimen: rifampin, ethambutol, clofazimine, and ciprofloxacin. *Annals of Internal Medicine*, **116**, 466–72.

Kent, R.J., Uttley, A.H.C., Stoker, N.G. *et al.* (1994) Transmission of tuberculosis in a British centre for patients infected with HIV. *British Medical Journal*, **309**, 639–40.

Klemens, S.P., DeStefano, M.S. and Cynamon, M.H. (1992) Activity of clarithromycin against *Mycobacterium avium* complex infection in beige mice. *Antimicrobial Agents and Chemotherapy*, **36**, 2413–7.

Masur, H. and the Public Health Service Task Force on Prophylaxis and Therapy for *Mycobacterium avium* complex. (1993) Recommendations on prophylaxis and therapy for disseminated *Mycobacterium avium* complex disease in patients infected with HIV. *New England Journal of Medicine*, **329**, 898–904.

Mayer, T., Vincent, V., Brel, F. *et al.* (1996) The French randomized clinical trial of combination therapy with clarithromycin for MAC bacteremia in AIDS patients: final results. 11th International Conference on AIDS July 1996, Vancouver, Abstract WeB 422.

Menzies, I.D., Fanning, A., Yuan, L. and Fitzgerald, M. (1995) Tuberculosis among health care workers. *New England Journal of Medicine*, **332**, 92–8.

Mitchell, I., Wendon, J., Fitt, S. and Williams R. (1995) Anti-tuberculous therapy and acute liver failure. *Lancet*, **345**, 555–6.

Mitchison, D.A., Ellard, G.A. and Grosset, J. (1988) New antibacterial drugs for the treatment of mycobacterial disease in man. *British Medical Bulletin*, **44**, 757–74.

Moreno, S., Baraia-Etxaburu, J., Bouza, E. *et al.* (1993) Risk for developing tuberculosis among anergic patients infected with HIV. *Annals of Internal Medicine*, **119**, 194–8.

Murray, C.J.L., De Jonghe, E., Chum, H.J. *et al.* (1991) Cost effectiveness of chemotherapy for pulmonary tuberculosis in three sub-Saharan African countries. *Lancet*, **338**, 1305–8.

Narang, P.K., Trapnell, C.B., Schoenfelder, J.R. *et al.* (1994) Fluconazole and enhanced effect of rifabutin prophylaxis. *New England Journal of Medicine*, **330**, 1316–17.

Nettleman, M.D., Fredrickson, M., Good, N.L. and Hunter, S.A. (1994) Tuberculosis control strategies: the cost of particulate respirators. *Annals of Internal Medicine*, **121**, 37–40.

Nightingale, S.D., Cameron, D.W., Gordin, F.M. *et al.* (1993) Two controlled trials of rifabutin prophylaxis against *Mycobacterium avium* complex infections in AIDS. *New England Journal of Medicine*, **329**, 828–33.

Nunn, P., Kibuga, D., Gathua, S. *et al.* (1991) Cutaneous hypersensitivity reactions due to thiacetazone in HIV-1 seropositive patients treated for tuberculosis. *Lancet*, **337**, 627–30.

Nunn, P., Mungai, M., Nyamwaya, J. *et al.* (1994) The effect of human immunodeficiency virus type 1 on the infectiousness of tuberculosis. *Tubercle and Lung Diseases*, **75**, 25–32.

O'Brien, R.J., Lyle, M.A. and Snider, D.E. Jr. (1987) Rifabutin (Ansamycin LM427): a new rifamycin S derivative for the treatment of mycobacterial diseases. *Reviews of Infectious Diseases*, **9**, 519–30.

O'Brien, R.J. and Perriëns, J.H. (1995) Preventive therapy for tuberculosis in HIV infection: the promise and the reality. *AIDS*, **9**, 665–73.

Okwera, A., Whalen, C., Byekwaso, F. *et al.* (1994)

Randomised trial of thiacetazone and rifampicin-containing regimens for pulmonary tuberculosis in HIV-infected Ugandans. *Lancet*, **344**, 1323–8.

Ormerod, L.P. for a subcommittee of the Joint Tuberculosis Committee (1990) Chemotherapy and management of tuberculosis in the United Kingdom: recommendations of the Joint Tuberculosis Committee of the British Thoracic Society. *Thorax*, **45**, 403–8.

Ormerod, L.P. for a subcommittee of the Joint Tuberculosis Committee (1992) Guidelines on the management of tuberculosis and HIV infection in the United Kingdom. *British Medical Journal*, **304**, 1231–3.

Ostroff, S.M., Speigel, R.A., Feinberg, J. *et al.* (1995) Preventing disseminated *Mycobacterium avium* complex disease in patients infected with human immunodeficiency virus. *Clinical Infectious Diseases*, **21** (suppl 1), S72–76.

Pape, J.W., Jean, S.S., Ho, J.L. *et al.* (1993) Effect of isoniazid prophylaxis on incidence of active tuberculosis and progression of HIV infection. *Lancet*, **342**, 268–72.

Parenti, F. (1989) New experimental drugs for the treatment of tuberculosis. *Reviews of Infectious Diseases*, **11**, S479–83.

Patel, K.B., Belmonte, R. and Crowe, H.M. (1995) Drug malabsorption and resistant tuberculosis in HIV-infected patients. *New England Journal of Medicine*, **332**, 336–7.

Pearson, M.L., Jareb, J.A., Frieden, T.R. *et al.* (1992) Nosocomial transmission of multidrug-resistant *Mycobacterium tuberculosis*. *Annals of Internal Medicine*, **117**, 191–6.

Perriëns, J.H., Colebunders, R.L., Karahunga, C. *et al.* (1991) Increased mortality and tuberculosis treatment failure rate among HIV seropositive compared with HIV seronegative patients with pulmonary tuberculosis treated with "standard" chemotherapy in Kinshasa, Zaire. *American Review of Respiratory Disease*, **144**, 750–5.

Perriëns, J.H., St. Louis, M.E., Mukadi, Y.B. *et al.* (1995) Pulmonary tuberculosis in HIV-infected patients in Zaire. *New England Journal of Medicine*, **332**, 779–84.

Perronne, C., Gikas, A., Truffot-Pernot, C. *et al.* (1990) Activities of clarithromycin, sulfisoxazole, and rifabutin against *Mycobacterium avium* complex. Multiplication within human macrophages. *Antimicrobial Agents and Chemotherapy*, **34**, 1508–11.

Peters, D.H. and Clissold, S.P. (1992) Clarithromycin – A review of its antimicrobial acitvity, pharmacokinetic properties and therapeutic potential. *Drugs*, **44**, 117–64.

Peters, M., Müller, C., Rüsch-Gerdes, S. *et al.* (1995) Isolation of atypical mycobacteria from tap water in hopitals and homes: Is this a possible source of disseminated MAC infection in AIDS patients? *Journal of Infection*, **31**, 39–44.

Pierce, M., Crampton, S., Henry, D. *et al.* (1996) A randomised trial of clarithromycin as prophylaxis against disseminated *Mycobacterium avium* complex infection in patients with advanced acquired immunodeficiency syndrome. *New England Journal of Medicine*, **355**, 384–91.

Porter, J.D.H. and McAdam, K.P.W.H. (1992) Aspects of tuberculosis in Africa 1 Tuberculosis in Africa in the AIDS era – the role of chemoprophylaxis. *Transactions of the Royal Society of Tropical Medicine and Hygiene*, **86**, 467–9.

Quinn, T.C. (1989) Interactions of the human immunodeficiency virus and tuberculosis and the implications for BCG vaccination. *Reviews of Infectious Diseases*, **11** (S2), S379–84.

Report (1991) Transmission of multidrug-resistant tuberculosis from an HIV-positive client in a residential substance-abuse treatment facility. Michigan. *Morbidity and Mortality Weekly Report*, **40**, 129–31.

Rieder, H.L. and Enarson, D.A. (1996) Rebuttal: time to call a halt to emotions in the assessment of thiacetazone. *Tubercle and Lung Disease*, **77**, 109–11.

Riley, R.L. (1982) Disease transmission and contagion control. *American Review of Respiratory Disease*, **125**, 16–19.

Rouillon, A. and Enarson, D.A., (1991) Treating tuberculosis in HIV-positive Africans. *Lancet*, **338**, 1140.

Saltzman, B.R., Motyl, M.R., Friedland, G.H. *et al.* (1986) *Mycobacterium tuberculosis* bacteremia in the acquired immunodeficiency syndrome. *Journal of the American Medical Association*, **256**, 390–1.

Saunders, N.A. (1995) State of the art: typing *Mycobacterium tuberculosis*. *Journal of Hospital Infection*, **29**, 169–76.

Selwyn, P.A., Hartel, D., Lewis, V.A. *et al.* (1989) A prospective study of the risk of tuberculosis among intravenous drug users with human immunodeficiency virus. *New England Journal of*

Medicine, **320**, 545–50.

Shafran, S.D., Deschênes, J., Miller, M. *et al.* (1994) Uveitis and pseudojaundice during a regimen of clarithromycin, rifabutin, and ethambutol. *New England Journal of Medicine*, **330**, 438–9.

Shafran, S.D., Singer, J., Zarowny, D.P. *et al* (1996) A comparison of two regimens for the treatment of *Mycobacterium avium* complex bacteremia in AIDS: rifabutin, ethambutol and clarithromycin versus rifampin, ehtambutol, clofazimine and ciprofloxacin. *New England Journal of Medicine*, **335**, 377–83.

Siddiqi, S.H., Hwangbo, C.C., Silcox, V. *et al.* (1984) Rapid radiometric methods to detect and differentiate *Mycobacterium tuberculosis/M. bovis* from other mycobacterial species. *American Review of Respiratory Disease*, **130**, 634–40.

Singh, N. and Yu, V.L. (1994) Potable water and *Mycobacterium avium* complex in HIV patients: is prevention possible? *Lancet*, **343**, 1110–37.

Skinner, C. and Joint Tuberculosis Committee of the British Thoracic Society (1994) Control and prevention of tuberculosis in the United Kingdom: code of practice 1994. *Thorax*, **49**, 1193–200.

Small, P.M., Schecter, G.F., Goodman, P.C. *et al.* (1991) Treatment of tuberculosis in patients with advanced human immunodeficiency virus infection. *New England Journal of Medicine*, **324**, 289–94.

Stead, W.W., Lofgren, J.P., Warren, E. and Thomas, C. (1985) Tuberculosis as an endemic and nosocomial infection among the elderly in nursing homes. *New England Journal of Medicine*, **312**, 1483–7.

Sullivan, E.A., Kreiswirth, B.N., Palumbo, L. *et al.* (1995) Emergence of fluoroquinolone-resistant tuberculosis in New York City. *Lancet*, **345**, 1148–50.

Sunderam, G., Mangura, B.T., Lombardo, J.M. and Reichman, L.B. (1987) Failure of 'optimal' four-drug short-course tuberculosis chemotherapy in a compliant patient with human immunodeficiency virus. *American Review of Respiratory Disease*, **136**, 1475–8.

ten Dam, H.G. (1990) BCG vaccination and HIV infection. *Bulletin of the International Union Against Tuberculosis and Lung Disease*, **65**, 38–9.

Vareldzis, B.P., Grosset, J., de Kantor, I. *et al.* (1994) Drug resistant tuberculosis: laboratory issues. *Tubercle and Lung Disease*, **75**, 1–7.

van Deutekom, H. (1990) Chemoprophylaxis and chemotherapy of tuberculosis in HIV infected patients. *Bulletin of the International Union against Tuberculosis and Lung Disease*, **65**, 84–91.

van Gorkom, J. and Kibuga, D.K. (1996) Cost-effectiveness and total costs of three alternative strategies for the prevention and management of severe skin reactions attributable to thiacetazone in the treatment of human immunodeficiency virus positive patients with tuberculosis in Kenya. *Tubercle and Lung Disease*, **77**, 30–6.

von Reyn, C.F., Maslow, J.N., Barber, T.W. *et al.* (1994) Persistent colonisation of potable water as a source of *Mycobacterium avium* infection in AIDS. *Lancet*, **343**, 1137–41.

Wadhawan, D., Hira, S., Mwansa, N. and Perrine, P. (1992) Preventive tuberculosis chemotherapy with isoniazid among patients infected with HIV1. VIII International Conference on AIDS, Amsterdam 1992, Abstract Tub0536.

Wallace, R.J., Brown, B.A., Griffith, D.E. *et al.* (1995) Reduced serum levels of clarithromycin in patients treated with multidrug regimens including rifampin or rifabutin for *Mycobacterium avium–M. intracellulare* infection. *Journal of Infectious Diseases*, **171**, 747–50.

Weber, A., Willeke, K., Marchioni R. *et al.* (1993) Aerosol penetration and leakage characteristics of masks used in the health care industry. *American Journal of Infection Control*, **21**, 167–73.

Weis, S.E., Slocum, P.C., Blais, F.X. *et al.* (1994) The effect of directly observed therapy on the rates of drug resistance and relapse in tuberculosis. *New England Journal of Medicine*, **330**, 1179–84.

Weltman, A.C. and Rose, D.N. (1993) The safety of bacille Calmette Guérin vaccination in HIV infection and AIDS. *AIDS*, **7**, 149–57.

Wenger, P.N., Otten, J., Breeden, A. *et al.* (1995) Control of nosocomial transmission of multidrug-resistant *Mycobacterium tuberculosis* among healthcare workers and HIV-infected patients. *Lancet*, **345**, 235–40.

Wilcox, M.H. (1995) Protection against hospital-acquired tuberculosis, American style: a report on the 4th Annual Meeting of the Society for Hospital Epidemiology of America (SHEA), New Orleans, 1994. *Journal of Hospital Infection*, **29**, 165–8.

Wilkinson, D. (1994) High-compliance tuberculosis treatment programme in a rural community. *Lancet*, **343**, 647–8.

World Health Organisation (1992) Severe hypersensitivity reactions among HIV seropositive patients with tuberculosis treated with thioacetazone. *Weekly Epidemiological Record*, **67**, 1–3.

World Health Organisation and International Union Against Tuberculosis and Lung Disease (1994) Joint statements on preventing tuberculosis. *Communicable Disease Report*, **4**, 37–38.

Yajko, D.M., Nassos, P.S. Sanders, C.A. and Hadley, W.K. (1989) Killing by antimycobacterial agents of AIDS-derived strains of *Mycobacterium avium* complex inside cells of the mouse macrophage cell line J774. *American Review of Respiratory Disease*, **140**, 1198–203.

Yajko, D.M., Nassos, P.S. Sanders, C.A. *et al.* (1992) Comparison of the intracellular activities of clarithromycin and erythromycin against *Mycobacterium avium* complex strains in J774 cells and in alveolar macrophages from human immunodeficiency virus type I-infected individuals. *Antimicrobial Agents and Chemotherapy*, **36**, 1163–5.

Young, L.S. (1988) *Mycobacterium avium* complex infection. *Journal of Infectious Diseases*, **157**, 863–6.

Young, L.S., Wiviott, L., Wu, M. *et al.* (1991) Azithromycin for treatment of *Mycobacterium avium-intracellulare* complex infection in patients with AIDS. *Lancet*, **338**, 1107–9.

Anton Pozniak

INTRODUCTION

Diseases caused by atypical mycobacteria were once obscure and of occasional interest to the clinician. Better laboratory techniques and heightened awareness of their clinical importance, focused by the HIV epidemic, have highlighted their potential as serious pathogens. No longer are they unclassified, anonymous or simply environmental. They are still grouped together, separately from *M. tuberculosis*. For this reason they will be referred to generically as 'nontuberculous' rather than 'atypical' as *M. tuberculosis* can present 'atypically' in the immunosuppressed. This chapter will concern itself with the diseases caused by these fascinating organisms, as well as their isolation and treatment. It will discuss in some detail individual mycobacteria that have caused disease in HIV-positive patients. The discussion is of course dominated by *M. avium*.

HISTORICAL PERSPECTIVE

The finding of nontuberculous acid-fast bacilli in human secretions dates back to 1885, three years after Koch's discovery of the tubercle bacillus. Although cases of nontuberculous infection were subsequently described and important contributions made over the next 50 years, it was not until 1948 with the discovery of *Mycobacterium ulcerans*

(MacCallum *et al.*, 1948) that these mycobacteria were clearly recognized as important pathogens for man. In 1949 a case of disseminated disease due to what is now known as *Mycobacterium intracellulare* (Cuttino and McCabe, 1949) was described. This was followed over the next five years by a flurry of papers describing diseases due variously to *Mycobacterium fortuitum, marinum, kansasii, avium* and *chelonae (abscessus)*.

The majority of nontuberculous mycobacteria cause localized pulmonary, lymph node or skin disease and until 1981 there had been a steady and relatively small number of cases of severe life-threatening disseminated infections described. With the advent of the HIV pandemic circumstances changed and there has been an almost exponential increase in the incidence of disseminated disease due to nontuberculous mycobacteria. This overall increase in the rate of nontuberculous mycobacterial diseases may be partly attributable both to improved laboratory methods for identification and increased awareness of mycobacteria as potential pathogens. As HIV-positive patients live longer with severe immunosuppression the more likely it is mycobacterial disease will occur, and nontuberculous mycobacteria have been reported in about 5.5% of reported AIDS cases. Postmortem studies suggest that these bacilli may be found in up to one half of AIDS patients having an

AIDS and Respiratory Medicine. Edited by A. Zumla, M.A. Johnson and R.F. Miller. Published in 1997 by Chapman & Hall, London. ISBN 0 412 60140 0

autopsy (Armstrong *et al.*, 1985) although the presence of mycobacteria does not necessarily mean the presence of disease. This fascinating interaction between mycobacteria and HIV infection has stimulated research in an otherwise little-investigated field. Consequently some of the mysteries surrounding the pathogenesis of these mycobacteria are being unravelled.

NOMENCLATURE AND CLASSIFICATION

Quite appropriately, *M. tuberculosis* has taken premier position in the mycobacterial hierarchy, *M. bovis*, *M. africanum*, and *M. BCG* being grouped in the same 'complex'. All other mycobacteria except *M. leprae* have been placed together in a single group and classified as 'atypical mycobacteria', 'environmental mycobacteria', 'non-tuberculous', or 'mycobacteria other than tuberculosis' (MOTT). This collection of names reflects the origin, low virulence and lack of transmittability from person to person of these mycobacteria. The distinction between *M. tuberculosis*, *M. leprae* and these other species lies not in the ability to cause serious disease but more in their differences in natural habitats and contagiousness. Consequently a new term, 'potential pathogenic environmental bacteria' (PPEM) has been proposed. Clinicians and scientists are moving away from these artificial homogeneous categories such as 'atypical' towards a more precise taxonomy, especially for *Mycobacterium avium* complex which, in some populations, has an even higher profile than *M. tuberculosis*.

The International Working Group on Mycobacterial Taxonomy have proposed several classification schemes. Apart from the usual culture, biochemical and enzymatic tests, thin layer chromatography of lipids, serology and analysis of mycobacterial antigens have all been used in classification. One classification in general usage by microbiologists is that proposed by Runyon

in 1959, based on pigment production, growth rates and colonial morphology of organisms (Runyon, 1959). His four main groups (groups 1–4) are the photochromogens, which produce yellow colonies when exposed to light; schotocromogens, which produce orange colonies independent of light exposure; nonphotochromogens, which produce little or no pigment, and rapid growers which produce little or no pigment, but where colonies appear in less than seven days. A major limitation of this classification is that there is no correlation between these groups and clinical syndromes.

Recently the use of molecular biological techniques has promised a rapid taxonomic classification. Sequencing of the 16S rRNA gene is a powerful technique for differentiating species but it is labor-intensive and may not be suitable for routine use in many laboratories. Amplified ribosomal DNA restriction analysis is an easier and more rapid technique which has the added advantage that it can be carried out in a day (Vaneechoutte *et al.*, 1993). The 65-kDa heat shock protein contains epitopes both common and unique to various species of mycobacteria. Evaluating the gene encoding for this protein by the polymerase chain reaction (PCR) can also allow differentiation to the species level in one working day (Telenti *et al.*, 1993).

16S ribosomal RNA nucleic acid isotopically labelled probes are available for the identification of *M. avium*, *M. kansasii* and *M. gordonae*. These are highly specific to a target nucleic acid sequence but unfortunately even a single base pair mismatch drastically affects stringency.

CLINICAL DIAGNOSTIC CRITERIA (Wallace *et al.*, 1990)

When mycobacteria are recovered from nonsterile anatomical sites such as the lung or gut it is important to be able to decide whether a patient is infected or colonized or whether the mycobacterium isolated is a contaminant. With this aim, diagnostic criteria have been suggested.

It is important to note that these criteria may not be applicable to immunodeficient patients.

CRITERIA USED FOR DIAGNOSING DISEASE DUE TO NON-TUBERCULOUS MYCOBACTERIA

Pulmonary disease

1. Patients with cavitation on the chest radiograph
   For patients with cavitation on their chest radiograph the diagnosis requires:

   (a) The presence of two or more sputa specimens or one sputum plus bronchial washings that are acid-fast smear positive and/or result in a moderate to heavy growth on culture; plus
   (b) Other reasonable causes for the disease process have been excluded such as tuberculosis and fungal disease.

2. Patients with non-cavitating infiltrate on the chest radiograph

   (a) The presence of two or more sputa specimens or one sputum plus bronchial washings that are acid fast smear-positive and/or produce moderate to heavy growth on culture.
   (b) If the isolate is *M. kansasii* or *M. avium*-complex, failure of the sputum to clear within two weeks of anti-mycobacterial drug therapy.
   (c) Other reasonable causes for disease process have been excluded.

3. Additional criteria
   In patients with or without cavities on the chest radiograph whose sputum is non-

diagnostic then the diagnosis can be made when:

   (a) A transbronchial or open-lung biopsy yields the organism on culture and shows typical histological features of mycobacterial disease.
   (b) The organism is not cultured from the biopsy but shows histological features of mycobacterial disease. Then in the absence of prior mycobacterial disease, two or more cultures of sputum or bronchial washings are positive even when light growths have been obtained and other reasonable causes have been excluded.

4. Gut disease
   Isolation from stool: this has a similar significance to that from sputum. Unless there are strong clinical features to suggest disease rather than colonization and/or evidence of histological changes on gut biopsy, most physicians would not embark on a course of treatment.

5. Other disease
   Isolation from sterile sites: isolation from bone marrow, blood or tissue biopsy should be considered indicative of infection and treatment offered.

GENERAL CONSIDERATIONS

The diagnosis of pulmonary disease in HIV-positive patients due to nontuberculous mycobacteria can be difficult. In patients who have had mycobacteria isolated from sterile sites such as blood the diagnosis is straightforward and any subsequent sputum isolation from such patients probably only reflects dissemination. Problems in clinical practice occur when patients have mycobacteria isolated only from non-sterile sites such as sputum alone or sputum and stool. Isolation of the organism from a single sputum with low numbers of organisms can occur as a consequence of colonization of the respiratory tract or from specimen contamination. In HIV-positive patients who may present with weight loss, fever, etc. due to HIV replication or other opportunistic diseases, the relevance of the isolation of these mycobacteria from non-sterile sites such as sputum has to be taken in the context of the whole clinical situation. As stated above, in HIV-negative patients the diagnosis of lung disease due to nontuberculous mycobacteria requires more than one positive sputum culture with a moderate to heavy growth. Some believe that one exception to this is when pulmonary disease due to *M. kansasii* is suspected where one positive sputum sample is usually adequate, as this organism is rarely a sputum contaminant. If there is doubt as to whether a mycobacterium may or may not be causing disease then transbronchial biopsy and bronchial lavage can be helpful.

LABORATORY ISOLATION OF ATYPICAL MYCOBACTERIA (Kiehn and Cammarata, 1986)

Most laboratories use at least two culture systems based on liquid and solid media. As respiratory and stool specimens can be contaminated they need to be processed to eliminate yeasts and rapidly-growing bacteria prior to culture. Blood can be cultured directly (unconcentrated) or centrifuged first (concentrated).

THE BACTEC SYSTEM

(Dickinson Diagnostic Instrument Systems Sparks MD)

BACTEC 12B System

Decontaminated specimens are inoculated into modified Middlebrook 7H9 liquid medium. This medium contains radioactively-labelled palmitic acid. Any mycobacteria growth will produce C^{14} labeled CO_2.

Detectable growth takes one to two weeks.

BACTEC 13A System

This is similar in principle to the 12B system but requires the use of a large volume (up to 5 ml) of unconcentrated blood inoculated directly into the medium.

Some mycobacteria such as MAC can grow in a BACTEC 6A non-radioactive system.

Solid media

Specimens can be inoculated using conventional methodology onto agar-based media such as Middlebrook 7H11 or an egg-based medium such as Lowenstein–Jensen medium. The isolation of some atypical mycobacteria such as MAC can be improved by lowering the pH to less than 6.5 and adding pyruvate or glycerol.

Biphasic systems such as the Septicheck AFB System is used in preference to others by some laboratories (Beckton Dickinson Microbiology Systems, Cockeysville, MD, USA).

Lysis centrifugation

Treating the blood with a lytic agent such as sodium deoxycholate improves the detection of mycobacteria in blood by lysing circulating macrophages which potentially contain high concentrations of mycobacteria. A commercial lysis centrifugation kit is available (Lysis Centrifugation Isolator, Wampole Laboratories, Cranberry, NJ, USA).

Quantification

Sequential quantification of mycobacterial load expressed as colony-forming units per ml is used in clinical trials of antimycobacterial treatment. This technique is labor-intensive and is not used routinely. It has been noted that the BACTEC 13A System can provide an approximation of the level of bacteremia as there is a correlation between the rate of growth (in terms of days to positive blood culture) and with the degree of bacteremia. Blood cultures that are positive in less than seven days usually have >400 colony-forming units per ml whereas those that were positive at twelve or more days had less than nine colony-forming units per ml (Havlir, Keyes and Davis, 1991).

Which system to use?

When these systems are compared (Agy *et al.*, 1989) the single most sensitive was the BACTEC 13A using 5 ml of blood collected in a vacutainer tube containing sodium polyanethol sulfonate. Mean time to detection with the 13A or 12B BACTEC System was 14 days and with the solid medium were 21–24 days.

Molecular techniques

Potentially both DNA probes and PCR can be used for diagnosis but at present are more suited to identification once growth has occurred. Oligonucleotide probes have been made to specific genes characteristic of a target organism. A commercially marketed oligonucleotide probe has been made to detect MAC. Unfortunately not all clinical isolates of *M. avium* are detected using these rRNA probes. By using specific sequences in the polymerase chain reaction followed by hybridization of labeled probes MAC could be detected rapidly and at the early stage of isolation of primary clinical samples (Thierry *et al.*, 1993). A PCR-based test for diagnosing MAC directly from blood specimens has been described with a specificity of 86% (Iralu *et al.*, 1993). Using molecular-based techniques it may be possible in the future not only to detect mycobacteria in a specimen but also to assign a species.

MYCOBACTERIUM AVIUM-COMPLEX

CLASSIFICATION OF MAC

Serotypes

MAC is a serological complex of 28 serovars containing *M. avium* and *M. intracellulare* and there are three additional serovars which belong to *M. scrofulatum*. The 'complex' referred to in most of the literature usually includes both *M. avium* and *M. intracellulare*. Serovar specificity is conferred by specific oligosaccharide residues linked to the cell wall glycopeptidolipid (Brennan, 1989). Serotyping can be done by thin layer chromatography or ELISA analysis as well as by conventional seroagglutination. Unfortunately the process of serotyping is complex, can be imprecise, and some strains are not typable. DNA homology studies combined with serovar studies appear to show that serovars 1–6 and 8–11 are *M. avium* whereas serovars 7 and 12–28 are *M. intracellulare* (Baess, 1983). Interestingly, in the US, the UK and Australia, strains from AIDS patients are predominantly serovars 1, 4, and 8, whereas in Sweden they are more commonly serovar 6. In order to improve classification other typing systems have been used such as multilocus enzyme electrophoresis (Wasem, McCarthy and Murray, 1991) but unfortunately this only separates the serovars into either *M. intracellulare* or *M. avium* clusters.

Genotypes

Based on restriction fragment length polymorphism (RFLP) analysis, 73% of MAC isolates recovered from individual patients with AIDS were found to be genetically indistinguishable (Hampson *et al.*, 1989). More recently, genotyping such isolates using pulsed field electrophoresis of restriction fragments shows that strains of *M. avium* are highly conserved and there has been an attempt to recover these particular strains from the environment. Interestingly, some patient isolates are indistinguishable from some of those found in drinking water, leading to the hypothesis that they were acquired from that source.

Phagotypes

Unfortunately this is not a useful typing system as only one third of clinical isolates are susceptible to mycobacterial phages (Crawford and Bates, 1985). This phenomenon may have an important bearing on the use of the luciferase phagemid system for the direct detection of MAC in clinical specimens.

Plasmid type

Only 50% of clinical isolates and 20% of environmental isolates of MAC carry plasmids (Meissner and Falkinham, 1986). However, plasmids seem to be more common in isolates from AIDS patients, perhaps because they are commoner in serovars 4 and 8. The carriage of certain plasmids might be associated with virulence though the data are conflicting. They may be important because of the association with antibiotic resistance (Inderlied, Kemper and Bermudez, 1993).

Colony type

There appear to be three colony variants: (1) smooth, opaque and domed; (2) smooth translucent and flat; and (3) a rough type. Translucent colonies appear to be more resistant to microbial agents and there is some evidence that this variant will more readily infect macrophages. In primary blood cultures isolates are frequently the smooth translucent type. Non-pigmented colony variants appear to be more resistant to antimicrobial agents than pigmented variants of the same strain (Stormer and Falkinham, 1989).

Environmental isolation

MAC may be isolated from both fresh and salt water sources (17–61% of samples). Recovery seems to be more frequent from waters of moderate salinity and from the southeast United States compared with the north-east (Falkinham, Parker and Gruft, 1980 and Gruft, Katz and Blanchard, 1975). It is also more commonly isolated from soil and water samples of relatively high acidity (pH 4.6–6.8) and lower altitude. MAC is found in aerosols in droplet sizes of 0.7–3.3 mm, sufficiently small to reach the alveolar space. In certain environments up to 18 organisms may be inspired by humans during a one-hour period of exposure (Wendt *et al.*, 1980). *M. avium* is an important cause of disease in birds and swine and the bacillus can persist in soil for long periods of time. There is disparity between genotype and phenotype from those isolates causing disease in animals and those from man, supporting the fact that direct transmission from animals to humans is probably very rare. MAC can also be isolated from cigarettes, plants and bedding material as well as house dust and water supplies. Drinking water contaminated with MAC was found in 32 of 141 rainwater tanks in Queensland, Australia although there was no relationship to human disease. Von Reyn has isolated strains of MAC from hospital water supplies that were indistinguishable from those causing bacteremia in patients (von Reyn *et al.*, 1994). Although this study implies possible nosocomial transmission larger scale prospective environmental studies are needed to test this hypothesis.

EPIDEMIOLOGY OF *MYCOBACTERIUM AVIUM* INFECTION

Geographic distribution

There are some data to suggest that exposure to MAC is similar in developed and developing countries from skin test studies of *Mycobacterium avium* sensitivities ranging from 7–12% of populations tested in the USA, Finland, Trinidad and Kenya (Huebner *et al.*, 1992). Disease caused by *M. avium* is diagnosed during life in about 30% of patients with AIDS in the USA (Pitchenic and Fertel, 1992). In contrast it occurs in only 10% of AIDS patients in Sweden. It has been postulated that the difference in incidence between the two countries is due to the use of BCG vaccination (Kallenius, Hoffner and Svenson, 1989) and there are some data from Haiti to suggest that BCG vaccination might afford some protection against pulmonary MAC disease in HIV-positive but not in HIV-negative persons. Clinical observations suggest that vaccination with BCG also protects against lymphadenitis caused by atypical mycobacteria. Disseminated MAC is also very rare in Africans in Africa (or elsewhere) (Gilks *et al.*, 1995) but this is not due to its environmental distribution (Colebunders *et al.*, 1990). An explanation for this is that Africans do not become severely immune-suppressed for long enough to develop MAC but develop disease due to the more pathogenic *Mycobacterium tuberculosis* instead.

There have been few CD4 data published from Africa and this hypothesis has little to support it. There is some evidence that certain environmental mycobacteria in Uganda are particularly effective in eliciting protective responses. By drinking or inhaling environmental bacteria a degree of immunity may be induced which prevents the establishment of foci of infection by MAC and other mycobacteria. Several other explanations for the difference in MAC epidemiology between countries have been proposed. One is that MAC disease is due to direct infection by pathogenic strains from contaminated drinking water or by inhalation of aerosol. These form long-standing silent foci of MAC in the lymphatic tissue of patients (Good, 1985) by crossing the epithelial lining of the pharynx

or GI tract, a process called translocation. It is thought that this process favors certain species, serotypes or genotypes of mycobacteria that might only be found in distinct geographical areas (Grange, 1994). The difference in epidemiology between the USA and Europe may, of course, be partly a temporal phenomenon. As the HIV epidemic started earlier on in the USA, cohorts of patients infected in the early 1980s have reached the stage of their HIV disease where they have become susceptible to MAC earlier than European patients.

Disseminated MAC in AIDS

Of all nontuberculous mycobacteria infecting AIDS patients 96–98% are found to be MAC. Progressive immunodeficiency appears to be the single most significant risk factor for disseminated disease. In the USA one year after a diagnosis of AIDS-disseminated MAC occurred in 21% of patients rising to 43% of patients at 2 years (Nightingale *et al.*, 1992) (CDC 1987 definition). The incidence of disseminated MAC at one year was 39% in patients with CD4 counts <10 cells m/L but only 3% in patients with counts between 100 and 200 (Horsburgh *et al.*, 1992). Although disseminated MAC may be an inevitable outcome for all HIV-infected patients who survive long-term, data so far suggest that MAC is more frequent in Caucasians and homosexual and bisexual men, and infrequent in children (Inderlied, Kemper and Bermudez, 1993).

Route of infection

There is great debate as to to how patients develop disseminated MAC. As Peyers patch and mesenteric lymph node involvement is a common histopathological finding in those patients with both MAC and chronic diarrhea it has been suggested that gastrointestinal colonization leads first to local infection and then dissemination (Bessesen *et al.*, 1990). Aerosol inhalation could also be a route of infection but, again, evidence is indirect and progression to disseminated disease occurs with equal frequency in those patients whose stool or sputum were initially positive for MAC (Horsburgh *et al.*, 1991b). About 75% of patients develop MAC mycobacteremia within one year of the isolation of MAC from respiratory secretions or stool. Conversely, of those patients who develop MAC bacteremia only 25% and 36% have had a preceding positive respiratory or stool culture respectively. In addition RFLP analysis has shown these stool and respiratory isolates may be genotypically different from those subsequently found in the blood. These data suggest that the methods available to screen for MAC lack sufficient sensitivity resulting in poor negative predictive values.

Immunology of MAC

In the presence of MAC activation of monocytes and macrophages is inadequate and monocyte macrophage intracellular killing is impaired. The results of studies examining the interaction between HIV and *M. avium* within macrophages are still preliminary. Lymphocyte proliferation and cytokine production are impaired in the presence of mycobacterial antigens. Although some cytotoxic T cells and NK cells kill mycobacterial-laden monocytes, activation of NK cells is impaired in patients with AIDS.

In *in vitro* models of MAC infection recombinant cytokines such as tumor necrosis factor alpha (TNFα), a granulocyte macrophage colony stimulating factor (GMCSF), can stimulate human and marine macrophages to inhibit and kill intracellular MAC. It is thought that MAC-infected macrophages have an impaired ability to produce and release cytokines such as this and this may lead to partial or complete unresponsiveness to this stimulation. Interestingly a com-

bination of GMCSF and either amikacin or azithromycin has been associated with a significant increase in killing of MAC both within cultured macrophages and in the beige mouse model (Bermudez *et al.*, 1994).

It has been proposed that exposure of MAC to small concentrations of ethanol may induce a stress-related response with a consequent increase in the synthesis of stress-related proteins (heat shock proteins). These proteins – especially the 65kD protein – inhibit superoxide production by macrophages (Bermudez *et al.*, 1993) and would in theory inhibit killing of mycobacteria.

CLINICAL DISEASE – NON HIV-INFECTED PULMONARY DISEASE

Pulmonary disease due to *M. avium* predominantly involves white males, 45–65 years of age, with pre-existing pulmonary disease such as chronic obstructive airways disease, bronchiectasis, chronic aspiration, recurrent pneumonia, active or inactive TB, pneumoconiosis, bronchial carcinoma or cystic fibrosis. There also appears to be a group of middle-aged women with no predisposing lung disease who develop pulmonary MAC (Reich and Johnson, 1992). Symptoms are similar to those of *M. tuberculosis* but fever and weight loss are less common. The chest radiograph usually shows apical cavitation but there is usually less surrounding infiltrate than is seen in *M. tuberculosis*. A solitary nodule can occur.

Immune-deficient patients, including those on cytotoxic therapy or who have had bone marrow, renal or cardiac transplantation, are at risk of pulmonary MAC. These patients commonly present with atypical radiographic features (Kurzrock *et al.*, 1984). Occasionally lung biopsies are required for diagnosis. Histology then shows caseating or non-caseating granulomatous necrosis but the granulomata are often ill-formed.

LYMPH NODE INFECTION

This is a common site of infection in children aged 1–5 years who present with insidious painless unilateral lymphadenitis, usually involving the cervical region (Grange, Yates and Pozniak, 1995). Surgical removal is often curative.

OTHER FOCAL SITES OF INFECTION

MAC has been found in many articular and periarticular infections with extension to the adjacent bone and soft tissues. Although the infections can be initiated by trauma or puncture wounds hematogenous dissemination is often the primary event. Osteomyelitis, urinary tract involvement, granulomatous prostatitis, skin disease, peritonitis, corneal ulceration and ENT infection have all been described.

Disseminated infection

Before AIDS, disseminated MAC disease was extremely rare. It usually occurred in patients with underlying malignancy or in those who were immunodeficient from another cause. Patients with hairy cell leukemia appeared to be particularly susceptible. Organisms have been isolated from the GI tract, respiratory system, skeletal system, skin and occasionally the brain, CSF or eye as well as the blood.

HIV-infected patients

The major problem for clinicians after isolating MAC from stool or sputum of patients with AIDS is in distinguishing between colonization and infection. This can be particularly difficult in asymptomatic patients. Sometimes there may only be a single positive culture from multiple specimens because of a transient or episodic excretion of organisms. Although the routine screening of stool and sputum specimens is not advocated, the finding of MAC in sputum or stool should lead to a search for evidence of either focal or disseminated disease.

Focal pulmonary infection (Modilevsky, Sattler and Barnes, 1989; Wallace *et al.*, 1990)

Focal pulmonary disease in HIV-positive patients is rare and accounts for less than 5% of all MAC in this group. The clinical presentation is similar to tuberculosis but is less severe. Patients have a persistent productive cough, breathlessness, fever, sweats and malaise. Hemoptysis is uncommon. The chest radiograph can show various abnormalities; diffuse interstitial or reticular nodular infiltrates occur in about half whereas alveolar infiltrates occur in 20%. Apical scarring or upper lobe involvement occurs in less than 10% of patients. In contrast to patients who are not HIV-infected, cavitatory disease is unusual, occurring in less than 5%. Pleural effusions and pleural reactions are rare.

MAC pulmonary disease can clinically resemble bacterial pneumonia, pneumocystosis, tuberculosis or fungal lung disease. In spite of isolation of MAC from sputum or bronchial lavage a search for other potential pathogens should always be made. In patients with a single sputum or BAL lavage culture positive for MAC, even if chest radiograph changes are present, a pathogen other than MAC is still more likely to be causing the pulmonary disease (Marinelli *et al.*, 1986). Transbronchial biopsy, needle biopsy or even open-lung biopsy may be necessary to make a definitive diagnosis.

When to treat focal disease

There is a lack of data to help guide the clinician in treating HIV-positive patients who have focal pulmonary disease. However, in those patients whose sputum is repeatedly culture-positive for MAC and who have symptoms and/or chest radiographic changes not attributable to other infections, antimycobacterial therapy should be considered. It is important to note that patients who have acid-fast bacilli in the sputum which has not been identified, regardless of prior BCG positive or a negative tuberculin test, should receive empiric therapy for *M. tuberculosis* until the identity of the organism can be established.

Focal lymph node disease

This is seen occasionally without evidence of disseminated disease and can be associated with cutaneous lesions (Figure 13.1a, b) (Barbaro, Orcutt and Coldiron, 1989). Some of these patients present with pyrexias of unknown origin. Gallium scanning can be useful in identifying infected intrathoracic or intra-abdominal lymph nodes which can then be biopsied. Needle cytology may be helpful. Until cultures are identified isolated lymphadenopathy should be treated as being due to *M. tuberculosis* if mycobacteria are seen on histology. In addition patients with histopathological evidence of granulomatous inflammation with or without acid-fast bacilli who are thought to have a mycobacterial infection should receive empiric anti-TB therapy. If cultures are negative in spite of positive histology or seeing acid-fast bacilli then the clinician should be aware that recently-recognized mycobacteria such as *Mycobacterium haemophilum* or *Mycobacterium genavense*, which grow under certain culture conditions, may have been missed.

DISSEMINATED INFECTION

Clinical features

This progressive illness is characterized by fevers, sweats, weakness, anorexia and weight loss. Of these patients, 40% will also have nausea or diarrhea and up to 20% will have vomiting sometimes associated with intractable crampy abdominal pain (Modilevsky, Sattler and Barnes, 1989). Hepatosplenomegaly is common but lymphadenopathy is unusual. Laboratory results often show increasing anemia or a markedly elevated alkaline phosphatase not always associated with comparable increases in hepatic transaminases (Kahn *et al.*, 1986). Almost any organ system can be involved as part of dissemination including the skin (Barbaro, Orcutt and Coldiron, 1989), bone joints (Blumenthal, Zucker and Hawkins, 1990), eyes, thyroid and adrenals (Hawkins *et al.*, 1986), large airways (Mehle *et al.*, 1989), testis (De Paepe, Guerrieri and Waxman, 1990), pericardium (Choo and McCormack, 1995) and brain (Dwork, Chin and Boyce, 1994). Isolation of *M. avium* from the CSF has been reported in some patients (Jacob *et al.*, 1991). Interestingly, patients who have histological evidence of GI involvement usually have disseminated disease (Poropatich, Labriola and Tuazon, 1987; Gray and Rabeneck, 1989) and upper GI MAC can be mistaken for lymphoma at endoscopy.

Early infection may be difficult to recognize and in the MAC rifabutin prophylaxis trials (Nightingale *et al.*, 1993) about one third of people who first develop MAC bacteremia had no signs of symptoms. Only 7% of patients had a classic syndrome of fevers, weight loss and anemia at the time bacteremia was first detected. Most do become symptomatic however within eight weeks.

Bacteremia occurs in up to 98% of patients with dissemination. When quantified most patients have counts of 1 to 3000 colony-forming units per ml of whole blood but occasionally up to a million per ml are found (Havlir *et al.*, 1991).

Bacterial load

The number of circulating mycobacteria has been used as a surrogate marker of efficacy of therapeutic agents. Although this may be of use in clinical trials there appears to be a

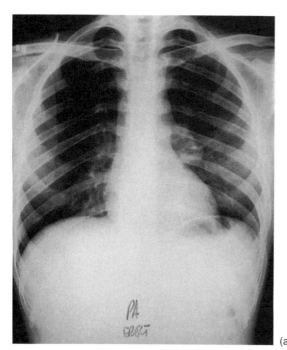

Fig. 13.1 Lymph node disease, without evidence of disseminated disease. (a) Infection of left hilar node due to *M. avium*. (b) CT scan demonstrating mass of abnormal tissue at left hilum.

(a)

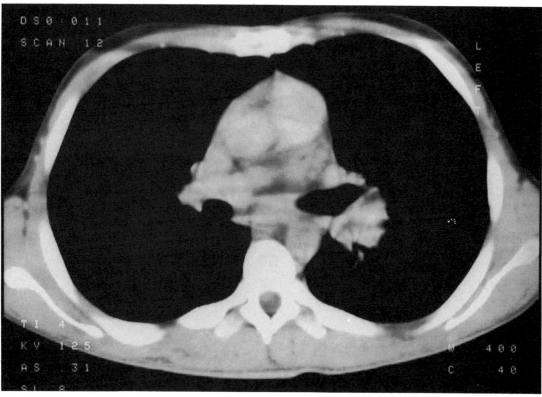

(b)

poor correlation between the level of infection in the tissues and the bacterial load in the bloodstream (Wiley *et al.*, 1992). In addition these colony counts do not take into account any diurnal variation in bacteremia. Some patients may have fluctuating low levels of mycobacteremia and consequently negative blood cultures. Other patients with established sites of infections in tissues may have their mycobacteria suppressed on therapy and then occasionally release showers of organisms into the bloodstream which may be at too low a level to be detected by the BACTEC culture system.

Some groups have used the detection of a 500 dB antigen specific to *M. avium* and *M. intracellulare* to predict dissemination of *M. avium* disease in AIDS patients. Although it had a specificity of 100%, sensitivity was only 64% and data are not sufficient to support its clinical application (Sippola *et al.*, 1993).

Histopathology

Organs involved are usually enlarged and yellow because of mycobacterial pigment and the tissues are filled with large numbers of histiocytes which are packed with acid-fast bacilli. The burden of organisms may be nearly 10^{10} colony-forming units per gram. Inflammatory reaction however is scant usually with minimal cellular infiltrate. Although a few patients do have a classic granulomatous response granulomas when present are often poorly formed. Poor granuloma formation probably reflects the inability of the host to mount an effective immune response.

Differentiating tuberculosis from MAC disease

The likelihood of isolating *M. tuberculosis* rather than MAC does depend to some degree on the patient's sex, ethnicity, HIV risk group and other factors, e.g. contact with someone with tuberculosis, country of origin or residence, recent travel, alcoholism, etc. Sputum smears are more likely to be positive in patients with *M. tuberculosis* than in those with MAC (83 versus 16%) but both are isolated with the same frequency from lymph nodes, bone marrow and stool specimen (Modilevsky, Sattler and Barnes, 1989). Positive blood cultures makes the diagnosis of TB less likely as blood cultures are positive in 86–98% of patients with disseminated MAC, usually within 14 days, but are rarely positive in patients with tuberculosis unless there is disseminated disease (Hawkins *et al.*, 1986; Modilevsky, Sattler and Barnes, 1986; Schluger *et al.*, 1994). The stage of HIV disease is important. Tuberculosis can occur at any stage of immunosuppression and it often precedes a diagnosis of AIDS. In contrast, most MAC occurs when the CD4 count is less then 75 cells/ml. Consequently in the USA only 15% of MAC infections represent the patient's first AIDS illness. Empiric therapy for TB should be given to patients with peripheral lymph node or clinical pulmonary disease when the mycobacterium has yet to be identified.

Survival

Untreated disseminated MAC infection can severely affect quality of life. Although one study has shown that developing disseminated MAC did not affect survival in patients with AIDS (Kuitert, Thomas and Ellis-Pegler, 1991), two case control and one longitudinal study identified MAC as an independent risk factor for early mortality (Chaisson and Levine, 1991; Horsburgh *et al.*, 1991a; Jacobson *et al.*, 1991). Treatment does have a positive survival effect. Median survival was only 4 months untreated versus 11 months if treatment was given (Horsburgh *et al.*, 1991a). A prospective study of 367 AIDS patients showed that MAC bacteremia was independently associated with an increase (almost twice) risk of death but those patients who were treated had a median survival of

263 versus 139 days for those who were not. Of these patients, 23% died within 28 days of diagnosis and a few of these were treated (Chin *et al.*, 1994).

A retrospective study suggests that high levels of mycobacteremia were associated with a shorter survival and that the use of antiretroviral or antimycobacterial therapy had protective effects (Horsburgh *et al.*, 1994). There are some data to suggest that early elimination of bacteremia is associated with a better survival.

Therapeutic agents

A large number of drugs have been tried both within and outside of clinical trials. On the basis of available *in vitro* and *in vivo* data the USA Task Force suggest a minimum of two agents, in particular, ethambutol plus one of the macrolides, clarithromycin or azithromycin. A third agent such as rifabutin, rifampicin, ciprofloxacin or another quinolone may be added to these. Amikacin may be reserved for patients who are intolerant of oral therapy or are failing on oral therapy. Zidovudine therapy should probably be continued whenever possible since this drug has been associated with clinical and microbiological improvement in patients with disseminated MAC (Bautista, Alcid and Gocke, 1991). There are some issues however which have still not been resolved in spite of these recommendations for treatment. Even if *in vitro* susceptibility and quantitative blood culture data are available, which might help selecting appropriate therapy, clinicians often offer empiric therapy. Reasons for this are that there is still no consensus about drug susceptibility testing methodology or how to interpret the data once it is obtained. Another issue is how long to treat. Most clinicians would continue lifelong therapy as discontinuation often results in recurrence of bacteremia (Kemper *et al.* 1992a). For some patients however there may be a period of time when, after stopping therapy, bac-teremia does not return (Kemper *et al.*, 1992a). A paradox is that although therapy may be associated with a prolonged clinical response ongoing MAC infection can still be found in those patients at postmortem (Kemper *et al.*, 1992b).

DRUG TREATMENT

MONOTHERAPY

In a short-term trial of clarithromycin given alone a small number of patients showed clearing of blood cultures (Dautzenberg *et al.*, 1991). In contrast patients randomized to placebo had the expected increase in MAC colony counts in the blood. Two multicenter prospective randomized studies have looked at the efficacy of clarithromycin. One (Chaisson *et al.*, 1994) looked at 154 patients with AIDS and mycobacteremia who in a double-blind trial received 500 mg, 1000 mg and 2000 mg of clarithromycin twice daily for 12 weeks. The median reduction in colony counts from base line range from 99.4% to 100%. There was a dose-dependent difference in the interval required for sterilization of blood with median intervals of 54, 43 and 29 days respectively for the three dosages given. There appeared to be a dose-dependent survival benefit favoring the 500 mg dose of clarithromycin but the largest dose was poorly tolerated because of GI side-effects. Patients reported improvements in fevers and night sweats as well as in quality of life.

In the other multicenter study 299 patients were randomized to receive either 500 mg or 1000 mg of clarithromycin daily and both doses gave similar microbiological and clinical responses (Gupta *et al.*, 1992). Azithromycin has shown similar activity in early clinical trials (Young *et al.*, 1991). Sparfloxacin and liposome-encapsulated gentamicin have been used as monotherapy but data are too few to make recommendations.

MULTIDRUG REGIMES

One of the first multidrug regimes was described by Chiu and colleagues (Chiu *et al.*, 1990) who used ethambutol, rifampicin, ciprofloxacin and amikacin. The main problem with the study was that a large proportion of patients prematurely discontinued therapy because of adverse events.

A prospective randomized placebo-controlled trial of only eight weeks' duration compared ethambutol and rifampicin and ciprofloxacin with placebo (Jacobson *et al.*, 1993). In spite of good microbiological effect 9 of 12 evaluable patients in the treatment arm experienced some dose-limiting toxicity due to one or more agents.

A randomized prospective comparative trial (ACTG135) of ciprofloxacin, ethambutol, rifampicin and clofazimine with or without amikacin, and/or ciprofloxacin or ofloxacin has been performed. Although 49 of 89 evaluable patients had an initial bacteriological response, relapse with clarithromycin-resistant organisms was documented in 14.

A trial is ongoing using rifabutin or placebo combined with ethambutol and clofazimine (Gordon *et al.*, 1993). In 27 patients treated with clofazimine, ciprofloxacin, ethambutol and rifampicin serum drug levels were below the expected range in 6 of the 7 whose mycobacteria were cleared and in 9 of 13 whose mycobacteria was not cleared. Low serum concentrations of these antimycobacterial drugs may be due to impaired drug absorption in patients with AIDS and disseminated MAC. Due to the intracellular nature of these infections serum drug levels may or may not be reliable in terms of response. A recently published comparison of rifampicin, ethanbutol, clofazimine and ciprofloxacin versus rifabutin, ethambutol and clarithromycin has shown the latter regimen to be superior in clearance of bacteremia and survival (Shafran *et al.*, 1996).

OTHER COMBINATIONS

Therapy using rifampicin, ethambutol, clofazimine and ciprofloxacin in combination can lead to a rapid reduction in symptoms and bacteremia as early as week two. In one study however colony counts rose dramatically after therapy was discontinued (Kemper *et al.*, 1992b). Another four-drug regime with rifabutin, clofazimine, isoniazid and ethambutol showed clearance of mycobacteremia in 22 of 25 patients. Eighteen patients experienced complete resolution of symptoms in spite of all 24 isolates being resistant *in vitro* to clofazimine, isoniazid and ethambutol and 16 of 24 resistant to rifabutin (Hoy *et al.*, 1990). Several other studies of MAC therapy are ongoing and have only been published in abstract (Table 13.1).

STEROIDS

These have been used alone or as an adjunct to treatment (Wormser, Horowitz and Dworkin, 1994) with symptomatic benefit. A large trial examining their use in 'end' stage AIDS is needed.

PROPHYLAXIS

Rifabutin (Nightingale *et al.*, 1993)

Two large concurrent double-blind placebo-controlled trials in patients who had AIDS and CD4 counts of <200 cells/ml have shown that daily rifabutin 300 mg orally reduced the frequency of MAC bacteremia by about 50%. The median duration of prophylaxis taken at analysis was 7.4 months. Combining the intention to treat analyses from both studies 48 of 566 patients (8.5%) who received drug developed at least one positive drug culture for MAC bacteremia compared with 102 of 580 (17.6%) of patients who received placebo. CD4 counts of less than 100 cells/ml at entry was the most important

Table 13.1 Unpublished drug trials in MAC disease

Trial name	Drugs				Provisional results
	Regimen 1		Regimen 2		
Canadian HIV Trials Network[b]	Rifampicin +Ethambutol +Clofazamine +Ciprofloxacin	(600 mg) (15 mg/kg) (100 mg) (1.5 g)	Clarithromycin vs Rifabutin +Ethambutol	(2 g) (300 mg) (15 mg/kg)	Regimen 2 better tolerated and clears bacteremia more effectively ? Better survival
CCTG Mac-Tx Study	Clarithromycin + Clofazamine	(2 g) (100 mg)	vs Clarithromycin + Clofazamine + Ethambutol	(2 g) (100 mg) (15 mg/kg)	Response rates similar Relapse rate less in regimen 2
Chaisson et al., 1994	Clarithromycin + Ethambutol	(2 g) (15 mg/kg)	vs Clarithromycin +Ethambutol +Clofazamine	(2 g) (15 mg/kg) (100 mg)	Response rate better in regimen 1. Increase in mortality in regimen 2
Curavium	Clarithromycin +Clofazamine	(2 or 1 g)	Clarithromycin Rifabutin Ethambutol	(2 or 1 g) (450 mg) (1.2 g)	Better response at 6 months for regimen 2. Less relapse for regimen 2
Swiss Mac-Tx Study	Clarithromycin +Rifabutin +Clofazamine	(2 to 1 g) (450 mg) (100 mg)			95% patients sterilized blood, at 1 month. 88% clinical response at 2 months
CPCRA027 Mac Tx[a] trial	Clarithromycin +Ethambutol +Rifabutin	(2 or 1 g) (15 mg/kg) (300 mg)	Clarithromycin vs +Ethambutol +Clofazamine	(2 to 1 g) (15 mg/kg) (100 mg)	High dose clarithromycin arms closed because of excess mortality (17 vs 7%)
ACTG 223 Mac Tx trial	Clarithromycin +Ethambutol	(1 g) (15 mg/kg)	vs Clarithromycin Rifabutin	(1 g) (450 mg)	Still recruiting
	vs Clarithromycin +Rifabutin +Ethambutol	(1 g) (450 mg) (15 mg/kg)			

[a]This is in fact 4 studies as patients randomized in each arm to high or low dose clarithromycin.
Note: Figures in parentheses are total daily doses.
[b]Now published (Shafran et al., 1996).

determinant of progression of bacteremia. Mycobacteremia occurred in 17.9% of those whose CD4 counts were less than 50 cells/ml, 13.5% of those whose CD4 counts were 50–99 cells/ml, but in only 5.6% of those with an initial CD4 count of between 100–200. A further analysis indicated that the clinical benefits of rifabutin were almost entirely limited to those with a CD4 count of less than 75 cells/ml at entry. Interestingly, 'long-term' use of rifabutin did not seem to result in resistance to rifabutin in those developing MAC bacteremia. Six patients developed TB during the study; three of these had received rifabutin. These three patients only had presumptive evidence of TB as cultures were negative. There appears to be a difference in overall survival between placebo and treatment arms (Moore and Chaisson, 1995) but the trial was not designed to examine this end point.

There are problems with such long-term prophylaxis. These include insuring compliance, the potential induction of rifampicin resistance in patients who develop TB (Bishai *et al.*, 1996) and potential for cumulative side effects from long-term prophylaxis. The study was of a relatively short duration and it is not known whether long-term rifabutin would either continue to be efficacious or be without any toxicity.

Clofazamine

In a randomized prospective open-label treatment versus no treatment community-based clinical trial of clofazimine as prophylaxis for MAC seven patients randomized to clofazimine developed disseminated MAC compared with six patients receiving no treatment. There were problems in study methodology, both in the calculation determining the numbers who may eventually go on to develop MAC and on length of time the prophylaxis needed to be taken.

Clarithromycin

Data from a recent randomized double-lined placebo-controlled trial of clarithromycin versus placebo in 684 patients have demonstrated the efficacy of this drug in the prevention of MAC (Pierce *et al.*, 1996). Of patients on placebo, 12.6% developed MAC compared with 4.5% on the drug. All causes of mortality were decreased by 30% in the prophylaxis group. Those patients on prophylaxis who developed breakthrough MAC had a 49% incidence of clarithromycin resistance.

Azithromycin

Recent data show that once weekly azithromycin is an effective prophylaxis and unfrequently (11%) selects for resistant isolates. Combination with daily rifabutin increases efficacy rates, but is not well tolerated (Havlir *et al.*, 1996).

Dapsone/pyrimethamine

This may have some effect in preventing MAC and has the advantage that it might prevent toxoplasmosis and *Pneumocystis* (Opravil *et al.*, 1995).

Drug susceptibility testing

There is no standardized reference method for susceptibility testing of MAC and there has not been any convincing data to suggest any correlation between the results of *in vitro* susceptibility testing and clinical efficacy in HIV positive patients, except for clarithromycin.

In the US and Canada the commonest technique employed is the indirect proportion method. This technique involves isolation and subculture of the organism before its inoculation in various dilutions into both drug-free media and into media containing appropriate concentrations of antimycobacterial drugs. The media is incubated at 37°C in 5–10% CO_2 and read weekly for three weeks. The control (drug-free media) plate should contain 50–200 individual mycobacteria colonies to which the number of surviving colonies in any drug-containing medium should be compared. The population of organisms is considered resistant when the number of colonies on drug-containing medium is greater than 1% of the number on drug-free medium. Using this method MAC isolates are usually resistant to all primary antimycobacterial drugs including isoniazid, streptomycin, rifampicin and pyrazinimide and are often resistant to ethambutol. MAC is often resistant to other drugs, including capriomycin, PAS, cycloserine, ethionamide and kanomycin. There is variable sensitivity to clofazimine, clarithromycin, ciprofloxacin, rifabutin and amikacin.

Susceptibility testing can be performed in liquid medium using the BACTEC system with minimal inhibitory concentration (MIC) calculated for both established and experimental drugs. This method compares the amount of radioactive labeled CO_2 released from drug-containing medium with the amount released from control medium. There are major problems with all these techniques however with intra- and inter-laboratory reproducibility and cost.

INTERPRETATION OF SUSCEPTIBILITY TESTING

In vitro sensitivity testing should be interpreted with caution as it is method-dependent and organisms can appear to be more sensitive in broth than on agar. Drug penetration into tissues and cells is probably a critical factor in the treatment of intracellular *M. avium* and some antibiotics are concentrated in cells resulting in greater efficacy than might be predicted on the basis of *in vitro* testing in cell-free systems. The ratio of the minimal

bactericidal concentration (MBC) to the minimal inhibitory concentration for some drugs such as rifabutin and clofazimine is >32 so that killing does not occur at any achievable serum level. The MIC 90 for azithromycin was 62 μg/ ml, far exceeding any achievable level in serum but the drug is concentrated in tissues, accounting for its *in vivo* activity (Girard *et al.*, 1987). Rifabutin is another drug with substantial accumulation in tissue and may explain its superior activity compared with rifampicin *in vitro*. *In vitro* testing lacks standardization although the BACTEC system appears to be more reproducible and convenient than others, though expensive. Isolates appear to be more sensitive to drugs when tested by this system when compared with the proportion method.

By the agar dilution method (Yajko, Nassos and Hadley, 1987) only 32% of AIDS patients were sensitive to ethambutol (50μg/ml), 27% to rifampicin (10μg/ml), 88% to clofazimine (1μg/ml) and 28% to rifabutin (0.5μg/ml). Using 2μg/ml of rifabutin 92% became susceptible. Most strains are sensitive to amikacin and the use of liposomal-encapsulated amikacin has demonstrated improved efficacy *in vitro* (Gangadharam *et al.*, 1988). About one third of *M. avium* isolates are sensitive to ciprofloxacin and both azithromycin and clarithromycin are also active *in vitro*.

Very little work has been done on combinations of agents to look for synergy although many drugs appear to show synergy when combined with ethambutol or ciprofloxacin or ethambutol plus ciprofloxacin or amikacin (Heifets, Iseman and Lindholm-Levy, 1988; Ozenna *et al.*, 1988; Baron and Young, 1986; Telles and Yates, 1994).

In conclusion, *in vitro* susceptibility of *M. avium* to antibiotics should be interpreted in the context of what is happening inside cells and the achievable tissue levels. MICs for betalactams and aminoglycoside which have limited penetration into tissues may over-estimate the utility of these drugs. For drugs concentrated in the tissues such as quinolones, macrolides and rifamycins, a drug may be active *in vivo* even though the MIC far exceeds achievable serum levels. The use of macrophage and animal models may help clarify this situation.

MYCOBACTERIUM SCROFULACEUM

This organism was included in the same 'complex' as *M. avium* and *M. intracellulare*. Only eight cases of disseminated infection have ever been reported. One patient with AIDS has developed disseminated chronically ulcerated and nodular skin lesions with probable lung cavitation. The organism was susceptible to clarithromycin, ethambutol and clofazimine (Sanders *et al.*, 1995).

MYCOBACTERIUM KANSASII

GENERAL FEATURES

This mycobacterium was first reported as a human pathogen 40 years ago when it was isolated from a patient hospitalized with pulmonary infection in Kansas City, Missouri. *M. kansasii* is widely distributed throughout the world and is found in soil, house dust and tap water and it may infect wild or domestic animals as well as humans. (Wolinsky, 1979). The highest rate of infection is found in the United States especially in the areas from Florida across to California and from Texas to Illinois. In some urban areas *M. kansasii* is more common than *Mycobacterium tuberculosis*. It is primarily a pulmonary pathogen but both localized extrapulmonary and disseminated disease have been reported. Although the definition of pulmonary disease recommended by the American Thoracic Society for Nontuberculous Mycobacteria (1990) are generally appropriate for *M. kansasii*, most clinicians believe that isolation of *M. kansasii* from only one, not two, respiratory cultures is enough.

Its isolation however can occasionally indicate colonization without invasive disease.

Before the HIV epidemic, patients with *M. kansasii* lung disease characteristically presented in their fifth to seventh decades of life and lived in urban environments rather than rural areas. They were usually cigarette smokers with one or more underlying pulmonary diseases including chronic obstructive pulmonary disease, lung cancer, prior TB, bronchiectasis or pneumoconiosis. The majority were white and any ethnic distribution corresponded to the geographic areas studied. Patients usually presented with cough, sputum production, hemoptysis, chest pain, fever, night sweats and weight loss. The chest radiograph mimicked that of *M. tuberculosis* with apical fibronodular infiltrates and cavitation being common.

LABORATORY FEATURES

Mycobacterium kansasii infection may be suspected when large cross-barred bacilli, characteristic of this species, are seen on an acid-fast smear of sputum. DNA probes such as ACUPROBE, an *M. kansasii* culture identification kit (Gen-Probe, San Diego, California), has dramatically simplified and shortened the procedures for its identification. Unfortunately a number of *M. kansasii* isolates fail to hybridize with ACUPROBE and the usual phenotypic methods have to be used. Some research groups have their own in-house PCR identification techniques and others have used methods such as biotyping using a panel of enzymatic activities (Tortoli *et al.*, 1994).

HIV disease

M. kansasii usually appears late in the course of HIV infection. Patients are usually profoundly immune suppressed and about 50% of patients will have disease localized to the lungs.

Respiratory tract disease in HIV

A study from the Johns Hopkins Hospital (Levine and Chaisson, 1991) reviewed 19 patients with *M. kansasii* seen from 1985–1990. Interestingly, 14 patients had exclusive pulmonary infection, 3 had pulmonary and extrapulmonary and 2 had exclusive extrapulmonary infection. At the time of diagnosis the median CD4 count was 49 cells/ml (range 0–198) and 16 of the patients had a previous AIDS diagnosis. The commonest chest radiograph abnormalities were focal upper lobe infiltrates or diffuse interstitial infiltrates (Figure 13.2). Nine patients also had thin-walled cavitatory lesions. Nine of the patients with pulmonary infection were treated with antituberculous chemotherapy with resolution of symptoms and improvement of their radiology together with sputum conversion. Two untreated patients developed progressive cavitatory pulmonary disease and died from *M. kansasii* pneumonia. Untreated pulmonary disease was rapidly fatal as 8 of 17 patients with exclusive pulmonary disease (almost 50%) died within 3 months of diagnosis and in half of these the disease was not recognized until death. Two patients with paranasal sinus infections have been reported, one with bacteremia. In spite of treatment the disease progressed in both (Naguib, Byers and Slater, 1994). Endobronchial infection presenting as a tumor can also occur (Quieffin *et al.*, 1994).

Disseminated disease

In those highly endemic areas of the southern and mid-western United States (Horsburgh and Selik, 1989) disseminated infection with *M. kansasii* develops in 0.44% of AIDS patients. Amongst AIDS patients *M. kansasii* is the second cause of disseminated mycobacteriosis after *M. avium* and accounts for 2.9% of reported cases (Horsburgh and Selik, 1989). Disseminated disease primarily affects

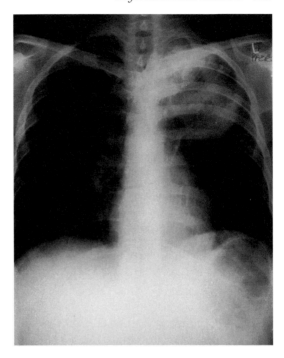

Fig. 13.2 Respiratory tract disease in an HIV patient showing rounded, cavitating consolidation in the left upper zone due to *M. kansasii* infection.

the lungs, lymph nodes, bones, joints and skin. The chest radiograph can be abnormal but it is unlikely to show typical cavitatory change. The distribution of any pulmonary infiltrate is variable and hilar adenopathy and mass lesions are more common.

M. kansasii can infect the CNS and there has been a case report of a patient with a central nervous system 'tuberculoma' (*kansasioma*) improving on treatment with isoniazid, rifampicin, ethambutol, with radiological resolution after three months.

In the study of 28 cases from Kansas City (Bamberger *et al.*, 1994) of *M. kansasii* infection the median CD4 count was only 12 cells/ml (range 0-90). Of these 28 patients, 11 had evidence of disseminated or extrapulmonary infection, and all but one had blood and/or bone marrow positive isolates. The frequency of disseminated cases was higher than that previously reported in HIV disease (Greene *et al.*, 1982; Hawkins *et al.*, 1986). Some of the discrepancies between studies may be related to differences and definitions of disease or in the frequency and/or methods of blood culture for mycobacteria.

DRUG TREATMENT AND SENSITIVITY

As with *M. tuberculosis*, *M. kansasii* demonstrates reliable *in vivo* susceptibility to antituberculous therapy such as isoniazid, rifampicin, ethambutol and streptomycin. In fact *M. kansasii* infection in the normal host closely resembles tuberculosis in its pathogenicity, clinical features and response to therapy, which is in marked contrast to infections caused by the other nontuberculous mycobacteria. In a recent study by a Research Committee of the British Thoracic Society (Research Committee, British Thoracic Society, 1994) 173 patients with pulmonary *M. kansasii* infection whose HIV status was unknown were treated with rifampicin and ethambutol in standard doses for nine months and studied over four years. There was a 9.7% relapse rate, a little higher than the rate acceptable in studies of *M. tuberculosis*. Twenty-three patients died during the study or follow-up period. These mortality data might suggest a high incidence of concomitant disease but the patients weren't tested for HIV antibodies. Although the treatment of non-HIV individuals in this trial cannot be extrapolated to HIV-infected patients, it might be a basis on which to develop treatment protocols.

Although the overall response to treatment in AIDS patients has been poor it appears that some patients with *M. kansasii* disease, even in the face of advanced HIV-related immunosuppression, may respond to standard antituberculous chemotherapy (Sherer *et al.*, 1986; Hirasuna, 1987). Of 11 patients with isolates of *M. kansasii* from blood, bone marrow or extrapulmonary tissue, 8 responded to therapy and survived for at

least 3 months, suggesting that disseminated disease can respond to appropriate therapy (Bamberger *et al.*, 1994). The majority of patients were treated with isoniazid, rifampicin and ethambutol but five were given rifampicin and ethambutol alone. The authors of this paper were unable to provide useful information regarding either the appropriate duration of therapy in HIV-infected patients or the likelihood of relapse. Two patients were on therapy for at least 12 months.

Rifampicin-resistant *M. kansasii* is increasing partly because of the HIV disease epidemic (Wallace *et al.*, 1994). Those patients with rifampicin-resistant isolation should be on a minimum of four drugs; clarithromycin 500 mg twice a day, high-dose isoniazid 900 mg a day with pyridoxine, streptomycin and ethambutol. Sulfamethoxazole, ciprofloxacin, ethionamide and cycloserine have also shown activity against *M. kansasii*. Rifabutin can also be active in spite of rifampicin resistance and might have a role in therapy.

MYCOBACTERIUM CELATUM

This is a recently-described species of mycobacteria (Butler *et al.*, 1993). It is similar to *M. avium* biochemically except that it has a mycolic acid pattern similar to *M. xenopi*. *M. celatum* has been further differentiated into types 1, 2, and 3 and has been described as causing pulmonary disease in HIV positive patients (Yakrus *et al.*, 1992). *M. celatum* is rarely isolated and of 13 500 laboratory isolates of mycobacteria over 5 years, only 24 isolates of *M. celatum* were found, an overall rate of 0.1%. Interestingly there is cross-reactivity of the DNA probe with this mycobacterium leading to false positive results for *M. tuberculosis*.

M. celatum has been isolated in an HIV-negative 15-month old boy with cervical lymphadenitis (Haase *et al.*, 1994) treated by excision. Histology showed granulomata, caseating necrosis and acid-fast bacilli. A slow-growing yellow pigmented mycobacteria was isolated, which on 16S rRNA gene sequencing was confirmed to be *M. celatum*.

There have been reports of *M. celatum* isolated from an AIDS patient with mycobacteremia (Piersimoni, Tortoli and De Sio, 1994; Bull *et al.*, 1995).

MYCOBACTERIUM FORTUITUM AND *MYCOBACTERIUM CHELONAE*

GENERAL FEATURES

These ubiquitous mycobacteria are rapidly-growing and are rare pathogens. Until recently most rapid growers belonged to the *M. fortuitum* complex and were subsequently divided between *M. fortuitum* and *M. chelonae*. New studies of DNA homology have clearly established the species status of *M. fortuitum*, *M. perigrinum*, *M. chelonae* and *M. abscessus* (Lévy-Frébault *et al.*, 1986; Kusunoki and Ezaki, 1992). Some would argue that *M. abscessus* is not a distinct species but belongs taxonomically to one of the two subspecies of *M. chelonae*, that is, *M. chelonae (abscessus)*. Pigmented rapid growers and *M. chelonae*-like organisms almost never cause lung disease but when they do the typical patient is a female non-smoker in her early sixties. Cough and sputum are the commonest symptoms and hemoptysis can occur. The chest X-ray shows bilateral interstitial infiltrates and cavitation is rare.

HIV disease

Disease due to *M. chelonae* has rarely been associated with immunosuppression but does occur in the setting of corticosteroid therapy. *Mycobacterium fortuitum* has caused multiple subcutaneous necrotizing nodules in an HIV-infected drug user (Sack, 1990). *M. fortuitum* has also caused a central venous catheter infection (Brady, Marcon and Maddux, 1987). Disseminated infections with both

M. fortuitum (Horsburgh and Selik, 1989) and *M. chelonae* have been reported in one pediatric case of AIDS. Unfortunately the species (subspecies) *M. chelonae (abscessus)* can be a contaminant in automated endoscopic washers (Maloney *et al.*, 1993; Fraser *et al.*, 1992) leading to false positive isolation from specimens.

Drug sensitivity and treatment

Drug susceptibility patterns of these organisms suggest that perhaps amikacin, rifampicin, cefoxitin and doxycyline may be useful. Clarithromycin has good activity against *M. chelonae* (Mushatt and Witzig, 1995) but most isolates were resistant to ciprofloxacin and doxycycline (Wallace, Brown and Onji, 1992). Some good results have been achieved using clarithromycin monotherapy for cutaneous and disseminated infection but more studies are required to examine treatment regimens more closely.

MYCOBACTERIUM GENAVENSE

GENERAL FEATURES

M. genavense was first discovered in 1990 by Hirschel and colleagues (Hirschel, Chang and Mach, 1990). They described disseminated infection caused by a slow-growing acid-fast organism which appeared to be a mycobacterium on both electron microscopy and chromatographic lipid analysis. Bottger and colleagues (Bottger *et al.*, 1992) reported 18 more cases and by using DNA analysis have confirmed the presence of a mycobacterial consensus sequence. They also developed a pair of PCR primers for use in the identification of *M. genavense* using the conserved portion of the 16S rRNA.

HIV infection

Disseminated *M. genavense* infection has been reported from several countries around the world and it is likely that this novel organism is widespread in the environment. About 30 cases of infection have been described in patients with advanced HIV disease (Hirschel, Chang and Mach, 1990; Bottger *et al.*, 1992; Wald *et al.*, 1992; Jackson *et al.*, 1992; Coyle *et al.*, 1992). The median survival for patients in the largest series was nine months if treated and only three months if untreated (Bottger *et al.*, 1992; Pechere *et al.*, 1995). The CD4 count of patients was $16/\mu l$, 87% had fever and weight loss. Anemia and diarrhea were also common.

Laboratory findings

Unless molecular techniques are used, recognition of *M. genavense* may be hampered by its slow growth and the low growth index achieved in the BACTEC system. Usually BACTEC samples are stained when the growth index exceeds 50–100 but to improve detection of *M. genavense* it may be important to stain samples even when the growth index is greater than 30.

It can be grown on M7, H11-MJ medium and a detailed review of its laboratory aspects has been described by Coyle and co-workers (Coyle *et al.*, 1992).

Drug sensitivity and treatment

In one series therapy with standard antimycobacterial drugs appears to have prolonged survival to 8 months compared with 2.5 months in untreated patients (Bottger *et al.*, 1992). Including clarithromycin in the treatment regimen was associated with a favorable clinical response with blood cultures becoming negative (Bessesen, Shlay and Stone-Venohr, 1993).

MYCOBACTERIUM GORDONAE

GENERAL FEATURES

M. gordonae is ubiquitous in the environment and is commonly isolated from water and

soil (Tsukamura, 1984). As it is found in hospital water it can contaminate bronchoscopy specimens (Steere, Corrales and von Graevenitz, 1979) and be included in clinical specimens during collection of processing. *M. gordonae* is considered to be one of the least pathogenic of the nontuberculous mycobacteria and in a literature review by Weinberger and colleagues only 24 cases of clinical disease were found up to 1992. Two of these occurred in patients with AIDS (Chan, McKitrick and Klein, 1984; Cárcaba *et al.*, 1989; Weinberger *et al.*, 1992).

In non-HIV infected patients soft tissue disease involving the extremities, peritoneum, cornea, endocardium, liver, bone marrow, kidney, CNS, lung and disseminated disease have all been reported. Lung disease usually occurs in males aged 40 to 76 years who have had previous pulmonary problems, for example, a history of *M. tuberculosis*, pulmonary carcinoma, pulmonary Hodgkin's disease or chronic obstructive airways disease with heavy smoking. Upper lobe disease, usually unilateral, is commonest and patients present with typical symptoms of mycobacterial disease. Bronchial biopsy may be useful in detecting granulomata in patients who are sputum positive for *M. gordonae* in order to document histologically invasive disease.

HIV infection

Of the two cases with AIDS reported by Weinberger, one was a 41-year-old intravenous drug user (IVDU) who had previous PCP (Weinberger *et al.*, 1992). He presented with weakness and fever and had *M. gordonae* in the lungs and bone marrow. He was treated with isoniazid, ethambutol, streptomycin, rifabutin and clofazimine but died nine months after diagnosis. The second case, another IVDU, a 28-year-old man with peritoneal infection presented with weight loss, abdominal pain and fever. He was treated with isoniazid, pyrazinamide, ethambutol and rifampicin. He later died from neurological disease unrelated to his *M. gordonae* infection. There have been further reports of patients with AIDS or severe HIV infection where *M. gordonae* has been isolated but the data published do not indicate whether these isolates were 'passengers' or 'pathogens'.

Drug treatment and sensitivity

M. gordonae is usually resistant to isoniazid but sensitive to ethambutol, rifampicin, cycloserine, kanamycin, ciprofloxacin, trimethoprim and sulfamethoxazole. Even with treatment none of the reported cases of pulmonary disease in HIV-negative patients were cured although the disease stabilized in about half.

MYCOBACTERIUM HAEMOPHILUM

CLINICAL FEATURES

M. haemophilum was first described by Sompolinsky and colleagues in 1978 after its isolation from subcutaneous abscesses of a 51-year-old Israeli woman who was receiving treatment for Hodgkin's lymphoma (Sompolinsky *et al.*, 1978). The 20 or so patients reported in the literature prior to the HIV pandemic have usually developed infection of skin or subcutaneous tissues. Only five were immunocompetent hosts. Of these five cases four were healthy young children with submandibular or cervical lymphadenitis without evidence of skin involvement and the remaining case was a 65-year-old woman who developed a right forearm cutaneous lesion following coronary artery bypass surgery (Males, West and Bartholomew, 1987). Most other patients with *M. haemophilum* infection were renal transplant recipients or patients immunosuppressed by cancer therapy.

The natural habitat of *M. haemophilum* and the route of infection is unknown. Patients have come from diverse geographic areas but the organism has not been cultured from the environment. Like *M. marinum* and *M. ulcerans* it can grow at low temperatures and this may explain the reason why it prefers skin extremities and joints. For some reason it seems to have a propensity to infect middle-aged women.

HIV infection

The first case of *Mycobacterium haemophilum* infecting a patient with AIDS was described in 1987 (Males, West and Bartholomew, 1987) and there have only been sporadic reports since then (Thibert, Lebel and Martineau, 1990; Rogers *et al.*, 1988; Armstrong *et al.*, 1991; Kristjansson, Bieluch and Byeff, 1991). Twenty-six cases of *M. haemophilum* in AIDS patients have been reported up until 1992, 13 from the New York City area (Becerer and Hopfer, 1992; Dever *et al.*, 1992; Holton, Nye and Miller, 1991; Straus *et al.*, 1994). All were profoundly immunosuppressed and responded poorly to treatment. In one study, 88% of those who had CD4 counts available had counts less than 25 cells/ml. Three of these patients with AIDS had disseminated *M. haemophilum*.

Little is known about the spectrum of illness caused by *M. haemophilum*. Presenting features have included fever, weight loss, subcutaneous and cutaneous lesions – particularly on the extremities and over joints – tenosynovitis, joint effusions and upper respiratory symptoms. Cutaneous lesions can vary greatly in appearance from erythematous and nodular to scaly plaques with the subsequent development of ulcers and pustular lesions. Because *M. haemophilum* prefers cooler areas of skin the distal extremities are most often affected and lesions can be misdiagnosed as Kaposi's sarcoma.

The organism has been recovered from a variety of sites in patients with AIDS including skin, lymph nodes, vitreous fluid, synovial fluid, sputum, bronchoalveolar lavage, lung tissue, bone, bone marrow and blood. Recovery of *M. haemophilum* from multiple sites suggests hematogenously disseminated infection.

Laboratory characteristics

Mycobacterium haemophilum is a fastidious slowly-growing mycobacterium which requires a low incubation temperature for growth. As it also requires heme- or ferric ammonium citrate-enriched media, it may not be isolated using standard techniques. When acid-fast bacilli are seen on histological samples they are usually associated with neutrophilic or mixed cellular infiltrates. Multinucleated giant cells are rare but areas of focal necrosis are often seen.

Drug sensitivity and treatment

For immunocompetent patients with localized infection surgical excision has been curative. In transplant recipients lesions can improve when the dosage of immunosuppressive therapy is decreased. Simple antimycobacterial regimes can be used and have included various combinations of first-line antituberculous treatment as well as ciprofloxacin, amikacin, minocycline, doxycycline, clarithromycin and clofazimine.

In AIDS patients there has been a disappointingly poor response to combination antimycobacterial therapy. Isoniazid, rifampicin, ethambutol and ciprofloxacin in combination has been a suggested regimen though recurrence of disease is common. Ciprofloxacin and perhaps azithromycin or clarithromycin might also be suitable to treat *M. haemophilum*. This use of multiple drug combinations is probably sensible but there is not enough experience to devise treatment protocols at present. Surgical debridement or excision may play a role, as may the addition of combination antiviral HIV therapy to any

drug regimen due to its possible action on improving cellular immunity.

MYCOBACTERIUM MALMOENSE

GENERAL FEATURES

M. malmoense was first described in 1977 by Schroder and Tumin (reported in Wayne and Sramek, 1992) in four patients with pulmonary disease from the Swedish city of Malmo. It has been isolated with increasing frequency ever since, mainly from Europe and occasionally from the United States. In a 22-year study among 221 Swedish patients, *M. malmoense* caused pulmonary infection in adults and cervical lymphadenopathy in children (Henriques *et al.*, 1994). There have been over 60 reported cases of extrapulmonary infection due to *M. malmoense* (Zaugg *et al.*, 1993).

M. malmoense is a slow-growing environmental non-chromogenic microaerophilic organism. It has been found in the stools of healthy individuals and it has been isolated from stream water. Presently it is most reliably distinguished from other mycobacteria by thin layer chromatography of its surface lipids (Jenkins, 1985).

In HIV-negative patients cough, fever and weight loss are the commonest symptoms of infection although patients can be asymptomatic (Roberts *et al.*, 1985). The chest radiograph usually shows unilateral changes which vary from patchy infiltrates to multiple thick-walled cavities in the upper and mid zones. A lacework pattern of thin-walled cysts with relatively little surrounding parenchymal infiltrate is said to be characteristic (Banks, Jenkins and Smith, 1985).

HIV-positive patients

M. malmoense has been rarely isolated from AIDS patients (Claydon, Coker and Harris, 1991; Willocks *et al.*, 1993; Yoganathan *et al.*,

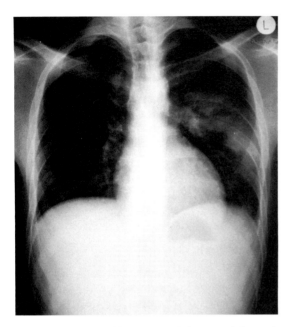

Fig. 13.3 Tumor-like mass in left upper lobe with central cavitation due to *M. malmoense* infection.

1994). It appears to occur at a late stage of HIV disease when the CD4 count is below 50 cells/ml. Claydon and colleagues (Claydon, Coker and Harris, 1991) reported two cases of pulmonary *M. malmoense* in HIV-positive patients who presented with productive cough and weight loss. Both had chest radiographs which showed diffuse bilateral soft shadows and one had co-existent mediastinal lymphadenopathy. Both had acid-fast bacilli in the sputum and one had *M. malmoense* in the stool. Standard antituberculous treatment was given but the patients died before any response could be assessed. Both deaths were considered to be unrelated to the *M. malmoense* infection. One case of *M. malmoense* presenting with a tumor-like mass has been reported (Figure 13.3) (Yoganathan *et al.*, 1994). The patient had been treated with anti-mycobacterial therapy for two years with good clinical but little radiological or bronchoscopic response, and eventually died of respiratory failure. Recently *M. malmoense*

bacteremia has been reported (Fakih *et al.*, 1996).

Drug treatment and sensitivity

There have been few reports describing response to treatment of pulmonary infection caused by *M. malmoense*.

In HIV-negative patients Banks and colleagues (Banks, Jenkins and Smith, 1985) obtained the best results with rifampicin, ethambutol and isoniazid for periods of between 18 and 24 months. Although the optimum treatment for HIV-positive patients has not been established the role of new macrolides and quinilones is undefined but were used with effect in the one patient (Yoganathan *et al.*, 1994). Surgical resection has been successful in four HIV-negative patients (Banks, Jenkins and Smith, 1985).

MYCOBACTERIUM MARINUM

GENERAL FEATURES

M. marinum typically causes a disease characterized by a self-limiting cutaneous infection known as 'swimming pool granuloma'.

HIV disease

M. marinum has caused multiple sores and boils on the face, chest and extremities of a 50-year-old man with HIV infection who kept a tropical freshwater aquarium (Ries, White and Murdock, 1990). As smears of the boils were AAFB positive he was treated as for TB with triple antituberculous therapy (isoniazid, rifampicin and ethambutol) and there was resolution of his lesions after several weeks. Culture confirmed *M. marinum* and the patient received five months of treatment. He had no recurrence after a year of follow-up. A sporotrichoid rash has also been reported (Hanau *et al.*, 1994) but this patient relapsed after treatment. Patients with AIDS may require prolonged treatment or suppressive therapy.

MYCOBACTERIUM SIMIAE

CLINICAL FEATURES

M. simiae is a photochromogenic acid-fast bacillus and was first described in monkeys imported from India in 1965. It may be recovered from water (Wolinsky, 1979), especially in Israel (Lavy and Yoshpe-Purer, 1982). *M. simiae* may colonize the upper respiratory tract without causing disease especially in patients who are middle-aged or older and have a history of tuberculosis. Sputum smears are then usually negative and few cultures are positive. This mycobacterium is rarely associated with human disease though there have been cases reported in non-immunocompromised patients from Europe and the United States (Bell *et al.*, 1983), especially monkey handlers. Most patients already have chronic lung disease although it can act as a primary pulmonary pathogen and cause chronic cavitatory lung disease (Krasnow and Gross, 1975). Chest radiographic changes include bilateral interstitial infiltrates, pleural effusions and apical cavities with surrounding infiltrates. Transbronchial biopsy can be helpful in determining whether invasive disease is present (Bell *et al.*, 1983). Osteomyelitis and renal involvement have both been reported (Rose *et al.*, 1982).

HIV-positive patients

To date, only four patients with AIDS have had infection with *Mycobacterium simiae* reported. Two were co-infected with *M. avium*-complex (Lévy-Frébault *et al.*, 1987; Torres *et al.*, 1991), one a Congolese and the other a Puerto Rican who lived in New York City. Two other patients have been reported from Israel; both had disseminated infection due to *M. simiae* (Huminer *et al.*, 1993). One

was a 21-year-old hemophiliac who had a normal chest radiograph and had two blood cultures that were positive for *M. simiae*. He died five days after the diagnosis was made. The other, also a hemophiliac, developed lung infiltrates and cavitation and *M. simiae* was isolated from nine sputum specimens, four blood cultures and an aspirate of bone marrow. In spite of treatment his blood cultures remained positive and he died three months after the diagnosis. Samples of tap water taken from this patient's house did not yield any mycobacteria.

Laboratory characteristics

M. simiae resembles *M. avium*-complex but has a distinct biochemical profile and may well be closely related to *M. genavense*. Investigation of the antigenic composition of several strains shows that there is some cross-reactivity between strains of *M. simiae* and *M. avium*-complex types 18 and 19.

Drug treatment and sensitivity

M. simiae is usually resistant to standard antituberculous chemotherapeutic agents. *In vitro* tests can demonstrate sensitivity to cycloserine, ethionamide, sulfamethoxozole and ciprofloxacin and treatment with ciprofloxacin 500 mg bd has been suggested. As initial therapy the American Thoracic Society suggest a four-drug regimen similar to that used in MAC. The efficacy of this regimen is not known.

MYCOBACTERIUM SZULGAI

GENERAL FEATURES

A case of pulmonary infection due to multi-drug resistant *M. szulgai* has been reported in a patient with AIDS (Newshan and Torres, 1994). A 42-year-old homosexual man with a CD4 count of 10 cells/ml had a 4 month history of weight loss, fatigue, fever and sweats. He had a nodule in the right upper lobe on chest radiograph. *M. szulgai* was isolated susceptible to ethambutol, rifampicin and ciprofloxacin. In HIV-negative patients *M. szulgai* causes a syndrome which is indistinguishable from *M. tuberculosis*. Middle-aged men with or without underlying lung disease are most prone; the chest radiograph shows apical infiltrates and cavitation rather than a solitary nodule.

MYCOBACTERIUM ULCERANS

GENERAL FEATURES

A case of *M. ulcerans* which causes Buruli ulcer has been described in an HIV-positive Zairean female. She was treated with rifampicin and clarithromycin rather than surgery and improved. She was not very immunosuppressed as her CD4 count was 500/μl, and it is possible her HIV disease was incidental to her developing Buruli ulcer (Delaporte *et al.*, 1994).

MYCOBACTERIUM XENOPI

GENERAL FEATURES

This organism derives its name from the toad from which it was first isolated in 1957 (Schwabacher, 1959). *M. xenopi* was recognized as a human pathogen eight years later. It has been found in both hot and cold water taps, hospital hot water generators, hospital shower water and storage tanks, and has been isolated from seabird and sparrow droppings and sewage sludge water (McSwiggan and Collins, 1974). In one report of nosocomially acquired *M. xenopi* infection in patients who were not immune-suppressed, the source of the organism was a hospital water cistern (Costrini *et al.*, 1981). In HIV-negative patients *M. xenopi* usually causes pulmonary disease in middle-aged or older men with pre-existing lung disease. Chronic cough, sputum and hemoptysis are common symptoms with cavitation, infiltrates and nodules commonly seen on the chest radiograph.

HIV infection (Schafer and Sierra, 1992; Tecson-Tumang and Bright, 1984; Ausina *et al.*, 1988)

The first reported case in an AIDS patient was in 1984 and although the organism was not found in the hospital's environmental water the suggestion was that it was acquired from a water source elsewhere such as a bathhouse. The patient had pulmonary and liver involvement and was treated with isoniazid and rifampicin with improvement (Eng *et al.*, 1984).

In one study *M. xenopi* was cultured from 23 of 33 patients (70%) with AIDS. One of the patients had bacteremia but in the remaining patients *M. xenopi* was only isolated from sputum or bronchoscopic specimens. Among these patients eight had concurrent *Pneumocystis carinii* pneumonia, four had active *M. tuberculosis* infection and five had other opportunistic infections. Six patients had transient pulmonary systems that abated without therapy and three had unexplained fevers and died before their condition was diagnosed. None of the patients were treated specifically for *M. xenopi* (Shafer and Sierra, 1992).

It is possible that many of the HIV-positive patients reported to have *M. xenopi* infection had either colonization or contaminated specimens. Contamination of specimens should not be expected however to be more common in HIV-positive compared with HIV-negative patients. Embarking on a course of treatment may be a difficult decision as it is often hard to differentiate colonization from slow progressive invasive disease.

Drug treatment and sensitivity

Optimal therapy is not known. With little correlation between *in vitro* susceptibility and clinical outcome. A multidrug regimen including a quinolone, rifampicin, ethambutol and a macrolide has been suggested as being appropriate. Lung surgery can be successful but has a high complication rate.

Mixed infections

There are several reports of patients having had more than one nontuberculous mycobacteria isolated at the same time, so-called mixed infections. Some of these include those with *M. genavense* and *M. avium* (Kirschner *et al.*, 1994), *M. simiae* and *M. avium* (Torres *et al.*, 1991), and *M. kansasii* and *M. avium* (Valainis, 1991). The clinical relevance of each component of these mixed infections is difficult to assess.

Mixed *M. avium* disease

Even amongst patients who have *M. avium* disease two or more different strains may be isolated from sequential cultures of various specimens. This reflects ongoing polyclonal infection (Slutsky *et al.*, 1994; Arbeit *et al.*, 1993). This genetic diversity was defined using pulsed-field gel electrophoresis which showed distinctive restriction fragment profiles for each strain. Identifying and understanding this phenomenon may be critical in developing effective treatments.

CONCLUSION

These mycobacteria, even those that still remain obscure, all have the potential for causing unusual and atypical disease in severely immunosuppressed patients. Although adequate prophylaxis, rapid diagnosis and effective treatment are being developed there is still much to be discovered about these enigmatic 'atypical' mycobacteria.

REFERENCES

Agy, M.B., Wallis, C.K., Plorde, J.J. *et al.* (1989) Evaluation of four mycobacterial blood culture media: Bactec 13A, Isolator/Bactec 12B, Isolator/Middlebrook agar and a biphasic medium. *Diagnostic Microbiology and Infectious Diseases*, **12**, 303–8.

Arbeit, R.D., Slutsky, A., Barber, T.W. *et al.* (1993) Genetic diversity among strains of *Mycobacterium avium* causing monoclonal and polyclonal bacteremia in patients with AIDS. *Journal of Infectious Diseases*, **167**, 1384–90.

Armstrong, D., Gold, J.W.M., Dryjanski, J. *et al.* (1985) Treatment of infections in patients with acquired immunodeficiency syndrome. *Annals of Internal Medicine*, **103**, 738–43.

Armstrong, D., Kiehn, T., Boone, N. *et al.* (1991) *Mycobacterium haemophilum* infections – New York City metropolitan area, 1990–91. *Morbidity and Mortality Weekly Reports*, **40**, 636–43.

Ausina, V., Barrio, J., Luquin, M. *et al.* (1988) *Mycobacterium xenopi* infections in the acquired immunodeficiency syndrone. *Annals of Internal Medicine*, **109**, 927–8.

Baess, I. (1983) Deoxyribonucleic acid relationships between different serovars of *Mycobacterium avium*, *Mycobacterium intracellulare*, and *Mycobacterium scrofulaceum*. *Acta Pathologica, Microbiologica, Immunologica Scandinavica*, **91**, 201–3.

Bamberger, D.M., Driks, MR., Gupta, M.R. *et al.* (1994) *Mycobacterium kansasii* among patients infected with human immunodeficiency virus in Kansas City. *Clinical Infectious Diseases*, **18**, 395–400.

Banks, J., Jenkins, P.A. and Smith, A.P. (1985) Pulmonary infection with *Mycobacterium malmoense*: a review of treatment and response. *Tubercle*, **66**, 197–203.

Barbaro, D.J., Orcutt, V.L. and Coldiron, B.M. (1989) *Mycobacterium avium-Mycobacterium intracellulare* infection limited to the skin and lymph nodes in patients with AIDS. *Review of Infectious Diseases*, **11**, 1145–8.

Baron, E.J. and Young, L.S. (1986) Amikacin, ethambutol and rifampin for treatment of disseminated *Mycobacterium avium-intracellulare* infections in patients with AIDS. *Diagnostic Microbiology and Infectious Diseases*, **5**, 215–20.

Bautista, G., Alcid, D. and Gocke, D. (1991) Quantitative blood culture for mycobacteria in patients with acquired immunodeficiency syndrome (abstract 242, p. 139). Program

Abstract. 31st Interscience Conference of Antimicrobial Agents and Chemotherapy. American Society for Microbiology, Washington DC.

Becherer, P. and Hopfer, R.L. (1992) Infection with *Mycobacterium haemophilum* [Letter]. *Clinical Infectious Diseases*, **14**, 793.

Bell, R.C., Higuchi, J.H., Donovan, W.N. *et al.* (1983) *Mycobacterium simiae*: clinical features and follow-up of twenty-four patients. *American Review of Respiratory Disease*, **127**, 35–8.

Bermudez, L.E., Martinelli, J., Petrofsky, M. *et al.* (1994) Recombinant granulocyte-macrophage colony-stimulating factor enhances the effects of antibiotics against *Mycobacterium avium* complex infection in the beige mouse model. *Journal of Infectious Diseases*, **169**, 575–80.

Bermudez, L.E., Young, L.S., Martinelli, J. *et al.* (1993). Exposure to ethanol up-regulates the expression of *Mycobacterium avium* complex proteins associated with bacterial virulence. *Journal of Infectious Diseases*, **168**, 961–8.

Bessesen, M.T., Berry, C.D., Johnson, M.A. *et al.* (1990) Site of origin of disseminated MAC infection in AIDS (abstract 1268, p. 297). Program Abstract. 31st Interscience Conference of Antimicrobial Agents and Chemotherapy. American Society for Microbiology, Washington DC.

Bessesen, M.T., Shlay, J., Stone-Venohr, B. (1993) Disseminated *Mycobacterium genavense* infection: clinical and microbiological features and response to therapy. *AIDS*, **7**, 1357–61.

Bishai, W.R., Graham, N.M.H., Harrington, S. *et al.* (1996) Rifampicin-resistant tuberculosis in a patient receiving rifabutin prophylaxis. *New England Journal of Medicine*, **334**, 1573–6.

Blumenthal, D.R., Zucker, J.R. and Hawkins, C.A. (1990) *Mycobacterium avium* complex-induced septic arthritis and osteomyelitis in a patient with the acquired immunodeficiency syndrome. *Arthritis and Rheumatism*, **33**, 757–8.

Bottger, E.C., Teske, A., Kirschner, P. *et al.* (1992) Disseminated *Mycobacterium genavense* infection in patients with AIDS. *Lancet*, **340**, 76–80.

Brady, M.T., Marcon, M.J. and Maddux, H. (1987) Broviac catheter-related infection due to *Mycobacterium fortuitum* in a patient with acquired immunodeficiency syndrome. *Pediatric Infectious Diseases*, **6**, 492–4.

Brennan, P.J. (1989) Structure of mycobacteria; recent developments in defining cell wall carbohydrates and proteins. *Review of Infectious Diseases*, **II**: S420–S430.

Bull, T.J., Shanson, D.C., Yates, M.D. *et al.* (1995) A new group (type 3) of *Mycobacterium celatum* isolated from AIDS patients in the London area. *International Journal of Systematic Bacteriology*, **45**, 861–2.

Butler, W.R., O'Connor, S.P., Yakrus, M.A. *et al.* (1993) *Mycobacterium celatum* sp. nov. *International Journal of Systematic Bacteriology*, **43**, 1540–50.

Cárcaba, V., Cartón, J.A., Fernández León, A. *et al.* (1989) Peritonitis por *Mycobacterium gordonae* en un paciente infectado por el virus de la immunodeficiencia humana. *Medicina Clinica (Barcelona)*, **93**, 598.

Chaisson, R.E. and Levine, B. (1991) *Mycobacterium kansasii* infection [letter]. *Annals of Internal Medicine*, **115**, 496–7.

Chaisson, R.E., Moore, R.D., Richman, D.D. *et al.* (1992) Incidence and natural history of *Mycobacterium avium*-complex infections in patients with acquired immunodeficiency virus disease treated with zidovudine. *American Review of Respiratory Disease*, **146**, 285–9.

Chaisson, R.E., Benson, C., Dube, M. *et al.* (1994) Clarithromycin therapy for bacteremic *Mycobacterium avium* complex disease in patients with AIDS. *Annals of Internal Medicine*, **121**, 905–11.

Chan, J., McKitrick, J.C. and Klein, R.S. (1984) *Mycobacterium gordonae* in the acquired immunodeficiency syndrome [letter]. *Annals of Internal Medicine*, **100**, 400.

Chin, D.P., Reingold, A.L., Stone, E.N. *et al.* (1994) The impact of *Mycobacterium avium* complex bacteremia and its treatment on survival of AIDS patients – a prospective study. *Journal of Infectious Diseases*, **170**, 578–84.

Chiu, J., Nussbaum, J., Bozzette, S. *et al.* (1990) Treatment of disseminated *Mycobacterium avium* complex infection in AIDS with amikacin, ethambutol, rifampin, and ciprofloxacin. *Annals of Internal Medicine*, **113**, 358–61.

Choo, P.S. and McCormack, J.G. (1995) *Mycobacterium avium*: a potentially treatable cause of pericardial effusions. *Journal of Infection*, **30**, 55–8.

Claydon, E.J., Coker, R.J. and Harris, J.R.W. (1991) *Mycobacterium malmoense* infection in HIV positive patients. *Journal of Infection*, **23**, 195–6.

Colebunders, R., Nambunzu, M., Portaels, F. *et al.* (1990) Isolation of mycobacteria from HIV seropositive and HIV seronegative patients with and without diarrhoea in Kinshasa, Zaire:

preliminary results. *Annales de la Société Belge de Medecine Tropicale*, **70**, 303–9.

Costrini, A.M., Mahler, D.A., Gross, W.M. *et al.* (1981) Clinical and roentgenographic features of nosocomial pulmonary disease due to *Mycobacterium xenopi*. *American Review of Respiratory Disease*, **123**, 105–9.

Coyle, M.B., Carlson, L.D.C., Wallis, C.K. *et al.* (1992) Laboratory aspects of *Mycobacterium genavense*, a proposed species isolated from AIDS patients. *Journal of Clinical Microbiology*, **30**, 3206–12.

Crawford, J.T. and Bates, J.H. (1985) Phage typing of the *Mycobacterium avium-intracellulare-scrofulaceum* complex: a study of strains of diverse geographic and host origin. *American Review of Respiratory Disease*, **132**, 386–9.

Cuttino, J.T. and McCabe, A.M. (1949) Pure granulomatous nocardiosis: A new fungus disease distinguished by intracellular parasitism. A description of a new disease in man due to a hitherto undescribed organism, *Nocardia intracellularis*, N. Sp., including a study of the biologic and pathogenic properties of this species. *American Journal of Pathology*, **25**, 1.

Dautzenberg, B., Truffot, C., Legris, S. *et al.* (1991) Activity of clarithromycin against *Mycobacterium avium* infection in patients with the acquired immune deficiency syndrome. A controlled clinical trial. *American Review of Respiratory Disease*, **144**, 564–9.

Delaporte, E., Savage, C., Alfandari, S. *et al.* (1994) Buruli Ulcer in a Zairian woman with HIV infection. *Annals of Dermatology and Venereology*, **121**, 557–60.

De Paepe, M.E., Guerrieri, C. and Waxman, M. (1990) Opportunistic infections of the testis in the acquired immunodeficiency syndrome. *Mt Sinai Journal of Medicine*, **57**, 25–9.

Dever, L.L., Martin, J.W., Seaworth, B. *et al.* (1992) Varied presentations and responses to treatment of infections caused by *Mycobacterium haemophilum* in patients with AIDS. *Clinical Infectious Diseases*, **14**, 1195–200.

Dwork, A.J., Chin, S. and Boyce, L. (1994) Intracerebral *Mycobacterium avium-intracellulare* in a child with acquired immune deficiency syndrome. *Journal of Paediatric Infectious Diseases*, **13**, 1149–51.

Eng, R.H.K., Forrester, C., Smith, S.M. *et al.* (1984) *Mycobacterium xenopi* infection in a patient with acquired immunodeficiency syndrome. *Chest*, **86**, 145–7.

Fakih, M., Chapalmadugu, S., Ricard, A. *et al.* (1996) *Mycobacterium malmoense* bacteremia in two AIDS patients. *Journal of Clinical Microbiology*, **34**, 731–3.

Falkinham, J.O. III, Parker, B.C. and Gruft, H. (1980) Epidemiology of infection by nontuberculous mycobacteria. *American Review of Respiratory Disease*, **121**, 931–7.

Fraser, V.J., Jones, M., Murray, P.R. *et al.* (1992) Contamination of flexible fiberoptic bronchoscopes with *Mycobacterium chelonae* linked to an automated bronchoscope disinfection machine. *American Review of Respiratory Disease*, **145**, 853–5.

Gangadharam, P.R., Perumal, V.K., Crawford, J.T. *et al.* (1988) Association of plasmids and virulence of *Mycobacterium avium* complex. *American Review of Respiratory Disease*, **137**, 212–4.

Gilks, C.F., Brindle, R.J., Mwachari, C. *et al.* (1995) Disseminated *Mycobacterium avium* infection among HIV-infected patients in Kenya. *Journal of Acquired Immune Deficiency Syndrome and Human Retrovirology*, **8**, 195–8.

Girard, A.E., Girard, D., English A.R. *et al.* (1987) Pharmacokinetic and *in vivo* studies with azithromycin (CP-62,993), a new macrolide with an extended half-life and excellent tissue distribution. *Antimicrobial Agents and Chemotherapy*, **31**, 1948–54.

Good, R. (1985) Opportunistic pathogens in the genus *Mycobacterium*. *Annual Review of Microbiology*, **39**, 347–69.

Gordon, S.M., Horsburgh, C.R. Jr, Peloquin, C.A. *et al.* (1993) Low serum levels of oral antimycobacterial agents in patients with disseminated *Mycobacterium avium* complex disease. *Journal of Infectious Diseases*, **168**, 1559–62.

Grange, J.M. (1994) Is the incidence of AIDS-associated *Mycobacterium avium-intracellulare* disease affected by previous exposure to BCG, *M. tuberculosis* or environmental bacteria? *Tubercle and Lung Disease*, **75**, 234–6.

Grange, J.M., Yates, M.D. and Pozniak, A. (1995) Bacteriologically confirmed non-tuberculous mycobacterial lymphadenitis in southeast England: A recent increase in the number of cases. *Archives of Disease in Childhood*, **72**, 516–7.

Gray, J.R. and Rabeneck, L. (1989) Atypical mycobacterial infection of the gastrointestinal tract in AIDS patients. *American Journal of Gastroenterology*, **84**, 1521–4.

Greene, J.B., Sidhu, G.S., Lewin, S. *et al.* (1982) *Mycobacterium avium-intracellulare*: a cause of disseminated life-threatening infection in homosexuals and drug abusers. *Annals of Internal Medicine*, **97**, 539–46.

Gruft, H., Katz, J. and Blanchard, D.C. (1975) Postulated source of *Mycobacterium intracellulare* (Battey) infection. *American Journal of Epidemiology*, **102**, 311–8.

Gupta, S., Blahunka, K., Dellerson, M. *et al.* (1992) Interim results of safety and efficacy of clarithromycin (C) in the treatment of disseminated *Mycobacterium avium* complex (MAC) infection in patients (Pts) with AIDS (abstract No. 892). Program Abstract. 32nd Interscience Conference of Antimicrobial Agents and Chemotherapy. American Society for Microbiology, Washington DC.

Haase, G. Skopnik, H. Batge, S. *et al.* (1994) Cervical lymphadenitis caused by *Mycobacterium celatum*. *Lancet*, **344**, 1020–1 [letter].

Hampson, S.J., Thompson, J., Moss, M.T. *et al.* (1989) DNA probes demonstrate a single highly conserved strain of *Mycobacterium avium* infecting AIDS patients. *Lancet*, **i**, 65–8.

Hanau, L.H., Leaf, A., Soeiro, R. *et al.* (1994) *Mycobacterium marinum* infection in a patient with the acquired immune deficiency syndrome. *CUTIS*, **54**, 103–5.

Havlir, D., Keyes, L. and Davis, C. (1991) Measurement of *Mycobacterium avium* bacteremia: quantitative Isolator lysis centrifugation versus BACTEC 13A blood culture systems, abstr 661, p. 209. Program Abstract. 32nd Interscience Conference of Antimicrobial Agents and Chemotherapy. American Society for Microbiology, Washington DC.

Hawkins, C.C., Gold, J.W., Whimbey, E. *et al.* (1986) *Mycobacterium avium* complex infections in patients with the acquired immunodeficiency syndrome. *Annals of Internal Medicine*, **105**, 184–8.

Heifets, L.B., Iseman, M.D. and Lindholm-Levy, P.J. (1988) Combination of rifampin or rifabutin plus ethambutol against *Mycobacterium avium* complex: bactericidal synergistic and bacteriostasis additive or synergistic effects. *American Review of Respiratory Disease*, **137**, 11–5.

Henriques, B., Hoffner, S.E., Petrini, B. *et al.* (1994) Infection with *Mycobacterium malmoense* in Sweden: report of 221 cases. *Clinical Infectious Diseases*, **18**, 596–600.

Hirasuna, J.D. (1987) Disseminated *Mycobac-terium kansasii* infection in the acquired immunodeficiency syndrome (AIDS). *Annals of Internal Medicine*, **107**, 784.

Hirschel, B., Chang, H.R., Mach, N. (1990) Fatal infection with a novel, unidentified mycobacterium in a man with AIDS. *New England Journal of Medicine*, **323**, 109–13.

Holton, J., Nye, P. and Miller, R. (1991) *Mycobacterium haemophilum* infection in a patient with AIDS. *Journal of Infection*, **32**, 303–6.

Horsburgh, C.R. Jr, Cohn, D.L., Roberts, R.B. *et al.* (1986) *Mycobacterium avium-M. intracellulare* isolates from patients with or without the acquired immunodeficiency syndrome. *Antimicrobial Agents and Chemotherapy*. **30**, 955–7.

Horsburgh, C.R. Jr, Metchock, B., Gordon, S.M. *et al.* (1994) Predictors of survival in patients with AIDS and disseminated *Mycobacterium avium* complex disease. *Journal of Infectious Disease*, **170**, 573–7.

Horsburgh, C.R. Jr, Wynne, B., Bianchine, J. *et al.* (1992) Epidemiology of *Mycobacterium avium* complex (MAC) bacteremia in patients enrolled in a placebo-controlled study (abstract PoB 3190, pB118). 8th Int. Conf. AIDS 1992.

Horsburgh, C.R. and Selik, R.M. (1989) The epidemiology of disseminated nontuberculous mycobacterial infection in the acquired immunodeficiency syndrome (AIDS). *American Review of Respiratory Disease*, **139**, 4–7.

Horsburgh, C.R. Jr, Havlik, J.A., Ellis, D.A. *et al.* (1991a) Survival of patients with acquired immunodeficiency syndrome and disseminated *Mycobacterium avium* complex infection with and without antimycobacterial chemotherapy. *American Review of Respiratory Disease*, **144**, 557–9 [A].

Horsburgh, C.R., Jr, Metchock, B.G., McGowan, J.E. *et al.* (1991b) Progression to disseminated infection in HIV-infected persons colonised with mycobacteria other than tuberculosis (MOTT). *American Review of Respiratory Disease*, **143**, A279 [B].

Hoy, J., Mijch, A., Sandland, M. *et al.* (1990) Quadruple-drug therapy for *Mycobacterium avium-intracellulare* bacteremia in AIDS patients. *Journal of Infectious Diseases*, **161**, 801–5.

Huebner, R.E., Schein, M.F., Cauthen, G.M. *et al.* (1992) Evaluation of the clinical usefulness of mycobacterial skin test antigens in adults with pulmonary mycobacterioses. *American Review of Respiratory Disease*, **145**, 1160–6.

Huminer, D., Schlomo, D., Zmira, S. *et al.* (1993)

Mycobacterium simiae infection in Israeli patients with AIDS. *Clinical Infectious Diseases*, **17**, 508–9.

Inderlied, C.B., Kemper, C.A. and Bermudez, L.E.M. (1993) The *Mycobacterium avium* complex. *Review of Clinical Microbiology*, **6**, 266–310.

Iralu, J.V., Sritharan, V.K., Pieciak, W.S. *et al.* (1993) Diagnosis of *Mycobacterium avium* bacteremia by polymerase chain reaction. *Journal of Clinical Microbiology*, **31**, 1811–4.

Jackson, K., Sievers, A., Ross, B.C. *et al.* (1992) Isolation of a fastidious *Mycobacterium* species from two AIDS patients. *Journal of Clinical Microbiology*, **30**, 2934–7.

Jacob, C., Henein, S., Heurich, A. *et al.* (1991) Nontuberculous mycobacterial meningitis in patients with AIDS. *American Review of Respiratory Disease*, **143**, 279A.

Jacobson, MA., Hopewell, P.C., Yajko, D.M. *et al.* (1991) Natural history of disseminated *Mycobacterium avium* complex infection in AIDS. *Journal of Infectious Disease*, **164**, 994–8.

Jacobson, MA., Yajko, D., Borthfeld, D. *et al.* (1993) Randomized, placebo-controlled trial of rifampin, ethambutol, and ciprofloxacin for patients with disseminated *Mycobacterium avium* complex infection. *Journal of Infectious Diseases*, **168**, 112–19.

Jenkins, P.A. (1985) *Mycobacterium malmoense*. *Tubercle*, **66**, 193–5.

Kahn, S.A., Saltzman, B.R., Klein, R.S. *et al.* (1986) Hepatic disorders in the acquired immunodeficiency syndrome: a clinical and pathological study. *American Journal of Gastroenterology*, **81**, 1145–8.

Kallenius, G., Hoffner, S.E. and Svenson, S.B. (1989) Does vaccination with the bacille Calmette-Guérin protect against AIDS? *Review of Infectious Diseases*, **11**, 349–51.

Kemper, C., Havlir, D., Bartok, A.E. *et al.* (1992a) Transient bacteremia due to *Mycobacterium avium* complex in patients with AIDS. Front. *Mycobacteriology*, **17** [A].

Kemper, C.A., Meng, T.-C., Nussbaum, J. *et al.* (1992b) Treatment of *Mycobacterium avium* complex bacteremia in AIDS with a four-drug oral regimen. *Annals of Internal Medicine*, **116**, 466–72 [B].

Kiehn, T.E. and Cammarata, R. (1986) Laboratory diagnosis of mycobacterial infections in patients with acquired immunodeficiency syndrome. *Journal of Clinical Microbiology*, **24**, 708–11.

Kirschner, P., Vogel, U., Hein, R. *et al.* (1994) Bias of culture techniques for diagnosing mixed *Mycobacterium genavense* and *Mycobacterium avium* infection in AIDS. *Journal of Clinical Microbiology*, **32**, 828–31.

Krasnow, I. and Gross, W. (1975) *Mycobacterium simiae* infection in the United States: a case report and discussion of the organism. *American Review of Respiratory Disease*, **111**, 357–60.

Kristjansson, M., Bieluch, V.M. and Byeff, P.D. (1991) *Mycobacterium haemophilum* infection in immunocompromised patients: case report and review of the literature. *Review of Infectious Diseases*, **13**, 906–10.

Kuitert, L.M., Thomas, M.G. and Ellis-Pegler, R.B. (1991) Outcome of untreated *Mycobacterium avium-intracellulare* complex infection in AIDS. *AIDS*, **5**, 1036–8.

Kurzrock, R., Zander, A., Vellekoop, L. (1984) Mycobacterial pulmonary infections after allogeneic bone marrow transplantation. *American Journal of Medicine*, **77**, 35–40.

Kusunoki, S. and Ezaki, T. (1992) Proposal of *Mycobacterium peregrinum* sp. nov., nom. rev., and elevation of *Mycobacterium chelonae* subsp. *abscessus* (Kubica *et al.*) to species status: *Mycobacterium abscessus* comb. nov. *International Journal of Systematic Bacteriology*, **42**, 240–5.

Lavy, A. and Yoshpe-Purer, Y. (1982) Isolation of *Mycobacterium simiae* from clinical specimens in Israel. *Tubercle*, **63**, 279–85.

Levine, B., and Chaisson, R.E. (1991) *Mycobacterium kansasii*: a cause of treatable pulmonary disease associated with advanced human immunodeficiency virus (HIV) infection. *Annals of Internal Medicine*, **114**, 861–8.

Lévy-Frébault, V., Grimont, F., Grimont, P. *et al.* (1986) Deoxyribonucleic acid relatedness study of the *Mycobacterium fortuitum-Mycobacterium chelonae* complex. *International Journal of Systematic Bacteriology*, **36**, 458–60.

Lévy-Frébault, V., Pagnon, B., Bure, A. *et al.* (1987) *Mycobacterium simiae* and *Mycobacterium avium-Mycobacterium intracellulare* mixed infection in acquired immunodeficiency syndrome. *Journal of Clinical Microbiology*, **25**, 154–7.

MacCallum, P., Tolhurst, J.C., Buckle, G. *et al.* (1948) A new mycobacterial infection in man. *Journal of Pathology and Bacteriology*, **60**, 93.

Males, B.M., West, T.E. and Bartholomew, W.R. (1987) *Mycobacterium haemophilum* infection in a patient with acquired immunodeficiency syndrome. *Journal of Clinical Microbiology*, **25**, 186–90.

Maloney, S., Welbel, S., Daves, B. *et al.* (1993) *Mycobacterium abscessus* pseudoinfection traced to an automated endoscope washer: utility of epidemiologic and laboratory investigation. *Journal of Infectious Diseases*, **169**, 1166–9.

Marinelli, D.L., Albelda, S.M., Williams, T.M. *et al.* (1986) Nontuberculous mycobacterial infection in AIDS: clinical, pathologic, and radiologic features. *Radiology*, **160**, 77–82.

McSwiggan, D.A. and Collins C.H. (1974) The isolation of *M. kansasii* and *M. xenopi* from water systems. *Tubercle*, **55**, 291–7.

Mehle, M.E., Adamo, J.P., Mehta, A.C. *et al.* (1989) Endobronchial *Mycobacterium avium-intracellulare* infection in a patient with AIDS. *Chest*, **96**, 199–201.

Meissner, P.S. and Falkinham, J.O. III (1986) Plasmid DNA profiles as epidemiological markers for clinical and environmental isolates of *Mycobacterium avium*, *Mycobacterium intracellulare*, and *Mycobacterium scrofulaceum*. *Journal of Infectious Diseases*, **153**, 325–31.

Modilevsky, T., Sattler, F.R. and Barnes, P.F. (1989) Mycobacterial disease in patients with human immunodeficiency virus infection. *Archives of Internal Medicine*, **149**, 2201–5.

Moore, R.D. and Chaisson, R.E. (1995) Survival analysis of two controlled trials of rifabutin prophylaxis against *Mycobacterium avium* complex in AIDS. *AIDS*, **9**, 1337–42.

Mushatt, D.M. and Witzig, R.S. (1995) Successful treatment of *Mycobacterium abscessus* infections with multidrug regimens containing clarithromycin [letter].

Naguib, MT., Byers, J.M. and Slater, L.N. (1994) Paranasal sinus infection due to atypical mycobacteria in two patients with AIDS. *Clinical Infectious Diseases*, **19**, 789–91.

Newshan, G. and Torres, R.A., (1994) Pulmonary infection due to a multidrug resistant *Mycobacterium szulgai* in a patient with AIDS. *Clinical Infectious Diseases*, **18**, 1022–3.

Nightingale, S.D., Byrd, L.T., Southern, P.M. *et al.* (1992) Incidence of *Mycobacterium avium-intracellulare* complex bacteremia in human immunodeficiency virus-positive patients. *Journal of Infectious Diseases*, **165**, 1082–5.

Nightingale, S.D., Cameron, D.W., Gordin, F.M. *et al.* (1993) Two controlled trials of rifabutin prophylaxis against *Mycobacterium avium* complex infection in AIDS. *New England Journal of Medicine*, **329**, 828–33.

Opravil, M., Pechere, M., Lazzarin, A. *et al.* (1995)

Dapsone/pyrimethamine may prevent mycobacterial disease in immunosuppressed patients infected with the human immunodeficiency virus. *Clinical Infectious Diseases*, **20**, 224–9.

Ozenna, G., Morel, A., Menard, J.F. *et al.* (1988) Susceptibility of *Mycobacterium avium* complex to various two-drug combinations of anti-tuberculous drugs. *American Review of Respiratory Disease*, **138**, 878–81.

Pechere, M., Opravil, M., Wald, A. *et al.* (1995) Clinical and epidemiologic features of infection with *Mycobacterium genavense*. Swiss HIV Cohort Study. *Archives of Internal Medicine*, **55**, 400–4.

Pierce, M., Crampton, S., Henry, D. *et al.* (1996) A randomized trial of clarithromycin as prophylaxis against disseminated *Mycobacterium avium* complex infection in patients with advanced acquired immunodeficiency syndrome. *New England Journal of Medicine*, **335**, 384–91.

Piersimoni, C., Tortoli, E., De Sio, G. (1994) Disseminated infection due to *Mycobacterium celatum* in patients with AIDS. *Lancet*, **344**, 332.

Pitchenik, A.E. and Fertel, D. (1992) Medical management of AIDS patients: tuberculosis and nontuberculous mycobacterial disease. *Medical Clinics of North America*, **76**, 121–71.

Poropatich, C.O., Labriola, A.M. and Tuazon, C.U. (1987) Acid-fast smear and culture of respiratory secretions, bone marrow, and stools as predictors of disseminated *Mycobacterium avium* complex infection. *Journal of Clinical Microbiology*, **25**, 929–30.

Quieffin, J., Poubeau, P., Laaban, J.P. *et al.* (1994) *Mycobacterium kansasii* infection presenting as an endobronchial tumor in a patient with the acquired immune deficiency syndrome. *Tubercle & Lung Disease*, **75**, 313–5.

Reich, J.M. and Johnson, R.E. (1992) *Mycobacterium avium* complex pulmonary disease presenting as an isolated lingula or middle lobe pattern. The Lady Windermere syndrome. *Chest*, **10**, 1605–9.

Research Committee, British Thoracic Scoiety (1994) *Mycobacterium kansasii* pulmonary infection: a prospective study of the results of nine months of treatment with rifampicin and ethambutol. *Thorax*, **49**, 442–5.

Ries, K.M., White, G.L. Jr, and Murdock, R.T. (1990) Atypical mycobacterial infection caused by *Mycobacterium marinum* [Letter]. *New England Journal of Medicine*, **322**, 633.

Roberts, C., Clague, H., Jenkins, P.A. *et al.* (1985)

Pulmonary infection with *Mycobacterium malmoense*: a report of four cases. *Tubercle*, **66**, 205–9.

Rogers, P.L., Walker, R.E., Lane, H.C. *et al.* (1988) Disseminated *Mycobacterium haemophilum* infection in two patients with the acquired immunodeficiency syndrome. *American Journal of Medicine*, **84**, 640–2.

Rose, H.D., Dorff, G.J., Lauwasser, M. *et al.* (1982) Pulmonary and disseminated *Mycobacterium simiae* infection in humans. *American Review of Respiratory Disease*, **126**, 1110–13.

Runyon, E.H. (1959) Anonymous mycobacteria in pulmonary disease. *Medical Clinics of North America*, **43**, 273.

Sack, J.B. (1990) Disseminated infection due to *Mycobacterium fortuitum* in a patient with AIDS. *Review of Infectious Diseases*, **12**, 961–3.

Sanders, J.W., Walsh, A.D., Snider, R.L. *et al.* (1995) Disseminated *Mycobacterium scrofulaceum* infection: a potentially treatable complication of AIDS.

Schluger, N.W., Condos, R., Lewis, S. *et al.* (1994) Amplification of DNA of *Mycobacterium tuberculosis* from peripheral blood of patients with pulmonary tuberculosis. *Lancet*, **344**, 232–3.

Schwabacher, H. (1959) A strain of mycobacterium isolated from skin lesions of a cold-blooded animal, *Xenopus laevis*, and its relation to atypical acid-fast bacilli occurring in man. *Journal of Hygiene (Cambridge)*, **57**, 57.

Shafer, R.W. and Sierra, M.F. (1992) *Mycobacterium xenopi*, *Mycobacterium fortuitum*, *Mycobacterium kansasii*, and other nontuberculous mycobacteria in an area of endemicity for AIDS. *Clinical Infectious Diseases*, **15**, 161–2.

Shafran, S.D., Singer, J., Zarowny, D.P. *et al.* (1996) A comparison of two regimens for the treatment of *Mycobacterium avium* complex bacteremia in AIDS: rifabutin, ethambutol and clarithromycin versus rifampicin, ethambutol, clofazamine and ciprofloxacin. *New England Journal of Medicine*, **335**, 377–83.

Sherer, R., Sable, R., Sonnenberg, M. *et al.* (1986) Disseminated infection with *Mycobacterium kansasii* in the acquired immunodeficiency syndrome. *Annals of Internal Medicine*, **105**, 710–12.

Sippola, A.A., Gillespie, S.L., Lewis, J.A. *et al.* (1993) *Mycobacterium avium* Antigenuria in patients with AIS and disseminated *M. avium* disease. *Journal of Infectious Diseases*, **168**, 466–8.

Slutsky, A.M., Arbeit, R.D., Barber, T.W. *et al.* (1994) Polyclonal infections due to *Mycobacterium avium* complex in patients with AIDS detected by pulsed-field gel electrophoresis of sequential clinical isolates. *Clinical Microbiology*, **32**, 1773–8.

Sompolinsky, D., Lagziel, A., Naveh, D. *et al.* (1978) *Mycobacterium haemophilum* sp. nov., a new pathogen of humans. *International Journal of Systematic Bacteriology*, **28**, 67–75.

Steere, A.C., Corrales, J. and von Graevenitz, A. (1979) A cluster of *Mycobacterium gordonae* isolates from bronchoscopy specimens. *American Review of Respiratory Disease*, **120**, 214–6.

Stormer, R.S. and Falkinham, J.O. III. (1989) Differences in antimicrobial susceptibility of pigmented and unpigmented colonial variants of *Mycobacterium avium*. *Journal of Clinical Microbiology*, **27**, 2459–65.

Straus, W.L., Ostroff, S.M., Jernigan, D.B. *et al.* (1994) Clinical and epidemiological characteristics of *Mycobacterium haemophilum*, an emerging pathogen in immunocompromised patients. *Annals of Internal Medicine*, **120**, 118–25.

Tecson-Tumang, F.T. and Bright, J.L. (1984) *Mycobacterium xenopi* and the acquired immunodeficiency syndrome. *Annals of Internal Medicine*, **100**, 461–2.

Telenti, A., Marchesi, F., Balz, M. *et al.* (1993) Rapid identification of mycobacteria to the species level by polymerase chain reaction and restriction enzyme analysis. *Journal of Clinical Microbiology*, **31**, 175–8.

Telles, M.A.S. and Yates, M.D. (1994) Single and double drug susceptibility testing of *Mycobacterium avium* complex and mycobacteria other than tubercle bacilli (MOTT) by a micro-dilution broth minimum inhibitory concentration (MIC) method. *Tubercle*, **75**, 286–90.

Thibert, L., Lebel, F. and Martineau, B. (1990) Two cases of *Mycobacterium haemophilum* infection in Canada. *Journal of Clinical Microbiology*, **28**, 621–3.

Thierry, D., Baugé, S., Poveda, J.-D. *et al.* (1993) Rapid identification of *Mycobacterium avium-intracellulare* complex strains: clinical practice evaluation of DT6 and DT1 probes. *Journal of Infectious Diseases*, **168**, 1337–8.

Torres, R.A., Nord, J., Feldman, R. *et al.* (1991) Disseminated mixed *Mycobacterium simiae-Mycobacterium avium* complex infection in acquired immunodeficiency syndrome. *Journal of Infectious Diseases*, **164**, 432–3.

Tortoli, E., Simonetti, T.M., Laccini, C. *et al.* (1994) Tentative evidence of AIDS-associated biotype of *Mycobacterium kansasii. Journal of Clinical Microbiology*, **32**, 1779–82.

Tsukamura, M. (1984) The 'non-pathogenic' species of mycobacteria: their distribution and ecology in non-living reservoirs, in *The Mycobacteria. A Sourcebook.* Park B (eds G.P. Kubica and L.G. Wayne), Marcel Dekker, New York, pp. 1339–59.

Valainis, G.T. (1991) *Mycobacterium kansasii* infection [letter]. *Annals of Internal Medicine*, **115**, 496–7.

Vaneechoutte, M., De Beenhouwer, H., Claeys, G. *et al.* (1993) Identification of *Mycobacterium* species by using amplified ribosomal DNA restriction analysis. *Journal of Clinical Microbiology*, **31**, 2061–5.

von Reyn, C.F., Maslow, J.N., Barber, T.W. *et al.* (1994) Persistent colonisation of potable water as a source of *Mycobacterium avium* infection in AIDS. *Lancet*, **343**, 1137–41.

Wald, A., Coyle, M.B., Carlson, L.C. *et al.* (1992) Infection with a fastidious mycobacterium resembling *Mycobacterium simiae* in seven patients with AIDS. *Annals of Internal Medicine*, **17**, 586–9.

Wallace, R.J. Jr, Dunbar, D., Brown, B.A. *et al.* (1994) Rifampin-resistant *Mycobacterium kansasii. Clinical Infectious Diseases*, **18**, 736–43.

Wallace, R.J., Brown, B.A. and Onyi, G.O. (1992) Skin, soft tissue, and bone infections due to *M. chelonae chelonae*: importance of prior corticosteroid therapy, frequency of disseminated infections, and resistance to oral antimicrobials other than clarithromycin. *Journal of Infectious Diseases*, **166**, 405–12.

Wallace, R.J., Jr, O'Brien, R., Glassroth, J. *et al.* (1990) Diagnosis and treatment of disease caused by nontuberculous mycobacteria. *American Review of Respiratory Disease*, **142**, 940–53.

Wasem, C.F., McCarthy, C.M. and Murray, L.W. (1991) Multilocus enzyme electrophoresis analysis of the *Mycobacterium avium* complex and other mycobacteria. *Journal of Clinical Microbiology*, **29**, 264–71.

Wayne, L.G. and Sramek, H.A. (1992) Agents of newly recognised or infrequently encountered mycobacterial diseases. *Clinical Microbiology Reviews*, **5**, 1–25.

Weinberger, M., Berg, S.L., Feuerstein, I.R. *et al.* (1992) Disseminated infection with *Mycobacterium gordonae*: report of a case and critical review of the literature. *Clinical Infectious Diseases*, **14**, 1229–39.

Wendt, S.L., George, K.L., Parker, B.C. *et al.* (1980) Epidemiology of infection by nontuberculous mycobacteria. III. Isolation of potentially pathogenic mycobacteria from aerosols. *American Review of Respiratory Disease*, **122**, 259–63.

Wiley, E.L., Perry, A., Nightingale, S.D. *et al.* (1992) Detection of *M. avium-intracellulare* using anti-BCG, anti-*M. duvalii*, Kenyon, and Fite stains in bone marrow biopsies (abstract PoB 3359, p.B146). 8th International Conference on AIDS.

Willocks, L., Leen, C.L.S., Brettle, R.P. *et al.* (1993) Isolation of *Mycobacterium malmoense* from HIV-positive patients [letter]. *Journal of Infection*, **26**, 345–6.

Wolinsky, E. (1979) Nontuberculous mycobacteria and associated diseases. *American Review of Respiratory Disease*, **119**, 107–59.

Wormser, G.P., Horowitz, H. and Dworkin, B. (1994) Low-dose dexamethasone as adjunctive therapy for disseminated *Mycobacterium avium* complex infections in AIDS patients. *Antimicrobial Agents in Chemotherapy*, **38**, 2215–17.

Yajko, D.M., Nassos, P.S. and Hadley, W.K. (1987) Broth microdilution testing of susceptibilities to 30 antimicrobial agents of *Mycobacterium avium* strains from patients with acquired immunodeficiency syndrome. *Antimicrobial Agents and Chemotherapy*, **31**, 1579–84.

Yakrus, M., Butler, W., Kilburn, J. *et al.* (1992) Characterization of a possible novel drug resistant species of mycobacteria associated with pulmonary disease is AIDS patients (Abstr U-24. p. 169) Abst. 92nd Gen. Meet. American Society of Microbiology 1992.

Yoganathan, K., Elliott, M.W., Moxham, J. *et al.* (1994) Pseudotumour of the lung caused by *Mycobacterium malmoense* infection in an HIV positive patient. *Thorax*, **49**, 179–80.

Young, L.S., Wiviott, L., Wu, M. *et al.* (1991) Azithromycin for treatment of *Mycobacterium avium* complex infection in patients with AIDS. *Lancet*, **338**, 1107–9.

Zaugg, M., Salfinger, M., Opravil, M. *et al.* (1993) Extrapulmonary and disseminated infections due to *Mycobacterium malmoense*: case report and review. *Clinical Infectious Diseases*, **16**, 540–9.

ACUTE BACTERIAL INFECTIONS

14

Charles F. Gilks

INTRODUCTION

As the AIDS epidemic developed in North America, it became clear to respiratory physicians that as well as seeing highly unusual opportunistic lung infections there was an important interaction between bacterial pneumonia and underlying HIV immunosuppression. The association was first described in male homosexuals with AIDS and whilst most patients responded well to antimicrobial therapy several then went on to develop recurrent pneumonia (Simberkoff *et al.*, 1984; Polsky *et al.*, 1986; White *et al.*, 1985).

Subsequently it was noted that HIV-positive intravenous drug users were also at increased risk of developing bacterial pneumonia; and that many cases were occurring early on in the course of HIV, before the individual had an AIDS-defining illness (Selwyn *et al.*, 1988). Coincident with the rise in cases of pneumonia and other serious bacterial infections a sharp rise in mortality was documented, suggesting that in inner city drug users pneumonia was a common HIV-related cause of death missed by standard surveillance for AIDS (Stoneburner *et al.*, 1988).

More recently, several European groups have described clinical series highlighting the importance of bacterial pneumonia in patients co-infected with HIV (Falco *et al.*, 1994; Jensen *et al.*, 1990; Magnenat *et al.*,

1991; Miller *et al.*, 1994; Willocks *et al.*, 1992). As in North America, drug users with HIV infection seem particularly liable to develop bacterial pneumonia. However with early detection and easy access to better medical care there does not appear to be any excess mortality from HIV-related pneumonia in drug-using populations (Mientjes *et al.*, 1992).

In the tropics, bacterial pneumonia has always been a major cause of disease and death, particularly for young adults living in poor and overcrowded urban areas. In Africa, as more comprehensive clinical studies have been undertaken, bacterial pneumonia is increasingly being appreciated as an important and early HIV-related problem (Gilks *et al.*, 1992, 1993; Kamanfu *et al.*, 1993; Pallangyo *et al.*, 1992). Indeed in one cohort study invasive pneumococcal disease was more common even than active tuberculosis (Gilks *et al.*, 1996).

Autopsy studies from industrialized and developing countries have shown that bacterial pneumonia is also common postmortem (Lucas *et al.*, 1993; McKenzie *et al.*, 1991; Monforte *et al.*, 1992; Nichols, Balogh and Silverman, 1990). Although in some patients the pneumonia is an agonal event that accompanies multiple opportunistic infections and organ failure, in many cases bacterial pneumonia can be considered the cause of death.

AIDS and Respiratory Medicine. Edited by A. Zumla, M.A. Johnson and R.F. Miller. Published in 1997 by Chapman & Hall, London. ISBN 0 412 60140 0

Pneumonia can present early on in the natural history of HIV and the incidence of pneumonia increases with the level of underlying immunosuppression (Farizo *et al.*, 1992). Although pneumonia is a relatively common diagnosis regardless of HIV status, and the usual causative bacteria are not considered opportunistic pathogens, multiple episodes of pneumonia are strongly associated with underlying immunosuppression. Thus in the 1993 revision of the CDC surveillance case definition for AIDS in adolescents and adults, recurrent pneumonia (two or more episodes in a one-year period) became an AIDS-defining condition (CDC, 1992).

In the USA it is now evident that bacterial pneumonia is the commonest major infectious disease that is not AIDS-defining in patients with underlying HIV (Farizo *et al.*, 1992; Hirschtick *et al.*, 1995). Most episodes of pneumonia are community-acquired although AIDS patients with indwelling catheters, lengthy hospital admissions for multiple opportunistic infections and drug-related neutropenia are also predisposed to nosocomial pneumonia. This means that many adults seen in hospital in North America with pneumonia will also have underlying HIV infection: the overall HIV seroprevalence in adults with pneumonia seen in 20 hospitals participating in the Sentinel Hospital HIV Surveillance System in 1989 was 11.5%, ranging from 0.9% to 48.6% (Janssen *et al.*, 1992).

Excluding AIDS-defining problems, pneumonia is also recognized as the leading cause of HIV-related morbidity and death in the USA (Buehler *et al.*, 1990; Chu *et al.*, 1990). There are as yet no comparable data from the UK or other industrialized countries.

With growing interest in and appreciation of the importance of non-opportunistic bacterial pneumonia in adults immunosuppressed with HIV several reviews have been published in the last five years (Caiaffa *et al.*,

1993; Chaisson, 1989; Cohn, 1991; Daley, 1994; Janoff *et al.*, 1992; Meduri and Stein, 1992; Murray and Mills, 1990). These reviews either deal exclusively with bacterial infections or highlight the importance of bacterial infections in HIV-related pulmonary disease. They should be consulted for more specific or detailed information and additional references.

CAUSES OF BACTERIAL PNEUMONIA

The pneumococcus (*Streptococcus pneumoniae*) is without doubt the commonest and most important of the bacterial pathogens to cause pneumonia in adults with underlying HIV immunosuppression (Janoff *et al.*, 1992). Although nosocomial infection, with penicillin-resistant pneumococci, has been described in AIDS patients (Blumberg and Rimland, 1989) most episodes are community-acquired. In general, serotypes isolated from HIV-infected adults are similar to those found in the general community and from 80–90% are vaccine types (Redd *et al.*, 1990). It appears from relatively limited cohort data that individuals with HIV or AIDS overall are about ten times more likely to develop pneumococcal pneumonia or bacteremia than seronegative adults (Caiaffa *et al.*, 1993). The risk increases with more advanced immunosuppression. Population-based surveillance data from New Jersey suggest that the attack rate for invasive pneumococcal disease in AIDS patients is more than 300 times the baseline rate (Schuchat *et al.*, 1991).

Haemophilus influenzae pneumonia is also clearly associated with HIV infection (Schlamm and Yankovitz, 1989; Moreno *et al.*, 1991) although epidemiological data are sparse (Caiaffa *et al.*, 1993). One study of New York drug addicts noted an annual rate for *H. influenzae* pneumonia, defined by positive sputum culture, of 42 per 1000 (Selwyn *et al.*, 1988). However, invasive disease is relatively infrequently seen (Steinhart *et al.*, 1992). Serotype b, other capsular types and nontypable strains have all been isolated. Recent data suggesting that drug users are at particular risk of developing pneumonia and *H. influenzae* type b bacteremia (Casadevall *et al.*, 1992) are in dispute (Rich, Sax and Kazanjian, 1993).

Of the other organisms *Staphylococcus aureus* is probably the next most important cause of community-acquired pneumonia in HIV-infected adults. It can often be recovered from respiratory tract cultures and may be indicative of underlying pneumonia in about 20% of cases (Levine, White and Fels, 1990). *S. aureus* usually figures prominently in case series of bacterial pneumonia (Cohn, 1991; Miller *et al.*, 1994) but may be infrequent (Falco *et al.*, 1994) or not even appear (Polsky *et al.*, 1986). These differences are not well explained and no good epidemiological data are available. *S. aureus* pneumonia can also occur as a secondary complication of indwelling catheters (Jacobson, Gellermann and Chambers, 1988), and is not uncommon at autopsy (Nichols, Balogh and Silverman, 1989) suggesting that nosocomial acquisition is important.

There are few data concerning the importance of Gram-negative bacteria (Enterobacteriaceae and *Pseudomonas aeruginosa*) in community-acquired pneumonia (Cohn, 1991). Recent case series suggest that they are more common with underlying HIV infection (Falco *et al.*, 1994; Miller *et al.*, 1994). Enterobacteriaceae appear to be the leading cause of nosocomial pneumonia in HIV-infected adults (Witt, Craven and McCabe, 1987) but the data are limited and no comprehensive case series has been reported. It is unclear whether *P. pseudomallei*, the cause of meliodosis, will emerge as an important HIV-associated pulmonary pathogen as the HIV epidemic extends into rural SE Asia (Daley, 1994).

Rhodococcus equi, a small Gram-positive coryneform, and *Nocardia asteroides*, a branching Gram-positive higher bacterium, are both uncommon opportunistic bacterial pathogens. Initially dismissed as a sputum contaminant, *R. equi* is now recognized as a rare cause of cavitary pneumonia in HIV seropositive patients (Drancourt *et al.*, 1992). Nocardiosis is now also recognized as an uncommon and often fatal complication of advanced HIV infection which usually presents as a chronic pneumonia which may also cavitate (Uttamchandani *et al.*, 1993).

There are case reports of other bacteria causing pneumonia in HIV-infected adults, including group A and group B streptococci, *Branhamella catarrhalis*, *Bordatella pertussis*, *Neisseria meningitidis*, *S. viridans* and various salmonellae (references in Caiaffa, Graham and Vlahov, 1993; Chaisson, 1989; Cohn, 1991; Murray and Mills, 1990). Their significance is uncertain and these may be chance associations. It is unlikely that these bacteria are important causes of pneumonia which HIV-immunosuppressed individuals are at particular risk of developing.

Atypical (bacterial) pneumonia does not appear significantly to be associated with HIV immunosuppression nor to occur at an increased rate in patients with HIV or AIDS. Bearing in mind that *Mycoplasma pneumoniae* is the commonest cause of atypical pneumonia in young immunocompetent adults, it is surprising how rarely it has been described in HIV-seropositive and AIDS patients (Fels, 1988). It is uncommon for *Legionella pneumophila* to cause serious disease even though it is a significant pathogen in other types of immunosuppression (Blatt *et al.*, 1994). One outbreak of *Chlamydia pneumoniae* has been reported, noted in a retrospective analysis of lower respiratory tract infection in Italian former drug users (Blasi *et al.*, 1994). Data suggesting a high seroprevalence for *Coxiella burnettii* in HIV-infected adults living in Marseilles (Raoult *et al.*, 1993) have not been confirmed in a serosurvey carried out in a Parisian hospital (Belec, Ekala and Gilquin, 1993).

Anaerobic bacteria causing pneumonia in HIV infection or AIDS has not been documented. This may be a problem of diagnosis because anaerobic cultures are not often set up on sputum and bacteremia is rare in anaerobic pneumonia (Cohn, 1991). Aspiration pneumonia appears to be no more common in patients with HIV infection, and there are no data to suggest that anaerobic infections in other sites are significantly associated with underlying HIV disease.

CLINICAL PRESENTATION

Community-acquired bacterial pneumonia usually presents acutely accompanied by the typical symptoms of cough, fever, chills, chest pain, shortness of breath and rapid breathing. The clinical signs are related to underlying lung consolidation: tachycardia, tachypnea, sweating, cyanosis, reduced percussion note, crackles and crepitations, bronchial breathing, use of accessory muscles of respiration and nasal flaring. There are no differences in the presentation of pneumonia between adults with underlying HIV and those who are seronegative (Chaisson, 1989). There are also no significant or consistent differences in the signs and symptoms caused by each specific bacterial pathogen or between typical or atypical pneumonias (Marrie, 1994).

Up to one half of patients may describe or have recently experienced an upper respiratory tract infection (URTI). Nevertheless, even in individuals with preceding URTI or underlying disease the onset of symptoms is relatively acute and can often be described clearly by the patient. The fever can be hectic, sustained or remittent and accompanied by sweats and rigors; there is no characteristic pattern and it may not always be present. The cough is generally productive of purulent sputum which can also be rusty or streaked with blood. Chest pain is usually pleuritic in nature and if severe may make the patient lie on the side of the pneumonia in an attempt to splint the thoracic cage and reduce movement. The clinical signs relate to the extent and severity of the underlying pneumonic process.

In addition to the specific symptoms up to a third of patients will also describe relatively non-specific symptoms such as headache, nausea, vomiting, abdominal pain, diarrhea, myalgia and arthralgia. A tender hepatomegaly, meningismus and jaundice may be clinically apparent. About 10% of patients may have on presentation or subsequently develop herpes labialis. In Nairobi we did not observe a significantly higher rate of herpes simplex in HIV infected compared to HIV seronegative patients with acute pneumonia (unpublished data).

Neither ethnic background nor gender appears to alter the risk of developing HIV-associated bacterial pneumonia although drug users are significantly more likely than homosexual men to develop bacterial pneumonia (Greenberg *et al.*, 1992).

Clinical presentation is therefore straightforward and in most cases it is relatively easy to identify a patient with pneumonia. In practice there are two issues of importance: whether the individual who presents with bacterial pneumonia has underlying HIV; and whether there is sufficient certainty to distinguish bacterial pneumonia from *Pneumocystis carinii* pneumonia (PCP).

IDENTIFICATION OF UNDERLYING HIV INFECTION

In areas where HIV is known to be prevalent, either in the general population or in specific risk groups such as drug users, community-acquired pneumonia is an early and often the first clinical manifestation of underlying HIV (Taelman *et al.*, 1992). As already discussed, HIV seroprevalence in cases of pneumonia seen in the 1989 Sentinel Hospital HIV Surveillance System ranged from 0.9% to 48.6% (Janssen *et al.*, 1992).

Certain features should increase clinical

awareness. These include oral candida, leukoplakia or other signs of underlying immunosuppression; being a member of a risk group; experiencing recurrent episodes; or having bacteremic disease (see below). However, many seropositive pneumonia patients will be without these indicators to alert the physician to possible underlying retroviral infection.

The course adopted will depend on local circumstances and policy. As a minimum it would seem sensible to counsel and offer HIV testing to all patients with (possible) recurrent pneumonia. This is indicative of marked immunosuppression and the patient may benefit from prophylaxis and antiretroviral therapy. Recurrent pneumonia is now an AIDS-defining problem (CDC, 1992), something which may have financial implications for the individual and institution.

DIFFERENTIATION OF PNEUMONIA FROM *PNEUMOCYSTIS*

There are several clinical features which can help discriminate between PCP and bacterial pneumonia. Together with the chest radiograph and initial laboratory evaluation (see below) it is often possible to distinguish with confidence the two diagnoses.

The onset of illness tends to be specific and acute in bacterial pneumonia and the length of reported symptoms is significantly shorter. Most patients with bacterial pneumonia will present within one week (Chaisson, 1989). In one study from Denmark HIV-infected patients with PCP had symptoms for nearly two weeks longer than patients with bacterial pneumonia. Dyspnea and a cough productive of sputum were also seen more frequently in patients with bacterial pneumonia (Nybo Jensen *et al.*, 1990). Pleuritic chest pain is uncommon in PCP but frequently reported by patients with bacterial pneumonia.

Physical examination of the lungs is usually either normal or only reveals bilateral fine crackles or wheezing in patients with PCP (Murray and Mills, 1990). In contrast clear signs of focal consolidation, such as coarse crepitations or bronchial breathing, will be present in over half the patients with bacterial pneumonia (Chaisson, 1989).

NATURAL HISTORY

Bacterial pneumonia can present early on in the normal course of HIV immunosuppression when there are few or no other features to suggest underlying HIV, as the first manifestation of HIV-related immunosuppression (Taelman *et al.*, 1992). Thus unless specifically looked for the underlying association with HIV will be missed unless specific serological testing is performed. This is of particular importance in tropical countries where many cases of pneumonia, and other acute bacterial infections, are often not recognized as HIV-related (Gilks, 1993a).

It is likely that most of the excess cases of pneumonia seen early on in HIV are pneumococcal, with the minority being due to *H. influenzae*. As already discussed, in all case series of HIV-related bacterial pneumonia the pneumococcus is the predominant pathogen identified. Furthermore, the interaction of *S. pneumoniae* and HIV can start early on in the course of infection, perhaps before any interaction with *H. influenzae*.

In a cohort of low-class female sex workers in Nairobi, where exposure to respiratory pathogens is high, we noted that the mean CD4 count in 54 episodes of invasive pneumococcal disease was 325/mm^3 and that nearly all episodes of community-acquired pneumonia were pneumococcal (Gilks, 1993). Where pathogen exposure is less intense *S. pneumoniae* may present relatively later; the mean CD4 count of (affluent) male patients in Denver seen with pneumococcal bacteremia was 132/mm^3 (Janoff *et al.*, 1993). In a review it was noted that the diagnosis of pneumococcal bacteremia precedes that of AIDS in 71% of cases evaluated (Janoff *et al.*, 1992).

Although there are few comparable data for invasive *H. influenzae* disease patients may in general be more immunosuppressed when they present. In one case series from Italy half the patients had CD4 counts below 200/mm^3 (Moreno *et al.*, 1991). In another series from New York over half the cases already had a diagnosis of AIDS at presentation (Casadevall *et al.*, 1992). However other case series emphasize that HIV-related *H. influenzae* can occur in many patients before the onset of AIDS (Schlamm and Yankowitz, 1989).

It is generally accepted that in the early stages of HIV the outcome of pneumococcal disease (Janoff *et al.*, 1992) and *H. influenzae* pneumonia (Schlamm and Yankowitz, 1989) can be excellent provided patients have good-quality health care. This is probably because most patients with HIV are relatively young with otherwise normal lungs and cardiovascular systems. The exception, at least in the USA, is the high excess mortality from bacterial pneumonia over and above that caused by AIDS noted in poor inner city areas in the USA (Stoneburner *et al.*, 1988). In the tropics substantial mortality occurs pre AIDS (Gilks, 1993a).

With advancing immunosuppression the risk of developing bacterial pneumonia clearly markedly increases (Hirschtick *et al.*, 1995). In pneumococcal disease the increase may be exponential rather than linear from a baseline risk in the USA of 17/100 000 to 510/100 000 median risk about 18 months before the development of AIDS to over 1000/100 000 in AIDS patients (Schuchat *et al.*, 1991). For *H. influenzae* the annual rate of invasive disease in HIV-infected adults without AIDS is about 15/100 000 and for adults with AIDS is about 80/100 000, with the background rate of about 3/100 000 (Steinhart *et al.*, 1992). The likelihood of developing disease seems to increase sharply and bacterial pneumonia is often now diagnosed together with a second virulent or opportunistic pathogen, in the lung or

elsewhere (Miller *et al.*, 1994).

One hallmark of bacterial pneumonia in HIV infection is the marked tendency to recur (Jordens *et al.*, 1995). This is indicative of more severe immunosuppression and is now classified as an AIDS-defining event if it occurs within one year. Few data have yet been published on the relapse rate of bacterial pneumonia in industrialized countries; of evaluable series the rate is about 13% within 6 months (Janoff *et al.*, 1992). In Nairobi we noted that 22% of women had recurrent pneumococcal disease, that the median time to recurrence was about 6 months and that most episodes were reinfection caused by a different serotype (Gilks, 1996). A series of recurrent pneumococcal pneumonias in one woman from this cohort study is shown in Figure 14.1.

Widespread use of co-trimoxazole prophylaxis for PCP may inadvertently be reducing substantially the actual number of cases of bacterial pneumonia that develop in individuals with AIDS. In a study of New York AIDS patients significantly fewer bacterial infections overall were noted in individuals receiving co-trimoxazole prophylaxis compared to inhaled pentamidine, with the most marked reduction seen in cases of bronchitis and pneumonia (Mayer *et al.*, 1993). Further data are required to evaluate this additional benefit of prophylaxis.

The risk of death with HIV-related pneumonia increases with more advanced immunosuppression. In the US some of the marked rise in the death rate from pneumonia in states with high HIV incidence is caused by disease in adults with low CD4 counts but who have not had an AIDS-defining illness rather than early pneumonia death in poor inner city dwellers (Buehler *et al.*, 1990). Many patients with AIDS are found to have pneumonia at autopsy (McKenzie *et al.*, 1991; Monforte *et al.*, 1992; Nichols, Balogh and Silverman, 1989). One study noted that in patients with

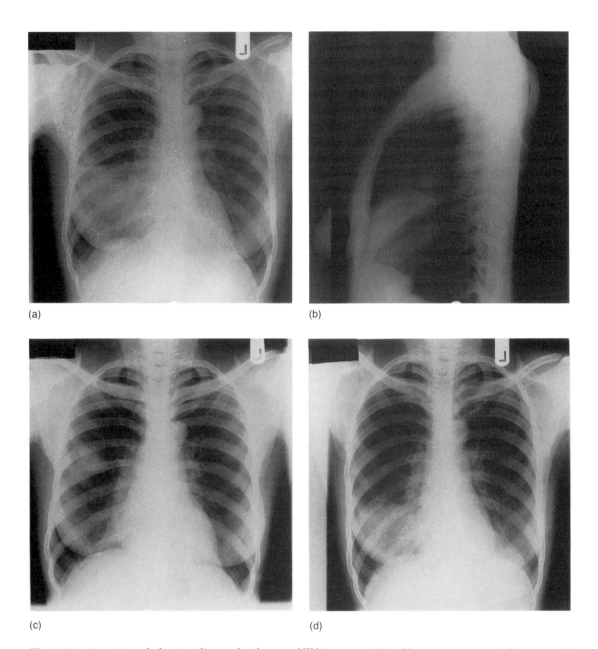

Fig. 14.1 A series of chest radiographs from a HIV-1 seropositive Kenyan woman with recurrent pneumococcal disease. (a) The initial episode. Uniform alveolar consolidation in the right middle lobe. *S. pneumoniae* serotype 7 isolated from blood and sputum cultures. (b) Lateral radiograph showing classical lobar consolidation. (c) The second episode, 8 months after the first. Subsegmental consolidation in the right lung; *S. pneumoniae* serotype 1 isolated from blood culture. (d) The third episode, 12 months after the first. Segmental consolidation in the right middle lobe; *S. pneumoniae* serotype 4 in blood culture but *M. tuberculosis* also grown from sputum culture.

AIDS and pneumococcal pneumonia with bacteremia, mortality was nearly 60%, significantly higher than elderly patients without HIV infection, and higher than HIV-infected patients without AIDS (Pesola and Charles, 1992).

RADIOGRAPHIC PRESENTATION

Patients who present acutely sick with signs and symptoms of pneumonia should have a chest radiograph taken on admission. Substantial information can be obtained from a standard postero-anterior view which can help to differentiate between an episode of bacterial or *Pneumocystis carinii* infection, suggest causative organism and play a critical role in determining initial patient management. The radiographic pattern of pulmonary disease in HIV infection has recently been extensively reviewed by McLoud and Naidich (1992).

In bacterial pneumonia the infection is usually focal, either in a segmental or subsegmental distribution, and can be unilateral or bilateral. The most classic appearance is of dense localized alveolar consolidation that is either lobar, segmental or occasionally nodular, features which are unusual in PCP (Amorosa *et al.*, 1990). In Switzerland 45% of HIV-seropositive patients with pneumonia had segmental or lobar alveolar consolidation patterns (Magnenat *et al.*, 1991). Figure 14.1 above shows three typical radiographs with lobar, segmental and subsegmental changes in a woman with recurrent pneumococcal pneumonia.

Such a radiographic appearance in immunocompetent young adults would be highly suggestive of pneumococcal disease and is probably so early on in HIV disease. However, with AIDS a wider range of pathogens can produce lobar pneumonia. In one series, whilst *S. pneumoniae* was still the commonest cause, *S. aureus*, *H. influenzae*, *P. aeruginosa* and *P. carinii* were also isolated; and in 30% of patients with an established etiological diagnosis multiple pathogens were isolated (Miller *et al.*, 1994). In Nairobi, we noted that 19% of HIV-infected adults and 8% of seronegative adults with pneumococcal pneumonia also had another pathogen isolated, either *M. tuberculosis*, *H. influenzae* or non-typhi salmonellae (Gilks *et al.*, 1993). (See also Figure 14.1d).

Bacterial pneumonia can also present with diffuse or localized reticulonodular shadowing. In one series 55% of episodes had a predominantly interstitial infiltrate which can be difficult to distinguish from PCP (Magnenat *et al.*, 1991). Such a diffuse appearance, if caused by a bacterial pathogen, may represent *H. influenzae* infection (Moreno *et al.*, 1991; Schlamm and Yancovitz, 1989) but other pathogens including *S. pneumoniae* can also cause such a radiographic appearance. Figure 14.2 shows the chest radiograph from a patient with widespread pneumococcal pneumonia and a predominantly interstitial infiltrate but also elements of more dense consolidation.

Pleural effusion is a relatively common finding in patients with bacterial pneumonia and is usually parapneumonic rather than an infected empyema. In one series from the US effusions were noted in 27% of AIDS patients and of these 31% were in association with bacterial pneumonia and 15% with PCP. If patients with obvious non-infectious causes such as hypoalbuminemia are excluded then nearly 50% of the effusions seen in association with HIV-related infections were associated with bacterial pneumonia; most were pneumococcal (Joseph, Strange and Sahn, 1993). Pleural effusions may also be common in *H. influenzae* pneumonia (Schlamm and Yancovitz, 1989). It is important always to consider tuberculosis in any patient with a pleural effusion, especially if it fails to resolve with broad-spectrum therapy. Figure 14.3 shows dense lobar consolidation and pleural effusion in a case of bacteremic pneumococcal pneumonia.

Cavitation may also occur in an acutely

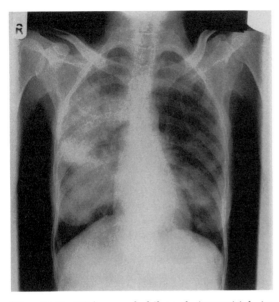

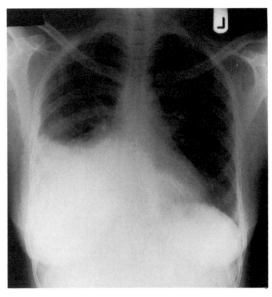

Fig. 14.2 Widespread bilateral interstitial infiltrates, particularly in the right lung, with an area of dense subsegmental consolidation. *S. pneumoniae* grown from sputum and blood culture.

Fig. 14.3 Uniform dense consolidation in the right middle and lower lobes with a parapneumonic pleural effusion. Both pneumonia and effusion cleared within 21 days after a one-week course of penicillin in standard dosage.

presenting bacterial pneumonia. It is most suggestive of *S. aureus*, *Klebsiella* or a mixed infection (Cohn, 1991). With a more chronic presentation, *R. equi* infection or nocardiosis should be considered although they are rare events. The radiological appearances of nocardia in AIDS have been reviewed (Kramer and Uttamchandani, 1990). More importantly, tuberculosis should always be considered in the differential diagnosis. Patients can present with relatively acute histories or have mixed infections and the consequences of missing a smear-positive, highly contagious case of open tuberculosis can be severe. Patients with lobar consolidation may also have cavitary lesions (Miller *et al.*, 1994) which can be visualized more easily with CT scanning (McLoud and Naidich, 1992).

Combined with accurate clinical information a chest radiograph should help to identify correctly a bacterial pneumonia in the majority of cases. In an important subset of patients it will still be unclear what the underlying pathology is. CT scanning or further radiological investigation probably has little to contribute at presentation but may be necessary in patients without a diagnosis and who fail to respond to antimicrobial therapy.

DIAGNOSIS

There are two steps in establishing the diagnosis of bacterial pneumonia in an adult with underlying HIV infection. The first is to decide whether the patient with pulmonary symptoms and an abnormal chest radiograph has bacterial pneumonia, or whether the pneumonia is likely to be caused by another pathogen. In most cases the differential will be with *Pneumocystis carinii*. The second step is to try to establish what bacterium is the likely etiological agent.

After clinical and radiological examination it should be apparent in over two-thirds of cases whether the patient has a typical bacterial pneumonia or another process. In those with relatively clear-cut bacterial pneumonia sputum specimens should be obtained for Gram stain and culture and for blood culture, preferably two or three samples each separated by at least ten minutes. In most straightforward cases it should not be necessary to proceed to other more invasive techniques to obtain diagnostic material.

Sputum Gram stain should confirm the presence of polymorphs and few squamous cells should be visible. Many sputum specimens are of poor quality and are unlikely to help in diagnosis (Woodhead *et al.*, 1991). Abundant Gram-positive lanceolate diplococci suggest pneumococcal pneumonia, Gram-positive cocci in clumps suggest staphylococcal pneumonia; Gram-negative coccobacilli *H. influenzae* pneumonia and Gram-negative rods a Gram-negative pneumonia. Culture of a diluted specimen will have a higher yield but be much less rapid. Overall sputum examination may yield a diagnosis in about 25% of cases.

Blood culture has high specificity but generally low sensitivity. High rates of bacteremia have been noted in HIV-seropositive patients with pneumococcal pneumonia (Janoff *et al.*, 1992) and may be found in other types of bacterial pneumonia. A positive blood culture confirms the diagnosis, or in a small number of cases identifies the organism as a co-infection.

It is best to start treatment after microbiology specimens have been collected. With correct treatment (see below) there should be a rapid clinical response in uncomplicated cases of bacterial pneumonia. The radiograph should also resolve rapidly in the majority of cases, confirming a clinical and therapeutic diagnosis in the absence of a firm bacteriological diagnosis. One study in Switzerland noted that when chest radiographs of HIV-infected patients with

bacterial pneumonia were repeated after 15 days that 72% had resolved, compared to only 8% of PCP patients (Magnenat *et al.*, 1991).

In the difficult minority in whom it is unclear what type of pneumonia is present, and in those patients who have failed to respond to appropriate treatment for bacterial pneumonia further investigations are required. Mixed infection with organisms such as *Pneumocystis carinii* or *M. tuberculosis* that will not respond to most antimicrobials can also occur in about 10% of cases (Gilks *et al.*, 1993; Schlamm and Yancovitz, 1989; Miller *et al.*, 1994). Some centers will first try induced sputum; others will proceed directly to bronchoscopy with bronchoalveolar lavage (BAL) (Coker and Mitchell, 1994).

Quantitative bacterial culture can be done on BAL fluid if the patient has previously received antibiotics and should identify the cause of over 80% of cases of bacterial pneumonia. Even if the patient has received antimicrobials one quarter of BAL cultures may still yield a bacterial pathogen (Magnenat *et al.*, 1991). Analysis of the BAL cellularity can also help in making a diagnosis. Cases of bacterial pneumonia have significantly more macrophages and neutrophils, and overall higher cell counts than PCP cases (Magnenat *et al.*, 1991).

Occasionally, AIDS patients will present with a chronic or sub-acute cough and fever and have cavitary or nodular consolidation on chest radiograph. A presumptive diagnosis of nocardiosis can be made by visualizing on sputum microscopy beaded, branching Gram-positive rods that are weakly acid fast on Ziehl-Neelsen staining. If Gram-positive, pleiomorphic rods are isolated from blood, sputum or BAL culture they should not immediately be disregarded as contaminating coryneforms; further identification may reveal *R. equi*.

Depending on how vigorous a diagnostic work-up is employed it may be possible to identify the causative organism(s) of bacterial pneumonia in over 70% of cases (Falco *et al.*, 1994; Willocks *et al.*, 1992). This is similar to the level achieved in a detailed study of community-acquired pneumonia in the UK in 1982–83 when HIV infection would have been at a very low level (British Thoracic Society, 1987). The remaining cases can confidently be diagnosed by the clinical response and radiological resolution if necessary.

TREATMENT

Despite the severity of many episodes of community-acquired bacterial pneumonia in HIV-infection and the high incidence of bacteremia the majority of patients respond to specific antimicrobial therapy. With prompt diagnosis and appropriate therapy only markedly immunosuppressed patients, usually already diagnosed with AIDS, should be at substantial risk of death (Pesola and Charles, 1992). Perhaps because there is such a good response in most cases to a relatively wide range of therapies no controlled trials have been undertaken; and the optimal duration of therapy, and route of administration, is unknown.

With an established etiological diagnosis therapy is relatively straightforward. The best therapy for pneumococcal pneumonia remains penicillin. In a cohort study in Nairobi we treated 79 episodes of invasive pneumococcal disease, 42 of which were bacteremic, with benzylpenicillin and had no deaths (Gilks *et al.*, 1996). 80% of patients should be afebrile by day five (Janoff *et al.*, 1992). There is no need to continue therapy beyond the standard 7 to 10 day course because most recurrent disease is reinfection rather than relapse. In penicillin-allergic patients erythromycin or co-trimoxazole can be used.

Penicillin-resistance may start to become a problem especially if it is associated with HIV infection (Bates *et al.*, 1992). In Nairobi where nearly 20% of isolates show intermediate resistance to penicillin (Bates *et al.*, 1992) we

still had good responses with standard dose penicillin therapy probably because alveolar penetration remains good and high levels of antibiotic are achieved. Vancomycin has been used with good effect (Blumberg and Rimland, 1989).

Haemophilus influenzae infections respond well to a wide range of antimicrobials. The first choice of many physicians is ampicillin. In areas where the prevalence of beta-lactamase-producing organisms is high then co-amoxiclav (amoxycillin plus clavulanic acid) should be used (Chaisson, 1989). Alternatives are co-trimoxazole, erythromycin and second- or third-generation cephalosporins (Schlamm and Yancovitz, 1989).

Proven *S. aureus* pneumonia should be treated with a penicillinase-resistant penicillin such as cloxacillin or flucloxacillin. In hospitals where methicillin-resistant organisms are a problem vancomycin should be used whilst awaiting sensitivity results (Levine, White and Fels, 1990). If the pneumonia is line-associated then the catheter will usually need to be replaced.

Gram-negative pneumonia, community-acquired or nosocomial, will need to be treated by broad-spectrum antimicrobials such as third-generation cephalosporins or a broad-spectrum semi-synthetic penicillin with an aminoglycoside. Blind therapy should include an antipseudomonal penicillin such as azlocillin or piperacillin if *P. aeruginosa* infection is a possibility. It is impossible to generalize and each case must be evaluated individually.

In HIV-negative patients with community-acquired pneumonia parenteral treatment can be switched to oral therapy when they have been afebrile for 24 hours, the respiratory rate is below 24 per minute, if oxygen saturation is 95% or more while breathing room air, if the chest radiograph is stable or improving and if oral medication is tolerated (Marrie, 1994). Such guidelines are sensible for HIV-seropositive patients.

For patients in whom concomitant *P. carinii* pneumonia is possible, or in whom the diagnosis is likely to be bacterial pneumonia but there is some doubt about whether it could be PCP, then high-dose co-trimoxazole can be used as empirical treatment. Fortunately this will provide effective cover for *S. pneumoniae* and *H. influenzae* and also be effective for most episodes of PCP.

The optimal therapy for nocardia in AIDS has not been determined. Sulphonamides (sulfisoxazole, co-trimoxazole or sulphadiazine) were effective in 78% of patients in one large series (Uttamchandani *et al.*, 1994). Also there are no guidelines published for therapy of *R. equi*. Rifampicin with erythromycin has proven disappointing whereas vancomycin has been effective in individual cases (Drancourt *et al.*, 1992).

It is worth remembering that although atypical pneumonias seem no more likely to occur in individuals immunosuppressed with HIV there is still a substantial background rate of such infections. In particular if there is high mycoplasma activity in the area then it may be sensible to use erythromycin more widely.

PREVENTION

Because bacterial pneumonia is such a frequent problem in HIV-infected individuals prevention could play a major role (Keller and Breiman, 1995). Given the morbidity, time off work, cost of effective therapy and days spent in hospital with each episode any effective preventive measure would seem to be highly cost-effective; and although mortality is relatively low except in the latter stages undoubtedly some premature deaths could be prevented.

Antimicrobial prophylaxis is one possibility and recent data support the efficacy of co-trimoxazole in reducing the incidence of bacterial pneumonia, and other bacterial infections, when being used to prevent *P. carinii* infection (Mayer *et al.*, 1993). It may

be difficult to persuade many individuals, particularly when asymptomatic and with high CD4 counts, to take regular antibiotics. Our experience in Nairobi is that compliance is a major problem even in patients with at least one prior episode of invasive pneumococcal disease (Gilks, 1993b). The possibility of monthly injections of long-acting penicillin will not be very popular as the injections can be painful and need to be given under supervision. It seems unlikely that any new strategies will be developed to widen the use of co-trimoxazole prophylaxis to cover bacterial infections such as pneumonia.

Vaccination is much more appealing as a preventive strategy and pneumococcal vaccine is highly effective in young immunocompetent adults (Austrian *et al.*, 1976). The current licenced vaccine contains capsular polysaccharide of 23 serotypes and covers about 90% of invasive episodes. It needs to be given only once, with booster shots every five years or so. Since 1989 adults with HIV infection and AIDS in the USA have been advised to have polysaccharide pneumococcal vaccine. Despite consistent recommendations for use, uptake has been poor; only 37% of more than 9000 potential recipients had received vaccination in one survey (Wortley and Farizo, 1994). There are no data for the UK or other industrialized countries where vaccination is also recommended. Levels are likely to be as low as in the USA.

This may be because of a general lack of appreciation of the importance of pneumococcal pneumonia in HIV, or because there has never been an efficacy study and physicians are skeptical about its value. The literature certainly contains several reports of vaccine failure (Simberkoff *et al.*, 1984).

Based on the argument that the vaccine may be effective, is safe and cheap, then perhaps uptake will increase in the next few years. It certainly seems sensible to offer vaccination to all HIV-infected adults and allow them the choice. Such a strategy is unaffordable in poor countries and a formal efficacy study is needed. We are at present conducting such a study in Uganda.

The rate of invasive *H. influenzae* infection is much less (Steinhart *et al.*, 1992) and the specific role of type b has been questioned (Rich, Sax and Kazanjian, 1993). There appears at present little role for conjugate *H. influenzae* type b (Hib) vaccination in adults with HIV infection.

RESEARCH PRIORITIES

Despite the undeniable importance of bacterial pneumonia as a cause of morbidity and mortality, many gaps exist in our basic knowledge of bacterial pneumonia in the context of HIV infection. It could be argued that bacterial infections in general, and pneumonia in particular, have been ignored by most investigators. One important priority must therefore be to raise the awareness and interest in the whole field.

In epidemiology and public health several critical lacunae exist in our knowledge and understanding. The basic descriptive epidemiology is woefully inadequate (Caiaffa, Graham and Vlahov, 1993) particularly since bacterial pneumonia is the commonest major infection that is not AIDS defining in adults with underlying HIV (Farizo *et al.*, 1992). Risk factors for developing pneumonia have not been assessed in any detail. The rate and importance of recurrent pneumonia have not yet been established and this is of importance now that this is an AIDS-defining condition (CDC, 1992). And perhaps most important of all, although many episodes of pneumococcal disease may be preventable by vaccination it is still not known how effective this may be nor how cost-effective such measures could be. And we have little idea why vaccine uptake is so poor.

On the basic science side several intriguing questions exist and there must be major research priorities. The reasons why adults immunosuppressed by HIV are particularly vulnerable to bacterial pneumonia have not been elucidated. Encapsulated bacteria like the pneumococcus and *H. influenzae* are classically B-cell rather than T-cell pathogens. It is quite unclear why in Nairobi the pneumococcus was the leading pathogen and the earliest to present, more so than even tuberculosis (Gilks, 1996). It has been suggested that abnormalities in humoral rather than cellular immunity are important (Janoff *et al.*, 1992) but these have not been defined.

Finally on the clinical side the most important priority is to produce better treatment guidelines based on controlled clinical trials. For such a common event it is very depressing not to be able to refer to well-conducted trials which have properly established the best antimicrobial therapy. In the future the global spread of penicillin-resistant pneumococci is worrying especially if our observations from Nairobi suggesting an association with HIV are borne out (Bates *et al.*, 1992).

It is unclear why acute pneumonia has been relatively neglected as an important study for clinical research and comparatively few data have been published. Hopefully the tide is now changing and in the next few years more widespread recognition will be given to this common clinical problem, and bacterial pneumonia will become a more active area of investigation.

REFERENCES

Amorosa, J.K., Nahass, R.G., Nosher, J.L. *et al.* (1990) Radiologic distinction of pyogenic pulmonary infection from *Pneumocystis carinii* pneumonia in AIDS patients. *Radiology*, **175**, 721–27.

Austrian, R., Douglas, R.M., Schiffman, G. *et al.* (1976) Prevention of pneumococcal pneumonia by vaccination. *Transactions of the American Association of Physicians*, **89**, 184–94.

Bates, J., Paul, J. Gilks, C.F. *et al.* (1992) Penicillin-resistant pneumococci: a common cause of infection in HIV-positive patients in Nairobi. *VIII International Conference on AIDS. Amsterdam, The Netherlands*, Abstract PoB 3752.

Belec, L., Ekala, M.-T. and Gilquin, J. (1993) *Coxiella burnetti* infection among HIV-1 infected people living in Paris, France. *AIDS*, **7**, 1136–37.

Blasi, F., Boschini, A., Cosentini, R. *et al.* (1994) Outbreak of *Chlamydia pneumoniae* infection in former injection-drug users. *Chest*, **105**, 812–15.

Blatt, S.P., Dolan, M.J., Hendrix, C.W. *et al.* (1994) Legionnaires' disease in HIV infected patients: eight cases and a review. *Clinical Infectious Diseases*, **18**, 227–32.

Blumberg, H.M. and Rimland, D. (1989) Nosocomial infection with penicillin-resistant pneumococci in patients with AIDS. *Journal of Infectious Diseases*, **160**, 725–26.

British Thoracic Society (1987) Community-acquired pneumonia in adults in British hospitals in 1982–1983: a survey of aetiology, mortality, prognostic factors and outcome. *Quarterly Journal of Medicine*, **62**, 195–220.

Buehler, J.W., Owen, J., Berkelman, R.L. *et al.* (1990) Impact of HIV epidemic on mortality trends in young men, United States. *American Journal of Public Health*, **80**, 1080–86.

Caiaffa, W.T., Graham, N.M.H. and Vlahov, D. (1993) Bacterial pneumonia in adult populations with HIV infection. *American Journal of Epidemiology*, **138**, 909–22.

Casadevall, A., Dobroszycki, J., Small, C. *et al.* (1992) *Haemophilus influenzae* type b bacteraemia in adults with AIDS and at risk of AIDS. *American Journal of Medicine*, **92**, 587–90.

Centers for Disease Control (1992) 1993 Revised classification system for HIV infection and expanded surveillance case definition for AIDS among adolescents and adults. *Morbidity and Mortality Weekly Report*, **41**, 1–19.

Chaisson, R.E. (1989) Bacterial pneumonia in patients with HIV infection. *Seminars in Respiratory Infections*, **4**, 133–38.

Chu, S.Y., Buehler, J.W. and Berkelman, R.L. (1990) Impact of the HIV epidemic on mortality in women of reproductive age, United States. *Journal of the American Medical Association*, **264** 225–29.

Cohn, D.L. (1991) Bacterial pneumonia in the HIV-infected patient. *Infectious Diseases Clinics of North America*, **5**, 485–507.

Coker, R.J. and Mitchell, D.M. (1994) The role of bronchoscopy in patients with HIV disease. *International Journal of STD and AIDS*, **5**, 172–76.

Daley, C.L. (1994) Pulmonary infections in the Tropics: impact of HIV infection. *Thorax*, **49**, 370–78.

Drancourt, M., Bonnet, E., Gallais, H. *et al.* (1992) *Rhodococcus equi* infection in patients with AIDS. *Journal of Infection*, **24**, 123–31.

Falco, V., de Sevilla, T.F., Alegre, J. *et al.* (1994) Bacterial pneumonia in HIV-infected patients: a prospective study of 68 episodes. *European Respiratory Journal*, **7**, 235–39.

Farizo, K.M., Buehler, J.W., Chamberland, M.E. *et al.* (1992) Spectrum of disease in persons with HIV infection in the United States. *Journal of the American Medical Association*, **267**, 1798–805.

Fels, A.O.S. (1988) Bacterial and fungal pneumonias. *Clinics in Chest Medicine*, **9**, 449–57.

Gilks, C.F. (1993a) The clinical challenge of the HIV epidemic in the developing world. *Lancet*, **342**, 1037–39.

Gilks, C.F. (1993b) Prophylaxis for HIV-associated infections in the developing world. *Journal of Antimicrobial Chemotherapy*, **31**, suppl.B, 119–28.

Gilks, C.F., Otieno, L.S., Brindle, R.J. *et al.* (1992) The presentation and outcome of HIV-related disease in Nairobi. *Quarterly Journal of Medicine*, **82**, 25–32.

Gilks, C.F., Mwachari, C., Simani, P. *et al.* (1993) A case-control study of HIV and pneumococcal pneumonia in Kenyatta Hospital, Nairobi. *IX International Conference on AIDS. Berlin, Germany*, Abstract WS-B08-2.

Gilks, C.F., Ojoo, S.A., Ojoo, J.C. *et al.* (1996) Invasive pneumococcal disease in a cohort of predominantly HIV-1 infected female sex workers in Nairobi, Kenya. *Lancet*, **347**, 718–23.

Greenberg, A.E., Thomas, P.A., Landesman, S.H. *et al.* (1992) The spectrum of HIV-1 related disease among outpatients in New York city. *AIDS*, **6**, 849–59.

Hirschtick, R.E., Glassroth J., Jordan, M.C. *et al.* (1995) Bacterial pneumonia in persons infected with the human immunodeficiency virus. *New England Journal of Medicine*, **333**, 845–51.

Jacobson, M.A., Gellerman, H. and Chambers, H. (1988) *Staphylococcus aureus* bacteraemia and recurrent staphylococcal infection in patients with AIDS and AIDS-related complex. *American*

Journal of Medicine, **85**, 172–6.

Janoff, E.N., Breiman, R.F., Daley, C.D. *et al.* (1992) Pneumococcal disease during HIV infection. *Annals of Internal Medicine*, **117**, 314–24.

Janoff, E.N., O'Brien, J., Thompson, P. *et al.* (1993) *Streptococcus pneumoniae* colonization, bacteraemia and immune response among persons with HIV infection. *Journal of Infectious Diseases*, **167**, 49–56.

Janssen, R.S., St Louis, M.E., Satten, G.A. *et al.* (1992) HIV infection among patients in U.S. acute care hospitals. *New England Journal of Medicine*, **327**, 445–52.

Jordens, Z.J., Paul, J., Bates, J., Beaumont, C., Kimari, J. and Gilks C. (1995) Characterisation of *Streptococcus pneumoniae* from human immunodeficiency virus - seropositive patients with acute and recurrent pneumonia. *Journal of Infectious Diseases*, **172**, 983–87.

Joseph, J., Strange, C. and Sahn, S.A. (1993) Pleural effusions in hospitalized patients with AIDS. *Annals of Internal Medicine*, **118**, 856–9.

Kamanfu, G., Mlika-Cabanne, N., Girard, P.M. *et al.* (1993) Pulmonary complications of HIV infected in Bujumbura, Burundi. *American Review of Respiratory Disease*, **147**, 658–63.

Keller, D.W., Breiman, R.F. (1995) Preventing bacterial respiratory tract infections among persons infected with human immunodeficiency virus. *Clinical Infectious Diseases*, **21**(suppl.) 577–83.

Kramer, M.R. and Uttamchandani, R.B. (1990) The radiographic appearance of pulmonary nocardiosis associated with AIDS. *AIDS*, **98**, 382–85.

Levine, S.J., White, D.A. and Fels, A.O.S. (1990) The incidence and significance of *Staphylococcus aureus* in respiratory cultures from patients infected with HIV. *American Review of Respiratory Disease*, **141**, 89–93.

Lucas, S.B., Hounnou, A., Peacock, C. *et al.* (1993) The mortality and pathology of HIV infection in a West African city. *AIDS*, **7**, 1569–79.

Magnenat, J.L., Nicod, L.P., Auckenthaler, R. *et al.* (1991) Mode of presentation and diagnosis of bacterial pneumonia in HIV-infected patients. *American Review of Respiratory Disease*, **144**, 917–22.

Marrie, T.J. (1994) Community-acquired pneumonia. *Clinical Infectious Diseases*, **18**, 501–15.

Mayer, H.B., Rose, D.N., Cohen, S. *et al.* (1993) The effect of *P. carinii* pneumonia prophylaxis regimens on the incidence of bacterial infections in HIV-infected patients. *AIDS*, **7**, 1687–89.

McKenzie, R., Travis, W.D., Dolan, S.A. *et al.* (1991) The cause of death in patients with HIV infection: a clinical and pathological study with emphasis on the role of pulmonary diseases. *Medicine*, **70**, 326–42.

McLoud, T.C. and Naidich, T.C. (1992) Thoracic disease in the immunocompromised patient. *Radiologic Clinics of North America*, **30**, 525–54.

Meduri, G.U. and Stein, D.S. (1992) Pulmonary manifestations of AIDS. *Clinical Infectious Diseases*, **14**, 98–113.

Mientjes, G.H., van Ameijden, E.J., van den Hoek, A.J.A.R. *et al.* (1992) Increased morbidity without rise in non-AIDS mortality among HIV-infected intravenous drug users in Amsterdam. *AIDS*, **6**, 207–12.

Miller, R.F., Foley, N.M., Kessel, D. *et al.* (1994) Community acquired lobar pneumonia in patients with HIV infection and AIDS. *Thorax*, **49**, 367–68.

Monforte, A.A., Vago, L., Lazzarin, A. *et al.* (1992) AIDS-defining diseases in 250 HIV-infected patients: comparative study of clinical and autopsy diagnoses. *AIDS*, **6**, 1159–64.

Moreno, S., Martinez, R., Borros, C. *et al.* (1991) Latent *Haemophilus influenzae* pneumonia in patients infected with HIV. *AIDS*, **5**, 967–70.

Murray, J.F. and Mills, J. (1990) Pulmonary infectious complications of HIV infection. Parts 1 and 2. *American Review of Respiratory Disease*, **141**, 1356–72 and 1582–98.

Nichols, L., Balogh, K. and Silverman, M. (1989) Bacterial infections in AIDS. *American Journal of Clinical Pathology*, **92**, 787–90.

Nybo Jensen, B., Gerstoft, J., Hojylyng, N. *et al.* (1990) Pulmonary pathogens in HIV-infected patients. *Scandinavian Journal of Infectious Diseases*, **22**, 413–20.

Pallangyo, K., Hakanson, A., Lema, L. *et al.* (1992) High HIV seroprevalence and increased HIV-associated mortality among hospitalized patients with deep bacterial infections in Dar es Salaam, Tanzania. *AIDS*, **6**, 971–76.

Pesola, G.R. and Charles, A. (1992) Pneumococcal bacteraemia with pneumonia. Mortality in AIDS. *Chest*, **101**, 150–55.

Pinching, A.J. (1991) Antibody responses in HIV infection. *Clinical Experimental Immunology*, **84**, 181–84.

Polsky, B., Gold, J.W.M., Whimbey, E. *et al.* (1986) Bacterial pneumonia in patients with AIDS.

Annals of Internal Medicine, **104**, 38–41.

Raoult, D., Levy, P.-Y., Dupont, H.T. *et al.* (1993) Q fever and HIV infection. *AIDS*, 1993, **7**, 81–6.

Redd, S.C., Rutherford, G.W., Sande, M.A. *et al.* (1990) The role of HIV infection in pneumococcal bacteraemia in San Francisco residents. *Journal of Infectious Diseases*, **162**, 1012–17.

Rich, J.D., Sax, P.E. and Kazanjian, P.H. (1993) Bacteraemic *H. influenzae* type b infections and HIV. *American Journal of Medicine*, **95**, 118–19.

Schlamm, H.T. and Yankovitz, S.R. (1989) *Haemophilus influenzae* pneumonia in young adults with AIDS, ARC or risk of AIDS. *American Journal of Medicine*, **86**, 11–14.

Schuchat, A., Broome, C.V., Hightower, A. *et al.* (1991) Use of surveillance for invasive pneumococcal disease to estimate the size of the immunosuppressed HIV-infected population. *Journal of the American Medical Association*, **265**, 3275–79.

Selwyn, P.A., Feingold, A.R., Hartel, D. *et al.* (1988) Increased risk of bacterial pneumonia in HIV-infected intravenous drug users without AIDS. *AIDS*, **2**, 267–72.

Simberkoff, M.S., Sadr, W.E., Schiffman, G. *et al.* (1984) *Streptococcus pneumoniae* infections and bacteraemia in patients with AIDS with a report of a pneumococcal vaccine failure. *American Review of Respiratory Disease*, **130**, 1174–76.

Steinhart, R., Reingold, A.L., Taylor, F. *et al.* (1992) Invasive *Haemophilus influenzae* infections in men with HIV infection. *Journal of the American Medical Association*, **268**, 3350–52.

Stoneburner, R.L., Des Jarlais, D.C., Benezra, D.

et al. (1988) A larger spectrum of severe HIV-1-related disease in intravenous drug users in New York City. *Science*, **242**, 916–19.

Taelman, H., Batungwanayo, J., Bogaerts, J. *et al.* (1992) Lobar pneumonia: an early indicator of HIV infection in Central Africa. *VIII International Conference on AIDS, Amsterdam, The Netherlands.* Abstract PoB 3141.

Uttamchandani, R.B., Daikos, G.L., Reyes, R.R. *et al.* (1994) Nocardiosis in 30 patients with advanced HIV infection: clinical features and outcome. *Clinical Infectious Diseases*, **18**, 348–53.

White, S., Tsou, E., Waldhorn, R.E. *et al.* (1985) Life-threatening bacterial pneumonia in male homosexuals with laboratory features of AIDS. *Chest*, **87**, 486–88.

Willocks, L., Cowan, F., Brettle, R.P. *et al.* (1992) The spectrum of chest infections in HIV positive patients in Edinburgh. *Journal of Infection*, **24**, 37–42.

Witt, D.J., Craven, D.E. and McCabe, W.R. (1987) Bacterial infections in adult patients with AIDS and AIDS-related complex. *American Journal of Medicine*, **82**, 900–6.

Woodhead, M.A., Arrowsmith, J., Chamberlain-Webber, R. *et al.* (1991) The value of routine microbiological investigation in community-acquired pneumonia. *Respiratory Medicine*, **85**, 313–17.

Wortley, P.M., Farizo, K.M. (1994) and the adult and adolescent spectrum of HIV disease project group (1994) Pneumococcal and influenza vaccine levels among HIV-infected adolescents and adults receiving medical care in the USA. *AIDS*, **8**, 941–44.

Girish Desai

INTRODUCTION

Empyema thoracis, defined as a collection of pus in the pleural space (Odell, 1994), was first described and treated using drainage by Hippocrates (Major, 1965). Whether the term 'empyema' should be defined as fluid which has pus on inspection or as fluid containing excess polymorphs is debatable. In the early phases of development of empyema, the fluid may not have a naked-eye appearance of pus. Tuberculous empyema may have cell counts which show a predominance (>50%) of lymphocytes, although polymorphs may dominate the early stages. Despite improved antimicrobial therapy and multiple options for drainage of the infected pleural space, empyema thoracis remains a condition with considerable morbidity and mortality in its treated and untreated forms (Kaplan, 1994; Desai and Mugala, 1992; LeMense, Strange and Sahn, 1995).

EPIDEMIOLOGICAL FEATURES

The prevalence and etiology of empyema vary with age and circumstances of the patient and with the part of the world in which the patient is living. In developing countries acute bacterial pneumonias and penetrating chest injuries were common causes of empyema prior to the advent of the AIDS epidemic. In the USA and Europe empyema usually develops without a history of pneumonia although many of these patients have an underlying predisposing factor such as alcoholism, carcinoma of the bronchus, inhalation or immunosuppression. There are very few reports of the occurrence of empyema thoracis in patients infected with the human immunodeficiency virus (HIV) in the USA and Europe (Mouroux *et al.*, 1995). Empyema thoracis appears to be relatively rare in adults infected with HIV despite the increased incidence of community-acquired respiratory bacterial infections (Coker, 1994). The reasons for the lack of associated empyema remain unclear. However, in Central African countries, the situation is quite different. Data now emerging show that the number of cases of empyema are steadily rising and these are closely associated with HIV infection (Desai, 1992; Hassan and Mabogunje, 1992; Bayley, 1990).

The HIV epidemic has reached epidemic proportions in all countries in Sub-Saharan Africa. The seroprevalence of HIV-1 among blood donors has been reported at 10% (Luo *et al.*, 1989) while 35% of all surgical admissions at the University Teaching Hospital (UTH), Lusaka, Zambia, are HIV-positive. The major mode of transmission of HIV in Zambia is heterosexual, affecting both males

AIDS and Respiratory Medicine. Edited by A. Zumla, M.A. Johnson and R.F. Miller. Published in 1997 by Chapman & Hall, London. ISBN 0 412 60140 0

Table 15.1 Age groups of 125 patients with empyema thoracis presenting to the University Teaching Hospital, Lusaka, Zambia, between 1990 and 1992

Age group (years)	Number (%)	HIV+ve (%)
0–5	15 (12)	10 (66)
6–15	4 (3)	1 (25)
16–40	94 (75)	69 (73)
41–60	10 (8)	4 (40)
61+	4 (2)	0 (0)
Total	125	84 (67)

and females approximately equally. In HIV-infected patients, acute bacterial chest infections and tuberculosis are two of the commonest causes of inpatient admissions in children and adults (Chintu *et al.*, 1995; Elliott *et al.*, 1990).

As a consequence of a rise in the number of these infections, there has been an exponential increase in the number of cases of empyema thoracis seen at UTH during the past 10 years (Desai, 1992). Prior to the HIV epidemic, empyema thoracis was an uncommon clinical problem in Africa. The number of cases presenting to the surgical inpatient wards at UTH has steadily increased from a total of 12 cases in 1980, 32 cases in 1983, 50 cases in 1985, 104 cases in 1990 to 158 in 1994. Both sexes and all age groups are affected (Table 15.1). The male:female sex ratio is 5:1 in adults while in children below 15 years of age the sex ratio is approximately equal (Desai, 1992).

The outcome of empyema thoracis is closely related to the degree of immunosuppression and prompt diagnosis and management; the latter two are usually delayed in developing countries. Published literature on empyema thoracis from Africa remains scanty. This chapter discusses the clinical features and management of empyema thoracis in a resource-poor setting of developing countries.

DEVELOPMENT OF EMPYEMA THORACIS

The development of empyema thoracis can be grouped into three stages (Odell, 1994; LeMense, Strange and Sahn, 1995). The first stage (exudative phase), is usually brief, lasting around 48 hours and is characterized by free-flowing exudate. Progression to the second stage (fibrinopurulent phase) results in the formation of septate fibrin strands throughout the purulent fluid with deposition of fibrin onto the visceral and parietal pleura, creating a multiloculated pleural space. In the third stage (organizational phase) fibroblasts grow into the exudate from both the visceral and parietal pleural surfaces to produce an inelastic membrane called the pleural peel or cortex. This may result in significant loss of lung volume and may restrict lung expansion even if the fluid is drained. Empyemas which become obvious when pus discharges spontaneously from the chest wall are called empyema necessitans or necessitatis (a pointing empyema). Complications of empyema thoracis include bronchopleural fistulae, esophagopleural fistulae, the formation of metastatic abscesses or development of amyloidosis.

The development of empyema thoracis in AIDS patients in the tropics appears to be an insidious process with the acute phase not being evident (Bayley, 1990; Desai and Mugala, 1992). The pus is usually thick by the time patients present to the surgeon, and the fibrinous reaction appears relatively slow and scant, resulting in the purulent fluid occupying the entire hemithorax or a large thin-walled cyst. Multiple loculation is comparatively less frequent. Most patients present with unilateral empyema; bilateral empyema thoracis is not a common feature in AIDS patients. Frozen chest with its sequelae is not seen. In children, presentation as empyema necessitatis is often seen (Figures 15.1 and 15.2). Extensive infective necrosis of the chest wall may also occur (Figure 15.3). Bronchopleural fistulae

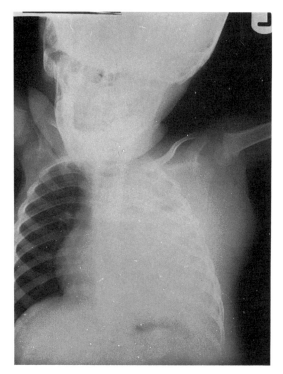

Fig. 15.1 An empyema necessitatis about to rupture on the surface on the left side of the chest in a child with AIDS.

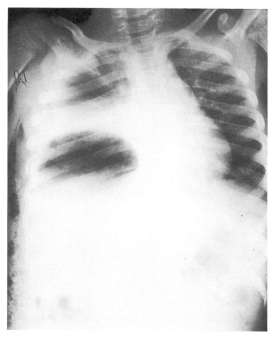

Fig. 15.2 An empyema necessitatis on the right side of the chest in a child with AIDS showing gas in the soft tissue of the chest wall.

are common complications while cerebral abscess and amyloidosis are rare.

PREDISPOSING FACTORS TO THE
DEVELOPMENT OF EMPYEMA THORACIS

The etiopathogenesis of empyema thoracis is usually determined by the nature of the patient population, the pattern of community-based chest infections (Ali and Unruh, 1990; Benfield, 1981), and the presence of risk factors such as immunodeficiency, alcoholism and diabetes (Desai, 1992; Mouroux *et al.*, 1995). An empyema is a consequence of infection of the structures surrounding the pleural space. In the lung, empyema commonly follows pneumonia but may also be associated with lung abscesses and bronchiectasis (Odell,

1994). It may also be associated with infection below the diaphragm, mediastinal infection or infection introduced post-trauma.

Table 15.2 shows the etiopathogenic factors underlying the development of empyema thoracis in a study of 125 patients presenting to the surgical wards of UTH in Lusaka over a 2-year period (1990–1992). Pulmonary TB (44%) and acute bacterial chest infections (36%) were the most common underlying etiological factors. Other underlying factors for development of empyema thoracis in our study at UTH included infection following chest trauma (10%); septicemia (4%); and peritonitis (4%). Of all empyema thoracis cases seen, 67% were seropositive for HIV compared to a seroprevalence rate of 11% in blood donors and 14% in surgical casualty attendances. All 10 patients with septicemia or peritonitis were HIV-seropositive. 72% of patients with underlying TB and 66% of

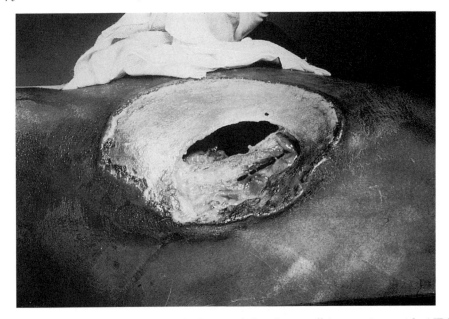

Fig. 15.3   Infective necrosis of the entire thickness of the chest wall in a patient with AIDS.

Table 15.2   Predisposing factors underlying empyema thoracis in 125 patients presenting to the University Teaching Hospital, Lusaka, Zambia between 1990 and 1992

Underlying condition	Number (%)	Number (%) HIV+ve
Pulmonary tuberculosis	55 (44)	40 (72)
Bacterial chest infections	45 (36)	30 (66)
Penetrating chest injuries	12 (10)	2 (16)
Secondary to septicemia	5 (4)	5 (100)
Secondary to peritonitis	5 (4)	5 (100)
Undetermined	3 (2)	1 (33)

patients with predisposing acute bacterial infection were HIV-positive. The TB figures are similar to those obtained in a study of tuberculous pleural disease in Zambian adults by Elliott *et al.*, (1990) in which HIV-positivity was 81% in those TB cases with pleural involvement compared to 49% HIV-seropositivity in those TB patients without pleural involvement.

CLINICAL PRESENTATION OF EMPYEMA THORACIS

Patients with empyema may have variable symptoms difficult to distinguish from those of the underlying predisposing factors such as pneumonia, abscess, subdiaphragmatic infection, or mediastinitis (Odell, 1994). The patient may be frankly toxic or virtually asymptomatic, depending upon the causal organisms, the volume of pus and the host defense system. Dyspnea is due to fluid in the pleural space or mediastinal displacement. A bronchopleural fistula presents with a characteristic history. Whenever the patient lies on the side opposite to the empyema he/she coughs excessively and the volume of pus produced on expectoration is large. A chest wall swelling caused by empyema necessitatis may be mistaken for a chest wall abscess.

The symptoms of empyema thoracis in AIDS patients vary from minimal discomfort to those of a severe toxic illness. These depend on the underlying condition, virulence of organisms, amount of purulent fluid present and stage of HIV disease. In AIDS patients there may be additional symptoms and signs of HIV disease and its complications. The development of empyema thoracis in AIDS patients is an insidious process. The mean duration of symptoms in HIV-positive patients presenting to the UTH is 60 days (range 14–150 days) as opposed to 5 days in HIV-negative patients (Desai, 1992). Table 15.3 shows the mode of presenta-

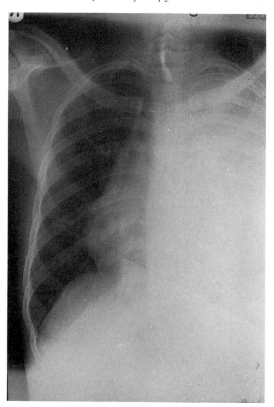

Fig. 15.4 An empyema thoracis of the left hemithorax causing a right shift of the mediastinum.

Table 15.3 Symptoms, signs and associated features of empyema thoracis in 125 patients seen at the University Teaching Hospital, Lusaka, Zambia, between 1990 and 1992

Symptom/sign	Number (%)
Dyspnea	97 (78)
Cough	80 (64)
Chest pain	75 (60)
Fever	55 (44)
Weight loss	52 (42)
Night sweats	10 (8)
Hemoptysis	6 (5)
Empyema – unilateral	122 (98)
– bilateral	3 (2)
Generalized lymphadenopathy	59 (47)
Oral candida	17 (14)
Empyema necessitatis	8 (6)
Kaposi's sarcoma (cutaneous)	6 (5)

tion of empyema thoracis in 125 consecutive patients seen over a 2-year period at UTH (1990–1992). 122 (98%) presented with unilateral empyema and 5% have associated Kaposi's sarcoma (Amadi, 1993). It is generally difficult to pinpoint the onset of empyema development.

DIAGNOSIS OF EMPYEMA THORACIS

The insidious nature of the presentation of empyema thoracis in AIDS patients makes the diagnosis a difficult one to make on history and physical examination alone. Lateral and PA chest radiograph views combined with diagnostic chest aspiration are important in making the diag-

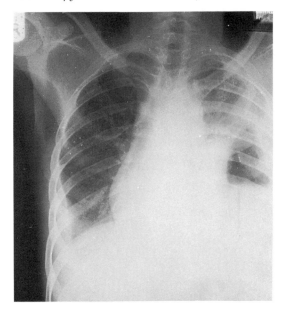

Fig. 15.5   A large encysted empyema thoracis on the left side in a patient with AIDS.

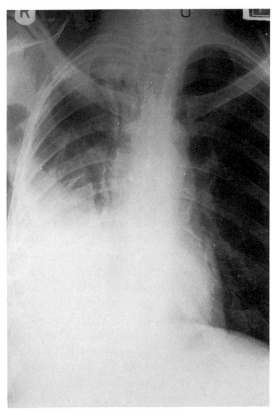

Fig. 15.6   A right-sided subpneumonic empyema thoracis secondary to infected tuberculous effusion in AIDS. There is also right apical consolidation.

nosis (DeMeester, 1983). By the time most patients with empyema present to the hospital the fluid is overtly purulent. Complete opacification of hemithorax with shift of mediastinum causing cardiorespiratory dysfunction (Figure 15.4) is a common radiological finding of empyema thoracis in AIDS patients. Multi-loculation is less common but a single large encysted collection frequently occurs (Figure 15.5). Another common radiological finding is a large sub-pneumonic opacification secondary to the infected effusion associated with tuberculous basal congestion of the lung (Figure 15.6). The presence of an air/fluid level in the pleural space with the production of copious purulent sputum by the patient is indicative of the development of a broncho-pleural fistula (Figure 15.7). In patients with no copious sputum, it may indicate that the empyema is infected by gas forming organisms. In a small proportion of cases it is difficult to diagnose underlying disease such as tuberculous cavitation, pneumonia and lung abscess which can be detected by CT imaging. In the absence of spiral CT scanning facilities it is useful to review previous case note records and to perform chest tomography.

MICROBIOLOGY OF EMPYEMA THORACIS

A wide spectrum of Gram-positive and Gram-negative aerobic and anaerobic bacteria, fungi, and mycobacteria have been isolated from patients with empyema thoracis in the USA and Europe (LeMense *et al.*, 1995). *Staphylococcus aureus* and *S. epidermidis* and *Streptococcus* spp appear to be common isolates. *Escherichia coli*, *Pseudomonas* spp, and

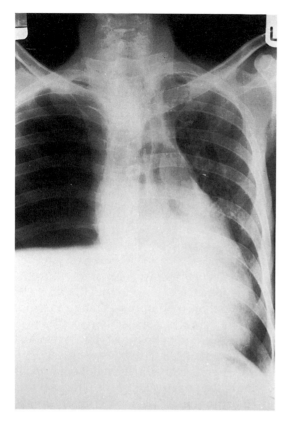

Fig. 15.7 A right-sided empyema thoracis with a broncho-pleural fistula showing air/fluid level (pyopneumothorax). This patient produced copious foul sputum.

Table 15.4 Microbiology of pleural aspirates from 125 patients presenting to University Teaching Hospital, Lusaka, with empyema thoracis

Organism isolated	Number (%)
Beta-hemolytic streptococcus spp	33 (20)
Staphylococcus aureus	33 (20)
Escherichia coli	15 (12)
Acinetobacter spp	15 (12)
Proteus spp	13 (10)
Salmonella spp	13 (10)
Streptococcus pneumoniae	9 (7)
Streptococcus faecalis	9 (7)
Mycobacterium tuberculosis	3 (2)

Note: 36 specimens had more than one pathogen isolated.

Haemophilus influenzae are other common isolates. The number of anaerobic organisms cultured has varied depending on the methods used for recovery (LeMense *et al.*, 1995). There are few comparative data from the tropics. Table 15.4 shows the microorganisms isolated from the aspirates of 125 cases of empyema thoracis seen at UTH in Lusaka during 1990–1992. The yield of microorganisms from pleural aspirates is rather low; 56 out of 125 (45%) of the aspirates were sterile. The administration of several courses of antibiotic therapy prior to presentation may account for the low microbial yield. Of the bacteria isolated, 80% were resistant to the routinely used antibiotics at this institution. In patients' pleural aspirates, 6% had mixed growths. While no obligatory anaerobes were isolated, this may be due to technical problems associated with collection and transportation of the aspirates (Bartlett *et al.*, 1974; Smith *et al.*, 1991). It is generally recognized that the yield of mycobacteria from pleural aspirate is low. Fungi and atypical mycobacteria do not appear to be as important as has been described elsewhere (Lucas, 1990; Okello *et al.*, 1990). As shown by our study, staining of the pleural fluid aspirate for acid- and alcohol-fast bacteria is seldom helpful.

To determine the microbiologic etiology of empyema, most surgeons in the tropics rely heavily on bacteriological examination of sputum in combination with chest radiography findings. Of the patients whose chest radiographs were suggestive of tuberculosis, over 60% had positive sputum for the *Mycobacterium tuberculosis* (Amadi, 1993; Elliott *et al.*, 1990). Pleural biopsy taken at the time of insertion of an intercostal drain or rib resection is also useful; 50% of the pleural biopsies showed tuberculous lesions in patients who had radiological evidence of tuberculosis (Amadi, 1993). Better cost-effective methods of diagnosing the presence of mycobacteria or mycobacterial antigens in pleural fluid are required for use in the tropics. The polymerase chain reaction and various serological antigen detection tests are currently under investigation.

MANAGEMENT OF EMPYEMA THORACIS

Various treatment modalities are available for the treatment of empyema thoracis and have recently been reviewed (Kaplan, 1994; LeMense et al., 1995; Odell, 1994). At present there is no definite consensus of opinion on the management of empyema thoracis, and this is even more so in immunocompromised patients. First principles dictate that the primary objective is to eradicate all infected material and to establish lung re-expansion by use of antimicrobial therapy and drainage of the pleural space. The underlying cause of the empyema should be treated at the same time as the empyema. Pneumonia and TB usually respond to appropriate antibiotics. A lung abscess may require separate drainage of the abscess and the empyema. Drainage, whether closed or open, is done at the most dependent site of the empyema collection.

Multiple drainage options are available: tube thoracostomy; image-directed catheters; intrapleural thrombolytics; thoracoscopic drainage; decortication and chronic open drainage. These have been used with success rates between 10% and 90% (LeMense et al., 1995). Recent studies show that intrapleural streptokinase may be effective in patients with multiloculated empyema which is refractory to antibiotics and intercostal tube drainage in HIV-negative patients (Bouros et al., 1994; Taylor et al., 1994) and HIV-infected patients (Miller and Severn, 1995).

The variable success rates of various management schedules, in part, can be attributable to the stage of the empyema at presentation. Lemmer and colleagues (Lemmer, Botham and Orringer, 1985) advocate early rib resection and drainage in immunosuppressed patients while Fishman and Ellerton (1987) suggest early decortication. Our earlier clinical experiences at the UTH in Lusaka of decortication in AIDS patients with empyema were associated with rapid deterioration of the patients and were associated with an unacceptably high mortality rate. Since we changed management in 1990, we have encountered no unexpected deaths and no adverse effects, such as lung collapse or mediastinal shift after rib resection in patients with AIDS, have been encountered in over 150 patients. No randomized clinical trials have been performed to date to compare the efficacy of any one of the treatments available for empyema thoracis. There are no data from the USA and Europe on the appropriate management of empyema thoracis in HIV-infected patients.

In resource-poor settings in developing countries, management has to be rationalized. Currently, our management objective is to render the patients non-toxic rather rapidly by emptying the empyema cavity as soon as possible and the use of appropriate antibiotics wherever indicated. Drainage of the empyema fluid in uncomplicated empyema thoracis depends on the consistency of the pleural exudate. The empyema is aspirated with a 10 ml syringe and a wide bore needle and the rate of flow of the purulent fluid is noted as 'easy' or 'difficult'; 'easy flow' is one that fills the syringe with one pull of the plunger and the 'difficult flow' requires two or more pulls. Patients with 'easy flow' are subject to management with intercostal under-water-seal drainage from the most dependent part (determined radiologically) using a thoracic tube of 1 cm diameter lumen and 7.5 cm length inside the chest. If after two weeks the drainage persists in these patients, an open drainage is carried out.

Patients with 'difficult flow' aspirates are immediately subjected to open drainage by resecting two ribs of 7.5 cm length each and all fibrinous and purulent material is sucked

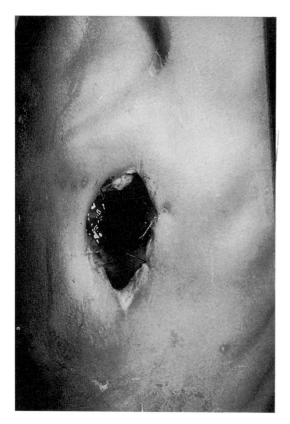

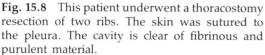

Fig. 15.8 This patient underwent a thoracostomy resection of two ribs. The skin was sutured to the pleura. The cavity is clear of fibrinous and purulent material.

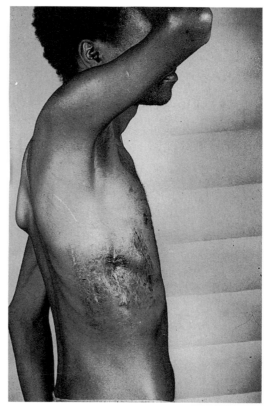

Fig. 15.9 A thoracostomy finally closed after mobilizing the surrounding skin around dried up sinuses.

out. The skin is sutured to the pleura as closely as possible without tension (Figure 15.8). Cutaneous flaps are made to facilitate flushing of the cavity post-operatively. Empyema necessitatis is managed by adequate incision and drainage. Patients with this condition are at a risk of developing fulminating infective necrosis of the chest wall after rib resection. Patients are encouraged to sit in bath tubs daily and flush the cavity with water. Several methods are employed to encourage drainage: chest physiotherapy; getting the patient to blow into surgical gloves; and to sleep on the side of the drainage.

PROGNOSIS AND FOLLOW-UP

At the UTH in Lusaka, 15% of AIDS patients who present with empyema die during the first hospital admission. The mean hospital stay for patients with empyema at our hospital is 8 days. About 50% of the patients dry up their sinuses after 8 weeks. If sinuses persist they can be closed by mobilizing and suturing the skin (Figure 15.9). The remainder of patients have intermittent discharge which is easily managed by the 'Home-Care Team'. Should a large collection occur, the sinus can be excised under local anesthesia and drainage re-established. This allows the patients to be sent home the next day. Overall, the prognosis of empyema thoracis in AIDS patients is poor and reasons for this are multifactorial. These include late presentation to hospital; the presence of immunodeficiency; other concomitant AIDS-associated illnesses; poor wound healing; and poor nutritional status. Follow-up studies show that one third of the patients die within 6 months of discharge from hospital (Desai and Mugala, 1992).

CONCLUSIONS

HIV infection predisposes patients to acquire serious and life-threatening chest infections. The sequelae of infections such as TB and acute bacterial sepsis sometimes present as empyema thoracis. In the tropics, the number of cases of empyema thoracis being seen as a result of the HIV epidemic is steadily rising. Early diagnosis and management of the condition are important in reducing inpatient mortality from this complication. Adequate and appropriate anti-microbial therapy in HIV-infected patients with chest infections could reduce the rising incidence of empyema thoracis.

REFERENCES

Ali, I. and Unruh, H. (1990) Management of empyema thoracis. *Ann. Thorac. Surg.*, **50**, 355–9.

Amadi, W.E. (1993) Prospective study of empyema thoracis at the University Teaching Hospital, Lusaka, Zambia. University of Zambia School of Medicine, Lusaka, Zambia dissertation.

Bartlett, J.G., Gorbach, S.L., Thadepalli, H. *et al.* (1974) Bacteriology of empyema. *Lancet*, **2**, 338–40.

Bayley, A.C. (1990) Surgical pathology of HIV infection: lesson from Africa. *Br. J. Surg.*, **77**, 863–8.

Benfield, G.F.A. (1981) Recent trends in empyema thoracis. *Br. J. Dis. Chest*, **75**, 358–65.

Bouros, D., Schiza, S., Panagon, P. *et al.* (1994) Role of streptokinase in the treatment of locu-lated parapneumonic pleural effusions and empyema. *Thorax*, **49**, 852–55.

Chintu, C., Luo, C., Bhatt, G. *et al.* (1995) Impact of HIV on common paediatric illnesses in Zambia. *J. Trop. Paediat.*, **41**, 348–53.

Coker, R.J. (1994) Empyema thoracis in AIDS (editorial). *J.R. Soc. Med.*, **87**, 2, 65–7.

DeMeester, T.R. (1983) The pleura in *Thoracic Surgery* (ed. D. Sabiston) W.B. Saunders, Philadelphia.

Desai, G.A. (1992) Empyema thoracis–open or closed drainage? (letter). *Trop. Doct.*, **22**, 2, 89.

Desai, G.A. and Mugala, D.D. (1992, Management of empyema thoracis at Lusaka, Zambia. *Br. J. Surg.*, **79**, 537–38.

Elliott, A.M., Luo, N., Tembo, G. *et al.* (1990) Impact of HIV on tuberculosis in Zambia: a cross sectional study. *Br. Med. J.*, **301**, 412–15.

Fishman, I.H. and Ellerton, D.G. (1987) Early pleural decortication for thoracic empyema in immune suppressed patients. *J. Thorac. Cardiovasc.*, **74**, 537–41.

Forbes, A.D., Marchioro, T.L., Schmidt, R.A. *et al.* (1994) Acquired immunodeficiency syndrome-related lymphoma of the lung presenting as empyema thoracis. *Ann. Thorac. Surg.*, **57**, 216–19.

Hassan, I. and Mabogunje, O. (1992) Paediatric empyema thoracis in Zaria, Nigeria. *Ann. Trop. Pedr.*, **12**, 3, 265–71.

Hornick, P. and Smith, P.L. (1994) Empyema thoracis in AIDS (letter). *J.R. Soc. Med.*, **87**, 570.

Kaplan, D.K. (1994) Treatment of empyema thoracis (editorial). *Thorax*, **49**, 845–6.

Kelly, J.W. and Morris, M.J. (1994) Empyema thoracis: medical aspects of evaluation and treatment. *South. Med. J.*, **87**, 1103–10.

LeMense, G.P., Strange, C. and Sahn, S.A. (1995) Empyema thoracis: therapeutic management and outcome. *Chest*, **107**, 6, 1532–37.

Lemmer, J.H., Botham, M.J. and Orringer, M.B. (1985) Modern management of adult empyema; *J. Thorac. Cardiovasc. Surg.*, **90**, 849–55.

Lucas, S.B. (1990) Missing infections in AIDS. *Trans. R. Soc. Trop. Med. Hyg.*, **84**(supp. 1, 34–38.

Luo, N.P., Dallas, A.B.C., Chipuka, G. *et al.* (1989) HIV sero-prevalence amongst healthy blood donors in 31 hospitals in Zambia. Fifth International Conference on AIDS Montreal, Ottawa; International Development Centre 1989, 246 (abstract).

Major, R.H. (1965) Hippocrates, in *Classic Description of Disease*. C.C. Thomas, Springfield, Illinois, pp. 568–69.

Miller, R.F. and Severn, A. (1995) Non surgical treatment of empyema thoracis with intrapleural streptokinase in a patient with AIDS. *Genitourin. Med.*, **71**, 259–61.

Mouroux, J., Riquet, M. and Padovani, B. (1995) Surgical management of thoracic manifestations in human immunodeficiency virus-positive patients: indications and results. *Br. J. Surg*, **82**, 39–43.

Odell, J.A. (1994) Management of empyema thoracis. *J. R. Soc. Med.*, **87**, 466–70.

Okello, D.O., Sewankambo, N., Goodgame, R. *et al.* (1990) Absence of bacteraemia with *Mycobacterium avium intracellulare* in Ugandan patients with AIDS. *J. Infect. Dis.*, **162**, 208–10.

Smith, J.A., Mullerworth, M.H., Westlake, G.W. *et al.* (1991) Empyema thoracis: 14 years experience in a teaching centre. *Ann. Thorac. Surg.*, **51**, 39–42.

Taylor, R.F.H., Rubens, M.B., Pearson, M.C. and Barnes, N.C. (1994) Intrapleural streptokinase in the management of empyema. *Thorax*, **49**, 856–57.

Rod J. Hay

INTRODUCTION

Fungal infections affecting the respiratory tract are important causes of disease in many immunocompromised, including AIDS, patients. In HIV-infected individuals mycoses which develop in patients with defective T lymphocyte-mediated immunity, such as histoplasmosis and cryptococcosis predominate (von Eiff *et al.*, 1994). In AIDS patients these infections, which in a healthy population are mainly subclinical, are more common because waning defense mechanisms fail either to contain disease after primary exposure or prevent reactivation of an occult focus of the primary infection. Their clinical presentations may also differ from those seen in other predisposed groups. Other opportunist fungal infections, including aspergillosis, may also occur in AIDS patients though less frequently. *Candida albicans* is only rarely found in pulmonary or systemic infections in AIDS but is a common cause of oropharyngeal disease. Finally, although genetically classified as a fungus, *Pneumocystis carinii* is discussed in chapters 6 and 7.

CANDIDOSIS

One of the commonest infectious complications of AIDS cited in the earliest reports (Gottlieb *et al.*, 1981) was oropharyngeal candidosis occurring either secondary to an ulcerative mucosal lesion or as a primary infection due to failure of the immune response. *Candida* infection has long been recognized as a complication seen in patients with defective T lymphocyte function (Odds, 1988) and in these immunodeficiency states is normally confined to the oral mucosa or skin. Vaginal or systemic infections may occur but are much less common in this group. Overall true pulmonary candidosis is uncommon in any predisposed group except as a feature of a rapidly disseminating systemic infection. Systemic candidosis is more typical of the neutropenic patient.

Oropharyngeal candidosis is a common problem in AIDS patients; in many published series it is cited as the most frequent infectious complication of the disease. In the normal healthy population the prevalence of oral carriage of *Candida albicans* is estimated to be between 2 and 41% (mean 16%) (Odds, 1988). Amongst HIV-positive individuals, carriage rates are generally higher. This has been confirmed by the finding that carriage rates are, for instance, greater in HIV-positive homosexual males (77.8%) than in a control group of HIV-negative homosexual men (Torssander *et al.*, 1987). In AIDS, colonization rates are higher in IV drug abusers, CDC group IV and in those with lymphopenia. In addition patients with CD4 cell depletion and those with elevated beta-2 microglobulin levels are also more likely to be carriers (Fetter *et al.*, 1993). The relationship between

AIDS and Respiratory Medicine. Edited by A. Zumla, M.A. Johnson and R.F. Miller. Published in 1997 by Chapman & Hall, London. ISBN 0 412 60140 0

CD4 counts, as a guide to disease progression, and oral candidosis in AIDS patients has been studied by a number of authors. The emergence of oral thrush does not predict the rate of decline in CD4 counts (Alcabes, Schoenbaum and Klein, 1993). However, some investigators have shown that overt *Candida* infection may provide some clues to the rate of progression to AIDS in HIV-positive men. Both hairy leukoplakia and oral candidosis are markers for increased rates of progression to AIDS in this group (Katz *et al.*, 1992). The presence of oral candidosis may also be a marker of survival in some patients. For instance HIV-positive patients with oral candidosis who have no other features of AIDS have a poorer survival rate than those without (Lin and Goodhart, 1993). Immunologically related events such as CD4 counts are not the only determinants of oral candidosis, and other factors such as the salivary flow rate are important.

Clinical features

The main clinical forms of oral candidosis include the acute and chronic plaque-types (pseudomembranous), acute and chronic atrophic oral candidosis, erythematous and hyperplastic candidosis (Samaranayake and Yaacob, 1990). AIDS patients may develop either the acute or chronic plaque or erythematous forms of oral candidosis (Greenspan, Greenspan and Winkler, 1988). Of these, the plaque type, presenting with white adherent patches on the buccal mucosa, is the best recognized. In AIDS patients infection is often extensive and may affect the dorsum of the tongue as well as other parts of the oral cavity. Pain, taste disturbance and altered touch sensation may all accompany plaque-type oral candidosis. Some AIDS patients develop the erythematous variety of infection. Here the changes are more subtle, often being confined to the palate and tongue, and patients complain of soreness, burning and

disturbed taste sensation. Sharp foods such as citrus fruits are difficult to tolerate. The mucosa appears inflamed and smooth with some loss of lingual papillae. These changes may persist into a chronic infection.

Secondary candidosis in the presence of other intraoral conditions such as hairy leukoplakia or herpetic ulceration is important to recognize because treatment responses are seldom long-lasting unless the underlying condition is eliminated. While the presence of *Candida* may be obvious because of the appearance of white plaques, at other times it is occult and has to be confirmed by microscopy and culture.

Spread of *Candida* infection beyond the oral cavity is a common occurrence but usually confined to the pharynx and esophagus. Esophageal condidosis may well be overlooked, although it usually accompanies oral infection. Symptomatic patients may present with dysphagia, reflux or pain on swallowing. Several investigators have shown that the presence of esophageal candidosis is not always accompanied by symptoms or oral candidosis (Pennazio *et al.*, 1992). Patients with esophageal candidosis have lower CD4 counts and CD4:CD8 ratios than those with oral infection alone suggesting that spread beyond the oral cavity may occur later in the disease (Lopez-Dupla *et al.*, 1992). However, in order to be certain of the extent of spread beyond the oral cavity, the diagnosis can be confirmed by endoscopy or barium swallow. Dual infections with herpes simplex virus (HSV) and *Candida* are common.

Systemic candidosis or invasion of the lower respiratory tract is uncommon in AIDS patients, although line-associated candidemia has been recorded.

Laboratory diagnosis

The methods used for the diagnosis of oropharyngeal candidosis in the AIDS patient do not differ substantially from those used in other patient groups. The main techniques are direct microscopy of oral smears and culture (Odds, 1988). Like other immunocompromised patients, positive mouth cultures may merely reflect colonization and laboratory findings have to be related to the symptoms and clinical appearances. Often the numbers of colonies obtained are very large and quantitative culture techniques have been advocated by some. In most AIDS patients *C. albicans* is the main pathogen although other species may be isolated and can, on occasions, cause disease. Examples include *Candida glabrata, C. tropicalis* and *C. krusei*.

Treatment

In non-immunocompromised patients the main treatments for oropharyngeal candidosis are topical nystatin or amphotericin B (which is available in Europe but not in USA), miconazole oral gel and clotrimazole troches (which are available in the USA but not in most European countries). There is very little to choose between these compounds in terms of treatment response although patients may find that some of the topical preparations such as nystatin suspension have an unpleasant taste. There is also considerable variation in the antifungal concentration in some of these topical preparations; nystatin vaginal tablets contain more drug than the conventional oral pastille and can be used to treat oral disease despite their unpleasant taste. Adjunctive measures such as denture care or oral antiseptic washes with chlorhexidine or povidone iodine may also be necessary (Greenspan, Greenspan and Winkler, 1988).

While these topical preparations may work in early HIV infection in most well-established AIDS cases, as with other conditions associated with severe immunodeficiency (Degregorio, Lee and Ries, 1982), it is necessary to use orally absorbed compounds such at ketoconazole, fluconazole and itraconazole. Ketoconazole is normally

effective in doses of 200 mg daily. However, there is evidence that absorption of ketoconazole may be reduced in some AIDS patients (Lake-Bakaar *et al.*, 1988) and therefore higher doses, 400 mg daily, are often used with success. Fluconazole is given in doses of 50–100 mg daily (Dupont and Drouhet, 1992). The clinical and mycological responses with this drug are generally rapid with significant reduction in oral *Candida* loads occurring after 4 days. Itraconazole is effective for oral candidosis in doses of 100 mg daily. Generally it is slower than fluconazole and in many AIDS patients it is advisable to use higher doses of 200 mg daily as absorption may be impaired in some (Grant and Clissold, 1989). A new oral solution of itraconazole may obviate these difficulties.

The most appropriate strategy for controlling symptomatic oral candidosis over long periods in the AIDS patient is still the subject of debate. Continuous administration of ketoconazole or fluconazole over weeks and months has been associated with breakthrough of infection or clinical tolerance and, in some cases, by the emergence of true drug resistance (Korting *et al.*, 1988; Dupont, 1992). The scientific basis for this phenomenon is not well understood nor is it known how and when resistance arises (Smith *et al.*, 1986). A recent study involving genotyping isolates taken from recurrent infections in HIV-positive patients showed that both infection with the same organism and infection with a new strain were possible explanations for re-emergence of infection (Powderly, Robinson and Keath, 1993).

Resistance has been reported most frequently with fluconazole and ketoconazole rather than itraconazole. This may be due to the fact that fewer AIDS patients have received long-term itraconazole, although it is also possible that there is an intrinsic difference in the facility with which the use of different azole drugs leads to microbial resistance. Whatever the reason, most physicians use a course of antifungal – oral or topical – to induce clinical remission and then, if possible, stop therapy while retreating each severe symptomatic relapse. There is no evidence that this policy is less likely to lead to relapse of infection or the emergence of antifungal resistance even though it seems a reasonable approach to management.

In esophageal candidosis, treatment with 10–30 days' fluconazole at 100 mg daily is often sufficient. Itraconazole 200 mg daily for 15–30 days or ketoconazole for similar periods is also effective. Intravenous therapy with amphotericin B is only rarely required.

CRYPTOCOCCOSIS

Cryptococcosis is an opportunistic fungal infection caused by the encapsulated yeast, *Cryptococcus neoformans*. There are two variants of this species known as the *neoformans* and *gattii* varieties respectively. They differ in their host preference, growth requirements and epidemiology (Swinne-Desgain and de Vroey, 1987). *Cryptococcus neoformans* var. *neoformans* is found in nature in pigeon excreta whereas the natural habitat of *C. neoformans* var. *gattii* is debris from certain species of Eucalyptus tree. Symptomatic infection occurs in both previously healthy individuals, usually in the tropics, and immunocompromised patients. The *gattii* variant is generally associated with infection in otherwise healthy individuals whereas the majority of patients with AIDS who develop cryptococcosis are infected with the *neoformans* form. It is one of the main infectious complications of HIV infection (Swinne-Desgain and de Vroey, 1987). Infection rates vary in different countries. In Zaire it is estimated that 12% of AIDS patients have cryptococcosis whereas in the USA 4–7% are infected with the organism (Dismukes, 1988); in the UK it is slightly fewer, 3–4%.

Cryptococcus invades the lungs after inhalation and is disseminated from this site causing fungemia and meningitis. A proportion of normal individuals are sensitized to this fungus, suggesting that subclinical exposure occurs in the community. In addition to AIDS patients, individuals with lymphoma, sarcoidosis and those receiving systemic corticosteroids are susceptible to infection.

A number of host immune defects, chiefly T lymphocyte-mediated abnormalities, predispose to infection. However, in addition, it appears that *Cryptococcus* may also possess factors which allow it to survive *in vivo*, for instance, by evading host defenses. Its mucopolysaccharide capsule is such a protective device (Bancroft, Rockett and Collins, 1992). The mechanisms of uptake of encapsulated versus nonencapsulated cryptococci by macrophages differ, with the latter being engulfed quicker and in greater numbers. Other potential virulence factors of *Cryptococcus neoformans* include diphenyl oxidase which is involved in the biosynthesis of fungal melanin.

Clinical features

The initial infection by *Cryptococcus neoformans* follows inhalation but the clinical features of pulmonary cryptococcosis are very variable. However, a significant proportion of AIDS patients with cryptococcosis may have asymptomatic or symptomatic lung infections. In a retrospective study of 31 patients in North Carolina 12 had pulmonary changes (Cameron *et al.*, 1991). Patients may present with fever, cough, dyspnea or chest pain. Even though some patients may present with respiratory symptoms, many either have or subsequently develop evidence of wider dissemination (Chechani and Kamholz, 1990). The radiological findings of pulmonary cryptococcosis in AIDS patients are also variable, but interstitial infiltrates and hilar lymphadenopathy are the two commonest features (Miller, Edelman and Miller, 1990) but in addition miliary nodules, pleural effusion or even widespread uni- or bilateral opacification can be found (Newman *et al.*, 1987; Wasser and Talvera, 1987). Unlike pulmonary cryptococcosis in the non-AIDS population large intrapulmonary nodules are uncommon in AIDS patients.

These observations should be viewed in the context of the sick patient and, generally, cryptococcosis is an uncommon cause of diffuse pneumonia in AIDS. More usually, lung involvement is discovered by chance on the chest radiograph in a patient with fungemia, meningitis or skin lesions due to *C. neoformans*. The symptoms of cryptococcal meningitis are often suppressed with patients developing a febrile episode together with headache and confusion. Loss of consciousness may also occur in the later stages of the disease. Focal cerebral signs and neck stiffness are less common in AIDS. The skin lesions of cryptococcosis resemble a variety of different entities from molluscum contagiosum to cellulitis or cold abscesses.

Laboratory diagnosis

The laboratory diagnosis is simplified by the fact that the cryptococcus can be seen by direct microscopy in clinical samples such as sputum or cerebrospinal fluid (CSF) by delineating the capsule with an opaque medium, India ink or Nigrosin. This is a useful test although it may be difficult at times to interpret if the organisms have a thin capsule. In the case of chest infection bronchoalveolar lavage fluid and pleural aspirates have both proved fruitful sources for positive microscopy and/or culture. Bronchial washings are a further method of diagnosis. Furthermore, rapid processing of smears from washings or lavage fluid is as useful as transbronchial biopsies for establishing a diagnosis; culture of transbronchial biopsies is inferior to isolation from material obtained using the other methods (Malabonga, Basti and Kam-

holz, 1991). *Cryptococcus neoformans* is readily grown in culture on Sabouraud's medium. Identification is not difficult using urease production or pigmentation on Niger seed agar. There is a rapid detection system for circulating cryptococcal antigen (capsular polysaccharide) using either latex agglutination or ELISA, both of which are accurate and positive in a very high percentage of cases. Antigen detection can also be used as a guide to prognosis as high initial or post-treatment titers indicate the likelihood of a poor response. False positive antigen tests are rare. There are a number of features which are unusual in the diagnosis of cryptococcal infection in patients with AIDS compared to other groups. These include:

1. high frequency of positive blood cultures;
2. high antigen titers in serum which are often greater than those in CSF;
3. slow fall of antigen levels with therapy.

Treatment

The strategy for treatment of cryptococcosis in patients with AIDS is also different to that employed in other groups of patients. Some estimate of the extent of infection can be obtained by positive blood cultures or CSF samples, the presence of disseminated cutaneous lesions, high antigen titers and pulmonary infiltrates, although the possibility that a second type of lung infection is present must be borne in mind. In each case it is important to exclude meningitis by examining and culturing CSF.

Current trends in the treatment of AIDS patients have been established by a number of clinical studies and observations. Most have specifically concentrated on patients with cryptococcal meningitis and the effect of therapy on pulmonary changes was not recorded. There are however certain principles of therapy which are applicable across a range of clinical presentations. Generally it is accepted that long-term suppressive therapy after an initial phase of treatment is necessary in order to prevent relapse. The choice of initial therapy is generally amphotericin B. One large study has shown that although the long-term remission rates are similar after induction therapy with both amphotericin B (0.3 mg/kg/day) and fluconazole (200–400 mg/day), a higher percentage of those dying in the first two weeks of therapy were receiving fluconazole (Saag et al., 1992). For this reason an initial phase of intravenous therapy with amphotericin B (AMB) at 0.4–0.6 mg/kg daily for 2–3 weeks is given in most centers. Some would also use the combination of AMB and flucytosine (5FC) although the value of using this drug combination in AIDS patients, unlike other groups, has not been formally published as yet in a large clinical trial. One smaller study in 20 evaluable patients found that none of the 6 patients receiving AMB 0.7 mg/kg daily for 1 week and 3 times weekly for 9 weeks plus flucytosine 150 mg/kg daily failed to achieve remission whereas 8 of 14 patients receiving 400 mg of fluconazole daily failed (Larsen, Leal and Chan, 1990). A potential disadvantage of using 5FC is the risk of drug-related bone marrow depression. Plasma 5FC levels should be monitored through treatment.

Fluconazole is often used as an alternative primary therapy. The comparative merits of this and other drugs or dosages in the initial phases of treatment are less clear. The dose of fluconazole employed in the study referred to previously (Saag et al., 1992) was 200–400 mg daily and it is not known how this drug would perform compared to AMB if the higher dose ranges used in other systemic fungal infections, 600–800 mg daily, were to be used. There are fewer studies of itraconazole as primary therapy for cryptococcosis in AIDS and at doses of 200 mg daily it is probably less effective than AMB and 5FC (Gans et al., 1992). Once again the role of higher doses of itraconazole, such as 400–600 mg daily, is unknown. Another alternative to AMB would be a lipid complex formulation containing amphotericin B such as the liposomal form (AmBisome) or the colloidal dispersion (ABCD). Preliminary data with AmBisome suggest that it is effective in cryptococcosis although its value compared to AMB is not known (Coker et al., 1992).

Whatever the initial choice of therapy the likely long-term outlook is not good and relapse occurs in over 50% of patients within 6 months. For this reason it is usual practice to continue therapy, after the initial 2–3-week phase of treatment, with an oral drug, commonly fluconazole in doses of 200–400 mg daily. Oral itraconazole at 400 mg daily and intermittent intravenous AMB 2–3 times weekly are alternatives. Some clue to course and outcome is given by following antigen titers and cultures. However with declining CD4 counts relapse occurs in some patients. Antifungal therapy should be continued indefinitely.

The management of AIDS patients with lung disease is not substantially different to those with other forms of cryptococcosis. However, as relapse is likely to be associated with the continued presence of extrapulmonary cryptococcosis, lung lesions should not be used as the sole criterion for monitoring progress. Monitoring serum and CSF antigen levels, blood and urine cultures and CT scans all play a role in assessing progress.

HISTOPLASMOSIS

Histoplasma capsulatum is a dimorphic fungus which is found in soil contaminated with bird or bat excreta. The disease caused by this organism is endemic in many parts of the world, although not in Europe. It is mainly confined to the Central and Eastern USA, Central and South America, Africa and the Far East. The fungus gains entry to the body through inhalation of spores (conidia). In the healthy host most infections are controlled by the immune system without the appearance of clinical disease, the only evidence of past infection being a positive delayed type skin test reaction to histoplasmin. Active infection may subsequently develop and involve the lung either in the form of chronic cavitary pulmonary disease, seen mainly in smokers or those with pre-existing lung disease, or as a disseminated infiltrative process, similar to miliary tuberculosis. Other forms of pulmonary presentation include a segmental infiltrate, with fever, chest pain and cough in the acute pulmonary form of the disease, which usually follows massive exposure to the organism, or as a solitary asymptomatic 'coin' lesion.

Estimates of exposure rates to *H. capsulatum* are based on the prevalence of positive reactions in the general population to intradermal histoplasmin tests. These range from over 80% in parts of Kentucky and Tennessee to about 60% in Trinidad to 20% or less in most African countries. As control of infection by the host is largely dependent on T lymphocyte responses it is to be anticipated that infection rates amongst the AIDS population would be high in endemic areas. This indeed appears to be the case. It is estimated that the prevalence of infection in the AIDS population in low endemic areas of the USA is 5% but may reach 75% in highly endemic regions (Sarosi and Johnson, 1990).

Clinical features

The chief symptoms of histoplasmosis in AIDS patients are fever, cough and weight loss (Neubauer and Bodensteiner, 1992). Splenomegaly, hepatomegaly or lymphadenopathy are common signs. There is often anemia, leukopenia and thrombocytopenia indicating bone marrow infiltration. Lung changes are usually micronodular (Negroni *et al.*, 1992) although less commonly other signs such as pleural effusion may occur (Marshall *et al.*, 1990). In AIDS patients the usual pattern of this disease is for the infection to spread rapidly

beyond the lungs (Graybill, 1988). Although in some, signs of lung disease are found, dyspnea is usually associated with diffuse pulmonary infiltrates (Wheat, Slama and Zeckel, 1985).

Laboratory diagnosis

The diagnosis is made by demonstrating the organisms in sputum, often difficult in view of their small size (2–4 μm) or by culture. Sputum, blood and bone marrow are all suitable sources. Serology (antibody detection) is generally positive in patients with active infections although the results of the immunodiffusion and complement fixation tests, which are commonly used, are variable in AIDS patients. A recent test for the detection of antigen from the fungal cell wall is highly useful but unfortunately not widely available. This can also be applied to the detection of antigen in BAL fluid and appears to be useful in a high proportion of cases with pulmonary disease (Wheat *et al.*, 1992).

Treatment

The treatment of histoplasmosis in AIDS patients has changed over the past few years and oral itraconazole is generally used, except in severely ill patients. Doses employed have ranged from 200–400 mg for primary therapy over 4–6 weeks and 100–200 mg daily as suppressive treatment (Negroni *et al.*, 1992; Sharkey-Mathis *et al.*, 1993). As with cryptococcosis, treatment should be continued indefinitely as permanent eradication of infection does not appear to be achievable. Fluconazole has been used in fewer patients and appears to be useful in some although probably not as active as itraconazole. Increase in fluconazole dosage from 100 to 400 or 800 mg daily did not appear to improve the responses in the small number of patients treated (Sharkey-Mathis, 1993). For very severely ill patients initial therapy with amphotericin B (0.6–1.0 mg/kg daily) is advised.

COCCIDIOIDOMYCOSIS

The soil fungus, *Coccidioides immitis*, which is found in the arid regions of North, Central and South America, is a respiratory pathogen. This includes parts of California, Texas, Arizona and New Mexico, Mexico, Argentina and Colombia. Infection is rarely acquired in other parts of Latin America. The pathogenesis of coccidioidomycosis is rather similar to that seen with histoplasmosis with the majority of exposed individuals remaining asymptomatic but developing positive skin tests. After primary infection pulmonary infiltrates, pleural effusion and hilar adenopathy may develop, together with erythema multiforme or nodosum. Chronic (cavitary) pulmonary, coin lesions and miliary pulmonary disease may all occur. In therapeutically immunocompromised patients such as solid organ transplant patients, progressive pneumonia may develop. The same is true of patients with AIDS. In endemic areas the risk of active infection is high with 1 in 5 of AIDS patients in Arizona having the infection (Bronniman *et al.*, 1987). Severity of infection parallels the decline in CD4 counts.

Clinical features

Clinical signs of infection in the AIDS patient vary, often with the stage of the disease (Bronniman *et al.*, 1987; Fish *et al.*, 1990). Focal pulmonary infiltrates or pneumonia may occur but many have a progressive pneumonia with increasing breathlessness, pleuritic pain and cough. On X-ray diffuse interstitial infiltrates may occur and hilar lymphadenopathy is common. Infection disseminated to other sites including meninges or skin may occur but AIDS patients may also have extensive infections involving the liver and spleen without obvious localizing signs.

Laboratory diagnosis

The disease is diagnosed by observing the typical spherules, large spore-containing structures 25–80 μm in diameter, of the organism in sputum, lavage or biopsy material. This fungus can be isolated easily but is highly infective in the laboratory and the diagnostic laboratory should be warned if this diagnosis is under consideration. Serology using immunodiffusion and complement fixation tests or immunoelectrophoresis is used for diagnosis; but as with histoplasmosis results of serodiagnosis are variable in AIDS patients.

Treatment

Treatment is difficult in this group of patients. Generally, intravenous amphotericin B (1 mg/kg daily) is used initially but subsequently oral itraconazole or fluconazole can be given for long-term suppression. There is less evidence of the efficacy of the latter drugs, as yet, as primary therapy in AIDS patients. Overall, at least 40% of patients may perish despite therapy.

INFECTION DUE TO *PENICILLIUM MARNEFFEI*

In 1959 a new fungal species was described as an isolate from a bamboo rat originating from Vietnam (Segretain, 1959). The organism, *Penicillium marneffei*, also caused an infection in a laboratory assistant. Subsequent case reports confirmed the existence of this infection in patients originating from or visiting South East Asia. Thailand and the southern provinces of China appeared to be the main foci of infection (Jayanetra *et al.*, 1984; Deng and Connor, 1985). The pathogenic form of the fungus multiplies in tissue as a small intracellular organism which resembles a yeast morphologically, but which divides by transverse fission. Previous cases had generally been misdiagnosed by histopathology as histoplasmosis. Subsequently cases have been described in patients with HIV infection (Peto *et al.*, 1988; Piehl, Kaplan and Haber, 1988; Viviani and Tortorano, 1990). In 1990, Viviani reviewed 7 cases in AIDS patients mainly from Europe, but who had travelled to SE Asia. With the spread of HIV infection in South East Asia a more serious problem has now emerged. In Thailand, for instance, *P. marneffei* has emerged as one of the major secondary infectious complications of AIDS, particularly in the north of the country. This suggests that exposure to the organisms is sufficiently great to ensure that a high proportion of immunocompromised patients develop active infections.

The portal of entry of *P. marneffei* is not known but infection is thought to follow inhalation in a similar way to that seen with the dimorphic fungal pathogens such as *Histoplasma capsulatum*. Symptomatic pulmonary infection is seen in patients with this infection. However, in the absence of an intradermal test, it is not known what proportion of the population is sensitized subclinically.

Clinical features

Most AIDS patients present with disseminated infection. This may be diagnosed on the basis of a solitary extra-pulmonary lesion often on the skin or oral mucosa or multiple infiltrates in the liver or spleen (hepatosplenomegaly) or bone marrow (pancytopenia). Alternatively, *P. marneffei* infections must be considered in the differential diagnosis of unexplained fever in patients who have travelled to an endemic area. The pulmonary changes are not diagnostic and in AIDS patients diffuse micronodular infiltrates may be the main sign of respiratory infection.

Laboratory diagnosis

The organisms of *P. marneffei* are small structures 2–4 μm in diameter. They are difficult to see but can be outlined by Giemsa stains in smears from bone marrow, skin lesions and in blood films. The organism can be grown on conventional media. The histopathological features such as septum formation can be shown best with methenamine silver or periodic acid Schiff (PAS) stains. Specific serological tests are not widely available.

Treatment

The main treatment for *P. marneffei* infection has been intravenous amphotericin B. However there is now evidence that oral itraconazole produces excellent results which in most patients are equivalent to those seen with amphotericin B (Supparatpinyo *et al.*, 1993); in addition, isolates of the fungus are generally sensitive to itraconazole *in vitro*. Fluconazole is less active *in vitro* and there is evidence of a higher rate of clinical failure in patients receiving this drug. Generally, itraconazole is probably the treatment of choice in AIDS, except in the acutely ill patient when amphotericin B is usually given. It is clear, though, that relapse generally follows stopping initial therapy after apparent clinical recovery and long-term suppression with itraconazole is used, as in histoplasmosis. Based on *in vitro* data intravenous miconazole or ketoconazole would be alternative drugs.

OTHER DIMORPHIC FUNGAL PATHOGENS

Other dimorphic fungal infections which affect the lungs such as blastomycosis and paracoccidioidomycosis (Goldani *et al.*, 1989; Herd *et al.*, 1990) have been infrequently recorded in AIDS patients. The reasons for this are not clear although the principal modes of host defense may not depend on

T lymphocytes in these infections. A further factor may be the low level of exposure to these organisms amongst the at-risk population.

ASPERGILLOSIS

Invasive infections due to aspergilli are most often seen in neutropenic subjects although for some years it has been recognized that other groups, including patients with multi-organ failure and solid organ, including heart transplant recipients, may develop invasive aspergillosis. There are various patterns of invasion seen in these groups, including rapidly progressive intrapulmonary, disseminated or paranasal invasion. It has been shown that invasive aspergillosis is an increasingly recognized, although uncommon, complication in AIDS. A recent paper reviewed 18 cases of *Aspergillus* infection in AIDS patients, with antemortem colonization being recorded in a somewhat larger number (Pursell, Telzak and Armstrong, 1992). A further study of 37 patients showed that in 18 the lung was the only site of infection and in a further 10 other sites were involved as well. Other sites of infection were the brain, heart, sinuses, kidney and skin (Minamoto, Barlam and Vander Els, 1992). Overall, a small percentage of AIDS patients have positive sputum cultures for aspergilli (usually *A. fumigatus*), 3% in one study as a single episode. Of these an estimated 20% had infection (Daleine *et al.*, 1993).

Clinical features

The clinical signs of invasion in AIDS patients are not substantially different to those seen in other patient groups, with invasive pulmonary disease being the main sign of disease. Tracheobronchial invasion may also occur. Usually the symptoms are non-specific and include fever, cough and dyspnea (Denning *et al.*, 1991; Miller *et al.*, 1994). Chest pain and hemoptysis can occur but

are less common. In many AIDS patients the progress of invasive pulmonary aspergillosis is not as rapid as that seen in the neutropenic group and the connection with colonization suggests that invasion may follow prolonged growth of aspergilli from pulmonary secretions. AIDS patients with aspergillosis are often in the later stages of infection and may also have received corticosteroid therapy or be neutropenic; in the latter case this may follow coincidental therapy such as zidovudine or ganciclovir. Other risk factors include administration of multiple antibiotics and alcohol abuse. X-ray changes include upper lobe cavitation which carries a high risk of severe hemoptysis. However, the air crescent sign, which is a common radiological feature of infection in neutropenic patients, is uncommon in this group (Miller *et al.*, 1994). Other patients have diffuse alveolar infiltration which may remain strikingly stable over a number of weeks. Another presentation is with atelectasis which may be transient. Such patients are likely to have tracheobronchial infection where masses of invading hyphae may clog airways. Pleural invasion with effusion can also occur. Occasionally, ill but radiologically normal patients may be found at postmortem to have aspergillosis.

Laboratory diagnosis

The diagnosis of invasive aspergillosis is difficult but can be established by the presence of aspergilli in sputum or BAL by culture. The microscopy of this material is suggestive but not diagnostic of aspergillosis. In addition some patients with the tracheobronchial form of this infection may expectorate casts which are positive for fungus by direct microscopy or histology. Transbronchial biopsies are more often negative. The isolation of *Aspergillus* species from sputum or lavage fluid should be regarded as a potentially sinister sign in AIDS patients and, if accompanied by appropriate clinical findings, an indication for therapy. As with other groups of patients serology is less helpful in the diagnosis of invasive aspergillosis. The choices rest between antibody and antigen detection tests (Rogers, Haynes and Barnes, 1990). While a single test may be positive it is often necessary to screen serial samples before a positive response is detected. At present there are few commercially available antibody or antigen detection systems and serology is best regarded as an adjunct to diagnosis. Newer methodologies such as the polymerase chain reaction are still in a development phase for the diagnosis of this condition (Tang *et al.*, 1993).

Treatment

There have been no comparative studies of itraconazole or amphotericin B as treatments in this group, although in other groups of patients both are active if treatment is initiated early in the course of infection. At present initial therapy with intravenous amphotericin B (1 mg/kg daily) should be used in severely ill patients, with itraconazole being the principal alternative. The latter can also be used in slowly progressive disease. There are few data at present on the value of long-term suppressive treatment after primary therapy. Unfortunately, many patients present with aspergillosis late in the course of AIDS and the mortality rate is high despite therapy.

CONCLUSION

Fungal infections of the respiratory system are seen regularly in patients with AIDS. In general these are confined to well-recognized conditions such as cryptococcosis, histoplasmosis and aspergillosis although rare pathogens can be involved. It is important carefully to consider fungal isolates from sputum or BLA in AIDS patients together with clinical features in order to make appropriate decisions on management.

As different immune defects are found in HIV disease so the range of possible lung pathogens is broad. Reports of other opportunistic fungal infections such as zygomycosis (mucormycosis) and pulmonary infection due to *Fusarium* are therefore not unexpected (del Palacio Hernanz *et al.*, 1989).

REFERENCES

Alcabes, P., Schoenbaum, E.E. and Klein, R.S. (1993) Correlates of the rate of decline of CD4$^+$ lymphocytes among injection drug users infected with the human immunodeficiency virus. *American Journal of Epidemiology*, **137**, 989–1000.

Bancroft, G.J., Rockett, E.R. and Collins, H.L. (1992) Capsule synthesis and immunity to *Cryptococcus neoformans*. In *New Strategies in Fungal Disease*. Churchill Livingstone, Edinburgh, pp. 179–91.

Bronniman, D.A., Adam, R.D. and Galgiani *et al.* (1987) Coccidioidomycosis in the acquired immunodeficiency syndrome. *Annals of Internal Medicine*, **106**, 372–79.

Cameron, M.L., Bartlett, J.A., Gallis, H.A. and Waskin, H.A. (1991) Manifestations of pulmonary cryptococcosis in patients with acquired immunodeficiency syndrome. *Reviews of Infectious Diseases*, **13**, 64–67.

Chechani, V. and Kamholz, S.L. (1990) Pulmonary manifestations of disseminated cryptococcosis in patients with AIDS. *Chest*, **98**, 1060–66.

Coker, R.J., Viviani, M., Gazzard, B.G. *et al.* (1993) Treatment of cryptococcosis with liposomal amphotericin B (Ambisome) in 23 patients with AIDS. *AIDS*, **7**, 829–35.

Daleine, G., Salmon, D., Lucet, J.F. *et al.* (1993) Frequency of bronchopulmonary isolation of *Aspergillus* species in patients infected with immunodeficiency virus. *Pathologie Biologie*, **41**, 237–41.

Degregorio, M.W., Lee, W.M.F. and Ries, C.A. (1982) *Candida* infections in patients with acute leukaemia: ineffectiveness of nystatin prophylaxis and relationship between oropharyngeal and systemic candidiasis. *Cancer*, **50**, 2780–84.

del Palacio Hernanz, A., Vera Casado, A., Fernandez Lopez, A. *et al.* (1989) Infeccion oportunista pulmonar por *Fusarium moniliforme* en paciente con SIDA. *Revista Iberica de Micologia*, **6**, 144–46.

Deng, Z. and Connor, D.H. (1985) Progressive disseminated penicilliosis caused by *Penicillium marneffei*: report of eight cases and differentiation of the causative organism from *Histoplasma capsulatum. American Journal of Clinical Pathology*, **84**, 323–27.

Denning, D.W., Follansbee, S.E., Scolaro, M. *et al.* (1991) Pulmonary aspergillosis in the acquired immunodeficiency syndrome. *New England Journal of Medicine*, **324**, 654–62.

Dismukes, W.E. (1988) Cryptococcal meningitis in patients with AIDS. *Journal of Infectious Diseases*, **157**, 624–27.

Dupont, B. (1992) Antifungal therapy in AIDS patients, in *New Strategies in Fungal Disease* (eds J.E. Bennett, R.J. Hay and P.K. Peterson), Churchill Livingstone, Edinburgh, pp. 290–300.

Dupont, B. and Drouhet, E. (1992) Fluconazole in the management of oropharyngeal candidosis in a predominantly HIV antibody positive group of patients. *Journal of Medical and Veterinary Mycology*, **26**, 67–71.

Fetter, A., Partisani, M., Koenig, H. *et al.* (1993) Asymptomatic oral *Candida albicans* carriage in HIV-infection: frequency and predisposing factors. *Journal of Oral Pathology and Medicine*, **22**, 57–59.

Fish, D.G., Ampel, N.M., Galgiani, J.N. *et al.* (1990) Coccidioidomycosis during human immunodeficiency virus infection. *Medicine*, **69** 384–98.

Gans, J. de, Portegies, Tiessens, G. *et al.* (1992) Itraconazole compared with amphotericin B plus flucytosine in AIDS patients with cryptococcal meningitis. *AIDS*, **6**, 185–90.

Goldani, L.S., Martinez, R., Landell, G.A.M. *et al.* (1989) Paracoccidioidomycosis in a patient with acquired immunodeficiency syndrome. *Mycopathologia*, **105**, 71–74.

Gottlieb, M.S., Schroff, R., Schanker, H.M. *et al.* (1981) *Pneumocystis carinii* pneumonia and mucosal candidiasis in previously healthy homosexual men. *New England Journal of Medicine*, **305**, 1425–30.

Grant, S.M. and Clissold, S.P. (1989) Itraconazole. A review of its pharmacodynamic and pharmocokinetic properties, and therapeutic use in superficial and systemic mycoses. *Drugs*, **37**, 310–44.

Graybill, J.R. (1988) Histoplasmosis in AIDS. *Journal of Infectious Diseases*, **1578**, 623–26.

Greenspan, J.S., Greenspan, D. and Winkler, J.R. (1988) Diagnosis and management of the oral manifestations of HIV infection and AIDS. *Infectious Disease Clinics of North America*, **9**, 99–96.

Herd, A.M., Greenfield, S.B., Thompson, G.W.S. and Brunham, R.C. (1990) Miliary blastomycosis and HIV infection. *Canadian Medical Association Journal*, **143**, 1329–31.

Jayanetra, P., Nitiyanant, P., Ajello, L. *et al.* (1984) *Penicilliosis marneffei* in Thailand: report of five human cases. *American Journal of Tropical Medicine and Hygiene*, **33**, 637–44.

Katz, M.H., Greenspan, D., Westenhouse, J. *et al.* (1992) Progression to AIDS in HIV-infected homosexual and bisexual men with hairy leucoplakia and oral candidiasis. *AIDS*, **6**, 95–100.

Korting, H.C., Ollert, M., Georgii, A. and Froschl, M. (1988) *In vitro* susceptibilities and biotypes of *Candida albicans* isolates from the oral cavities of patients infected with human immunodeficiency virus. *Journal of Clinical Microbiology*, **26**, 2626–31.

Lake-Bakaar, G., Tom, W., Lake-Bakaar, D. *et al.* (1988) Gastropathy and ketoconazole malabsorption in the acquired immunodeficiency syndrome. (AIDS). *Annals of Internal Medicine*, **109**, 471–75.

Larsen, R.A., Leal, M.A. and Chan, L.S. (1990) Fluconazole compared with amphotericin B plus flucytosine for cryptococcal meningitis in AIDS: a randomised trial. *Annals of Internal Medicine*, **113**, 183–87.

Lin, R.Y. and Goodhart, P. (1993) The role of oral candidiasis in survival and hospitalization patterns: analysis of an inner city hospital immunodeficiency virus/acquired immune deficiency syndrome registry. *American Journal of Medical Science*, **306**, 345–53.

Lopez-Dupla, M., Mora Sanz, P., Pintado Garcia, V. *et al.* (1992) Clinical, endoscopic, immunologic and therapeutic aspects of oropharyngeal and esophageal candidiasis in HIV-infected patients: a survey of 114 cases. *American Journal of Gastroenterology*, **87**, 1771–76.

Malabonga, V.M., Basti, J. and Kamholz, S.L. (1991) Utility of bronchoscopic sampling techniques for cryptococcal disease in AIDS. *Chest*, **99**, 370–72.

Marshall, B.C., Cox, J.K., Carroll, K.C. and Morrison, R.E. (1990) Histoplasmosis as a cause of pleural effusion in the acquired immunodeficiency syndrome. *American Journal of Medical Science*, **300**, 98–101.

Miller, W.T., Edelman, J.M. and Miller, W.T. (1990) Cryptococcal pulmonary infection in patients with AIDS: radiological appearance. *Radiology*, **175**, 725–28.

Miller, W.T., Sais, G.J., Frank, I. *et al.* (1994) Pulmonary aspergillosis in patients with AIDS. Clinical and radiographic correlations. *Chest*, **105**, 37–44.

Minamoto, G.Y., Barlam, T.F. and Vander Els, N.J. (1992) Invasive aspergillosis in patients with AIDS. *Clinics in Infectious Disease*, **14**, 66–74.

Negroni, R., Taborda, A., Robies, A.M. and Archevala, A. (1992) Itraconazole in the treatment of histoplasmosis associated with AIDS. *Mycoses*, **35**, 281–87.

Neubauer, M.A. and Bodensteiner, D.C. (1992) Disseminated histoplasmosis in patients with AIDS. *Southern Medical Journal*, **85**, 1166–70.

Newman, T.G., Soni, A., Acaron, S. and Huang, C.T. (1987) Pleural cryptococcosis in the acquired immunodeficiency syndrome. *Chest*, **91**, 459–61.

Odds, F.C. (1988) *Candida and candidosis*. Baillière Tindall, London.

Pennazio, M., Arrigoni, A., Spandra, M. *et al.* (1992) Endoscopy to detect oral and oesophageal candidiasis in acquired immune deficiency syndrome. *Italian Journal of Gastroenterology*, **24**, 324–27.

Peto, T.E.A., Bull, R., Millard, P.R. *et al.* (1988) Systemic mycosis due to *Penicillium marneffei* in a patient with antibody to human immunodeficiency virus. *Journal of Infection*, **16**, 285–88.

Piehl, M.R., Kaplan, R.L. and Haber, M.H. (1988) Disseminated penicilliosis in a patient with acquired immunodeficiency syndrome. *Archives of Pathology and Laboratory Medicine*, **112**, 1262–65.

Powderly, W.G., Robinson, K. and Keath, E.J. (1993) Molecular epidemiology of recurrent oral candidiasis in human immunodeficiency virus-positive patients; evidence for two patterns of recurrence. *Journal of Infectious Diseases*, **168**, 463–66.

Pursell, K.J., Telzak, E.E. and Armstrong, D. (1992) *Aspergillus* species colonization and invasive disease in patients with AIDS. *Clinics in Infectious Disease*, **14**, 141–48.

Rogers, T.R., Haynes, K.A. and Barnes, R.A. (1990) Value of antigen detection in predicting invasive pulmonary aspergillosis. *Lancet*, **336**, 1210–13.

Saag, M.E., Powderly, W.G., Cloud, G.A. *et al.* (1992) Comparison of amphotericin B with fluconazole in the treatment of acute AIDS-associated cryptococcal meningitis. *New England Journal of Medicine*, **326**, 83–100.

Samaranayake, L.P. and Yaacob, H.B. (1990) Classification of oral candidosis, in *Oral Candidosis* (eds L.P. Samaranayake and T.W. MacFarlane) Wright, London, pp. 124–32.

Sarosi, G.A. and Johnson, P.C. (1990) Progressive disseminated histoplasmosis in the acquired immunodeficiency syndrome: a model for disseminated disease. *Seminars in Respiratory Disease*, **5**, 146–50.

Segretain, G. (1959) Description d'une nouvelle espece de penicillium: *Penicillium marneffei* n.sp. *Bulletin de la Société de Mycologie Française*, **75**, 412–16.

Sharkey-Mathis, P.K., Velez, J., Fetchick, R. and Graybill, J.R. (1993) Histoplasmosis in the acquired immunodeficiency syndrome (AIDS): treatment with itraconazole and fluconazole. *Journal of the Acquired Immunodeficiency Syndromes*, **6**, 809–19.

Smith, K.J., Warnock, D.W., Kennedy, C.T.C. *et al.* (1986) Azole resistance in *Candida albicans*. *Journal of Medical and Veterinary Mycology*, **24**, 133–44.

Supparatpinyo, K., Nelson, K.E., Merz, W.G. *et al.* (1993) Response to antifungal therapy by human immuno-deficiency virus infected patients with disseminated *Penicillium marneffei* infections and *in vitro* susceptibilities of isolates from clinical specimens. *Antimicrobial Agents and Chemotherapy*, **37**, 2407–11.

Swinne-Desgain, D. and de Vroey, C. (1987) Epidemiologie de la cryptoccose. *Revista Iberica de Micologia*, **4**, 77–83.

Tang, C.M., Holden, D.W., Aufauvre-Brown, A. and Cohen, J. (1993) The detection of *Aspergillus* spp by the polymerase chain reaction and its evaluation in bronchoalveolar lavage fluid. *American Review of Respiratory Disease*, **148**, 1313–17.

Torssander, J., Morfeldt-Manson, L., Biberfeld, G. *et al.* (1987) Oral *Candida albicans* in HIV infection. *Scandinavian Journal of Infectious Diseases*, **19**, 291–95.

Viviani, M.A. and Tortorano, A.M. (1990) Unusual mycoses in AIDS patients, in *Mycoses in AIDS Patients* (eds H. Van den Bossche, D.W.R. Mackenzie, G. Cauwenbergh, J. Van Cutsem, E. Drouhet and B. Dupont). Plenum Press, New

York, pp. 147–53.

von-Eiff, M., Roos, N., Fegeter, W., von-Eiff, C. *et al.* (1994) Pulmonary fungal infections in immunocompromised patients: incidence and risk factors. *Mycoses*, **37**(9–10), 329–35.

Wasser, L. and Talvera, W. (1987) Pulmonary cryptococcosis in AIDS. *Chest*, **92**, 692–5.

Wheat, L.J., Connolly-Stringfield, P., Williams, B. *et al.* (1992) Diagnosis of histoplasmosis in patients with the acquired immunodeficiency syndrome by detection of *Histoplasma capsulatum* polysaccharide antigen in bronchoalveolar lavage fluid. *American Journal of Respiratory Disease*, **145**, 1421–24.

Wheat, L.J., Slama, T.G. and Zeckel, M. (1985) Histoplasmosis in the acquired immunodeficiency syndrome. *American Journal of Medicine*, **78**, 203–10.

Barry S. Peters

This chapter deals with three different genuses of parasite, two protozoal and one nematode, that can cause pulmonary disease in patients with HIV infection and AIDS. These organisms are *Toxoplasma gondii*, *Cryptosporidium* sp. and *Strongyloides stercoralis*. Lung disease due to these organisms is usually only found in immunosuppressed individuals, for example, those with advanced HIV disease or AIDS.

TOXOPLASMA LUNG INFECTION

Toxoplasma gondii is an obligate intracellular protozoan. It is a common disease in birds and mammals, and is common in humans whether they are immunocompetent or immunosuppressed. Most cases of primary toxoplasma infection among the immunocompetent are asymptomatic, although a pyrexial illness with lymphadenopathy is the classical 'seroconversion illness'. Specific organ involvement can also rarely occur involving, for example, the lungs, liver, myocardium and pericardium.

Most cases of toxoplasmosis in immunosuppressed patients, such as those with AIDS, are due to reactivation of primary infection. Patients are invariably systemically unwell, with an accompanying pyrexia. The most common manifestation in AIDS patients is central nervous system (CNS) involvement with headache, confusion – which inevitably leads to coma if untreated – fitting and focal neurological signs. Toxoplasmosis in patients with AIDS is a fulminant and rapidly fatal condition if left untreated.

In patients with cancer, multisystem involvement, particularly of the lungs and heart, is common (Gleason and Hamlin, 1974). Multisystem disease is uncommon in AIDS, despite the fact that patients with AIDS have a high incidence of evidence of past infection with toxoplasmosis (Luft and Remington, 1988), and approximately a third of these develop CNS disease. For example, Navia and colleagues found that in 27 patients with cerebral toxoplasmosis, only 3 had evidence of disease outside of the CNS at autopsy (in the heart, lungs and prostate gland) (Navia *et al.*, 1986).

Pulmonary toxoplasmosis is, however, an increasingly reported complication of AIDS, and the lungs are the second commonest site of infection with *Toxoplasma gondii* (Marche *et al.*, 1989). The incidence of toxoplasma pneumonia is unknown, but varies from 4% (7/169) of AIDS patients who underwent bronchoscopy in one French series (Derouin *et al.*, 1990), to <1% (1/441) of AIDS patients with pneumonia in the USA (Murray *et al.*, 1984). This might partly reflect the increased prevalence of toxoplasma infection in France, and the fact that the investigation from the

AIDS and Respiratory Medicine. Edited by A. Zumla, M.A. Johnson and R.F. Miller. Published in 1997 by Chapman & Hall, London. ISBN 0 412 60140 0

USA was in the early years of the AIDS epidemic when there was less experience of diagnosing toxoplasma lung infection.

Although patients with lung involvement often also have CNS toxoplasmosis, pulmonary disease can also occur in the absence of neurological disease. For example, in one series of 13 HIV-infected patients with toxoplasma pneumonia, 10 had no evidence of CNS involvement (Oksenhendler *et al.*, 1990). Another series describes 6 patients with pulmonary toxoplasmosis but no neurological disease (Schnapp *et al.*, 1992).

After reviewing reported cases, Pomeroy and Filice have suggested a terminology for *Toxoplasma gondii* infection of the lungs (Pomeroy and Felice, 1992). They suggest that the term 'toxoplasma pneumonia' be restricted to cases in which the clinical features of pneumonia are the main presentation. They use the term 'pulmonary toxoplasmosis' to refer to the entire spectrum of pulmonary disease caused by *Toxoplasma gondii*, whether clinically apparent or not.

There is little to distinguish toxoplasma pneumonia clinically from *Pneumocystis carinii* pneumonia (PCP) (Schnapp *et al.*, 1992; Pomeroy and Felice, 1992). Hence cough and dyspnea are the commonest reported symptoms, and the physical signs in the chest are the same as for PCP. The cough in toxoplasma pneumonia is non-productive in the absence of other concomitant chest infections. Compared to patients immunosuppressed due to other causes, AIDS patients with pulmonary toxoplasmosis appear less likely to have lymphadenopathy or hepatosplenomegaly.

The chest radiograph is also non-specific and the most common appearance, diffuse interstitial infiltrates, is indistinguishable from PCP. Other radiological appearances have been reported, including micronodular infiltrates (Oksenhendler *et al.*, 1990; Tawney *et al.*, 1986; Prosmanne *et al.*, 1984), a predominantly coarse nodular pattern (Good-man and Schnapp, 1992), cavitation and lobar pneumonia (Cohen *et al.*, 1984).

Specific diagnosis is best achieved by means of bronchoalveolar lavage (Maguire *et al.*, 1986). *Toxoplasma gondii* trophozoites, pseudocysts and cysts are then best visualized on hematoxylin and eosin and Giemsa-stained cytospin preparations of bronchoalveolar lavage (BAL) fluid. Polymerase chain reaction (PCR) of BAL fluid is a much more sensitive technique for revealing toxoplasma in the lungs and might be positive for many cases of pulmonary toxoplasmosis that are not clinically apparent. For example, in one study the prevalence of pulmonary toxoplasmosis was assessed by a prospective analysis of 144 bronchoalveolar lavage (BAL) samples using competitive polymerase chain reaction (PCR) (Bretagne *et al.*, 1993). None of the samples from the 37 immunocompetent patients and only 1 sample (1.7%) from the 59 immunocompromised patients without human immunodeficiency virus infection were PCR-positive.

In contrast, *Toxoplasma gondii* DNA was found in 6 (14%) of 42 samples from patients with AIDS. In these 6 patients with AIDS, cerebral toxoplasmosis was also present, and clinical lung disease was not a feature in most of the cases.

In another study BAL fluid from 47 immunocompromised patients (26 with AIDS and 21 patients on immunosuppressive therapy) was analysed for the presence of *Toxoplasma gondii* DNA by means of PCR. *Toxoplasma gondii* was detected in BAL fluids from 3 patients with AIDS (6.4%). Pneumonia as the presenting feature of disseminated toxoplasmosis was confirmed by both clinical findings and by detection of *Toxoplasma gondii* DNA in blood obtained from two patients. The findings of this study indicate that PCR has potential value in the detection of *Toxoplasma gondii* as an etiologic agent of pneumonia in immunocompromised patients.

First-line therapy for toxoplasmosis is usually a combination of intravenous sulfadiazine and oral pyrimethamine (Peters *et al.*, 1994); both are folate antagonists which act synergistically to inhibit nucleic acid synthesis. In patients unable to tolerate sulfadiazine, clindamycin and pyrimethamine with calcium folinate is an effective alternative (Dannemann *et al.*, 1992), and other combinations include pyrethamine and clarithromycin (Fernandez-Martin *et al.*, 1991). Current therapies are inactive against the cyst form and so lifelong maintenance is necessary to reduce the likelihood of relapse. Atovoquone has been shown to be an effective alternative therapy (Kovacs, 1992; Araujo *et al.*, 1992) and is thought to be active against the cyst form. Atovoquone is licenced for use against *Pneumocystis carinii* pneumonia but is still being investigated for use in toxoplasmosis.

CRYPTOSPORIDIOSIS

Cryptosporidium belongs to the class Sporozoa, and because the number of species belonging to this genus has not been fully described, the organism is usually referred to as *Cryptosporidium* sp. The parasite undergoes its complete life-cycle within the intestine, although it may occasionally occur in other sites, such as the lung. The main symptom is a non-inflammatory diarrhea, which may prove intractable and life-threatening in the immunosuppressed patient. Although infection in man was originally thought to be zoonotic in origin, spread can occur from person to person either directly or indirectly, for example, through infected water sources.

Cryptosporidium infection of the respiratory tract is a rare manifestation that occurs in a variety of immunosuppressed states, including patients undergoing bone marrow transplantation (Kibbler *et al.*, 1987), patients with malignant lymphoma (Travis *et al.*, 1990), and children with severe combined immune deficiency (Kocoshis *et al.*, 1984). Cryptosporidium lung infection has also been described in AIDS, and although it appears to be rare, with relatively few reported cases in the literature, this condition is undoubtedly underdiagnosed.

Clinically, cryptosporidium infection of the lung appears indistinguishable from other causes of pneumonia in HIV-positive patients (Hojlyng and Jensen, 1988). The most frequent symptoms described in a recent review of cases were cough, 91%, dyspnea, 64%, and fever, 59% (Brea-Hernando *et al.*, 1993). Bowel disease due to cryptosporidium, usually with diarrhea, has accompanied most of the cases of respiratory cryptosporidiosis so far described. It is important to note, however, that there have been several cases where there have been no bowel symptoms whatsoever.

The majority of cases of cryptosporidial lung disease have concomitant pulmonary infection with other organisms, for example, *Pneumocystis carinii*, cytomegalovirus and pathogenic bacteria including mycobacteria. It is difficult in these cases to evaluate the significance of pulmonary cryptosporidial disease. In a series of 6 HIV-positive patients with cryptosporidium respiratory disease, however, cryptosporidium was the sole identifiable pathogen in 4 of the cases (Hojlyng and Jensen, 1988). These 4 patients were all alive at least 9 months after the diagnosis of their lung disease and this corroborates other evidence that cryptosporidial lung disease is usually not severe (Travis *et al.*, 1990).

Cryptosporidium in the lung is usually diagnosed by a Ziehl-Neelsen technique, or auramine stain, applied to lavage or biopsy material. These direct staining techniques may have a low sensitivity when compared with immunofluorescence or ELISA tests, and some authors suggest that these latter tests should be used preferentially (Hojlyng and Jensen, 1988). Cryptosporidium has not been grown on artificial media, and although cell culture techniques do exist (Current and Haynes, 1984), these are not suitable for routine diagnostics.

There is no widely accepted effective therapy for cryptosporidium. There have been several reports suggesting therapeutic value for various agents, for example, azithromycin (Dunne, 1993), letrazuril (Walach *et al.*, 1993) and paromomycin (Bissuel *et al.*, 1993), but their use in clinical practice is frequently disappointing and there are no large-scale trials demonstrating the effectiveness of these or other compounds.

Disseminated microsporidiosis due to *Encephalitozoon hellum* may give a clinical picture similar to disseminated cryptosporidiosis, and pulmonary involvement has been documented (Weber *et al.*, 1993).

STRONGYLOIDIASIS

Strongyloides stercoralis is a nematode that is endemic in warm countries throughout the world. This organism is unusual for a helminth in that it can reproduce parthogenetically in the gastrointestinal tract without the need for repeated exposure to new infection; this process is known as autoinfection. The infection can also be sexually transmitted.

Symptoms are rarely severe in immunocompetent individuals; in these cases, the patient may be symptomatic or present with abdominal pain, bloating, or rectal bleeding. In patients who are immunosuppressed with a defective cell-mediated immunity, the autoinfective capacity of the parasite is enhanced, and the organism completes its life-cycle and multiplies many times without the need for further infection. This leads to a great increase in the worm load and a hyperinfective state can result. In this state massive, acute disseminated infection with *Strongyloides* can occur in the lungs, brain, kidneys and pancreas.

Although infection with *Strongyloides* might be more severe in patients with immunosuppression, it does not appear to be more common in patients with HIV infection, and there have been very few cases of disseminated infection reported in this group. Extra-intestinal *Strongyloides* infection has therefore been removed from the revised classification of AIDS (Gachot *et al.*, 1990).

It is still important to have a high index of suspicion of hyper-infection with *Strongyloides* in any ill HIV-positive or immunosuppressed patient and to offer immediate management for this medical emergency. For example, if a pyrexial moribund patient with respiratory failure presents to the ward, and he has travelled or lived in a country endemic for *Strongyloides*, then disseminated infection with this organism must be considered. The patient might be shocked, with secondary bacterial septicemia or disseminated intravascular coagulation (DIC). The patient will probably urgently need infusion with plasma expanders, broad spectrum antibiotics and also fresh frozen plasma if there is DIC, as well as specific therapy against *Strongyloides*. There is a high early mortality from this condition, and it appears to be higher in HIV infection than other immunosuppressed states, with the majority of patients failing to survive the episode (Gompels *et al.*, 1991).

The main significance of pulmonary infection with *Strongyloides* is that it can occur in HIV-positive patients in the absence of marked symptoms elsewhere. In these cases lung infection with *Strongyloides* might be a forerunner of disseminated infection and therefore requires prompt diagnosis and treatment (Zumla and James, 1991). The pulmonary signs and symptoms of *Strongyloides* infection of the lung are non-specific, and should therefore be considered in any patient with HIV infection who has lived in, or traveled to, an endemic area. Although examination of the sputum might reveal the parasite in cases of pneumonia (Maayan *et al.*, 1987), bronchoscopy is a more sensitive technique for diagnosis; this is illustrated by the case in which I was involved where involvement of *Strongyloides* in the lungs was only discovered when bronchoscopy was performed (Gompels *et al.*, 1991).

Treatment of *Strongyloides stercoralis* infection is with thiabendazole, but there is a greater risk of treatment failure in HIV-positive patients (Lessnau, Can and Talavera, 1993). For this reason prolonged courses of treatment followed by maintenance regimens should be considered in patients with HIV infection. Ivermectin is a promising alternative treatment to thiabendazole. An open trial of ivermectin in HIV patients with *Strongyloides* bowel disease demonstrated a sustained clinical and parasitological cure in all 7 patients who took multiple doses of the drug therapy (Torres *et al.*, 1993); single dose therapy was less effective. However, we are not aware of any trials comparing the efficacy of drugs for the treatment of *Strongyloides* in AIDS.

REFERENCES

Araujo, F.G., Huskinson, M.J., Gutteridge, W.E. and Remington, J.S. (1992) *In vitro* and *in vivo* activities of the hydroxynaphthoquinone 566C80 against the cyst form of *Toxoplasma gondii*. *Antimicrobial Agents and Chemotherapy*, **36**, 326–30.

Bissuel, F., Cotte, L., Rabodonirina, M. *et al.* (1993) Paromomycin therapy for cryptosporidial diarrhoea in 24 AIDS patients. IX International Conference on AIDS, Berlin, **1**, 56 (abstract WS-B 13-6).

Brea-Hernando, A.J., Bandres-Franco, E., Mosquera-Lozano, J.D. *et al.* (1993) Criptosporidiasis pulmonary AIDS. Presentacion de un caso y revision de la literatura. *An. Med. Interna.*, **10**, 232–6.

Bretagne, S., Costa, J.M., Vidaud, M. *et al.* (1993) Detection of *Toxoplasma gondii* by competitive DNA amplification of bronchoalveolar lavage samples. *J. Infect. Dis.*, **168**, 1585–8.

Cohen, B.A., Pomeranz, S., Rabinowitz, J.G. *et al.* (1984) Pulmonary complications and AIDS: radiologic features. *AJR*, **143**, 115–22.

Current, W.L. and Haynes, T.B. (1984) Complete development of *Cryptosporidium* in cell culture. *Science*, **224**, 603–5.

Dannemann, B., McCutchan, J.A., Israelski, D. *et al.* (1992) The California collaborative treatment group. Treatment of toxoplasmic encephalitis in patients with AIDS. A randomised trial comparing pyrimethamine plus clindamycin to pyrimethamine plus sulphadiazine. *Ann. Intern. Med.*, **116**, 33–43.

Derouin, F., Sarfati, C., Beauvais, B. *et al.* (1990) Prevalence of pulmonary toxoplasmosis in HIV-infected patients. *AIDS*, **4**, 1036.

Dunne, M.W. (1993) Open-label azithromycin in the treatment of cryptosporidiosis. IX International Conference on AIDS, Berlin, **1**, 385 (abstract PO-B10-1500).

Fernandez-Martin, J., Leport, C., Morlat, P. *et al.* (1991) Pyrimethamine-clarithromycin combination for therapy of acute toxoplasma encephalitis in patients with AIDS. *Antimicrobial Agents and Chemotherapy*, **35**, 2049–52.

Gachot, B., Bouvet, E., Bure, A. *et al.* (1990) Infection VIH et anguillulose "maligne". *Rev. Pract.*, **40**, 2129–30.

Gleason, T. and Hamlin, W. (1974) Disseminated toxoplasmosis in the compromised host. *Arch. Intern. Med.*, **134**, 1059–62.

Gompels, M.M., Todd, J., Peters, B.S. *et al.* (1991) Disseminated strongyloidiasis: uncommon but important. *AIDS*, **5**, 329–32.

Goodman, P.C. and Schnapp, L.M. (1992) Pulmonary toxoplasmosis in AIDS. *Radiology*, **184**, 791–3.

Hojlyng, N. and Jensen, B.N. (1988) Respiratory cryptosporidiosis in HIV-positive patients. *Lancet*, **12**,(1)590–1.

Kibbler, C.C., Smith, A., Hamilton-Dutoit, S.J. *et al.* (1987) Pulmonary cryptosporidiosis occurring in a bone marrow transplant patient. *Scand. J. Infect. Dis.*, **19**, 581–4.

Kocoshis, S.A., Cibull, M.L., Davis, T.E. *et al.* (1984) Intestinal and pulmonary cryptosporidiosis in an infant with severe combined immune deficiency. *J. Pediatr. Gastroenterol. Nutr.*, **3**(1), 149–57.

Kovacs, J.A. (1992) NIAID-Clinical Center Intramural AIDS Program. Efficacy of atovaquone in treatment of toxoplasmosis in patients with AIDS. *Lancet*, **340**, 637–8.

Lessnau, K.D., Can, S. and Talavera, W. (1993) Disseminated *Strongyloides stercoralis* in human immunodeficiency virus-infected patients. Treatment failure and a review of the literature. *Chest*, **104**, 119–22.

Luft, B. and Remington, J. (1988) Toxoplasmic encephalitis. *J. Infect. Dis.*, **157**, 1–6.

Maayan, S., Wormser, G.P., Widerhom, J. *et al.* (1987) *Strongyloides stercoralis* hyperinfection in a patient with the acquired immune deficiency syndrome. *Am. J. Med.*, **83**, 945–8.

Maguire, G.P., Tatz, J., Giosa, R. and Ahmed, T. (1986) Diagnosis of pulmonary toxoplasmosis by bronchoalveolar lavage. *N.Y. State J. Med.*, **86**, 204–5.

Marche, C., Wolff, M., Mayorga, R. *et al.* (1989) Toxoplasmose pulmonaire au cours du SIDA [abstract no. WBP 23]. V International Conference on AIDS Montreal, Canada.

Murray, J.F., Felton, C.P., Garay, S.M. *et al.* (1984) Pulmonary complications of the acquired immunodeficiency syndrome. *N. Engl. J. Med.*, **310**, 1682–8.

Navia, B., Petito, C., Gold, J. *et al.* (1986) Cerebral toxoplasmosis complicating the acquired immune deficiency syndrome: clinical and neuropathological findings in 27 patients. *Ann. Neurol.*, **19**, 224–38.

Oksenhendler, E., Cadranel, J., Sarfati, C. and Katlama, C. (1990) *Toxoplasma gondii* pneumonia in patients with the acquired immunodeficiency syndrome. *Am. J. Med.*, **88**(5N), 18N–21N.

Peters, B.S., Carlin, E., Weston, R.J. *et al.* (1994) Adverse effects of drugs used in the management of opportunistic infections associated with HIV infection. *Drug Safety*, **10**, 439–54.

Pomeroy, C. and Filice, G.A. (1992) Pulmonary toxoplasmosis: a review. *Clin. Infect. Dis.*, **14**, 863–70.

Prosmanne, O., Chalaoui, J., Sylvestre, J. and Lefebvre, R. (1984) Small nodular pattern in the lungs due to opportunistic toxoplasmosis. *J. Can. Assoc. Radiol.*, **35**, 186–8.

Roth, A., Roth, B., Hoffken, G. *et al.* (1992) Application of the polymerase chain reaction in the diagnosis of pulmonary toxoplasmosis in immunocompromised patients. *Eur. J. Clin. Microbiol. Infect. Dis.*, **11**, 1177–81.

Schnapp, L.M., Geaghan, S.M., Campagna, A. *et al.* (1992) *Toxoplasma gondii* pneumonitis in patients infected with the human immunodeficiency virus. *Arch. Intern. Med.*, **152**(5), 1073–7.

Tawney, S., Masci, J., Berger, H.W. *et al.*, (1986) Pulmonary toxoplasmosis: an unusual nodular radiographic pattern in a patient with AIDS. *Mt Sinai J. Med.*, **53**, 683–5.

Torres, J.R., Isturiz, R., Murillo, J. *et al.* (1993) Efficacy of ivermectin in the treatment of strongyloidiasis complicating AIDS. *Clin. Infect. Dis.*, Nov; **17**, 900–2.

Travis, W.D., Schmidt, K., MacLowry, J.D. *et al.* (1990) Respiratory cryptosporidiosis in a patient with malignant lymphoma. Report of a case and review of the literature. *Arch. Pathol. Lab. Med.*, **114**, 519–22.

Walach, C., Loeb, M., Phillips J. *et al.* (1993) Use of letrazuril in refractory cryptosporidiosis in AIDS. IX International Conference on AIDS, Berlin, **1**, 380 (abstract PO-B10-1472).

Weber, R., Kuster, H., Visvesvara, G.S. *et al.* (1993) Disseminated microsporidiosis due to *Encephalitozoan hellum*: pulmonary colonization, microhaematuria and mild conjunctivitis in a patient with AIDS. *Clin. Infect. Dis.*, **17**, 415–19.

Zumla, A. and James, D.G. (1991) Lung immunology in the tropics, in *Lung Disease in the Tropics* (ed. O.P. Sharma), Marcel Dekker, New York, pp. 1–64.

Arshi S. Denton and Margaret F. Spittle

Pulmonary Kaposi's sarcoma is a frequent complication of human immunodeficiency virus (HIV) infection. This chapter will discuss pulmonary Kaposi's sarcoma in the context of HIV disease in terms of epidemiology, pathogenesis, presentation and diagnosis. Current therapeutic approaches will also be outlined as will new potential treatments that may supercede our present management of this difficult condition.

INTRODUCTION

Since the identification of Kaposi's sarcoma (KS) in 1872, the rather rare condition has emerged from obscurity to being a common problem amongst the HIV-infected community. Four clinical varieties of KS have been described.

1. Classical KS affects mainly elderly Mediterraneans or eastern Europeans of Jewish ancestry producing a slowly progressive course with only occasional visceral involvement.
2. African or endemic KS occurs in the Sub-Saharan region of Africa, especially among young black adult males and children. In this type there are a range of presentations from an indolent course with rare visceral involvement to

an aggressive infiltrating and lymphadenopathic type which is more common in children, with frequent involvement of the viscera and rapid dissemination. Those cases occurring in women may lead to vertical transmission. A fifth form of African KS, associated with AIDS, has been recognized since 1983 and has primarily heterosexual transmission. This form of KS is more clinically aggressive than that seen in the developed world.
3. Transplant-associated KS affects a much wider age group with variable progression of disease and frequent improvement after discontinuation of the iatrogenic immunosuppression.
4. Epidemic or AIDS-related KS also affects a wide age group but is distinguished by a high incidence of visceral involvement, with a rapidly progressive course. HIV infection is associated with a 7000-fold increase in the incidence of KS. The classification of KS is listed in Table 18.1 (Hood and Farmer, 1993).

All these subtypes have in common a male predominance which is most striking in the AIDS subtype. Differences in geographical distribution and ethnicity may account for this variation.

AIDS and Respiratory Medicine. Edited by A. Zumla, M.A. Johnson and R.F. Miller. Published in 1997 by Chapman & Hall, London. ISBN 0 412 60140 0

Table 18.1 Types of Kaposi's sarcoma

Type	Age	M/F ratio
Classical	50–80	8–17:1
African		
Nodular	25–40	
Florid	25–40	17:1
Infiltrating/aggressive	25–40	17:1
Lymphadenopathic	1–15	1–3:1
AIDS-associated-African KS age and M/F ratio not established		
Iatrogenic immunosuppressive	12–80	2:1
Epidemic	18–65	50–100:1

The occurrence of KS in young male homosexuals and bisexuals was first reported in 1981 when KS became one of the first AIDS-defining diagnoses and was the presenting feature in more than 30% of cases. Although the incidence at diagnosis has fallen to 15%, in a 1990 report from the Centers for Disease Control and Prevention (CDC), it continues to affect approximately one-third of HIV-infected male homosexuals at some stage in their disease (Hoover *et al.*, 1993). KS remains the commonest malignancy associated with HIV infection, with increasing prevalence as improved management of HIV-related problems leads to longer survival in this population.

The cutaneous manifestations of KS (Figure 18.1) can be most distressing and

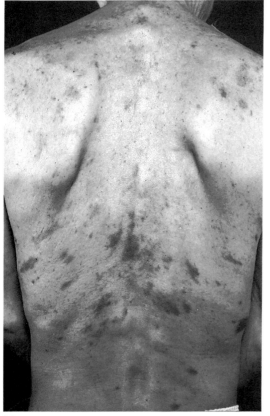

(a)

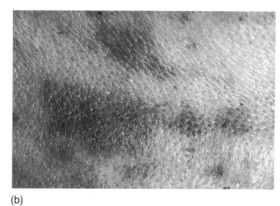

(b)

Fig. 18.1 (a) The typical pattern for multiple cutaneous lesions of Kaposi's sarcoma. (b) Close-up view of cutaneous KS lesions.

cause social isolation due to associated stigmatization, but it is the visceral involvement that is ultimately life threatening. Pulmonary KS, due to atypical presentation and concurrent disease, is often not diagnosed in life and postmortem examinations have revealed that nearly 50% of HIV-infected individuals with cutaneous disease have co-existing intrathoracic involvement (Meduri *et al.*, 1986). Pulmonary KS accounts for at least one-third of respiratory episodes in patients requiring evaluation with established cutaneous lesions (White and Matthay, 1989) and without treatment has a median survival of six months from diagnosis (Gill *et al.*, 1990). To date, treatment of this difficult problem is palliative, although it is hoped that alternative approaches may emerge which may improve survival of AIDS patients.

PATHOGENESIS

Kaposi's sarcoma is a rare multicentric, multiorgan neoplasm which occurs 20 times more frequently in homosexual or bisexual men with AIDS than in hemophiliacs with this condition (Beral *et al.*, 1990). Epidemiological data suggest that an infectious agent is involved in the pathogenesis of this lesion in both AIDS and non-AIDS forms of KS. Several agents had been implicated in the past, the most frequent being cytomegalovirus (CMV) (Gallant *et al.*, 1994) and human papillomavirus-16 (HPV16) (Huang *et al.*, 1992). However, recent data have emerged confirming the association of a previously unidentified human herpesvirus, now called Kaposi's sarcoma herpesvirus (KSHV), in these lesions (Chang *et al.*, 1994). As KSHV has homology to Epstein-Barr virus (EBV), which is implicated in neoplastic processes, it is speculated that this new agent may have a critical role in the transformation that results in KS lesions.

With the ability to culture KS cells *in vitro*, several cytokines present in the supernatant of human retrovirus-infected T cell lines have been identified and shown to promote the growth of KS cells (Ensoli *et al.*, 1989). It has been proposed that growth factors and cytokines from HIV-infected or immune activated cells are expressed and released following interaction with an infectious cofactor in the context of immunosuppression (Ensoli *et al.*, 1992). The HIV transactivating gene (*tat*) and its product (Tat) are retroviral regulatory factors which may pay a role in the process of transformation and KS cell growth, through dysregulated cytokine production (Ensoli *et al.*, 1990). This cooperative interaction may then result in the lesions of KS by inducing normal vascular progenitor cells to acquire features of the KS phenotype, with spindle cell morphology and growth responsiveness to the mitogenic effect of HIV-1 Tat protein. A hypothetical model for pathogenesis is illustrated in Figure 18.2.

Various cytokines and growth factors have been implicated in the pathogenesis of KS. Oncostatin M, a mitogen regulating the growth and differentiation of AIDS-KS cells in tissue culture, has been shown to be essential for long-term growth (Nair *et al.*, 1992), perhaps through its effects on other cytokines such as interleukin-6 (IL-6). Other cytokines which have been shown to sustain the growth of these cells *in vitro* include tumor necrosis factor (TNF), acidic and basic fibrobast growth factor (aFGF and bFGF), vascular endothelial cell growth factor (VEGF), platelet-derived growth factor, (PDGF) and granulocyte colony stimulating factor (GCSF) (Barillari *et al.*, 1992).

All these cytokines have been shown to exhibit significant effects on vascular progenitor cells. bFGF and aFGF are known to promote the growth of endothelial cells, smooth muscle cells and fibroblasts, in addition to promoting neovascularization (Burgess and Macaig, 1989). Interleukin-1 (IL-1) may induce angiogenesis by interacting with cells of the immune system, and is

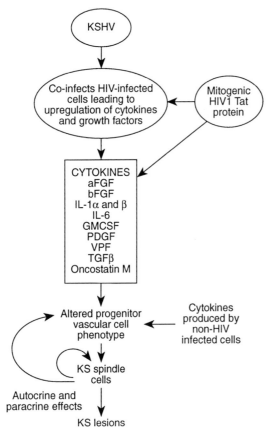

Fig. 18.2 Model for pathogenesis of Kaposi's sarcoma.

capable of inducing PDGF, resulting in the growth of fibroblast and smooth muscle growth (Dinarello, 1991). IL-1 also activates endothelial cells, smooth muscle cells and fibroblasts to produce GCSF and IL-6, which are multifunctional cytokines capable of effects on the vascular, immune and hemopoietic systems. In turn GCSF together with IL-1, IL-6 and vascular permeability factor (VPF) can mediate the inflammatory cell infiltration and edema observed in early KS lesions (Bussolino *et al.*, 1991). Both GCSF and VPF can induce endothelial cell growth. Transforming growth factor (TGF) induces chemotaxis and activation of monocytes, and promotes angiogenesis *in vivo* (Ensoli *et al.*, 1992).

An autocrine or paracrine stimulation of angiogenesis has been postulated in the pathogenesis of these lesions (Weindel *et al.*, 1992). Examination of the release of some of these cytokines suggests that major increases in serum circulating levels are closely aligned with the development of opportunistic infections, explaining the dramatic increase in rate of growth of KS at times of opportunistic infections (Ammann *et al.*, 1987).

In summary, KS is a cytokine-mediated disease and inflammatory and angiogenic cytokines cooperate with KSHV in its induction and progression in HIV-1 infected individuals. Exposure to HIV in the presence of KSHV appears to alter the morphology and growth regulation of the KS progenitor cells by expression of different cytokine receptors and autocrine and paracrine growth loops.

HISTOLOGY

KS is a relatively well differentiated tumor, but as the extent and rate of progression vary considerably among patients, with considerable tumor heterogeneity and multifocality, it has been postulated that KS may be a reactive tumor rather than a true malignancy (Friedman-Kien, 1984). Hence disseminated disease may represent either widespread metastasis or multifocal primary tumors.

The individual lesions of KS are bands of spindle cells, with nuclear pleomorphism, within proliferations of aberrant vascular structures, lined by abnormal endothelial cells and extravasated erythrocytes with a mononuclear cell infiltrate. Its malignant potential is conferred by the spindle cell, which is a tumor cell of mesenchymal origin and lies between the vascular structures (Zhang *et al.*, 1994). The patterns of cells have been described as inflammatory, granulomatous, angiomatous, mixed cellularity and anaplastic and are characterized by early angiomatous and later sarcomatous appearances. The histology of skin lesions is remarkably similar to lesions of the viscera including the respiratory system; the appearance of pulmonary KS is shown in Figure 18.3. Cutaneous lesions are divided into patch, plaque, and nodular stages, characterized by the following features (Martin, Hood and Farmer, 1993):

Patch stage

1. proliferation of ectatic jagged, irregularly branching superficial blood vessels around appendages and normal appearing blood vessels, dissecting between reticular fibers;
2. extravasated red blood cells;
3. hemosiderophages.

Plaque stage

1. spindle cells between vascular spaces forming fascicles;
2. prominent endothelial/spindle cell mitoses and nuclear abnormalities;
3. extravasated red blood cells;
4. hemosiderin/hemosiderophages;
5. occasional spindle cell esinophilic inclusions.

Nodular stage

1. fascicles of well-defined densely packed spindle cells and vascular slits;
2. mitotic figures;
3. extravasated red blood cells;
4. obvious hemosiderin/hemosiderophages;
5. spindle cells with esinophilic hyaline body inclusions.

Recent evaluations of the histological appearance of KS have suggested that nodular histology and the presence of spindle cell nodules may be associated with a slower progression of disease and improved prognosis (Niedt *et al.*, 1992).

Classical and African KS have similar clinical and histological patterns. The histology of epidemic KS lesions does not necessarily correlate with the clinical appearance, therefore any attempt to identify clear cut histological variants of epidemic KS may be misleading (Santucci *et al.*, 1988). Establishing a tissue diagnosis of pulmonary KS by endoscopic, transbronchial, or CT guided biopsy may have diagnostic limitations, in addition to technical difficulties such as accessing an adequate biopsy sample, crush artifact, the risk of hemorrhage, and the danger of aerosolized blood to the operator during the procedure.

The predominant dissemination of KS in the lung is along lymphatic routes. The pattern of involvement varies from multifocal interstitial infiltrates involving the pulmonary interstitium, bronchovascular sheaths, interlobular septa and pleura, to nodular masses obliterating the underlying pulmonary tissue. Pathological assessment of lung tissue in patients with AIDS and KS involving the lung reveals characteristic findings that explain the various pulmonary abnormalities seen radiographically. Interstitial linear and nodular accumulations of spindle cells that form vascular slits containing erythrocytes are noted and areas of fresh pulmonary hemorrhage are common.

CLINICAL FEATURES

Cutaneous lesions can vary in size and are often raised. Characteristically they are violaceous and may coalesce to form plaques which can ulcerate and bleed with associated edema. In the lung KS lesions are similar and have the potential to increase in size, bleed and cause obstruction.

Most commonly, the presence of visceral KS is an extension of cutaneous disease, although this is not always the case as visceral involvement can occur in the absence of any skin disease. In general, therefore, it is important to assess skin involvement

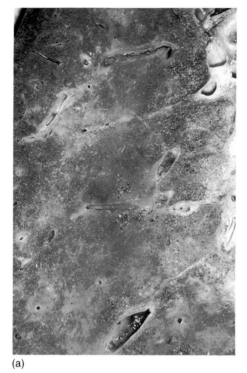

(a)

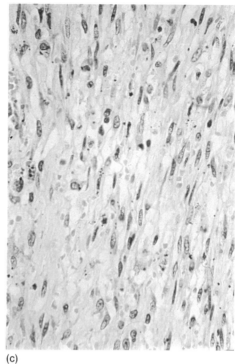

(c)

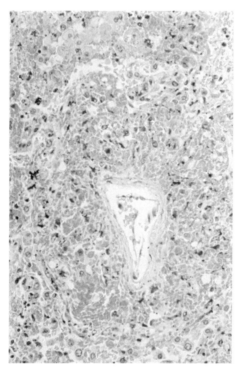

(b)

Fig. 18.3 (a) Postmortem lung showing pulmonary Kaposi's sarcoma; massive tumor is replacing normal lung tissue. (b) Kaposi's sarcoma around a blood vessel in the lung (hematoxylin and eosin × 40). (c) At high power the tumor is seen to be composed of spindle cells and vascular slits, many of which are not lined by endothelial cells (hematoxylin and eosin × 200). (From Denton, A.S., Miller, R.F. and Spittle, M.F. (1995) The management of pulmonary Kaposi's sarcoma; new perspectives, *BJHM*, **53**, (7), 344-50, reproduced with permission.)

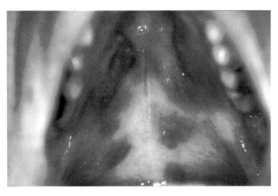

Fig. 18.4 The appearance of palatal Kaposi's sarcoma which is a strong predictor of pulmonary KS.

and to be suspicious of new respiratory symptoms in the context of progressive mucocutaneous disease. Palatal KS (Figure 18.4) is thought to be an indicator of the presence of pulmonary involvement (Moss *et al.*, 1989) and so questions relating to the oropharynx must always be incorporated into an assessment.

Epidemic KS may cause nonspecific features, termed B symptoms by analogy to lymphoma staging. These include >10% involuntary weight loss, diarrhea persisting more than 2 weeks, lethargy and persistent fevers or night sweats. Of course, in the context of HIV infection, these features are not exclusive to KS but they may be used to assess the effect on the immune system as prognostic indicators. The association of KS with immune function is variable and it has been noted that exacerbations of KS are often related to opportunistic infections and falls in the CD4 count. Nevertheless, limited cutaneous disease can also co-exist with a relatively well preserved immune system and, especially early in the AIDS epidemic, was therefore the AIDS-defining diagnosis with the best prognosis. It is necessary to assess the extent of HIV-related disease with the following information, in order to tailor treatment appropriately.

History

- date of HIV infection;
- AIDS-defining diagnosis;
- mode of transmission;
- details of opportunistic infections;
- last CD4 count;
- antiretroviral treatment;
- oral involvement resulting in dental manifestations or pain;
- date of first skin lesions, distribution and subsequent progression;
- Karnofsky performance status.

Manifestations of pulmonary KS are diverse and often non-specific. The presentation may resemble that of an infective episode and sometimes these two processes are concurrent. If symptoms persist once the infective component has been treated, there should be a high index of suspicion of the presence of pulmonary KS. The patient may also be asymptomatic. Symptoms, where present, often depend on the site and extent of involvement (Table 18.2).

EXAMINATION

The degree of mucocutaneous KS often reflects the extent of visceral involvement, as described above, and palatal KS may predict development of pulmonary lesions (Moss *et al.*, 1989). Serial documentation of cutaneous tumors is valuable for assessing disease progression. Findings on respiratory examination can be nonspecific and again may relate to the degree of involvement as shown in Table 18.3. However, it must be emphasized that the degree of tumor burden does not always correlate with the clinical or radiological findings.

INVESTIGATIONS

In addition to establishing the diagnosis, an initial assessment of the general condition and respiratory performance should be made

Table 18.2 Some symptoms of pulmonary KS

Stridor
Dyspnea
Non-productive cough
Fever in the absence of an infective episode
Hemoptysis
Wheezing
Pleuritic-type chest pain
Progression to respiratory failure

which can be compared serially to monitor improvement or deterioration in response to therapy.

Blood and sputum and pleural fluid analysis

A baseline hematological and biochemical screen are of value in assessing bone marrow reserve, coagulation abnormalities that may exacerbate hemoptysis and/or pulmonary hemorrhage and other co-existing disease processes. Other relevant indices are:

- CD4 count to detect level of immunosuppression;
- cultures for bacterial, viral or fungal pathogens which may complicate or mask pulmonary KS;
- arterial blood gases to assess level of oxygenation at rest and following exercise;
- sputum samples should be sent for culture

and microscopic analysis, including cytology.

When pleural effusions occur, biochemical analysis of the aspirate is generally unhelpful as both transudates and exudates are found, reflecting concurrent cardiogenic pathology or hypoalbuminemia from other causes. Stains and cultures for bacteria, fungus and mycobacteria are often negative. Pleural biopsy specimens are rarely diagnostic but will often show reactive mesothelial cells without evidence of neoplasm.

Pulmonary function tests

This investigation should be performed on dedicated equipment and corrections made for age, gender, race, anemia and smoking history. Results may vary according to the presence of localized or widespread pulmonary KS. Localized disease occurs when lesions are observed only in the segmental bronchus of a single lobe or on the wall of the trachea. Widespread disease occurs when both a single lobe and the trachea are affected or if the segmental bronchi of two or more lobes are affected. FEV_1 (forced expiratory volume) and FVC (forced vital capacity) are relatively preserved in localized disease but fall in widespread involvement, giving an obstructive defect with reduced peak expiratory flow rate (PEFR) and an FEV_1/FVC ratio of less than 75%. Carbon monoxide

Table 18.3 Physical signs associated with pulmonary KS

Examination site	*Findings*
Lower larynx	Stridor suggesting significant airway obstruction
Endobronchial	Pulmonary consolidation
	Bronchial obstruction leading to lobar collapse
Mediastinal	Pulmonary edema secondary to lymphatic obstruction from the involvement of mediastinal nodes in advanced pulmonary KS
Pleural	Rapidly forming bilateral pleural effusions may occur in advanced pulmonary KS

Table 18.4 Chest X-ray features of pulmonary KS

Examination site	Findings
Parenchyma	Reticulonodular shadowing due to tumor nodules Diffuse interstitial infiltrates or linear/septal angiomatous involvement (these may be non-specific and could represent old or concurrent opportunistic infection) Focal consolidation or collapse Pulmonary edema due to lymphatic or nodal obstruction Parenchymal lesions may not be apparent on radiographs, particularly in the early stages
Pleura	Rapidly accumulating, often bilateral effusions which can occur in relation to subpleural or visceral involvement and often reaccumulate following drainage
Mediastinum	10% demonstrate mediastinal lymphadenopathy in the advanced stages of KS

transfer factor (TLCO) and transfer coefficient (KCO) are reduced in both localized and widespread pulmonary KS and provide a sensitive indicator of pulmonary involvement (Miller *et al.*, 1992).

IMAGING

1. CXR;
2. bronchoscopy and tissue diagnosis;
3. CT;
4. radionuclide scanning.

CXR

This is frequently the first investigation performed. As abnormalities can potentially lie at the level of the parenchyma, pleura and mediastinum, a variety of appearances may be present according to the stage and severity of the disease (Meduri and Stein, 1992) (Table 18.4). However, radiographic images do not always parallel clinical features in pulmonary KS; moreover, chest radiography is difficult to interpret due to the frequency of multiple processes in these patients. Nevertheless, several chest radiographic findings suggest the presence of KS even in the setting of known opportunistic infection. Nodular lung densities and linear infiltrates are commonly seen in pulmonary KS but are not typical of opportunistic lung infection alone. Also, pleural effusions can be seen in patients with isolated *Pneumocystis carinii* pneumonia, but are more common in those with KS, either alone or superimposed on *P. carinii* pneumonia (PCP). A change in the radiographic pattern of lung disease in a patient known to have *P. carinii* pneumonia or another opportunistic infection should prompt re-investigation, especially when there is development of parenchymal nodules, linear infiltrates, pleural effusion, or mediastinal or hilar lymphadenopathy (Figure 18.5).

Bronchoscopy

Direct inspection of lesions with fibre-optic bronchoscopy is the most sensitive technique available for establishing a diagnosis of pulmonary KS. However, even with this procedure, only 45% have endobronchial lesions which can be identified and which have

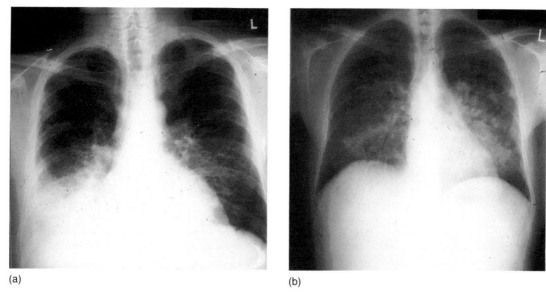

(a)   (b)

Fig. 18.5 (a) The appearance of pulmonary KS producing a right-sided pleural effusion, bilateral hilar lymphadenopathy and coarse infiltrates. (b) Pulmonary Kaposi's sarcoma mimicking the appearance of *Pneumocystis carinii* pneumonia.

the typical appearance of red/purple plaques located at segmental orifices in the main trachea or bronchi (Mitchell and Miller, 1992). Parenchymal lesions may occur in the absence of tracheobronchial lesions and hence may be missed on bronchoscopy.

Although endobronchial and transbronchial biopsies can be performed, they are often considered unnecessary in lesions with a typical appearance. However, in the presence of typical lesions or in rare cases when there are no cutaneous manifestations of KS, bronchial biopsy may be indicated although one series reported a 30% incidence of significant hemorrhage (Meduri *et al.*, 1986). Both procedures have a diagnostic yield of 10–20% because of the patchy submucous nature of the lesions. Histological identification is difficult because the lesions are composed of spindle cells and blood vessels, some of which may appear to be entirely normal (Broderick and Krinsley, 1990). Because of the paucity of malignant

features, biopsies are often reported as reactive fibrous tissue. Open lung biopsy has a high diagnostic yield of approximately 75% but is a much more invasive procedure which should be avoided if possible in this group of patients in view of their poor prognosis.

Occult alveolar hemorrhage from bronchoalveolar lavage was once thought to be a sensitive indicator of the presence of pulmonary KS; subsequent work has demonstrated that this is a non-specific finding and reflects a host of infective and non-infective HIV-associated disease in the lung (Hughes-Davies *et al.*, 1992).

CT

CT is particularly useful when the chest X-ray is abnormal yet bronchoscopy fails to identify endobronchial lesions, thus suggesting that parenchymal disease is present. As stated above, some parenchymal lesions may appear normal on CXR. However, in cross-

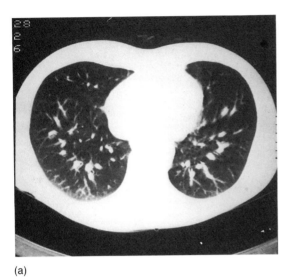
(a)

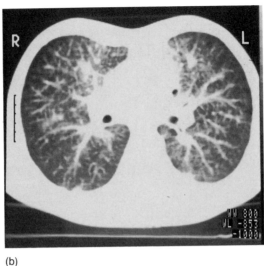
(b)

Fig. 18.6 (a) CT of the chest with lung windows through the lower lobes showing coarse nodular infiltrates. (b) CT of the chest with lung windows below the hila demonstrating coarse nodular infiltrates.

section, infiltrates are bronchocentric or angiocentric and sub-pleural nodules are easier to identify. A review of the literature shows that CT gives a higher detection of lymphadenopathies and peri-bronchovascular distribution of opaque areas in situations where X-rays are inconclusive. In addition, pleural and parenchymal disease are noted more frequently on CT with a higher pick-up of extrapulmonary involvement (Wolff *et al.*, 1993). The technique of spiral CT scanning has advantages for imaging breathless patients and is often the preferred modality in this group (Figure 18.6).

Nuclear medicine studies

These techniques are of value when infection co-exists with pulmonary KS so that conventional imaging fails to distinguish changes of infection from those of KS. [67]Gallium scintigraphy can localize infection and unsuspected lymphoma (Wassie *et al.*, 1992). [111]Indium-labeled polyclonal human immunoglobulin

identifies the presence and extent of infection, with the advantage that it does not accumulate in lymphoma (Buscombe *et al.*, 1993).

An algorithm of the method of diagnostic processes involved in pulmonary KS is demonstrated in Figure 18.7.

DIFFERENTIAL DIAGNOSIS

Essentially, evaluation of pathology in the AIDS-lung involves making the distinction between infective and non-infective processes. The previous section has outlined the principal methods used. It is notable that in African KS the main differential diagnosis is tuberculosis, exemplifying that racial and geographical factors may have a significant effect on co-existing disease processes.

STAGING

A staging system must be effective for evaluation of therapeutic regimens and give meaningful information regarding the patient's ultimate prognosis.

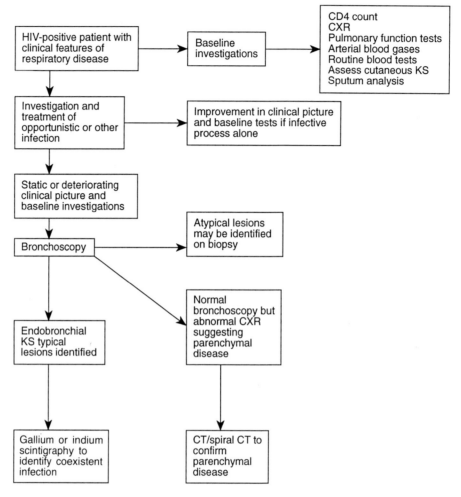

Fig. 18.7 Algorithm demonstrating the method of investigation in pulmonary Kaposi's sarcoma. (From Denton, A.S., Miller, R.F. and Spittle, M.F. (1995) The management of pulmonary Kaposi's sarcoma: new perspectives, *BJHM*, **53**, (7), 344-50, reproduced with permission.)

The most widely used classification for KS defines:

stage 1   cutaneous, locally indolent or classical KS;

stage 2   locally aggressive cutaneous KS with or without regional lymph nodes (as is characteristically seen in African KS);

stage 3   generalized mucocutaneous and/or lymph node involvement;

stage 4   visceral KS.

These stages are further subtyped by the absence (A), or presence (B) of B symptoms. Although this system is useful for classifying all forms of KS it is limited to a 2-stage system in AIDS-related KS as patients generally present with stages 3 and 4. In addition there is no assessment of the severity of immunosuppression (Krigel *et al.*, 1983).

Several other staging systems have been proposed for AIDS-related KS that have used extent of tumor, clinical symptoms of HIV

Table 18.5 ACTG staging classification

	Good risk (0)	Poor risk (1)
Tumor (T)	Confined to skin and/or lymph nodes and/or min. oral disease	Tumor-associated edema or ulceration Extensive oral KS GI KS or in non-nodal areas
Immune system (I)	CD4 > 200	CD4 < 200
Systemic illness (S)	No Hx of OI/thrush No B symptoms KPS > 70%	Hx of OI and/or thrush B symptoms KPS < 70% Other HIV-related illness

OI = Opportunistic infection.

disease and various other prognostic indicators. A recent review of staging systems concluded that the importance of CD4, prognostic factors such as a history of opportunistic infections, and the presence of B symptoms, are critical in predicting survival in this group of patients (Antinorri *et al.*, 1992). To better characterize patients before entry onto therapeutic clinical trials the AIDS clinical trials group (ACTG) have developed a proposal for evaluation, staging, and response assessment of patients with KS (Table 18.5) (Krown *et al.*, 1989). This includes a standardized format for documenting the extent of KS on initial and subsequent evaluations, response definitions that include assessment of the lesion's nodularity and tumor-associated edema in addition to the more traditional method of tumor, immune status, and other AIDS-related manifestations.

TREATMENT

Management of pulmonary KS involves treatment of specific pulmonary complications such as pleural effusion or pneumothorax; local and systemic anti-tumor therapy and

the complications of such therapies. Treatment of pulmonary KS is essential in a well patient because of its severely debilitating and rapidly fatal nature if left untreated. The condition is not curable in strict oncological terms, in direct contrast to classical KS and transplant-associated KS, where withdrawal of immunosuppressive agents may be followed by regression of the tumor; spontaneous regression has also been recorded. The aims of treatment and potential side effects should be clearly defined to avoid unrealistic expectations by the patient and relatives and be primarily directed toward improvement in quality of life. In addition, of course, informed consent is mandatory before any therapy can be instituted.

Treatment should be tailored according to the severity of symptoms, the extent of pulmonary involvement (tumor burden), the degree of immunosuppression and the general health of the patient. No clear survival advantage has been demonstrated and its diagnosis implies a very poor prognosis. Gill *et al.* (1990) have reported a series in which survival was 6 months for non-responders and 12 months for those who responded to treatment.

Local treatment of specific PKS problems

1. Medical or surgical pleurodesis for recurrent pleural effusions is rarely effective but can be attempted.
2. Laser for obstructive endobronchial lesions can provide local control and symptomatic relief; however, the hazards of aerosolized infected blood should not be overlooked (Nathan *et al.*, 1990).
3. Early radiotherapeutic intervention may provide palliation and delay the onset of respiratory distress. It is of particular value in the treatment of laryngeal KS. In this situation critical lesions may produce stridor and obstruction. They can be treated effectively with localized radiotherapy at a dose of 16 Gray (Gy) delivered in 8 fractions, although hoarseness and mucositis are recognized complications. KS is relatively radiosensitive and the dose required is much less than that necessary for squamous laryngeal tumors.
4. Localized radiotherapy may be of use in lobar disease, causing significant hemoptysis, and in nodal mediastinal disease. A total dose of 10.5–15 Gy (150 cGy per fraction) can be supplemented by an increased dose to a coned-down field. Again, this dose is much smaller than for other bronchial neoplasms, because of the radioresponsive nature of the tumor.

Meyer and colleagues have shown a transient improvement in a proportion of their study group and a sustained response in 50% in terms of symptom control and radiological changes (Meyer, 1993). In clinical practice, however, irradiation of the lung is not commonly used in this context and is of questionable value, especially as it may exacerbate pre-existing pleural effusions.

Systemic treatment – CD4 count greater than 200/mm^3

If the CD 4 count exceeds 200/mm^3, biological response modifiers can be successful in controlling early disease which is asymptomatic. In certain cases this can lead to a long-term remission and stabilization of the overall clinical picture. Treatment regimens include a combination of α-interferon and zidovudine (AZT) which has the advantage of producing both an anti-tumor and an anti-viral response. Low doses of interferon are initially administered thrice weekly, with progressive dose intensification and increased frequency depending on the individual's ability to tolerate the side effects (Krown *et al.*, 1992). A drawback of this treatment is that interferon is administered subcutaneously; however, recently a new formulation of human natural α-IFN, stabilized for oral administration, in a complex polysaccharide carrier, has been developed (Koech and Obel, 1990). The side effects of IFN treatment include myelosuppression and 'flu like symptoms which may be difficult to tolerate for long periods. This approach is contraindicated in advanced disease as a period of 6–8 weeks is required before improvement is noted and a period of 6 months is required for optimal benefit.

Systemic treatment – CD4 count less than 200/mm^3

If the CD4 count is below 200/mm^3 interferon will not be effective and chemotherapy is recommended. In view of the myelosuppressive toxicity, PCP prophylaxis is required and the need for hematological support with GCSF may arise. In the past a number of single agent therapies have been attempted with variable results. These include vinblastine, vincristine, etoposide, bleomycin, epirubicin and Adriamycin. These have been superceded by liposomal agents and combination therapy as listed in Table 18.6, and the currently used regimens in practice will be discussed.

Bleomycin and vincristine is an effective standard chemotherapy regimen. Gompels

Table 18.6 Cytotoxic regimens ever used in the treatment of AIDS-related KS

Treatment regimen	Specific drug(s) used
Single agent	Vincristine, vinblastine Vinblastine/vincristine alternating weeks Etoposide Bleomycin Adriamycin Epirubicin

Combination treatment	Adriamycin, bleomycin, vinblastine
	  Adriamycin, bleomycin, vincristine,
	  MTX and vinblastine
	Etoposide, Adriamycin, bleomycin and vinblastine
	
	Vinblastine and Adriamycin or etoposide and Adriamycin, alternating
	  with bleomycin and vincristine
	
	Actinomycin D, vincristine, DTIC alternating with Adriamycin,
	  bleomycin and vinblastine

Commonly used regimens	Adriamycin, bleomycin and vincristine (ABV) Bleomycin and vincristine (BV) Liposomal doxorubicin and daunorubicin

and colleagues reported a partial response in 57% and disease progression was arrested in a further 35% (Gompels *et al.*, 1992) and this has superceded combinations of Adriamycin, bleomycin and vincristine, which though more effective produce greater toxicity, notably alopecia (Ireland-Gill *et al.*, 1991). The concern that bleomycin might accelerate lung fibrosis has been investigated with serial pulmonary function tests (Denton *et al.*, 1996). The authors concluded that none of the patients in their series developed significant pulmonary toxicity although close monitoring is warranted with cumulative doses of this drug. Most recently a regimen using continuous bleomycin has been reported to be effective (Remmick *et al.*, 1994). Also of note is the fact that there have been reports that the use of bleomycin can induce Raynaud's phenomenon and digital gangrene (Gunton,

Roth and Von Roem, 1993). Vincristine has been long associated with the development of peripheral neuropathy and if this is progressive then vinblastine could be substituted. In addition there have been reports of loss of retinal ganglion cells associated with vincristine.

Liposomal doxorubicin is an anthracycline derivative surrounded by a phospholipid membrane and its use in this form has been associated with fewer side effects and higher intralesional levels than in the conventional method of administration. This type of chemotherapy is well tolerated and generally safe and effective with a 90% partial response rate. However, myelosuppression may occur and hepatotoxicity and liver failure have been reported (Simpson, Miller and Spittle, 1993). Similarly, liposomal daunorubicin is well tolerated with minimal toxicity. Published response rates are comparable to stan-

Table 18.7　Therapeutic options in pulmonary KS

Treatment option		Type of intervention
Local		Management of pleural effusions
		Endobronchial laser of obstructive lesions
		RT to laryngeal KS
		localized pulmonary KS
		whole lung for widespread lesions
Systemic	CD4 > 200/mm^3	alpha-interferon sc using dose escalation to 10 MU once daily
	CD4 < 200/mm^3	chemotherapy
		– bleomycin and vincristine vs Adriamycin, bleomycin and vincristine
		– continuous bleomycin
		– L doxorubicin
		– L daunorubicin

L = Liposomal formulation.

dard chemotherapy regimes, suggesting that this form of chemotherapy may be effective even in patients resistant to other treatments (Money-Kyrle *et al.*, 1993). The current therapeutic options are summarized in Table 18.7 and administration regimens are listed in Table 18.8.

All the chemotherapeutic regimens quoted have in common an effective tumor response but remissions tend to be short with inevitable relapse following withdrawal of treatment. In general, bleomycin-containing regimens are used as first-line chemotherapy to achieve a partial response. Upon relapse or progression liposomal anthracyclines can be used as second-line agents. The aim of all these treatments is to reduce the pulmonary burden, relieve obstruction and to improve oxygenation. It should be appreciated that treatment of this condition is very difficult because it represents an advanced stage of an aggressive disease occurring in a weakened host.

The administration of myelosuppressive regimens to an already immunocompromised host is associated with a variety of complications as listed in Table 18.9.

POTENTIAL NEW TREATMENTS

In general, immunotherapy and chemotherapy are the main tools available for the control of pulmonary KS. New and specific treatments are being developed, mainly directed towards cytokines, growth factors and other targets involved in the pathogenesis of KS. However the best approach to reducing AIDS-related KS will ultimately involve eradication of HIV infection so that promotion of existing health initiatives should be supported. These include the following:

Sulfated polysaccharide peptidoglycans: AIDS-KS is a highly vascularized tumor that overproduces bFGF, hence sulfated polysaccharide peptidoglycans, structural analogs of heparin, such as pentosan, may have potential usefulness because it prevents binding of bFGF to its receptor on the endothelial cell and inhibits tumor growth by cutting off the blood supply (Pluda *et al.*, 1993; Schwartsmann *et al.*, 1995). Objective antitumor activity with low toxicity has been recorded and such agents are currently being evaluated in KS and include derivatives of

Table 18.8   Administration of chemotherapy (3 weekly cycles – all intravenous drugs)

Specific drug(s) used	Dose
Bleomycin and vincristine	Bleomycin 30 units in 250 ml normal saline over 30 minutes Vincristine 1.4 mg/m^2 (max, 2 mg) i.v. bolus or vinblastine 2.5–5.0 mg bolus Hydrocortisone 100 mg i.v. bolus
Adriamycin Bleomycin Vincristine	Doxorubicin 10–20 mg/m^2 bolus Bleomycin 10 units/m^2 infusion as above Vincristine 1.4 mg/m^2 (max 2 mg) bolus
Continuous bleomycin	Bleomycin 20 mg/m^2 in 1 L normal saline over 24 hours for 3 days
Liposomal doxorubicin	Liposomal doxorubicin 10–20 mg/m^2 in 250 ml 5% dextrose over 30 minutes (2–3 weekly)
Liposomal daunorubicin	Liposomal daunorubicin 40 mg/m^2 in 250 ml 5% dextrose over 30 minutes (2 weekly)

Table 18.9   Treatment-related complications

Treatment type	Associated complications
IF	Reversible elevation in transaminases Myalgia, severe flu-like symptoms, anemia and occasional hypotension
RT larynx/lung	Mucositis and pneumonitis
Chemotherapy	General: problems of stomatitis, alopecia and nausea Poor bone marrow reserve causing prolonged myelosuppression, anemia, thrombocytopenia and infection Specific: – bleomycin – pulmonary fibrosis in cumulative doses and Raynaud's phenomenon – vinca alkaloids – peripheral neuropathy and destruction of retinal ganglion cells accelerated by DDI/DDC – anthracyclines – cardiotoxicity liposomal anthracyclines – cardiotoxocity in cumulative doses, monitored by serial ECG, measurement of left ventricular ejection fraction on echo or MUGA scan

IF = interferons.

fumagillin (Pluda *et al.*, 1994).

Interleukin-4 (IL-4): this is a potent inhibitor of IL-6 expression and subsequently reduces proliferation of AIDS-KS cells *in vitro*. This agent is currently undergoing evaluation with a focus on whether alteration in cytokine levels will result in tumor regression. Other inhibitors of cytokines, or receptor antagonists of HIV-Tat, IL-1 (Krown *et al.*, 1995) or TNF or antisense oligonucleotides may also have biological activity in patients with AIDS-KS. Early trials are in progress.

Recombinant platelet factor 4 (rPF4): this is a normal constituent of platelet alpha granules and has angiostatic activity in several cell types including KS. Phase 1/11 trials are assessing its safety and efficacy (Northfelt *et al.*, 1995).

Retinoic compounds: retinoic compounds such as All-trans-retinoic acid are thought to have an anti-proliferative effect on KS lesions by reducing growth and differentiation as demonstrated in many cell lines (Corbeil *et al.*, 1994). The postulated mechanism is by reduction of IL-6. Initial results have been promising and further evaluation in combination with interferon is planned.

Taxol: this agent stabilizes microtubule polymers and has been found to be cytostatic in KS-derived spindle cell lines. Preliminary data suggest that taxol has substantial activity in AIDS-related KS and may be a useful therapeutic agent (Saville *et al.*, 1995).

Photodynamic therapy: this is a new approach for cutaneous AIDS-KS based on light activation of a photosensitizer accumulating in the lesions. This may in the future be extended to pulmonary KS (Bernstein *et al.*, 1995).

Autologous activated cytotoxic lymphocytes: another novel approach may be the use of the patient's own lymphocytes. HIV-specific cytotoxic lymphocytes bearing the CD8 marker can recognize viral-infected cells and are capable of suppressing HIV-replication in a dose-dependent manner requiring IL2. Continued HIV-replication can induce various growth factors which promote KS cell growth and the use of *ex-vivo* expanded

autologous CD8 cells and IL2 in AIDS-KS has shown evidence of tumor regression (Kilmas, 1992).

Future treatments: in view of the recent identification of KSHV in these lesions one could potentially anticipate that in the future treatment approaches might include the use of a KSHV vaccine or specific antiviral agent directed against this pathogen.

CONCLUSIONS

One of the main problems in establishing the diagnosis of pulmonary KS is that the clinical picture is not specific for this condition. Hence a high index of suspicion is indicated which would then be supported by the results of further confirmatory investigations.

Another confounding issue is that the severity of the condition does not parallel the radiographic picture and indeed the lesions can be missed on bronchoscopic identification and tissue biopsy.

Of the various treatment options available no clear survival advantage has been demonstrated; however, a significant degree of palliation can be achieved with either chemotherapy or radiotherapy. In addition, the recent identification of KSHV as an infective cofactor potentially involved in the pathogenesis of KS may lead to new targeted approaches for both treatment and prophylaxis.

As the treatment of HIV improves, patients are demonstrating increased incidence of late complications such as malignancy. Until the treatment of pulmonary KS advances the diagnosis of this complication will continue to be associated with a poor prognosis.

REFERENCES

Ammann, A.J., Palladino, MA., Voldberding, P. *et al.*, (1987) Alpha and beta tumour necrosis factor in acquired immunodeficiency syndrome and the AIDS related complex. *Journal of Clinical Immunology*, **7**, 481–5.

Antinorri, A., Immacolata, I., Ammassari, A. *et al.* (1992) Evaluation of different staging systems of Kaposi's sarcoma in HIV infected patients. *Journal of Cancer Research Clinical Oncology*, **118**, 635–6.

Barillari, G., Buonagura, L., Fiorelli, V. *et al.* (1992) Cytokines from activated immune cells on vascular cell growth and genome expression. *Journal of Immunology*, **149**, 3727–34.

Bernstein, Z.P., Wilson, D., Summers, K. *et al.* (1995) Pilot/Phase I study of photodynamic therapy in the treatment of AIDS related Kaposi's sarcoma. *Proceedings of ASCO*, **14**, 289.

Beral, V., Peterman, T.A., Berkelman, R.L. and Jaffe, H.W. (1990) Kaposi's sarcoma among persons with AIDS: a sexually transmitted infection? *Lancet*, **335**, 123–8.

Broderick, P.A., and Krinsley, J.S. (1990) Transbronchial biopsy in Kaposi's sarcoma. *Connecticut Medicine*, **54**, 555–7.

Burgess, W.H. and Macaig, T. (1989) The heparin binding (fibroblast) growth factor family of proteins. *Annual Review of Biochemistry*, **58**, 575–62.

Buscombe, J.R., Oyen, W.J.G., Grant, A. *et al.* (1993) Indium-111 labeled polyclonal human immunoglobulin: Identifying focal infection in patients positive for HIV. *Journal of Nuclear Medicine*, **34**, 1621–25.

Bussolino, F., Ziche, M., Wang, J.M. *et al.* (1991) *In vitro* and *in vivo* activation of endothelial cells by colony stimulating factors. *Journal of Clinical Investigation*, **87**, 986–95.

Chang, Y., Cesarman, E., Pessin, M.S. *et al.* (1994) Identification of herpesvirus like sequences in AIDS associated Kaposi's sarcoma. *Science*, **266**, 1865–9.

Corbeil, J., Rappaport, E., Richman, D.D., Cooney, D.J. *et al.* (1994) Anti-proliferative effect of retinoid compounds in Kaposi's sarcoma. *Journal of Clinical Investigation*, **93**, 1981–6.

Dinarello, C.A. (1991) Interleukin1 and intereukin1 antagonism. *Blood*, **77**, 1627–34.

Denton, A.S., Miller, R.F. and Spittle, M.F. (1995) Management of pulmonary Kaposi's sarcoma: new perspectives. *British Journal of Hospital Medicine*, **53**, 344–50.

Denton, A.S., Simpson, J.K., Hallam, M.H. *et al.* (1996) Effects on pulmonary function of two regimens of chemotherapy for AIDS related Kaposi's sarcoma. *Clinical Oncology*, **8**, 48–50.

Ensoli, B., Nakamura, S., Salahuddin, S.Z. *et al.* (1989) AIDS-Kaposi's sarcoma derived cells express cytokines with autocrine and paracrine growth effects. *Science*, **243**, 223–6.

Ensoli, B., Barillari, G., Salahuddin, S.Z. *et al.* (1990) The tat protein of HIV 1 stimulates growth of cells derived from Kaposi's sarcoma lesions of AIDS patients. *Nature*, **345**, 84–86.

Ensoli, B., Barillari, G. and Gallo, R.C. (1992) Cytokines and growth factors in the pathogenesis of AIDS associated Kaposi's sarcoma. *Immunological Reviews*, **127**, 147–55.

Friedman-Kien, A.E. (1984) Kaposi's sarcoma is an opportunistic neoplasm. *Journal of Investigative Dermatology*, **82**, 446–48.

Gill, P.S., Rarick, M.U., Montgomery, T. *et al.* (1990) Acquired immunodeficiency syndrome related Kaposi's sarcoma. *Cancer*, **65**, 1074–8.

Gallant, J.E., Moore, R.D., Richman, D.D. *et al.* (1994) Risk factors for Kaposi's sarcoma in patients with advanced HIV treated with zidovudine: zidovudine epidemiology study group. *Archives of Internal Medicine*, **154**, 566–72.

Gompels, M.M., Hill, A., Jenkins, P. *et al.* (1992) Kaposi's sarcoma in HIV infection treated with bleomycin and vincristine. *AIDS*, **6**, 1175–80.

Gunton, C.F., Roth, E.L. and Von Roem, J.H. (1993) Raynaud's phenomenon in bleomycin containing chemotherapies. *Cancer*, **72**, 2004–6.

Huang, Y.Q., Li, J.J., Rush, M.G. *et al.* (1992) Human papilloma virus type 16-related DNA sequences in Kaposi's sarcoma. *Lancet*, **339**, 515–18.

Hoover, D.R., Black, C., Jacobson, L.P. *et al.* (1993) Analysis of Kaposi's sarcoma as an early or late outcome in HIV affected men. *American Journal of Epidemiology*, **138**, 226–78.

Hughes-Davies, L., Kocjan, G., Spittle, M.F. and Miller, R.F. (1992) Occult alveolar haemorrhage in pulmonary Kaposi's sarcoma. *Journal of Clinical Pathology*, **45**, 536–7.

Ireland-Gill, A., Espina, B.M., Akil, B. and Gill, P.K. (1991) Treatment of AIDS related Kaposi's sarcoma containing bleomycin in various regimens. *Seminars in Oncology*, **19**, Suppl 5, 32–39.

Kilmas, N.G. (1992) Clinical impact of adoptive therapy with purified CD8 cells in HIV infection. *Seminars in Haematology*, **29**, (supplement 1), 40–43.

Koech, D.K. and Obel, A.O. (1990) Efficiency of low dose oral natural human interferon alpha in the management of HIV1 infection in AIDS. *East African Medical Journal*, **67**, 64–68.

Krigel, R., Laubenstein, L., Muggia, F. *et al.* (1983) Kaposi's sarcoma: a new staging classification. *Cancer Treatment Reports*, **67**, 531–4.

Krown, S.E., Metroka, C., Wernz, J.C. *et al.* (1989) AIDS Clinical Trials Group oncology committee: Kaposi's sarcoma in the acquired immune deficiency syndrome; A proposal for uniform evaluation, response and staging criteria. *Journal of Clinical Oncology*, **7**, 1201–7.

Krown, S.E., Paredes, J., Bundow, D. *et al.* (1992) Alpha-IFN, AZT and GMCSF; a phase 1 clinical trial in Kaposi's sarcoma associated with AIDS. *Journal of Clinical Oncology*, **10**, 1344–51.

Krown, S.E., Paredes, J., Polsky, B. *et al.* (1995) Phase I/II trial of soluble recombinant interleukin 1 receptor in patients with HIV infection. *Proceedings of ASCO*, **14**, 292.

Martin, R.W., Hood, A.F. and Farmer, E.R. (1993) Kaposi's sarcoma. *Medicine*, **72**(4)1, 245–61.

Meduri, G.U. and Stein, D.S. (1992) Pulmonary manifestations of acquired immune deficiency syndrome. *Clinical Infectious Diseases*, **14**, 98–113.

Meduri, G.U., Stover, D.E., Lee, M. *et al.* (1986) Pulmonary Kaposi's sarcoma in acquired immunodeficiency syndrome. *American Journal of Medicine*, **81**, 11–18.

Meyer, J.H. (1993) Whole lung radiotherapy in pulmonary Kaposi's sarcoma. *American Journal of Clinical Oncology*, **16**, 372–6.

Miller, R.F., Tomlinson, M.C., Cottril, C.P. *et al.* (1992) Bronchopulmonary Kaposi's sarcoma in patients with AIDS. *Thorax*, **47**, 721–25.

Mitchell, D.M. and Miller, R.F. (1992) Developments in the management of pulmonary complications of HIV disease. *Thorax*, **47**, 381–90.

Money-Kyrle, J.F., Bates, F., Ready, J. *et al.* (1993) Efficacy of liposomal daunorubicin in the treatment of AIDS related Kaposi's sarcoma. *Clinical Oncology*, **5**, 367–71.

Moss, F., Flemming, J., Nelson, J. *et al.* (1989) Palatal KS is a strong predictor of pulmonary involvement. *Thorax*, **44**, 326P.

Nair, B.C., DeVico, A.L., Nakamura, S. *et al.* (1992) Identification of a major growth factor for AIDS Kaposi's sarcoma cells as oncostatin M. *Science*, **255**, 1430–2.

Nathan, S., Vaghaiwalla, R., Monsenfor, Z. *et al.* (1990) Use of the Nd:YAG laser in endobronchial Kaposi's sarcoma. *Chest*, **98**, 1299–300.

Niedt, G.W., Myskowsky, P.L., Urmacher, C. *et al.* (1992) Histological predictors of survival in Kaposi's sarcoma. *Human Pathology*, **23**, 1419–26.

Northfelt, D.W., Robles, R., Lang, W. *et al.* (1995) Phase I/II study of intravenous recombinant PF4 in AIDS related Kaposi's sarcoma. *Proceedings of ASCO*, **14**, 289.

Pluda, J.M., Shay, L.E., Foly, N.K. *et al.* (1993) Administration of pentosan to HIV related Kaposi's sarcoma. *Journal of the National Cancer Institute*, **85**, 1585–92.

Pluda, J.M., Wyvill, K., Figg, W.D. *et al.* (1994) A phase 1 study of angiogenesis inhibition with TNP470 administered to HIV patients with associated Kaposi's sarcoma. *Proceedings of ASCO*, **13**, 51.

Remmick, S.C., Reddy, M. and Hermin, D. *et al.* (1994) Infusional bleomycin as a treatment for AIDS related Kaposi's sarcoma. *Journal of Clinical Oncology*, **12**, 1130–6.

Santucci, M., Pimpinelli, N., Moretti, S. *et al.* (1988) Classical and immunodeficiency associated Kaposi's sarcoma. Clinical histological and immunological correlations. *Archives of Pathology and Laboratory Medicine*, **112**, 1214–20.

Schwartzmann, G., Mans, D.R.A., Machado, V.L. *et al.* (1995) Phase II study of bFGF inhibiting agent pentosan polysulphate in patients with AIDS related Kaposi's sarcoma. *Proceedings of ASCO*, **14**, 290.

Saville, M.W., Pluda, J.M., Fenerstein, I. *et al.* (1995) Treatment of HIV associated Kaposi's sarcoma with paclitaxel (Taxol). *Lancet*, **346**, 26–28.

Simpson, J.K., Miller, R.F. and Spittle, M.F. (1993) Liposomal doxorubicin in the treatment of AIDS related Kaposi's sarcoma. *Clinical Oncology*, **5**, 372–4.

Wassie, E., Buscombe, J.R., Miller, R.F. and Ell, P.J. (1992) Ga scintigraphy in HIV positive patients: a review of its clinical usefulness. *British Journal of Radiology*, **67**, 349–52.

Weindel, K., Marme, D., Weich, H.A. *et al.* (1992) AID-associated Kaposi's sarcoma cells in culture express vascular endothelial growth factor. *Biochemical and Biophysical Research Communications*, **183**, 167–74.

White, D.A. and Matthay, R.A. (1989) Non infectious pulmonary complications of infection with the human immunodeficiency virus. *American*

Review of Respiratory Disease, **140**, 1763–87.

Wolff, S.D., Kuhlman, J.E., Fishman, E.K. *et al.* (1993) CT findings of Thoracic Kaposi's sarcoma in acquired immune deficiency syndrome. *Journal of Computer Assisted Tomography*, **17**, 60–62.

Zhang, Y.M., Backmann, S., Hemmer, C. *et al.* (1994) Vascular origin of Kaposi's sarcoma. *American Journal of Pathology*, **144**, 51–59.

Thomas F. Schulz

INTRODUCTION

First described by the Austro-Hungarian dermatologist Moritz Kaposi just over 100 years ago (Kaposi, 1872), Kaposi's sarcoma (KS) was, until recently, considered a rare, slowly progressive tumor of elderly males. In this 'classical' form of KS, lesions are mainly confined to the skin and localized preferentially on the extremities. In the early 1960s it emerged that KS was endemic in central Africa, particularly Zaire, and that four different clinical variants of 'endemic KS' could be distinguished (reviewed in Buchbinder and Friedman-Kien, 1991; see also Chapter 18). These are (1) benign disease with few lesions reminiscent of classical KS; (2) aggressive disease mainly localized to extremities with local invasions and destruction; (3) widely disseminated disease with visceral involvement; and (4) a lymphadenopathic form with preferential involvement of lymph nodes and visceral organs but minimal mucocutaneous lesions. In addition, KS occurs in iatrogenically immunosuppressed individuals ('iatrogenic KS'). However, in developed countries, KS is now most commonly associated with HIV infection, and this variant, termed 'epidemic KS', is characterized by widely distributed lesions, visceral as well as lymph node involvement and a rapidly progressive course. These clinical aspects of KS are discussed in more detail in Chapter 18.

The features of KS discussed below indicate that, at least in its early stages, it is not a truly malignant neoplasm but more akin to a proliferative lesion whose growth is maintained by a cascade of growth factors secreted by, and acting on, cells of different lineage. While HIV may have a direct role in the pathogenesis of epidemic KS, there is also evidence for the involvement of an independently transmitted 'KS agent'. The recently discovered gamma-herpes virus, KSHV/HHV-8 (Chang *et al.*, 1994), which is consistently found in all forms of KS (Moore and Chang, 1995; Boshoff *et al.*, 1995; Dupin *et al.*, 1995; Lebbé *et al.*, 1995; Ambroziak *et al.*, 1995; Huang *et al.*, 1995; Chang *et al.*, 1996; Schalling *et al.*, 1995), is a good candidate for the 'KS agent' but its precise role in the pathogenesis of KS remains to be defined.

THE KS LESION: HISTOLOGICAL FEATURES

KS skin lesions develop from the early 'patch' stage to the 'plaque' and 'nodular' stage (reviewed in Cockerell, 1991). The early patch stage is characterized by pink macular

AIDS and Respiratory Medicine. Edited by A. Zumla, M.A. Johnson and R.F. Miller. Published in 1997 by Chapman & Hall, London. ISBN 0 412 60140 0

lesions. Histologically, these are characterized by an increased number of slit-like vascular spaces situated in the dermis between collagen bundles. These vascular spaces are lined by flattened endothelial cells and lack any of the other histological features of small vessels (hence the 'slit-like' appearance). Normal vessels may be located immediately adjacent to these vascular spaces and protrude into them ('promontory sign'). A cellular infiltrate of lymphocytes and plasma cells is often present and can, when combined with aggregated endothelial cells, contribute to the 'pseudogranulomatous' character of some of these lesions.

Once the proliferation of these atypical vessels becomes more extensive and spreads to the whole of the dermis as well as the underlying layers of subcutaneous fat, the clinical appearance of the lesion is that of a plaque or papule. The atypical thin-walled vessels are numerous and have a jagged appearance. The accompanying cellular infiltrate is much more pronounced and there are many extravasated erythrocytes and their remnants, hyaline deposits.

With the progression of KS lesions to nodules and tumors, a spindle-like morphology of the abnormal endothelial cells dominates the histological appearance and numerous interweaving spindle cells, surrounding extravasated erythrocytes and hyaline deposits make up the characteristic appearance of these advanced lesions.

ORIGIN OF KS SPINDLE CELLS

Although KS lesions, particularly in the early stages, contain a variety of different cell types, the hallmark of the advanced KS lesion is the spindle cell surrounding slit-like spaces. Most of the available evidence suggests an endothelial origin of these spindle cells (either vascular or lymphatic endothelium), but cells from venous lymphatic junctions, fibroblasts, smooth muscle cells, dermal dendrocytes, have all been proposed as progenitors of KS spindle cells (reviewed in Roth, Brandstetter and Stürzl, 1992; Stürzl, 1992a). A relationship with lymphatic endothelium is suggested by their expression of the En-4 antigen (which is normally found on vascular and lymphatic endothelium) but lack of the Pal-E antigen, expressed on blood vessel but not lymphatic endothelial cells (Rappersberger et al., 1991). However, other markers for blood vessel endothelium (OKM-5 and factor VIII related antigen (von Willebrand factor; vWF)) are expressed on KS endothelial or spindle cells, although slightly varying results have been reported by different laboratories (Nadji et al., 1981; Modlin et al., 1983; Little et al., 1986; Rappersberger et al., 1991; further references in Roth, Brandstetter and Stürzl, 1992). *Ulex europaeus* agglutinin 1 (UEA-1), another marker for endothelial cells, has also produced contradictory results. Ultrastructural examination failed to show the presence of Weibel-Palade bodies, the storage vesicles for vWF and therefore a characteristic feature of vascular endothelium, in spindle cells from KS lesions (Rappersberger et al., 1991). Staining with monoclonal antibody BMA 120, detecting an antigen specific for endothelial cells, lends support to an endothelial origin of KS cells (Roth et al., 1988). KS spindle cells and endothelia lining vascular spaces in lesions express LAM-1 (leukocyte adhesion molecule 1) and thrombomodulin which are markers of lymphokine-activated endothelial cells (Zhang et al., 1994). This observation supports the notion that KS spindle cells are of endothelial origin and are activated by growth factors (see below).

The staining (observed by some laboratories but not by others) of spindle cells with antibodies to CD14 and factor XIIIa has been interpreted to reflect a possible link between KS spindle cells and cells of the monocyte/macrophage lineage, possibly dermal dendrocytes (Nickoloff and Griffiths, 1989; Rappersberger et al., 1991). These cells are distinct from Langerhans cells (Nickoloff and Griffiths, 1989). Similar histochemical data have been interpreted to suggest a relationship with smooth muscle cells or myofibroblast (reviewed in Roth, Brandstetter and Stürzl, 1992). These discrepant results could suggest that cells of different lineage can adopt a spindle cell like morphology when present in KS lesions.

IN VITRO CULTURES DERIVED FROM KS LESIONS

A number of laboratories have cultured cells expressing markers characteristic for vascular or lymphatic endothelium from KS lesions (Delli Bovi *et al.*, 1986; Nakamura *et al.*, 1988; Roth *et al.*, 1988; Siegal *et al.*, 1990; Corbeil *et al.*, 1991; Herndier *et al.*, 1994), but cultures related to smooth muscle cells (Albini *et al.*, 1988; Wittek *et al.*, 1991) as well as mixed populations (Siegal *et al.*, 1990; further references in Roth, Brandstetter and Stürzl, 1992) have also been reported. The lineage of cultured cells has been defined by staining for similar markers as in the *in situ* studies: vimentin and cytokeratin, endothelial markers such as vWF, Pal E, OKM-5, BMA 120 (typical for blood vessel endothelium), En4 and UEA-I lectin (reactive with blood vessel and lymphatic endothelium), CD14 and factor XIIIa (indicating cells of the monocyte/macrophage lineage), SMC α-actin (smooth muscle and myofibroblast) and others (reviewed in Roth, Brandstetter and Stürzl, 1992; Stürzl, Brandstetter and Roth, 1992a).

Two stable, fully transformed and tumorigenic cell lines have been reported: a cell line expressing endothelial markers, established by Siegal and colleagues (Siegal *et al.*, 1990; Herndier *et al.*, 1994) induced KS-like tumors of human origin in nude mice. This cell line had a normal diploid karyotype, expressed the endothelial markers factor VIII, EN-4 and UEA-I lectin. In addition, it produced high levels of urokinase plasminogen activator (uPA) and plasminogen

activator inhibitor (PAI-1; Herndier *et al.*, 1994). Interestingly, plasminogen activator has been shown to be involved in the development of endothelial tumors in mice transgenic for the polyoma middle T protein (Montesano *et al.*, 1990). More recently, a second cell line capable of causing tumors of human origin in nude mice has been described (Lunardi-Iskander *et al.*, 1995). The growth of these lesions in nude mice is inhibited by β-HCG (Lunardi-Iskander *et al.*, 1995) and first attempts are presently being undertaken to exploit this observation for therapeutic use (Harris, 1995).

In contrast, a few KS cell cultures, also of an endothelial phenotype, induce the growth of 'KS like' lesions of *murine* origin, when inoculated into nude mice (Nakamura *et al.*, 1988; Salahuddin *et al.*, 1988). Spindle-shaped cells showing a moderate expression of endothelial antigens were also cultured from peripheral blood of KS patients and have been reported to induce angiogenesis in nude mice (Browning *et al.*, 1994). This observation, along with other *in vitro* findings (see below), suggested that growth factors produced by these cultures could induce mouse cells to proliferate and develop into such KS-like lesions.

Most other cell cultures, including some which are capable of acidic LDL uptake and express the endothelial marker BMA 120, did not induce tumor formation in nude mice, were not capable of growing in soft agar, and only showed a slightly reduced serum dependence (Roth *et al.*, 1988). Similarly, cultures expressing the endothelial marker OKM-5 were not tumorigenic in nude mice (Delli Bovi *et al.*, 1986). Cell cultures of smooth muscle origin do not induce KS-like lesions *in vivo* but are capable of local invasion in muscle organ cultures and through artificial basal membranes (Albini *et al.*, 1988; Wittek *et al.*, 1991). The reason for these differences is not clear but may be linked to differences in the cytokine profile secreted by these different cultures (see below).

GROWTH FACTORS INVOLVED IN THE PROLIFERATION OF SPINDLE CELLS

Several laboratories have examined the role that particular lymphokines might play during the development of a KS tumor and in the growth of KS-derived cells *in vitro*.

Fibroblast growth factors

Ensoli *et al.* (1989) reported that basic fibroblast growth factor (bFGF) was secreted by, and may have promoted the growth of, KS cultures expressing endothelial cell markers. Other groups, working with KS cultures of either an endothelial phenotype (Corbeil *et al.*, 1991) or mixed fibroblastoid/endothelial appearance (Werner *et al.*, 1989) also found an FGF like activity in supernatants of their KS cultures which stimulated the growth of normal fibroblasts and endothelial cells.

Members of the FGF family, including bFGF and ECFG (endothelial cell growth factor), stimulate the growth of normal endothelial cells, and cultured KS cells with endothelial characteristics have been shown to induce transient neoangiogenesis in nude mice (Nakamura *et al.*, 1988). The FGF family of cytokines may thus play a crucial role during the development of KS lesions. In KS lesions, the expression of bFGF and FGF5 in spindle cells has been shown by *in situ* hybridization (Xerri *et al.*, 1991). Acidic FGF and FGF6 are also expressed in KS lesions (Li *et al.*, 1993), but the cell type(s) secreting these two members of the FGF family is not known. The importance of bFGF in the development of experimental 'KS-like' lesions is further supported by the report that a bFGF specific antisense oligonucleotide can inhibit the angiogenic effect of cultured KS cells in nude mice (Ensoli *et al.*, 1994b).

Platelet derived growth factor (PDGF)

Normal endothelial cells (Roth *et al.*, 1989; Ensoli *et al.*, 1989) as well as some KS cell cultures with endothelial characteristics (Ensoli *et al.*, 1989) produce and are thus independent of exogenous PDGF (Ensoli *et al.*, 1989; Corbeil *et al.*, 1991). However, PDGF has been found to be essential for the propagation *in vitro* of other KS cell cultures which express mRNA for the receptors for PDGFα and PDGFβ (Roth *et al.*, 1989; Werner *et al.*, 1990). KS spindle cells *in vivo* express mRNA for PDGF-β receptor whereas mRNA for PDGF-α and PDGF-β were expressed on some tumor cells localized in the vicinity of slit-like spaces (Stürzl, Brandsetter and Zietz, 1992b). These findings could suggest that some cells in the KS lesion produce PDGF which is required for the growth of other cell types, thus highlighting the interdependence of the different cell lineages found in a KS lesion.

IL-1

Il-1 has also been reported to be secreted by KS cultures of an endothelial phenotype (Ensoli *et al.*, 1989; Corbeil *et al.*, 1991) and to have a potent stimulatory effect on cultured KS cells with an endothelial phenotype (Nakamura *et al.*, 1988).

IL-6

KS cultures of an endothelial phenotype secrete, and proliferate in response to, IL-6 (Miles *et al.*, 1990; Corbeil *et al.*, 1991). The expression of receptors for IL-6 on cultured KS cells has also been reported (Miles *et al.*, 1990) and *in vivo* KS cells expressed IL-6 mRNA (Gillitzer and Berger, 1991). However, KS cell cultures expressing the endothelial marker BMA 130 did not express receptors for IL-6 (Roth, Brandstetter and Stürzl, 1992). Thus IL-6 may play a role in the proliferation of at least some of the cell lineages present in a KS lesion, again presumably in a paracrine fashion.

TNF-α

TNF-α has a potent stimulatory effect on some KS cell cultures (Nakamura *et al.*, 1988) but whether it is produced by KS cultures with endothelial characteristics is controversial (Ensoli *et al.*, 1989; Corbeil *et al.*, 1991). *In vivo*, TNF-α has been reported to be expressed by KS cells in low amounts but was mainly found in epidermal cells adjacent to the tumor (Gillitzer and Berger, 1991), indicating a possible paracrine role of TNF-α.

Miscellaneous

Secretion of GM-CSF and TGF-β by KS cell cultures with endothelial characteristics, but not by normal endothelial cells, has been reported (Ensoli *et al.*, 1989). TGF-β1 also promotes the growth of cultured KS cells and, in KS lesions, is mainly found in macrophage-like cells, but not in spindle cells, suggesting a paracrine role for this cytokine (Williams *et al.*, 1995). Hepatocyte growth factor (scatter factor) also promotes the growth of cultured KS cells and may thus play a role in KS pathogenesis (Naidu *et al.*, 1994).

Taken together, these findings from different laboratories all suggest that different cell lineages (endothelial cells, fibroblasts, epithelial cells) are present in a KS lesion, can adopt a spindle-cell-like morphology, and may depend on each other for certain growth factors acting in a paracrine fashion. Some of the cytokines discussed above may also have an autocrine effect and some may be required for the maintenance of KS cells in culture.

CLONALITY OF KS LESIONS

The effect of these different cytokines, and some viral factors (see below), may go beyond promoting the polyclonal proliferation and/or differentiation of endothelial cells in KS lesions. Individual KS nodules have been shown to contain monoclonal cell populations (Rabkin *et al.*, 1995). Short-term cultures of KS biopsies have been noted to contain chromosomal rearrangements but no consistent pattern has emerged so far (Delli-Bovi *et al.*, 1986).

THE ROLE OF HIV-1 TAT IN PROMOTING KS LESIONS

Experimental evidence suggests that the Tat protein of HIV-1 can enhance the growth of cultured 'endothelial' KS cells (Ensoli *et al.*, 1990). In this *in vitro* model, Tat is thought to cooperate with bFGF to enhance KS cell proliferation. The effect of Tat seems to be mediated by its binding to $\alpha_5 \beta_1$ and $\alpha_v \beta_3$ integrins via an RGD sequence element in a manner similar to, and replaceable by, their physiological ligands fibronectin and vitronectin (Ensoli *et al.*, 1994a; Barillari *et al.*, 1993). On other KS cell cultures the effect of Tat was found to be inconsistent (Roth, Brandstetter and Stürzl, 1992).

Several cytokines, including TNF, IL-1 and gamma-interferon, can render normal endothelial and smooth muscle cells susceptible to the growth promoting effect of Tat (Barillari *et al.*, 1993), possibly by increasing the expression of integrin receptors which interact with Tat (Ensoli *et al.*, 1994a; Barillari *et al.*, 1993). Injection of Tat into nude mice (Ensoli *et al.*, 1994a), or immunocompetent C57/BL mice (after incorporation into Matrigel (Albini *et al.*, 1994)), induces angiogenes and this effect is potentiated by bFGF (Ensoli *et al.*, 1994a) or heparin (Albini *et al.*, 1994). This Tat- and heparin-induced neoangiogenesis can be inhibited by the matrix metalloproteinase inhibitor TIMP-2 (Albini *et al.*, 1994), and Tat and bFGF synergize to increase the expression of collagenase IV in nude mice (Ensoli *et al.*, 1994a). These studies suggest the involvement of tissue proteinases in the development of KS lesions.

Several groups have investigated the angiogenic properties of HIV-1 *tat* in transgenic mice. Vogel and colleagues reported the emergence of KS-like lesions in mice transgenic for HIV-1 *tat* (Vogel *et al.*, 1988) and Corallini and colleagues, including the early region of BK virus in an LTR-*tat* transgenic construct, also observed 'KS-like' lesions in addition to other malignancies (Corallini *et al.*, 1993). However, other lines of transgenic mice, carrying the complete HIV-1 genome, failed to develop similar lesions (Leonard *et al.*, 1988). In *tat*-transgenic mice which did develop KS-like lesions, the expression of *tat* was not found in spindle cells but in neighboring keratinocytes (Vogel *et al.*, 1988), suggesting that secreted Tat could be responsible for the angiogenic effect. Ensoli *et al.* (1994a), using immunohistochemical techniques, reported that in human AIDS-KS biopsies, Tat, presumably released from infected mononuclear cells, could be found on spindle cells.

Thus, the ability of HIV-1 Tat to induce neoangiogenesis in concert with other factors has been demonstrated in several experimental systems. However, this property may not be unique to HIV-1 infection, as supernatants from T-cell lines infected with HTLV-II have been shown to enable the propagation of KS-derived cells *in vitro*. The lymphokine responsible for this growth enhancing effect has been identified as oncostatin M (Nakamura *et al.*, 1988; Nair *et al.*, 1992; Miles *et al.*, 1992). This suggests that infection by other human retroviruses can result in the production of lymphokines which promote the growth of cells found in KS lesions. In view of the non-human retroviruses that have been shown to induce KS-like lesions in several animal models (see below), as well as of a report that mice transgenic for the middle T gene of polyomavirus develop endothelial cell tumors (Bautch *et al.*, 1987), it is conceivable that different infectious organisms could inititate such a cascade of events.

AN INFECTIOUS AGENT AS A CAUSE OF KS?

There is strong epidemiological evidence for the involvement of an infectious agent, distinct from HIV-1, in the pathogenesis of Kaposi's sarcoma: KS is much more common in homosexual or bisexual men with AIDS than in other risk groups for HIV (Beral *et al.*, 1990; reviewed in Beral, 1991). In the US, the incidence of KS among HIV-infected homosexuals is highest on the East and West coast, but much lower in other federal states (Beral, 1991) and homosexual or bisexual men with KS are more likely to have had sexual partners from geographic areas where KS is relatively common (Archibald *et al.*, 1990; Beral, 1991). KS has been reported in HIV-negative homosexual patients in whom it may be clinically more benign (Friedman-Kien *et al.*, 1990). KS is strongly associated with promiscuity and a variety of past sexually transmitted infections (Jacobson *et al.*, 1990).

These findings suggest the involvement of a most likely sexually transmitted agent, which is distinct from HIV-1. Exposure to this agent may have preceded exposure to HIV-1 (Jacobson *et al.*, 1990). The decrease in KS incidence in homosexuals over the last 10 years may thus reflect decreased transmission of the 'KS agent' following the adoption of 'safe sex' practices (Beral, 1990). Further evidence suggests that the putative 'KS agent' might be more easily, but not exclusively, transmitted via a fecal–oral route as KS incidence was associated with sexual practices involving oral–anal contact (Beral *et al.*, 1992; Darrow *et al.*, 1992; Peterman *et al.*, 1992). However, this effect has not been observed in other cohort studies (Elford, Tindall and Sharkey, 1992; Page-Bodkin *et al.*, 1992).

Among HIV-infected individuals, KS is particularly rare in hemophiliacs, rarer than in recipients of blood transfusions or IVDUs

(Beral *et al.*, 1990). This suggests that parenteral transmission of the putative KS agent may occur rarely, and that in this case it is preferentially transmitted with cellular blood components.

HIV-negative, iatrogenically immunosuppressed individuals have an increased risk of developing KS (Kinlen, 1982). The frequency of transplant-associated KS varies considerably in different geographic areas, as illustrated by the observation that in Saudi Arabia KS is a common tumor occurring after transplantation (Quinibi *et al.*, 1988) whereas transplant-associated KS is rarer in Britain, USA or Australia (Kinlen, 1982; further references in Beral, 1991). These observations, as well as reports of localized foci of KS in Europe (Rappersberger *et al.*, 1991) and the existence of HIV-negative KS in Africa all suggest that the putative 'KS agent' is likely to have a wide, but uneven, geographic distribution.

Although suggested initially (Haverkos *et al.*, 1985; Archibald *et al.*, 1990), inhalation of nitrites ('poppers') has not been found to be associated with an increased incidence of KS in most studies (Beral *et al.*, 1992; Darrow *et al.*, 1992; Jacobson *et al.*, 1990; Lifson *et al.*, 1990).

THE SEARCH FOR A KS AGENT

In view of the strong epidemiological evidence for the involvement of an infectious agent in the pathogenesis of KS, extensive efforts have been made over the last 25 years to identify such an agent. Serological studies looking for antibodies to known viruses have not shown any convincing association with KS (e.g. Holmberg, 1990; further references in Roth, Brandstetter and Stürzl, 1992). Antibodies to HIV-1 gp41 (the transmembrane portion of the envelope protein complex) and *nef* (one of the accessory proteins of HIV-1) have been described in an otherwise serologically negative patient with KS (Bowden *et al.*, 1991), but the implications of this report are still uncertain.

Several laboratories have tried to isolate viruses from KS lesions, so far without success. However, virus particles have been reported in KS lesions *in vivo* by several groups. C-type retroviruses were described in KS biopsies from a group of HIV-negative KS patients from a distinct region on the Southern Peloponnesus in Greece (Rappersberger *et al.*, 1991). Interestingly, some of the clinical features of KS in this group of patients (involvement of oral and genital mucosa and gastrointestinal tract; extensive involvement of facial skin) were reminiscent of African or AIDS-associated KS rather than 'classical' KS. Retroviral particles have also been described in KS biopsies from patients with AIDS (Gyorkey *et al.*, 1984; Schenk, 1986); however, in at least one report (Schenk, 1986) the morphological features of these retroviral particles were suggestive of HIV and it is therefore uncertain whether they could represent the 'KS agent'.

Further, albeit indirect, evidence supporting a possible role of retroviruses in the pathogenesis of KS, comes from several animal models. Macaque monkeys infected with the D-type simian retrovirus type 2 (SRV-2) develop retroperitoneal and subcutaneous fibrosis with progressive fibrovascular proliferation, reminiscent of, but not identical with, KS lesions. Cell cultures could be established from these lesions and induced self-limited, transient spindle cell proliferation, accompanied by pronounced vascularization, when inoculated into nude mice (Tsai *et al.*, 1990). In fowl, some strains of avian leukosis virus can, in addition to lymphoma, induce disseminated hemangiomatosis characterized by a progression from early patch-like lesions with predominant endothelial cell proliferation to hemangiosarcoma (Victor and Jarplid, 1988). In Balb/c mice, a strain of Moloney murine sarcoma virus (MMSV 349), containing the *mos* oncogene, induces lesions that resemble human KS both on the basis of histopathology and electron microscopy (Stoica, Hoffman and Yuen, 1990). The *mos* oncogene does not seem to be sufficient to induce these lesions as another strain of MMSV, also containing the *mos* oncogene, does not induce similar lesions (Stoica, Hoffman and Yuen, 1990). In addition to the HIV-1 *tat* transgenic mice developing KS-like lesions (see above), mice transgenic for the middle T antigen of polyomavirus develop endothelial tumors (Bautch *et al.*, 1987).

Therefore, several infectious agents or their proteins can induce vascular proliferation which bears some resemblance to KS lesions and it is therefore difficult to extrapolate from these animal models to a candidate for an infectious agent involved in the pathogenesis of human KS.

Herpes virus-like particles has been observed in short-term cultures from KS lesions from African patients (Giraldo, Beth and Hagenau, 1972), and in KS biopsies (Walter *et al.*, 1984), but their identity remains unresolved. Although a series of earlier studies, based on serology, Southern blot analysis of KS biopsies as well as *in situ* hybridization suggested a possible involvement of cytomegalovirus (CMV) in the pathogenesis of KS (reviewed in Roth, Brandstetter and Stürzl, 1992), other groups failed to obtain similar results and some of the positive hybridization results may have been due to cross-reactions with normal cullular DNA (Rüger, Colimon and Fleckenstein, 1984). Human papillomavirus HPV-16 was detected by PCR in a proportion of skin biopsies from AIDS-associated, as well as HIV-negative KS and in several cultures established from KS biopsies or pleural effusions (Huang *et al.*, 1992). Dermal dendrocytes within, as well as in the vicinity of, KS lesions expressed HPV-related antigens in a proportion of cases (Nickoloff *et al.*, 1992). However, others could also detect 'high risk' HPV-types (HPV-18, -33) in normal skin of HIV-infected individuals without KS and HIV-negative control subjects (Adams *et al.*, 1995). Although a sexually transmitted agent, the relatively widespread

distribution of 'high risk' HPVs could not explain the characteristic epidemiology of KS. In addition to these viruses, small 40–50 nm particles have been observed in a culture derived from a KS biopsy (Siegal *et al.*, 1990), but have not been identified.

Non-viral transmissible agents have also been considered. Early work reported the isolation of a mycoplasma from NIH 3T3 cells transformed with human DNA from KS lesions (Lo *et al.*, 1989). This mycoplasma was subsequently identified as a strain of *Mycoplasma fermentans* (strain *incognitus*). However, using PCR, *Mycoplasma fermentans* (*incognitus* strain) can be found in both HIV-positive and HIV-negative individuals (Katseni *et al.*, 1993). Although both the HIV-positive and HIV-negative group in this study consisted mainly of homosexual males, *M. fermentans* was found with comparable frequency in samples from HIV-negative, heterosexual women, indicating that there does not seem to be a correlation between the presence of *M. fermentans* and groups known to be at particular risk for KS (Katseni *et al.*, 1993). Another mycoplasma, *M. penetrans* (Lo *et al.*, 1991), seems to be more common in HIV-infected than in HIV-negative individuals as shown by the prevalence of antibodies to this organism (Wang *et al.*, 1992). Serological evidence would suggest that *M. penetrans* might be more common in HIV-infected homosexuals, but not in intravenous drug users or hemophiliacs, thus suggesting a link to those patient groups known to be at an increased risk for KS (Wang *et al.*, 1993). However, only about a third of homosexual men with KS had antibodies to *M. penetrans* (Wang *et al.*, 1993).

THE ROLE OF KAPOSI'S SARCOMA ASSOCIATED HERPESVIRUS (KSHV/HHV 8)

The recently discovered new human gammaherpesvirus (Chang *et al.*, 1994), provisionally termed Kaposi's sarcoma-associated herpesvirus (KSHV) (Chang *et al.*, 1994) or HHV 8 (Schulz and Weiss, 1995), is a strong candidate for the 'KS agent'. Work from several laboratories has shown that it is consistently found in the vast majority (>95%) of biopsies from AIDS-associated KS (Chang *et al.*, 1994; Boshoff *et al.*, 1995a; Huang *et al.*, 1995; Lebbé *et al.*, 1995), classical Mediterranean KS (Boshoff *et al.*, 1995a; Moore and Chang, 1995; Buonaguro *et al.*, 1996), post-transplant KS (Boshoff *et al.*, 1995a; Buonaguro *et al.*, 1996) and African endemic KS (Chang *et al.*, 1996a; Schalling *et al.*, 1995; Buonaguro *et al.*, 1996). Detection of KSHV/HHV 8 in broncho-alveolar lavage fluid is diagnostic for the presence of pulmonary KS. KSHV/HHV 8 is present in the flat endothelial cells lining ectatic vascular spaces, as well as in spindle cells, of KS lesions (Boshoff *et al.*, 1995b). These two cell types represent the bulk of proliferating cells in KS lesions and this observation is therefore compatible with a causative role of this virus in the development of KS lesions. However, primary cultures established from KS biopsies lose KSHV/HHV 8 after a few passages, and established KS cell cultures, including permanent cell lines (see above), are negative for this virus (Ambroziak *et al.*, 1995; Lebbé *et al.*, 1995). The implications of this observation are not yet clear: KSHV/HHV 8 might not be required for the development of KS lesions *in vivo* and only infect, and/or replicate preferentially in, already established KS endothelial or spindle cells; alternatively, the murine angioproliferative lesions induced by KS cell cultures in nude mice and the human tumorigenic cell lines (see above) may not be an adequate model for KS or parts of the KSHV/HHV8 genome may be lost from stable cell lines.

In view of the characteristic epidemiology of KS, the prevalence of KSHV/HHV 8 in different populations is presently the subject of intense investigation. Using PCR, KSHV/HHV 8 can be detected in peripheral blood mononuclear cells from about 50% of KS patients (Collandre *et al.*, 1995; Ambroziak *et al.*, 1995; Whitby *et al.*, 1995), but not (Ambroziak *et al.*, 1995; Whitby *et al.*, 1995; Moore *et al.*, 1996a) or only in 9% (Bigoni *et al.*, 1996) of healthy blood donors. In asymptomatic HIV-infected individuals, detection of KSHV/HHV 8 in peripheral blood predicts progression to KS (Whitby *et al.*, 1995; Moore *et al.*, 1996a). These findings suggest that KSHV/HHV 8 only has a limited distribution in Western populations and are supportive of its causative role in the pathogenesis of KS. However, two groups have found KSHV/HHV 8 in semen samples and prostate of healthy HIV-1 seronegative individuals (Lin *et al.*, 1995; Monini *et al.*, 1996), whereas others have not made this observation (Li, Huang and Friedman-Kien, 1995; Ambroziak *et al.*, 1995, Gupta *et al.*, 1996; Howard, personal communication). On the other hand, the first available serological data suggest that antibodies to several proteins of KSHV/HHV 8 can be detected in the majority of KS patients, but less commonly in HIV-1 infected individuals without KS and infrequently in the general population of Western countries (Miller *et al.*, 1996; Kedes *et al.*, 1996; Gao *et al.*, 1996; Simpson *et al.*, 1996). Therefore, several laboratories have found a strong association between detecting KSHV/HHV 8 by either PCR or serology and the presence of, or increased risk for, KS, and this observation supports a causative role of this virus in KS pathogenesis.

KSHV/HHV 8 belongs to the γ-2-subgroup of herpesviruses and is, so far, most closely related to herpesvirus *saimiri* (HVS), a potently lymphomagenic virus of squirrel monkeys (Moore *et al.*, 1996b). Its genomic organization, as known so far (Moore *et al.*, 1996b), is also similar, and in some parts, highly homologous to Epstein-Barr virus (EBV). Like HVS, KSHV/HHV 8 contains a homologue of the human cyclin D gene and a member of the family of G-protein coupled receptors (Cesarman *et al.*,

1995a). The KSHV/HHV 8 D-type cyclin homologue is active in abrogating the function of the retinoblastoma tumor suppressor protein (Chang *et al.*, 1996b) and could thus be involved in dysregulating cellular proliferation/differentiation.

Like its relative EBV, KSHV/HHV 8 infects peripheral blood B-cells (Ambroziak *et al.*, 1995) and establishes a latent infection in some B-cell lymphoma cell lines (Renne *et al.*, 1996). Its detection in peripheral blood correlates inversely with the number of CD4 T-cells, thus suggesting that its replication is under immunological control (Whitby *et al.*, 1995). It is also found in a rare form of AIDS-associated B-cell lymphoma, 'body-cavity associated' lymphoma (Cesarman *et al.*, 1995b), in a proportion of AIDS-associated primary CNS lymphomas (Boshoff *et al.*, 1996), and in some cases of both HIV-related and unrelated multicentric Castleman's disease (Soulier *et al.*, 1995).

Thus, all the evidence available at present suggests that KSHV/HHV 8 is a strong candidate for the long sought after 'KS agent'. However, how it contributes to the development of KS lesions and what its distribution is in different geographic areas remains to be determined. In addition, KSHV/HHV 8 may contribute to some rare AIDS-related B-cell lymphomas.

SUMMARY

The experimental and epidemiological evidence available today suggests that KS is not, or only exceptionally, a true malignancy. KS lesions are made up of different cellular lineages, probably mainly endothelial cells and fibroblastoid cells, which proliferate in response to several growth factors acting in an autocrine and paracrine fashion. The cascade of events leading to the production of these growth factors and to the proliferation of fibroblastoid and epithelial cells is most likely triggered by an infectious agent. The recently discovered new human

γ herpesvirus KSHV/HHV 8 seems the best candidate reported so far, but its precise role in the pathogenesis of KS, as well as of some AIDS-related B-cell lymphomas, remains to be established.

ACKNOWLEDGMENT

I would like to thank Denise Whitby for her help with this chapter and her critical reading of the manuscript.

REFERENCES

Adams, V., Kempf, W., Hassam, S. *et al.* (1995) Detection of several types of human papilloma viruses in AIDS-associated Kaposi's sarcoma. *J. Med. Virol.*, **46**, 189–93.

Albini, A., Mitchell, C.D., Thompson, E.W. *et al.* (1988) Invasive activity and chemotactic response to growth factors by Kaposi's sarcoma cells. *J. Cell. Biochem.*, **36**, 369–76.

Albini, A., Fontanini, G., Masiello, L. *et al.* (1994) Angiogenic potential *in vivo* by Kaposi's sarcoma cell-free supernatants and HIV-1 *tat* product: inhibition of KS-like lesions by tissue inhibitor of metalloproteinase-2. *AIDS*, **8**, 1237–44.

Ambroziak, J.A., Blackbourn, D.J., Herndier, B.G. *et al.* (1995) Herpes-like sequences in HIV-infected and uninfected Kaposi's sarcoma patients. *Science*, **268**, 582–83.

Archibald, C.P., Schechter, MT., Craib, K.J.P. *et al.* (1990) Risk factors for Kaposi's sarcoma in the Vancouver lymphadenopathy – AIDS study *J. AIDS*, **3** (suppl. 1), S18–S23.

Barillari, G., Gendelman, R., Gallo, R.C. and Ensoli, B. (1993) The Tat protein of human immunodeficiency virus type 1, a growth factor for AIDS Kaposi's sarcoma and cytokine-activated vascular cells, induces adhesion of the same cell types by using integrin receptors recognizing the RGD amino acid sequence. *Proc. Natl. Acad. Sci. USA*, **90**, 7941–5.

Bauer, F.A., Wear, D.J., Angritt, P. and Lo, S.-C. (1991) *Mycoplasma fermentans* (*incognitus* strain) infection in the kidneys of patients with acquired immunodeficiency syndrome and associated nephropathy: a light microscopic, immunohistochemical and ultrastructural study. *Hum. Pathol.*, **22**, 63–69.

Bautch, V.L., Toda, S., Hassel, J.A. and Hanahan,

D. (1987) Endothelial cell tumours develop in transgenic mice carrying polyomavirus middle T oncogene. *Cell*, **51**, 529–38.

Beral, V., Peterman, T.A., Berkelman, R.L. and Jaffe, H.W. (1990) Kaposi's sarcoma among persons with AIDS: a sexually transmitted infection? *Lancet*, **335**, 123–28.

Beral, V. (1991) Epidemiology of Kaposi's sarcoma, in *Cancer, HIV and AIDS*. (eds V. Beral, H.W. Jaffe and R.A. Weiss). *Cancer Surv.*, **10**, 5–22. Cold Spring Harbor Laboratory Press, MT.

Beral, V., Bull, D., Darby, S. *et al.* (1992) Risk of Kaposi's sarcoma and sexual practices associated with faecal contact in homosexual or bisexual men with AIDS. *Lancet*, **339**, 632–35.

Bigoni, B., Dolcetti, R., de Lellis, L. *et al.* (1996) Human herpesvirus 8 is present in the lymphoid system of healthy persons and can reactivate in the course of AIDS. *J. Infect. Dis.*, **173**, 542–54.

Boshoff, C., Whitby, D., Hatziioannou, T. *et al.* (1995a) Kaposi's sarcoma associated herpesvirus in HIV-negative Kaposi's sarcoma. *Lancet*, **345**, 1043–44.

Boshoff, C., Schulz, T.F., Kennedy, M.M. *et al.* (1995b) Kaposi's sarcoma-associated herpes virus (KSHV) infects endothelial and spindle cells. *Nature Med.*, **1**, 1274–8.

Boshoff, C., O'Leary, J.J., Thomas, A. *et al.* (1996) Presence of Kaposi's sarcoma-associated herpesvirus (KSHV) in AIDS-related CNS lymphomas. Submitted for publication.

Bowden, F.J., McPhee, D.A., Deacon, N.J. *et al.* (1991) Antibodies to gp41 and *nef* in otherwise HIV-negative homosexual man with Kaposi's sarcoma. *Lancet*, **337**, 1313–14.

Browning, P.J., Sechler, J.M.G., Kaplan, M. *et al.* (1994) Indentification and culture of Kaposi's sarcoma-like spindle cells from the peripheral blood of human immunodeficiency virus-1-infected individuals and normal controls. *Blood*, **84**, 2711–20.

Buchbinder, A., Friedman-Kien, A.E. (1991) Clinical aspects of epidemic Kaposi's sarcoma, in *Cancer, HIV and AIDS*. (eds V. Beral, H.W. Jaffe and R.A. Weiss). *Cancer Surv.*, **10**, 39–52.

Buonaguoro, F.M., Tornesello, M.L., Beth-Giraldo, E. *et al.* (1996) Herpes virus-like DNA sequences detected in endemic, classic, iatrogenic and epidemic Kaposi's sarcoma (KS) biopsies. *Int. J. Cancer*, **65**, 25–28.

Campioni, D., Corallini, A., Zauli, G. *et al.* (1995)

HIV type 1 extracellular *tat* protein stimulates growth and protect cells of BK virus/*tat* transgenic mice from apoptosis. *AIDS Res. Hum. Retrovirus.*, **11**, 1039–48.

Cesarman, E., Chang, Y., Moore, P.S. *et al.* (1995a) Kaposi's sarcoma-associated herpesvirus-like DNA sequences in AIDS-related body-cavity-based lymphomas. *N. Engl. J. Med.*, **332**, 1186–91.

Cesarman, E., Nador, R., Chang, Y. *et al.*, (1995b) Characterization of Kaposi's sarcoma associated herpesvirus-like (KSHV) DNA in AIDS-related lymphoma cell lines and sequence analysis of a 12 kb region of KSHV. *AIDS Res. Hum. Retrovirus.*, **11** (suppl. 1), S68 (abstract).

Chang, Y., Cesarman, E., Pessin, M.S. *et al.* (1994) Identification of herpesvirus-like DNA sequences in AIDS-associated Kaposi's sarcoma. *Science*, **266**, 1865–69.

Chang, Y., Ziegler, J., Wabinga, H. *et al.* (1996a) Kaposi's sarcoma-associated herpesvirus DNA sequences are present in African endemic and AIDS-associated Kaposi's sarcoma. *Arch. Intern. Med.*, **156**, 202–4.

Chang, Y., Moore, P.S., Talbot, S.J. *et al.*, (1996b) Cyclin encoded by KS herpesvirus. *Nature*, **382**, 410.

Cockerell, C.J. (1991) Histopathological features of Kaposi's sarcoma in HIV infected individuals, in *Cancer, HIV and AIDS*. (eds V. Beral, H.W. Jaffe and R.A. Weiss). *Cancer Surv.*, **10**, 39–52.

Collandre, H., Ferris, S., Grau, O. *et al.* (1995) Kaposi's sarcoma and new herpesvirus. *Lancet*, **345**, 1043.

Corbeil, J., Evans, L.A., Vasak, E. *et al.* (1991) Culture and properties of cells derived from Kaposi's sarcoma. *J. Immunol.*, **146**, 2972–76.

Corralini, A., Altavilla, G., Possi, L. *et al.* (1993) Systemic expression of HIV-1 *tat* gene in transgenic mice induces endothelial proliferation and tumors of different histotypes. *Cancer Res.*, **53**, 5569–75.

Darrow, W.W., Peterman, T.A., Jaffe, H.W. *et al.* (1992) Kaposi's sarcoma and exposure to faeces. *Lancet*, **339**, 685.

Delli-Bovi, P., Donti, E., Knowles, D.M. *et al.* (1986) Presence of chromosomal abnormalities and lack of AIDS retrovirus DNA sequences in AIDS-associated Kaposi's sarcoma. *Cancer Res.*, **46**, 6333–8.

Dupin, N., Grandadam, M., Calvez, V *et al.* (1995) Herpesvirus-like DNA sequences in patients with Mediterranean Kaposi's sarcoma. *Lancet*,

345, 761–2.

Elford, J., Tindall, B. and Sharkey, T. (1992) Kaposi's sarcoma and insertive rimming. *Lancet*, **339**, 938.

Ensoli, B., Nakamura, S., Salahuddin, S.Z. *et al.* (1989) AIDS-Kaposi's sarcoma-derived cells express cytokines with autocrine and partacrine growth effects. *Science*, **243**, 223–26.

Ensoli, B., Barillari, G., Salahuddin, S.Z. *et al.* (1990) Tat protein of HIV-1 stimulates growth of cells derived from Kaposi's sarcoma lesions of AIDS patients. *Nature*, **345**, 84–86.

Ensoli, B., Gendelman, R., Markham, P. *et al.* (1994a) Synergy between basic fibroblast growth factor and HIV-1 tat protein in induction of Kaposi's sarcoma. *Nature*, **371**, 674–80.

Ensoli, B., Markham, P., Kao, V. *et al.* (1994b) Block of AIDS-Kaposi's sarcoma (KS) cell growth, angiogenesis, and lesion formation in nude mice by antisense oligonucleotide targeting basic fibroblast growth factor. *J. Clin. Invest.*, **94**, 1736–46.

Friedman-Kien, A.E., Saltzman, B.R., Cao, Y. *et al.* (1990) Kaposi's sarcoma in HIV-negative homosexual men. *Lancet*, **I**, 168–69.

Gao, S.J., Kingsley, L., Li, M. *et al.* (1996) Seroprevalence of KSHV antibodies among North Americans, Italians, and Ugandans with and without Kaposi's sarcoma. *Nature Med.*, **2**, 925–8.

Gillitzer, R., Berger, R. (1991). High levels of macrophage chemotactic protein 1 and IL-6 in lesions of Kaposi's sarcoma *in situ*. *J. Cell. Biochem.*, suppl. **15F**, 249.

Giraldo, G., Beth, E., and Hagenau, F. (1972) Herpes-type virus particles in tissue culture of Kaposi's sarcoma from different geographic regions. *J. Natl. Cancer Inst.*, **49**, 1509–26.

Gupta, P., Mandaleshwer, D.S., Rinaldo, C. *et al.* (1996) Detection of Kaposi's sarcoma herpesvirus DNA in semen of homosexual men with Kaposi's sarcoma. *AIDS* (in press).

Gyorkey, F., Sinkovics, J.G., Melnick, L. and Gyorkey, P. (1984) Retroviruses in Kaposi's sarcoma cells in AIDS. *N. Engl. J. Med.*, **311**, 1183–84.

Harris, P.J., (1995) Treatment of Kaposi's sarcoma and other manifestations of AIDS with human chorionic gonadotropin. *Lancet*, **346**, 118–19.

Haverkos, H.W., Pinsky, P.F., Drotman, P. and Bregmen, D.J. (1985) Disease manifestation among homosexual men with acquired immunodeficiency syndrome: a possible role of nitrites in Kaposi's sarcoma. *Sexually Transm. Dis.*, **12**, 203–208.

Herndier, B.G., Werner, A., Arnstein, P. *et al.* (1994) Characterization of a human Kaposi's sarcoma cell line that induces angiogenic tumours in animals. *AIDS*, **8**, 575–81.

Holmberg, S.D. (1990) Possible cofactors for the development of AIDS-related neoplasms. *Cancer Detect. Prev.*, **14**, 331–36.

Howard, M., Brink, N., Miller, R. and Tedder, R.S. (1995) Association of human herpesvirus with pulmonary Kaposi's sarcoma. *Lancet*, **346**, 712.

Huang, Y.Q., Li, J.J., Rush, M.G. *et al.* (1992) HPV-16-related sequences in Kaposi's sarcoma. *Lancet*, **339**, 515–18.

Huang, Y.Q., Li, J.J., Kaplan, M.H. *et al.* (1995) *Lancet*, **345**, 759–61.

Jacobson, L.P., Muñoz, A., Fox, R. *et al.* (1990) Incidence of Kaposi's sarcoma in a cohort of homosexual men infected with the human immunodeficiency virus type 1. *J. AIDS*, **3**, (suppl. 1) S24–S31.

Kaposi, M. (1872) Idiopathisches Multiples Pigmentsarkon der Haut. *Arch. Dermatol. Syphil.*, **4**, 742–49.

Katseni, V.L., Gilroy, C.B., Ryait, B.K. *et al.* (1993) *Mycoplasma fermentans* in individuals seropositive and seronegative for HIV-1. *Lancet*, **341**, 271–73.

Kedes, D.H., Operskalski, E., Busch, M. *et al.* (1996) The seroprevalence of human herpesvirus 8(Kaposi's sarcoma-associated herpesvirus): Distribution of infection in KS risk groups and evidence for sexual transmission. *Nature Med.*, **2**, 918–24.

Kinlen, L.J. (1982) Immunosuppressive therapy and cancer. *Cancer Surv.*, **1**, 565–83.

Lebbé, C., De Cremoux, P., Rybojad, M. *et al.* (1995) Kaposi's sarcoma and new herpesvirus. *Lancet*, **345**, 1180.

Leonard, J.M., Abramczuk, J.W., Pezen, D.S. *et al.* (1988) Development of disease and virus recovery in transgenic mice containing HIV proviral DNA. *Science*, **242**, 1665–70.

Lifson, A.R., Darrow, W.W., Hessol, N.A. *et al.* (1990) Kaposi's sarcoma in a cohort of homosexual and bisexual men. *Am. J. Epidemiol.*, **131**, 221–31.

Little, D., Said, W., Siegel, R.J. *et al.* (1986) Endothelial cell markers in vascular neoplasms: an immunohistochemical study comparing factor VIII-related antigen, blood group specific antigens, 6-keto-PGF1-α, and *Ulex europaeus* 1 lectin. *Am. J. Pathol.*, **149**, 89–95.

Li, J.J., Huang, Y.Q., Moscatelli, D. *et al.* (1993) Expression of fibroblast growth factors and their receptors in acquired immunodeficiency syndrome-associated Kaposi's sarcoma tissue and derived cells. *Cancer*, **72**, 2253–62.

Li, J.J., Huang, Y.Q. and Friedman-Kien, A.E. (1995) Detection of DNA sequences of KSHV in peripheral blood, semen, KS tumor, and uninvolved skin of KS patients. *AIDS Res. Hum. Retrovirus.*, **11**, (suppl. 1): S98 (Abstract).

Lin, J.C., Lin, S.C., Mar, E.C. *et al.* (1995) Is Kaposi's sarcoma-associated herpesvirus detectable in semen of HIV-infected homosexual men? *Lancet*, **346**, 1601–2.

Little, D., Said, W., Siegel, R.J. *et al.* (1986) Endothelial cell markers in vascular neoplasms: an immunohistochemical study comparing factor VIII-related antigen, blood group specific antigens, 6-keto-PGF1-α, and *Ulex europaeus* 1 lectin. *Am. J. Pathol.*, **149**, 89–95.

Lo, S.-C., Shih, J.W.-K., Yang, N.-Y *et al.* (1989) A novel virus-like infectious agent in patients with AIDS. *Am. J. Trop. Med. Hyg.*, **40**, 213–16.

Lo, S.-C., Hayes, M.M., Wang, R.Y.-H. *et al.* (1991) Newly discovered mycoplasma isolated from patients infected with HIV. *Lancet*, **338**, 1415–18.

Lunardi-Iskandar, Y., Bryant, J.L., Zeman, R.A. *et al.* (1995) Tumorigenesis and metastasis of neoplastic Kaposi's sarcoma cell line in immunodeficient mice blocked by a human pregnancy hormone. *Nature*, **375**, 64–68.

Miles, S.A., Rezai, A.R., Salazar-Gonzalez, J.F. *et al.* (1990) AIDS-Kaposi's sarcoma-derived cells produce and respond to interleukin 6. *Proc. Natl. Acad. Sci. USA*, **87**, 4068–72.

Miles, S.A., Martinez-Maza, O., Rezai, A. *et al.* (1992) Oncostatin M as a potent mitogen for AIDS-Kaposi's sarcoma-derived cells. *Science*, **255**, 1432–30.

Miller, G., Rigsby, M.O., Heston, L. *et al.* (1996) Antibodies to butyrate-inducible antigens of Kaposi's sarcoma-associated herpesvirus in patients with HIV-1 infection. *N. Engl. J. Med.*, **334**, 1292–97.

Modlin, R.L., Hofman, F.M., Kempf, R.A. *et al.* (1983) Kaposi's sarcoma in homosexual men: an immunohistochemical study. *J. Am. Acad. Dermatol.*, **8**, 620–27.

Monini, P., de Lellis, L., Fabris, M. *et al.* (1996) Kaposi's sarcoma–associated herpesvirus DNA sequences in prostate tissue and human semen. *N. Engl. J. Med.*, **334**, 1168–72.

Montesano, R., Pepper, M.S., Mohle-Steinlein, U. *et al.* (1990) Increased proteolytic activity is responsible for the aberrant morphogenetic behaviour of endothelial cells expressing the middle T oncogene. *Cell*, **62**, 435–55.

Moore, P.S. and Chang, Y. (1995) Detection of herpesvirus-like DNA sequences in Kaposi's sarcoma in patients with and without HIV infection. *N. Engl. J. Med.*, **332**, 1181–85.

Moore, P.S., Kingsley, L.A., Holmberg, S.D. *et al.* (1996a) KSHV infection prior to onset of Kaposi's sarcoma. *AIDS*, **10**, 175–80.

Moore, P.S., Gao, S.-J., Dominguez, G. *et al.* (1996) Primary characterization of a herpesvirus agent associated with Kaposi's sarcoma. *J. Virol.*, **70**, 549–58.

Nadji, M., Morales, A.R., Ziegler-Weissman, J. and Penneys, N.S. (1981) Kaposi's sarcoma: immunohistological evidence for an endothelial origin. *Arch. Pathol. Lab. Med.*, **105**, 274–75.

Naidu, Y.M., Rosen, E.M., Zitnick, R. *et al.* (1994) Role of scatter factor in the pathogenesis of AIDS-related Kaposi's sarcoma. *Proc. Natl. Acad. Sc. USA*, **91**, 5281–85.

Nair, B.C., DeVico, A.L., Nakamura, S. *et al.* (1992) Identification of a major growth factor for AIDS-Kaposi's sarcoma cells as oncostatin M. *Science*, **255**, 1430–32.

Nakamura, S., Salahuddin, S.Z., Biberfeld, P. *et al.* (1988) Kaposi's sarcoma cells: Long-term culture with growth factor from retrovirus-infected CD4$^+$ T cells. *Science*, **242**, 426–30.

Nickoloff, B.J. and Griffiths, C.E.M. (1989) Factor XIIIa-expressing dermal dendrocytes in AIDS-associated cutaneous Kaposi's sarcoma. *Science*, **243**, 1736–37.

Nickoloff, B.J., Huang, Y.Q., Li, J.J. and Friedman-Kien, A.E. (1992) Immunohistochemical detection of papillomavirus antigens in Kaposi's sarcoma. *Lancet*, **339**, 548–49.

Page-Bodkin, K., Tappero, J., Samuel, M. and Winkelstein, W. (1992) Kaposi's sarcoma and faecal-oral exposure. *Lancet*, **339**, 1490.

Peterman, T.A., Friedman-Kien, A.E., Jaffe, H.W. and Beral, V. (1992) Kaposi's sarcoma and exposure to faeces. *Lancet*, **339**, 685–86.

Qunibi, W., Akhtar, M., Sheth, K. *et al.* (1988) Kaposi's sarcoma: the most common tumour after renal transplantation in Saudi Arabia. *Am. J. Med.*, **84**, 225–32.

Rabkin, C.S., Bedi, G., Musaba, E. *et al.* (1995) AIDS-related Kaposi's sarcoma is a clonal neoplasm. *Clin. Cancer Res.*, **1**, 257–60.

Rappersberger, K., Tschachler, E., Zonzit, E. *et al.* (1991) Endemic Kaposi's sarcoma in human immunodeficiency virus type I-seronegative persons: demonstration of retrovirus-like particles in cutaneous lesions. *J. Invest. Dermatol.*, **95**, 371–81.

Renne, R., Zhong, W., Herndier, B. *et al.* (1993) Lytic growth of Kaposi's sarcoma-associated herpesvirus (human herpesvirus 8) in culture. *Nature Med.*, **2**, 342–46.

Roth, W.K., Werner, S., Risau, W. *et al.* (1988) Cultured, AIDS-related Kaposi's sarcoma cells express endothelial cell markers and are weakly malignant *in vitro*. *Int. J. Cancer*, **42**, 767–73.

Roth, W.K., Werner, S., Schirren, C.G. and Hofschneider, P.H. (1989) Depletion of PDGF from serum inhibits growth of AIDS-related and sporadic Kaposi's sarcoma cells in culture. *Oncogene*, **4**, 483–87.

Roth, W.K., Brandstetter, H. and Stürzl, M. (1992) Cellular and molecular features of HIV-associated Kaposi's sarcoma. *AIDS*, **6**, 895–913.

Rüger, R., Colimon, R. and Fleckenstein, B. (1984) Search for DNA sequences of human cytomegalovirus in Kaposi's sarcoma tissues with cloned probes. *Antibiot. Chemother.*, **32**, 43.

Salahuddin, S.Z., Nakamura, S., Biberpeld, P. *et al.* (1988) Angiogenic properties of Kaposi's sarcoma-derived cells after long-term culture *in vitro*. *Science*, **242**, 430–33.

Schalling, M., Eukman, M., Kaaya, E.E. *et al.* (1995) A role for a new Herpesvirus (KSHV) in different forms of Kaposi's sarcoma. *Nature Med.*, **1**, 707–708.

Schenk, P. (1986) Retroviruses in Kaposi's sarcoma in acquired immunodeficiency syndrome (AIDS). *Acta Otolaryngol.*, *(Stockh)*, **101**, 295–98.

Schulz, T.F. and Weiss, R.A. (1995) Kaposi's sarcoma: A finger on the culprit. *Nature*, **373**, 17–18.

Siegal, B., Levinton-Kriss, S., Schiffer, A. *et al.* (1990) Kaposi's sarcoma in immunosuppression possibly the result of a dual infection. *Cancer*, **65**, 492–98.

Simpson, G.R., Schulz, T.F., Whitby, D. *et al.* (1996) Prevalence of KSHV infection measured by antibodies to a recombinant capsid protein and a latent immunofluorescence antigen. *Lancet*, **348**, 1133–38.

Soulier, J., Grollet, L., Oksenhendler, E. *et al.* (1995) Kaposi's sarcoma-associated herpesvirus-like DNA sequences in multicentric Castleman's disease. *Blood*, **86**, 1276–80.

Stoica, G., Hoffman, J. and Yuen, P.H. (1990) Moloney murine sarcoma virus 349 induces Kaposi's sarcoma-like lesions in Balb/c mice. *Am. J. Pathol.*, **136**, 933–47.

Stürzl, M., Brandstetter, H. and Roth, W.K. (1992a) Kaposi's sarcoma: a review of gene expression and ultrastructure of KS spindle cells *in vivo*. *AIDS Res. Hum. Retrovirus*, **8**, 1765–75.

Stürzl, M., Roth, W.K., Brockmayer, N.H. *et al.* (1992b) Expression of platelet-derived growth factor and its receptor in AIDS-related Kaposi's sarcoma *in vivo* suggests paracrine and autocrine mechanisms of tumor maintenance. *Proc. Natl Acad. Sci. USA*, **89**, 7046–50.

Tsai, C.C., Tsai, C.-C., Roodman, S.T. and Woon, M.-D. (1990) Mesenchymo-proliferative disorders (MPD) in simian AIDS associated with SRV-2 infection. *J. Med. Primatol.*, **19**, 189–202.

Victor, M. and Jarplid, B. (1988) The cause of Kaposi's sarcoma: an avian retroviral analog. *J. Am. Acad. Dermatol.*, **18**, 398–402.

Vogel, J., Hinrichs, S.H., Reynolds, R.K. *et al.* (1988) The HIV *tat* gene induces dermal lesions resembling Kaposi's sarcoma in transgenic mice. *Nature*, **335**, 601–11.

Walter, P.R., Philippe, E., Nguemby-Mbina, C. and Chamlian, A. (1984) Kaposi's sarcoma: presence of herpes-type particles in a tumour specimen. *Hum. Pathol.*, **15**, 1145–46.

Wang, R.Y.-H., Shih, J.W.-K., Grandinetti, T. *et al.* (1992) High frequency of antibodies to *Mycoplasma penetrans* in HIV-infected patients. *Lancet*, **340**, 1312–16.

Wang, R.Y., Shih, J.W., Weiss, S.H. *et al.* (1993) *Mycoplasma penetrans* infection in male homosexuals with AIDS: high seroprevalence and association with Kaposi's sarcoma. *Clin. Infect. Dis.*, **17**, 724–29.

Weich, H.A., Salahuddin, S.Z., Gill, P. *et al.* (1991) AIDS-associated Kaposi's sarcoma-derived cells in long term culture express and synthesize smooth muscle alpha-actin. *Am. J. Pathol.*, **139**, 1251–58.

Werner, S., Hofschneider, P.H., Stürzl, M. *et al.* (1989) Cytochemical and molecular properties of simian virus 40 transformed Kaposi's sarcoma-derived cells: evidence for the secretion of a member of the fibroblast growth factor family. *J. Cell. Physiol.*, **141**, 490–502.

Werner, S., Hofschneider, P.H., Heldin, C.H. *et al.* (1990) Cultured Kaposi's sarcoma-derived cells express functional PDGF A-type and B-type receptors. *Exp. Cell. Res.*, **187**, 98–103.

Whitby, D., Howard, M.R., Tenant-Flowers, M. *et al.* (1995) Detection of Kaposi's sarcoma-associated herpesvirus (KSHV) in peripheral blood of HIV-infected individuals and progression to Kaposi's sarcoma. *Lancet*, **346**, 799–802.

Williams, A.O., Ward, J.M., Li, J.F. *et al.* (1995) Immunochemical localization of transforming growth factor-β1 in Kaposi's sarcoma. *Hum. Pathol.*, **26**, 469–73.

Wittek, A.E., Mitchell, D., Armstrong, G.R. *et al.* (1991) Propagation and properties of Kaposi's sarcoma-derived cell lines obtained from patients with AIDS: similarity of cultured cells to smooth muscle cells *AIDS*, **5**, 1485–1.

Xerri, L., Hassoun, J., Planche, J. *et al.* (1991) Fibroblast growth factor gene expression in AIDS-Kaposi's sarcoma detected by *in situ* hybridisation. *Am. J. Pathol.*, **138**, 9–15.

Zhang, Y.-M., Bachmann, S., Hemmer, C. *et al.* (1994) Vascular origin of Kaposi's sarcoma: expression of leukocyte adhesion molecule-1, thrombomodulin, and tissue factor. *Am. J. Pathol.*, **144**, 51–59.

Matthias Schrappe

EPIDEMIOLOGY

In HIV-infected patients, non Hodgkin's (NHL) and Hodgkin's lymphomas (HD) are increased by a factor of 30–60 (NHL) and 5 (HD) in comparison to the HIV-negative population (Beral *et al.*, 1991; Hessol *et al.*, 1992; Rabkin *et al.*, 1992). HIV-associated NHLs represent the second most common opportunistic tumor after Kaposi's sarcoma and are listed, together with invasive cervical carcinoma, as AIDS-defining conditions (Centers for Disease Control, 1992). The association of Hodgkin's disease with HIV-infection is well established but its role as AIDS-defining manifestation is still under discussion (Reynolds *et al.*, 1993).

Non Hodgkin's lymphomas are reported as index diagnoses in 3% of all AIDS-cases, without exhibiting as strong epidemiological correlations with gender or risk group (Beral *et al.*, 1991) as is the case in Kaposi's sarcoma, for which a second sexually transmitted infectious agent besides HIV is under discussion (Elford, McDonald and Kaldor, 1993). In general, it is suggested that malignant lymphomas are increasing in frequency, but estimations are hampered by the fact that in most cohorts lymphomas are only documented as an AIDS index diagnosis, possibly underscoring an increase during the patient's later course, when up to 10% of all patients will experience such a tumor (Rabkin *et al.*,

1992). There is no difference in time from infection or in the $CD4^+$ cell count (if corrected for time since HIV seroconversion) between patients with NHL as index diagnosis and patients with other initial AIDS manifestations (Beral *et al.*, 1991; Rabkin *et al.*, 1992). Antiretroviral treatment was thought to play a causal role in pathogenesis (Pluda *et al.*, 1990), but later analyses did not confirm this hypothesis (Moore *et al.*, 1991).

CLINICAL PRESENTATION

Non Hodgkin's lymphomas of HIV-infected patients (HIV-NHL) present with high- grade malignancy and disseminated tumor localization (reviewed in Levine, 1992). The same is true for Hodgkin's lymphomas, which show preponderance of mixed cullularity and lymphocyte depletion (Errante *et al.*, 1994a; Serraino *et al.*, 1993). Although NHL of intermediate and low malignancy (including CLL) as well as T-cell lymphomas have also been described, in general HIV–NHLs should be regarded as B-cell tumors. Of 2824 AIDS patients with HIV–NHL registered by the CDC in the USA, 1686 patients (60%) had an immunoblastic and 590 patients (21%) a Burkitt lymphoma (Beral *et al.*, 1991).

The majority of cases exhibit an extranodal involvement on diagnosis (Ziegler *et al.*, 1984); even primary extranodal manifestation

AIDS and Respiratory Medicine. Edited by A. Zumla, M.A. Johnson and R.F. Miller. Published in 1997 by Chapman & Hall, London. ISBN 0 412 60140 0

Table 20.1 Prevalence of secondary and primary pulmonary NHL

	Secondary involvement	Primary pulmonary NHL
Bermudez et al., 1989	4/31 (13%)	
Cologne (unpublished)	3/60 (5%)	
Di Carlo et al., 1986	2/30 (7%)	
Gill et al., 1987		0/22
Ioachim, 1992		1/100 (1%)
Kalter et al., 1985	2/14 (14%)	
Kaplan et al., 1989	5/84 (6%)	
Knowles et al., 1988		0/89
Lamb et al., 1990	4/25 (16%)	
Loureiro et al., 1988	8/9[a]	
Tirelli et al., 1992a	6/37 (16%)	
Ziegler et al., 1984	8/80 (10%)	

[a]postmortem.

is very common in immunoblastic and large cell lymphomas (41 and 35% (Roithmann et al., 1991)). Up to 74% of patients have gastrointestinal tract manifestation (Bermudez et al., 1989) and between 7 and 66% CNS manifestation (Beral et al., 1991; Loureiro et al., 1988; Levine, 1990a). Disseminated, extranodal and atypical presentation is also seen in most patients with HIV-associated Hodgkin's disease (Andrieu et al., 1993; Pelstring et al., 1991).

While extranodal manifestation is a common condition in HIV–NHL and HIV–HD, something which characterizes these HIV-associated tumors and represents a substantial difference compared to their HIV-negative analogues, is that there is no increase in primary or secondary involvement of the lung.

In HIV-negative patients, the prevalence of clinically diagnosed lung involvement of NHLs is well below 10% (L'Hoste et al., 1984; Doran et al., 1991; Mentzer et al., 1993). In the Danish population-based NHL-registry, 24 primary NHLs of the lung were detected in the total group of 1257 newly diagnosed NHLs (1.9%) (D'Amore et al., 1991). From the information available, the prevalence in HIV-infected patients is in the same range (Irwin and Kaplan, 1993). More information about the prevalence in clinical and pathological studies is given in Table 20.1. Although the above-mentioned characteristics of HIV–NHLs in regard to manifestation and dissemination favor the hypothesis that primary lymphomas of the lung are more common in HIV-infected patients than in HIV-negative patients, data are not sufficient to prove this assumption.

Pulmonary involvement or primary lung manifestation of Hodgkin's disease is extremely rare in HIV-negative patients (Radin, 1990), and there are only scattered reports in HIV-infected patients (Fajac et al., 1992; Anchisi, Pugin and Baur, 1993). In regard to mediastinal involvement, HIV-infected patients seem to exhibit this feature less commonly than HIV-negative patients (Roithmann et al., 1992).

Some series in the literature, which provide information on histology in primary extranodal pulmonary NHL in HIV-negative patients, demonstrate that the majority of tumors are of low-grade malignancy (L'Hoste et al., 1984). Keeping in mind that HIV-related NHLs are of high-grade malignancy

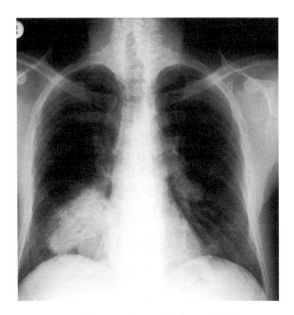

Fig. 20.1 Chest radiograph from HIV-negative patient showing large tumor in lower lobe of right lung.

in the majority of cases, the small number of cases reported does not permit comparisons between immunocompetent and HIV-infected patients in regard to histological presentation. The same is true for the clinical appearance of lung involvement.

DIFFERENTIAL DIAGNOSIS

In HIV-negative patients, pulmonary involvement shows nodular and alveolar infiltration as well as mass-like consolidation and pleural effusions (Cordier *et al.*, 1993). The diagnosis largely depends on employing sensitive methods to detect small nodules of less than 1 cm diameter (Lewis, Casky and Fishman, 1991) and, to get definitive information, on histology (Campbell *et al.*, 1989). In AIDS patients, all these forms may be observed, and NHL has to be considered even in the differential diagnosis of interstitial pneumonia (Teuscher *et al.*, 1992). In 58 patients with HIV–NHL treated at Cologne University Clinic since 1986, 3 patients had

pulmonary manifestations, all of a secondary nature. Two patients showed multilocular nodular infiltrates, one patient a large tumor in the lower lobe of the right lung (Figure 20.1), and all were of high-grade malignancy (Teuscher *et al.*, 1992).

As a consequence, malignant lymphoma of the lung and pulmonary involvement of systemic lymphoma can apparently mimic all kinds of pulmonary manifestation in HIV-infected patients. These include:

- nodular infiltrates: other tumors (testicular carcinoma), atypical mycobacterioses, invasive mycoses;
- patchy lymphangitic infiltrates: pulmonary involvement by Kaposi's sarcoma, bronchopneumonias of other etiology, atypical *Pneumocystis carinii* pneumonia;
- pulmonary infiltrates: *Pneumocystis carinii* pneumonia, *Mycobacterium tuberculosis*, Kaposi's sarcoma, atypical mycobacteria, bacterial and fungal infections;
- alveolar infiltrates: lobar or bronchopneumonia (i.e. pneumococci);
- interstitial infiltrates: *Pneumocystis carinii* pneumonia, CMV pneumonia;
- mass-like consolidation: other tumors, invasive mycoses, bacterial pneumonia;
- pleural effusion: all kinds of pneumonia and tumors, Kaposi's sarcoma, *M. tuberculosis*, *Mycobacterium-avium-intracellulare*.

PATHOGENESIS

Theories about the pathogenesis of HIV-associated lymphomas are based on abundant B-cell stimulation on the background of profound impairment of $CD4^+$ T-helper cell control. The polyclonal B-cell proliferation is in part driven by viral co-infections (i.e. EBV); protein components of HIV and certain cytokines like interleukin 6 (Emilie *et al.*, 1992). This proliferation predisposes to translocations, e.g. of the *c-myc* gene (t(8:14), t(8:2) t(8:22)) in the region of the immunoglobulin genes (reviewed in Levine, 1990b).

One of the characteristics of HIV-associated NHLs is the high frequency of extranodal and gastrointestinal manifestations and involvement, despite the profound lymphoid depletion observed in the compartments of the gut-associated lymphocytic tissue, which develops in late HIV-infection and is caused by $CD4^+$ T-cell loss as well as IgA-producing plasma cells (Schrappe-Bächer *et al.*, 1990). It would be very attractive to integrate stepwise proliferation-induced lymphomagenesis of HIV-associated NHLs into the so-called MALToma concept, which describes a certain subgroup of low-grade lymphomatous tumors deriving from the mucosa-associated lymphoid tissue of the gastrointestinal tract, the respiratory tract and the ductal mucosa of the parotid and breast (Isaacson and Spencer, 1987). Furthermore, the question of how to explain the low frequency of pulmonary lymphomas in comparison to the huge number of gastrointestinal lymphomas in HIV-infected patients remains unsolved, since there is no difference at all in regard to other manifestations of HIV-infection and AIDS, neither to those of infectious etiology nor to Kaposi's sarcoma.

PROGNOSIS AND TREATMENT

Treatment of HIV-associated malignant lymphomas is complicated by the following:

- high rate of treatment failures;
- short survival times;
- common intercurrent opportunistic manifestations during therapy;
- severe hematotoxicity.

With this background, the most important consideration in treating these patients is to identify the subgroup of patients which experiences more benefit in terms of survival time and quality of life as opposed to treatment-induced adverse effects and long hospitalization periods. As long as it is not possible to abrogate the underlying immune deficiency, the treatment of HIV-related opportunistic tumors is based on the concept of pretreatment risk factor stratification, and all data support the assumption that host-related risk factors describing the degree of immunodeficiency are overriding the traditional risk factors such as tumor stage and histology (Levine, 1991b).

HIV-ASSOCIATED NON HODGKIN'S LYMPHOMAS

If unselected patients are considered, the median survival time of HIV-infected patients with NHL does not exceed 6 months (Levine, 1990a; Cottrill *et al.*, 1992), the poorest survival of all initial AIDS manifestations. During the last 10 years, no improvement in survival has so far been observed, in contrast to most other complications. 20–70% of patients with HIV–NHL die as a result of opportunistic infections and 35–55% as a result of the progression of the HIV–NHL (Levine, 1990a; Roithmann *et al.*, 1991). The response rates and complete remissions (CR) of standard induction regimes (i.e. CHOP) are between 40 and 70% and 10 and 56% respectively. Of treated patients with HIV–NHL, 10–20% survive more than one year and can be regarded as long-term survivors (Roithmann *et al.*, 1991).

In large retrospective analyses of cohort studies and treatment protocols, general condition, immunological status and preexisting AIDS, tumor stage and – to a minor degree – histology were identified as the main risk factors (Ziegler *et al.*, 1984; Kaplan *et al.*, 1989; Levine, 1991a; Roithmann *et al.*, 1991; Gisselbrecht *et al.*, 1993). As yet, these have not been considered as stratification parameters in prospective studies.

The immunological status is described in the most appropriate way by the threshold of 100 $CD4^+$ T cells per μl (Kaplan *et al.*, 1989; Gisselbrecht *et al.*, 1993) or 200 $CD4^+/\mu$l (Levine, 1991a). In the French–Italian cooperative trial, there was also a trend towards

Table 20.2 AIDS as a negative risk factor in HIV–NHL, an overview of the literature

	n	AIDS	Non-AIDS PGL Asymptomatic
Gisselbrecht *et al.*, 1993	141	15%[4]	26%[4]
Kaplan *et al.*, 1989	84	2.2 ± 0.8[1]	8.3 ± 1.5[1]
Levine *et al.*, 1991a	35	2/8[2]	14/27[2]
Roithmann *et al.*, 1991	131	3 mo.[1]	8 mo.[1]
Ziegler *et al.*, 1984	66	19/21[3]	26/33[3] 5/12[3]

[1]median survival (months); [2]proportion with CR; [3]proportion of death or illness; [4]2 years' survival.

a better prognosis for p24 antigen-negative patients (CR 64%, survival 2 years 32%) in comparison to p24 antigen-positive patients (CR 54%, survival 2 years 27%) (Gisselbrecht *et al.*, 1993). The prognosis for patients with HIV–NHL is also negatively and independently influenced by the presence of prior AIDS manifestations on diagnosis (Table 20.2).

Among traditional risk factors, tumor stage has an appreciable effect on the survival time, particularly stage IV with bone marrow involvement (Gill *et al.*, 1987; Levine, 1991a, b; Roithmann *et al.*, 1991; Gisselbrecht *et al.*, 1993), although in the analyses of Ziegler *et al.* (1984) and Cottrill *et al.* (1992) this could not be demonstrated. There is a trend towards a poorer prognosis with extranodal manifestations (Kaplan *et al.*, 1989; Gisselbrecht *et al.*, 1993). A worse prognosis is given for patients with primary brain involvement, in most cases immunoblastic and EBV-containing (Ziegler *et al.*, 1991). If secondary leptomeningeal involvement is regarded separately, the sparse data existing so far favor a comparable response (65% CR without vs 55% CR with leptomeningeal manifestation) and survival rate (30% estimated 2 years' survival in both groups), if 12 mg MTX is given intrathecally twice a week up to 9 times or until sterilization of CSF (Gisselbrecht *et al.*, 1993).

Histology is probably the least important

prognostic tumor parameter for highly malignant HIV–NHL. Investigations by Knowles *et al.* (1988) and Roithmann *et al.* (1991) reveal on retrospective analysis that the prognosis for immunoblastic lymphomas is comparatively poor. In the prospective study of the French–Italian group, immunoblastic NHL had a lower 2-year survival rate (16%; small non-cleaved 40%, anaplastic large cell 50%) (Gisselbrecht *et al.*, 1993). The prognostic importance of histology is not yet considered to be settled, and further analysis is warranted as, for example, in regard to the distribution of CNS–NHLs, which tend to be immunoblastic and will severely influence the survival of the immunoblastic subgroup (Ziegler *et al.*, 1991).

One of the most powerful prognostic parameters in tumor therapy is represented by general condition, and the investigations carried out until now show that this is also true in HIV-related NHLs (Bermudez *et al.*, 1989; Kaplan *et al.*, 1989; Levine, 1991a, b; Gisselbrecht *et al.*, 1993). Conversely, general condition is even more difficult to assess as an objective risk factor in HIV-infected, patients than in other tumor patients, if the large array of opportunistic infections and their systemic manifestations (i.e. mycobacterioses; wasting syndrome) are taken into account.

The ongoing controlled trial of the EORTC (No. 70931) on the treatment of HIV–NHLs

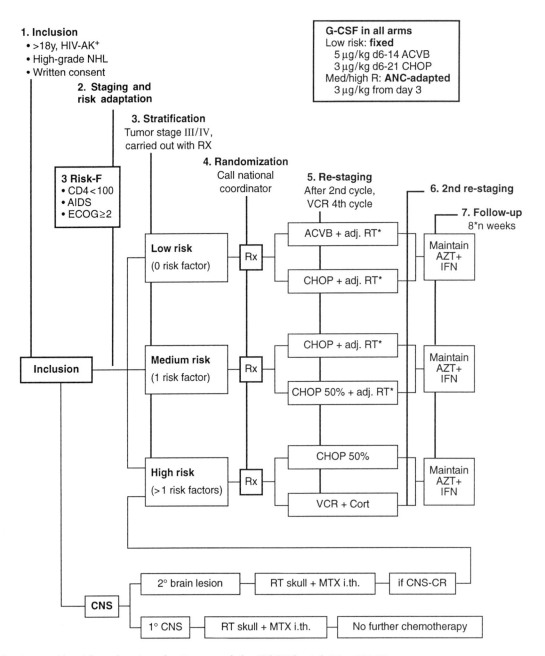

Fig. 20.2 Algorithm showing the 7 arms of the EORTC trial (No. 70933).

ACVB = cyclophosphamide 1200 mg/m² iv day 1; Adriamycin 75 mg/m² iv day 1; vindesine 2 mg/m² iv day 1 + 5; bleomycin 10 mg iv day 1 + 5 and prednisolone 40 mg/m² po days 1-5, to be repeated at day 15 and at day 30 (3 cycles). Standard CHOP is given 4 times every three weeks.

LD-CHOP = cyclophosphamide 400 mg/m² iv day 1; Adriamycin 25 mg/m² iv day 1; vincristine 1.4 mg/m² iv day 1 and prednisolone 40 mg/m² po days 1-5 to be repeated at day 22, 43, 64 (4 cycles).

VS = vincristine 2 mg iv day 1; prednisolone 50 mg/m² po days 1-5 to be repeated day 15, 30 (every 2 weeks).

is, as a consequence, based on a pretreatment stratification by 3 risk factors (general condition; pre-existing AIDS; and CD4$^+$ cell count $<100/\mu l$), thus forming 3 risk groups (low risk: no risk factor; medium risk: 1 risk factor, high risk: more than 1 risk factor) (Figure 20.2). In each risk group, patients are randomized either to treatment with higher dose intensity (i.e. CHOP; ACVB) or to treatment with lower dose intensity (low dose CHOP; vincristine plus steroids in the high risk group), in order to give an answer to the above-mentioned question – whether aggressive treatment is superior in regard to survival time, and in the light of the high rate of complications, to treatment with lower dose intensity. The following modalities should be considered:

1. Prophylaxis against *Pneumocystis carinii* pneumonia with co-trimoxazole or pentamidine inhalations should be instituted, although PCP cannot be prevented in all cases (Levine, 1991a).
2. Intercurrent cytomegalovirus infection is very common and should be carefully evaluated (i.e. with regular ophthalmoscopic examination).
3. Tumor stage IA: due to the high tendency towards early dissemination, chemotherapy is recommended.
4. CNS-prophylaxis (i.e. methotrexate 15 mg i.th.) is strongly recommended during initial diagnostic lumbar puncture and before each following chemotherapy cycle (Levine, 1991a).
5. In primary CNS-lymphoma, no further chemotherapy is recommended. In secondary leptomeningeal CNS-involvement, methotrexate is given until sterilization of CSF.
6. Because of the severe hematotoxicity of chemotherapy in HIV-infected patients, hematopoietic growth factors should be used if indicated (Kaplan *et al.*, 1991).
7. Antiretroviral treatment during chemotherapy may result in greater toxicity and may have to be interrupted until chemotherapy is terminated.
8. Maintenance therapy has not been proven to prolong survival.

HIV-ASSOCIATED HODGKIN'S LYMPHOMAS

In Hodgkin's disease, knowledge about risk factors and treatment regimens is less advanced than in HIV-NHLs. In general, HD is emerging in HIV-infected patients with more favorable immune status than NHLs (Roithmann *et al.*, 1992), resulting in better overall response rates and longer survival than in the latter. Complete response (CR) can be achieved in more than half such patients, and CR is maintained for substantial periods of time (i.e. median 20 months (Errante *et al.*, 1994b) with an overall 2-year survival of 41% (Roithmann *et al.*, 1992)).

Opportunistic infections were the most common cause of death (Roithmann *et al.*, 1992), particularly with standard chemotherapy with MOPP or alternating MOPP-ABVD when these are complicated by a high proportion of these events during treatment and follow-up (Tirelli *et al.*, 1992b). A regimen containing epirubicin, vinblastine and bleomycin (EBV) showed fewer complications (Errante *et al.*, 1994b).

The following risk factors have been identified up to now and are associated with a poor prognosis (Roithmann *et al.*, 1992; Errante, 1994a):

- low CD4$^+$ cell count ($<250/\mu l$ or $<300/\mu l$);
- previous AIDS-manifestations;
- 'B-symptoms' (i.e. systemic symptoms).

The first trial using these risk factors for stratification has been published (Errante, 1994b). In addition, the combination of antineoplastic chemotherapy and antiretroviral therapy has been used in HIV-related Hodgkin's disease (Errante *et al.*, 1994b; Sparano *et al.*, 1994). Hampered by the low incidence of HIV-associated Hodgkin's disease, a definition of standard treatment can only be achieved by large multinational trials, such as those ongoing in the EORTC tumor study group (Chairman Dr U. Tirelli, Aviano, Italy).

REFERENCES

Anchisi, S., Pugin, P., Baur, A. (1993) Primary Hodgkin disease of the lung. *Schweiz. Med. Wochenschr.*, **123**, 65–6.

Andrieu, J.M., Roithmann, S., Tourani, J.M. *et al.* (1993) Hodgkin's disease during HIV-1 infection: the French registry experience. *Ann. Oncol.*, **4**, 635–41.

Beral, V., Peterman, T., Berkelman, R. and Jaffe, H. (1991) AIDS-associated non-Hodgkin's lymphoma. *Lancet*, **337**, 805–9.

Bermudez, M.A., Grant, K.M., Rodvien, R. and Mendes, F. (1989) Non-Hodgkin's lymphoma in a population with or at risk for acquired immunodeficiency syndrome: indications for intensive chemotherapy. *Am. J. Med.*, **86**, 71–6.

Campbell, J.H., Raina, V., Banham, S.W. *et al.* (1989) Pulmonary infiltrates – diagnostic problems in lymphoma. *Postgrad. Med. J.*, **65**, 881–84.

Centers for Disease Control (1992) 1993 Revised classification system for HIV-infection and expanded surveillance case definition for AIDS among adolescents and adults. *MMWR*, **41**, 1–19.

Cordier, J.F., Chailleux, E., Lauque, D. *et al.* (1993) Primary pulmonary lymphomas. A clinical study of 70 cases in nonimmunocompromised patients. *Chest*, **103**, 201–8.

Cottrill, C.P., Young, T.E., Bottomley, D. *et al.* (1992) HIV-associated non-Hodgkin's lymphoma (NHL): the experience of the United Kingdom AIDS oncology group. In: 3rd European Conference on Clinical Aspects and Treatment of HIV Infection, March 12–13, 1992, Paris, p.61.

D'Amore, F., Christensen, B.E., Brincker, H. *et al.* (1991) Clinicopathological features and prognostic factors in extranodal non-Hodgkin lymphomas. *Eur. J. Cancer*, **27**, 1201–8.

Di Carlo, E.F., Amberson, J.B., Metroka, C.E. *et al.* (1986) Malignant lymphomas and the acquired immunodeficiency syndrome. *Arch. Pathol. Lab. Med.*, **110**, 1012–16.

Doran, H.M., Sheppard, M.N., Collins, P.W. *et al.* (1991) Pathology of the lung in leukaemia and lymphoma: a study of 87 Autopsies. *Histopath.*, **18**, 211–19.

Elford, J., McDonald, A. and Kaldor, J. (1993) Kaposi's sarcoma as a sexually transmissible infection: an analysis of Australian AIDS surveillance data. The National HIV Surveillance Committee. *AIDS*, **7**, 1667–71.

Emilie, D., Coumbaras, J., Raphael, M. *et al.* (1992) Interleukin-6 production in high-grade B lymphomas: correlation with the presence of malignant immunoblasts in acquired immunodeficiency syndrome and in human immunodeficiency virus-seronegative patients. *Blood*, **80**, 498–504.

Errante, D., Tirelli, U., Serraino, D. *et al.* (1994a) Epidemiological, virological and clinico-pathological data from 114 patients with Hodgkin's disease and HIV-infection: evidence of significant relation to Epstein-Barr virus, increase of mixed cellularity and lymphocyte depletion subtypes and feasibility of combined treatment with chemotherapy and zidovudine. *Proc. ASCO*, **13**, 55.

Errante, D., Tirelli, U., Gastaldi, R. *et al.* (1994b) Combined antineoplastic and antiretroviral therapy for patients with Hodgkin's disease and human immunodeficiency virus infection. A prospective study of 17 patients. The Italian Cooperative Group on AIDS and Tumors (GICAT). *Cancer*, **73**, 437–44.

Fajac, I., Cadranel, J.L., Mariette, X. *et al.* (1992) Pulmonary Hodgkin's disease in HIV-infected patient. Diagnosis by bronchoalveolar lavage. *Chest*, **102**, 1913–14.

Gill, P.S., Levine, A.M., Karailo, M. *et al.* (1987) AIDS-related malignant lymphoma: results of prospective treatment trials. *J. Clin. Oncol.*, **5**, 1322–28.

Gisselbrecht, C., Oksenhendler, E., Tirelli, U. *et al.* (1993) Human immunodeficiency virus-related lymphoma. Treatment with intensive combination chemotherapy. French-Italian Cooperative Group. *Am. J. Med.*, **95**, 188–96.

Hessol, N.A., Katz, M.H., Liu, J.Y. *et al.* (1992) Increased incidence of Hodgkin disease in homosexual men with HIV infection. *Ann. Intern. Med.*, **15**, 309–11.

Ioachim, H.L. (1992) Lymphoma: an opportunistic neoplasia of AIDS. *Leukemia*, **6**, Suppl. 3, 30–3.

Irwin, D.H. and Kaplan, L.D. (1993) Pulmonary manifestations of acquired immunodeficiency syndrome-associated malignancies. *Sem. Respir.*

Infect., **8**, 139–48.

Isaacson, P.G. and Spencer, J. (1987) Malignant lymphoma of mucosa-associated lymphoid tissue. *Histopathol.*, **11**, 445–62.

Kalter, S.P., Riggs, S.A., Cabanillas, F. *et al.* (1985) Aggressive non-hodgkin's lymphomas in immunocompromised homosexual males. *Blood*, **66**, 655–59.

Kaplan, L.D., Abrams, D.I., Feigal, E. *et al.* (1989) AIDS-associated non-Hodgkin's lymphoma in San Francisco. *JAMA*, **261**, 719–24.

Kaplan, L.D., Kahn, J.O., Crowe, S. *et al.* (1991) Clinical and virologic effects of recombinant human granulocyte-macrophage colony-stimulating factor in patients receiving chemotherapy for human immunodeficiency virus-associated non-Hodgkin's lymphoma: results of a randomized trial. *J. Clin. Oncol.*, **9**, 929–40.

Knowles, D.M., Chamulak, G.A., Subar, M. *et al.* (1988) Lymphoid neoplasia associated with the acquired immunodeficiency syndrome (AIDS). *Ann. Intern. Med.*, **108**, 744–53.

Lamb, R., Gonzalez, R., Myers, A. *et al.* (1990) Aggressive non-Hodgkin's lymphomas in AIDS: the University of Colorado experience. *Am. J. Med. Sci.*, **300**, 345–9.

Levine, A.M. (1990a) Therapeutic approaches to neoplasms in AIDS. *Rev. Infect. Dis.*, **12**, Suppl. 5, 938–43.

Levine, A.M. (1990b) Lymphoma in acquired immunodeficiency syndrome. *Semin. Oncol.*, **17**, 104–12.

Levine, A.M., Wernz, J.C., Kaplan, L. *et al.* (1991a) Low-dose chemotherapy with central nervous system prophylaxis and zidovudine maintenance in AIDS-related lymphoma. A prospective, multi-institutional trial. *JAMA*, **266**, 84–8.

Levine, A.M., Sullivan-Halley, J., Pike, M.C. *et al.* (1991b) Human immunodeficiency virus-related lymphoma. Prognostic factors predictive of survival. *Cancer*, **68**, 2466–72.

Levine, A.M. (1992) Acquired immunodeficiency syndrome-related lymphoma. *Blood*, **80**, 8–20.

Lewis, E.R., Caskey, C.I. and Fishman, E.K. (1991) Lymphoma of the lung: CT findings in 31 patients. *Am. J. Roentgenol.*, **156**, 711–14.

L'Hoste, R.J., Filippa, D.A., Lieberman, P.H. and Bretsky, S. (1984) Primary pulmonary lymphomas. A clinicopathologic analysis of 36 cases. *Cancer*, **54**, 1397–406.

Loureiro, C., Gill, P.S., Meyer, P.R. *et al.* (1988) Autopsy findings in AIDS-related lymphoma.

Cancer, **62**, 735–9.

Mentzer, S.J., Reilly, J.J., Skarin, A.T. and Sugarbaker, D.J. (1993) Patterns of lung involvement by malignant lymphoma. *Surgery*, **113**, 507–14.

Moore, R.D., Kessler, H., Richman, D.D. *et al.* (1991) Non-Hodgkin's lymphoma in patients with advanced HIV infection treated with zidovudine. *JAMA*, **265**, 2208–11.

Pelstring, R.J., Zellmer, R.B., Suolak, L.R. *et al.* (1991) Hodgkin's disease in association with human immunodeficiency virus infection. *Cancer*, **67**, 1865–73.

Pluda, J.M., Yarchoan, R., Jaffe, E.S. *et al.* (1990) Development of non-Hodgkin's lymphoma in a cohort of patients with severe human immunodeficiency virus (HIV) infection on long-term antiretroviral therapy. *Ann. Intern. Med.*, **113**, 276–82.

Rabkin, C.S., Hilgartner, M.W., Hedberg, K.W. *et al.* (1992) Incidence of lymphomas and other cancers in HIV-infected and HIV-uninfected patients with hemophilia. *JAMA*, **267**, 1090–4.

Radin, A.I. (1990) Primary pulmonary Hodgkin's disease. *Cancer*, **65**, 550–63.

Reynolds, P., Saunders, L.D., Layefsky, M.E. and Lemp, G.F. (1993) The spectrum of acquired immunodeficiency syndrome (AIDS)-associated malignancies in San Francisco, 1980–1987. *Am. J. Epidemiol.*, **137**, 19–30.

Roithmann, S., Toledano, M., Tourani, J.M. *et al.* (1991) HIV-associated non-Hodgkin's lymphomas: clinical characteristics and outcome. *Ann. Oncol.*, **2**, 289–95.

Roithmann, S., Tourani, J.M., Gastaut, J.A. *et al.* (1992) Hodgkin's disease associated with HIV infection: clinical characteristics and development. French registry of tumors associated with HIV infection. *Bull. Cancer (Paris)* **79**, 873–82.

Schrappe-Bächer, M., Salzberger, B., Fätkenheuer, G. *et al.* (1990) T-lymphocyte subsets in the duodenal lamina propria of patients infected with human-immunodeficiency-virus 1 and influence of high-dose immunoglobulin therapy. *AIDS.*, **3**, 238–43.

Serraino, D., Carbone, A., Franceschi, S. and Tirelli, U. (1993) Increased frequency of lymphocyte depletion and mixed cellularity subtypes of Hodgkin's disease in HIV-infected patients. Italian Cooperative Group on AIDS and Tumours. *Eur. J. Cancer*, **29A**, 1948–50.

Sparano, J.A., Wiernik, P.H., Dutcher, J.P. *et al.* (1994) A pilot trial of infusional cyclophosphamide, doxorubicin, and etoposid (CDE) plus didanosine (DDI) in HIV-related non-Hodgkin's lymphoma (NHL). *Proc. ASCO*, **13**, 51.

Teuscher, A.U., Opravil, M., Speich, R. *et al.* (1992) Diagnosis and course of patients with HIV infections and exclusion of *Pneumocystis carinii* pneumonia. *Dtsch. Med. Wochenschr.*, **117**, 1052–56.

Tirelli, U., Errante, D., Oksenhendler, E. *et al.* (1992a) Prospective study with combined low-dose chemotherapy and zidovudine in 37 patients with poor-prognosis AIDS-related non-Hodgkin's lymphoma. French-Italian Cooperative Study Group. *Ann. Oncol.*, **3**, 843–7.

Tirelli, U., Errante, D., Vaccher, E. *et al.* (1992b) Hodgkin's disease in 92 patients with HIV infection: the Italian experience. GICAT (Italian Cooperative Group on AIDS & Tumors). *Ann. Oncol.*, **3** (Suppl. 4), 69–72.

Ziegler, J.L., Beckstead, J.A., Volberding, P.A. *et al.* (1984) Non-Hodgkin's lymphomas in 90 homosexual men. *N. Engl. J. Med.*, **311**, 565–70.

Ziegler, J.L. (1991) ''Biologic'' differences in acquired immune deficiency syndrome-associated non-Hodgkin's lymphomas? *J. Clin. Oncol.*, **9**, 1329–31.

LYMPHOCYTIC INTERSTITIAL PNEUMONITIS

Jussi J. Saukkonen and Harrison W. Farber

Interstitial lung disease in HIV-infected individuals is commonly due to infection or malignancy. However, in some patients non-infectious inflammatory interstitial lung disease, either **lymphocytic interstitial pneumonitis** (LIP) or **non-specific interstitial pneumonitis** (NSIP), occurs. Although the etiology and pathogenesis of these inflammatory processes are unknown, they have raised controversies regarding the role of retroviruses and their elicited immune responses in causing pulmonary injury.

LYMPHOCYTIC INTERSTITIAL PNEUMONIA

INTRODUCTION

LIP in the pre-AIDS era

Two decades before the appearance of the AIDS epidemic Carrington and Liebow (1966) provided the first description of the clinicopathologic entity of LIP. An uncommon disease, LIP is characterized by chronic fevers, cough, and dyspnea; bibasilar interstitial or consolidative infiltrates; and prominent lymphoplasmacytic pulmonary septal infiltration.

LIP has been reported in association with a variety of autoimmune and lymphoproliferative disorders, including lymphoma, rheumatoid arthritis, Hashimoto's thyroiditis (Strimlan *et al.*, 1978), myasthenia gravis (Montes, Tomasi and Noehren, 1968), pernicious anemia (Levinson *et al.*, 1976), autoerythrocyte sensitization syndrome (DeCoteau *et al.*, 1974), chronic active hepatitis (Helman, Keeton and Benatar, 1977), common variable immunodeficiency (Popa, 1988), and, most frequently, Sjögren's syndrome (Strimlan *et al.*, 1976, 1978). The association of LIP with Sjögren's syndrome is interesting since a similar syndrome occurs in some HIV-infected individuals. Although the majority of LIP patients have evidence of B cell dysfunction, as evidenced by polyclonal hypergammaglobulinemia (Strimlan *et al.*, 1978; Greenberg *et al.*, 1973; Kradin and Mark, 1983), it is unclear whether the lymphocytes infiltrating the pulmonary interstitium are predominantly B cells (Greenberg *et al.*, 1973; Banerjee and Ahmed, 1982) or T cells (Kaufmann, 1977). Although the lymphocytic infiltrate is polyclonal, malignant transformation or association with lymphoid malignancy has been reported (Kradin and Mark, 1983; Strimlan *et al.*, 1976; Banerjee and Ahmed, 1982; Kaufman and Long, 1977; Kamholz *et al.*, 1987).

AIDS and Respiratory Medicine. Edited by A. Zumla, M.A. Johnson and R.F. Miller. Published in 1997 by Chapman & Hall, London. ISBN 0 412 60140 0

The majority of symptomatic patients have been treated with corticosteroids, with approximately half improving (Strimlan *et al.*, 1978; Greenberg *et al.*, 1973). Chlorambucil or cyclophosphamide with or without corticosteroids has also been used with inconclusive results (Strimlan *et al.*, 1978; Essig *et al.*, 1974). The Mayo Clinic experience suggests there is a high mortality associated with this disease, at least in older patients (Strimlan *et al.*, 1978). In some instances end-stage fibrosis may occur despite treatment (Liebow and Carrington, 1973; McFarlane and Davies, 1973).

LIP and the human immunodeficiency virus-1 (HIV-1)

In 1983 the first reports appeared describing HIV-infected children and adults with clinicopathologic findings similar to those of classic LIP (Oleske *et al.*, 1983; Rubinstein *et al.*, 1983; Saldana, Montes and Buck, 1983). As additional reports appeared, interesting demographic findings emerged. LIP, previously rare in children, was found commonly in the pediatric HIV population, occurring in 22–75% of children with pulmonary disease (Pahwa *et al.*, 1986; Scott *et al.*, 1984; Joshi *et al.*, 1987). In contrast, LIP remains uncommon among adult HIV patients, accounting for 3% of adult HIV-related pulmonary pathology (Marchevsky *et al.*, 1985). It is unclear why HIV-infected children are predisposed to the development of LIP. Interestingly, however, hemophiliac children infected with HIV are less commonly affected by LIP, having an incidence of LIP approximating that of adults, although age-matched pediatric populations have not been studied (Jason *et al.*, 1988). LIP has been found in every HIV risk group, but appears to be increased among individuals of African ancestry (Oleske *et al.*, 1983; Rubinstein *et al.*, 1983; Solal-Celigny *et al.*, 1985; Saldana, Montes and Buck, 1983; Lin *et al.*, 1988; White and Matthay, 1989). In adults LIP develops

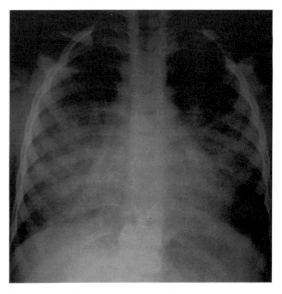

Fig. 21.1 Chronic interstitial infiltrates in an HIV-infected child consistent with LIP.

prior to the appearance of AIDS (Grieco and Chinoy-Acharya, 1986; Saldana, Montes and Buck, 1983; Ziza *et al.*, 1985; Couderç *et al.*, 1987; Bach, 1987; Itescu *et al.*, 1990), whereas in children LIP was previously designated an AIDS-defining illness by the Centers for Disease Control (CDC, 1985).

HIV-related LIP is, in many patients, part of a spectrum of HIV-associated infiltrative immune disorders (Figures 21.1–3). In HIV-infected children, LIP often co-exists with pulmonary lymphoid hyperplasia (PLH), occurring in sites of pre-existing bronchus-associated lymphoid tissue (White and Matthey, 1989). Among HIV-infected adults, lymphocytic alveolitis, which may represent a *forme fruste* of LIP, is a common finding (Guillon *et al.*, 1988). HIV-infected patients who are HLA DR5[+] and HLA DR6[+] are predisposed to developing a diffuse visceral lymphocytosis syndrome with LIP (Itescu *et al.*, 1990, 1993). Thus, LIP may be part of a continuum of lymphocytic infiltrative syndromes associated with HIV.

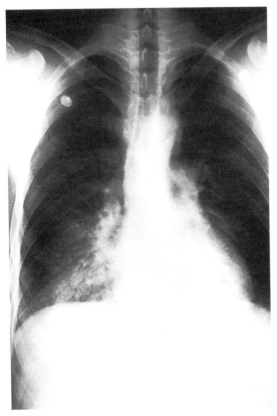

Fig. 21.2 Bibasilar interstitial infiltrates in an HIV-infected adult with LIP.

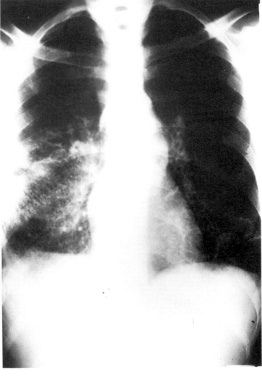

Fig. 21.3 Fibrotic changes on the chest radiograph of an HIV-infected individual with a protracted course of LIP.

Clinical features

The most common clinical manifestations of LIP include gradually progressive dyspnea, chronic cough, weight loss, malaise, and fever. Pleuritic chest pain and hemoptysis are infrequent (Lin *et al.*, 1988). Among pediatric LIP patients clubbing, hepatosplenomegaly and parotid enlargement are common features (Oleske *et al.*, 1983; Rubinstein *et al.*, 1983). In contrast, clubbing has not been reported in adults, while hepatosplenomegaly and parotid enlargement are seen in one third of cases (White and Matthay, 1989; Lin *et al.*, 1988). Râles are usually present in adults, but may be a less prominent feature in children (Rubinstein *et al.*, 1983; Lin *et al.*, 1988).

Systemic lymphadenopathy is common in both adults and children with LIP (Rubinstein *et al.*, 1983; Lin *et al.*, 1988).

Some HIV patients suffer from a Sjögren-like sicca syndrome often associated with LIP. This is manifested by xerophthalmia and/or xerostomia, parotid infiltration and visceral organ lymphocytic infiltration (Gordon, Golbus and Kurtides, 1984; Morris *et al.*, 1987; Couderç *et al.*, 1987; Itescu *et al.*, 1990). In contrast to the female predominance of classic Sjögren's sicca complex, HIV-associated sicca syndrome is largely a male entity. Auto-antibodies are usually undetectable or present in low titer. (Couderç *et al.*, 1987; Itescu *et al.*, 1990). The presence of sicca symptoms, parotid enlargement and/or uveitis in an HIV-positive individual with

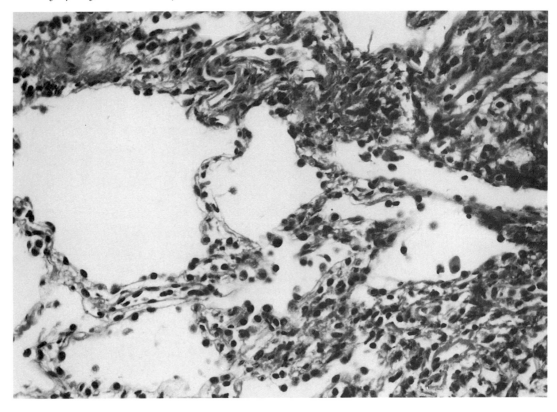

Fig. 21.4 Histopathologic section from an individual with LIP, demonstrating lymphoid cells infiltrating the pulmonary interstitium.

interstitial infiltrates is highly suggestive of LIP (White and Matthey, 1989).

Etiology and pathogenesis

The etiology and pathogenesis of HIV-related LIP are poorly understood. Accumulation of lymphocytes in the pulmonary interstitium may result from (1) an *in situ* lymphoproliferative response to chronically presented viral antigens or to locally elaborated cytokines; and/or (2) from recruitment of circulating lymphocytes to the lung in response to chemoattractants.

With respect to the first hypothesis, it is possible that a single virus or a viral cofactor acting with HIV is responsible for the development of LIP. Epstein-Barr virus

(EBV) is a putative viral etiologic agent for LIP. EBV DNA has been detected in lung biopsy specimens from 8/10 pediatric LIP patients, but not in lung tissue from HIV-infected controls, although controls were not well matched. The children with LIP tended to have higher concentrations of EBV antibody than did controls (Andiman *et al.*, 1985). A follow-up case-control study (Katz, Berkman and Shapiro, 1992) correlated the presence of EBV viral DNA in LIP tissue with serologic evidence of active infection. Only pediatric patients with EBV-positive lung tissue were studied, but all seven of these patients had evidence of primary or reactivation EBV infection at the time of biopsy. Investigators in these studies suggested that EBV replication may be occurring in the lung and that the lymphocytes infiltrating pulmonary tissue may consist of EBV-infected cells with reactive mononuclear cells. Elevated titers of antibodies directed against EBV have been reported in adult patients with LIP (Kramer *et al.*, 1992). In contrast, EBV RNA was not detected by *in situ* hybridization in lung specimens from four adult cases of LIP (Travis *et al.*, 1992). The role of EBV in the etiology and pathogenesis of LIP is still unclear, but it may be one of several possible viral cofactors that contribute to the development of this pulmonary lesion.

LIP is associated with retroviral infections, including HIV-1, human T cell leukemia virus (HTLV)-1 (Setoguchi, Takahashi and Nokwa, 1991), and ovine visna (maedi) virus (VV) (Lairmore *et al.*, 1986). The latter two retroviruses share an ability to induce a lymphocytic infiltrative pulmonary lesion, followed by the eventual development of opportunistic respiratory infections. Understanding the pathogenesis of LIP in HTLV-1 and VV infection may provide models for understanding this process in HIV-infected individuals.

Visna virus can cause multiorgan lymphocytic infiltration in sheep, but predominantly affects the lungs. VV-infected sheep develop $CD8^+$ lymphocytic alveolitis and LIP, manifested as dyspnea, cough, constitutional symptoms, and, eventually, opportunistic infections (DeMartini *et al.*, 1993). The severity of VV-associated LIP appears to correlate with the viral load, with the most compromised sheep demonstrating increased serum viral capsid antigenemia and antibodies to viral surface antigens. By polymerase chain reaction viral DNA amplification, visna provirus is detectable in these animals in as many as 1 of 200 alveolar macrophages. Co-infection with common ovine respiratory pathogens, including corynebacteria and mycoplasma, may contribute to development of pulmonary lymphoid lesions and to enhancement of local viral replication via induction of tumor

necrosis factor-alpha (TNF-α). Thus, ovine VV-associated LIP provides an attractive model for the study of HIV-related LIP (DeMartini *et al.*, 1993).

HTLV-1 is associated with a spectrum of pulmonary lymphoproliferative syndromes, including LIP. Recently, five of six patients with LIP from an area of Japan non-endemic for HTLV-1 had circulating antibodies to HTLV-1, while none was seropositive for HIV or Epstein-Barr virus (Setoguchi, Takahashi and Nokwa, 1991). Patients with HTLV-1-associated adult T cell leukemia frequently develop leukemic pulmonary infiltrates (Yoshioka *et al.*, 1985), while patients with HTLV-associated myelopathy (HAM), tropical spastic paraparesis (H-TSP), and uveitis commonly have a lymphocytic alveolitis (Semenzato and Agostini, 1989; Sugimoto *et al.*, 1993). The lymphocytic alveolitis of H-TSP is composed mainly of $CD8^+$ T cells, while that of HAM patients is comprised of both $CD4^+$ and $CD8^+$ T cells. Healthy HTLV-1 carriers have a $CD4^+$ lymphocytic alveolitis (Semenzato and Agostini, 1989).

The transactivating protein of HTLV-1, $p40^{Tax}$, is capable of activating the genes for interleukin (IL)-2 and the high affinity-alpha chain of the IL2 receptor (IL2R) (Yodoi and Uchiyama, 1992), perhaps explaining the polyclonal T cell proliferation seen in early stages of HTLV-1 infection. Furthermore, increased soluble IL2R levels are detectable in bronchoalveolar lavage (BAL) fluid and serum from HAM patients, correlating with spontaneous pulmonary lymphocyte proliferation (Sugimoto *et al.*, 1989). Thus, IL-2-driven lymphocyte proliferation could explain HTLV-1-related lymphoproliferative pulmonary lesions. Whether or not such viral antigen-driven lymphocyte proliferation accounts for HIV-related LIP is unclear. Preliminary evidence points to spontaneous production of IL-2 by alveolar lymphocytes from HIV-infected individuals (Spain *et al.*, 1994).

The evidence for HIV itself as an etiologic

agent in LIP is intriguing but circumstantial. By *in situ* hybridization large amounts of HIV RNA have been detected within pulmonary macrophages in germinal centers in one adult patient with LIP, while only occasional cells expressing HIV RNA were found in two additional patients with LIP (Travis *et al.*, 1992). However, the presence of HIV in the lung in LIP patients is a non-specific finding. Whether patients with LIP have a higher HIV-1 load in the lung is unclear, since there is considerable controversy as to the extent of the pulmonary viral load in HIV-infected individuals (Chayt *et al.*, 1986; Dean *et al.*, 1988; Linneman *et al.*, 1989; Mayaud and Cadranel, 1993).

Thus, several questions remain unanswered regarding the etiology and pathogenesis of HIV-associated LIP. It is unclear whether a single viral agent or, more likely, an array of viral cofactors may be instrumental in eliciting the lesion of LIP.

Natural history

The natural history of LIP in HIV-infected individuals, as in non-infected patients, is variable. It has been reported to have a duration ranging from 1 month to 11 years, may remain stable for months without treatment (Solal-Celigny *et al.*, 1985; Lin *et al.*, 1988; Morris *et al.*, 1987; Itescu *et al.*, 1990) or may spontaneously improve (Grieco and Chinoy-Acharya, 1986). Mortality data are inexact due to lack of reported follow-up. Symptoms are often recurrent, and in some instances end-stage fibrosis (Teirstein and Rosen, 1988) or bronchiectasis (Amorosa *et al.*, 1992; McGuiness *et al.*, 1993) may occur.

Diagnosis

Although the combination of clinical and diagnostic data is often highly suggestive of LIP, such information is non-specific. Thus, the diagnosis ultimately rests on tissue diagnosis. However, in the pediatric population empiric treatment for LIP is often initiated based on the presence of insidiously developing dyspnea, mild hypoxemia, and clubbing (Rubinstein, 1986). In adults the clinical features of LIP are not sufficiently characteristic to make this diagnosis without a lung biopsy. Infection must be excluded in the evaluation of the patient, since LIP may mimic pulmonary infections and because patients with LIP are prone to frequent bacterial infections (Lin *et al.*, 1988).

The chest radiograph in adults usually demonstrates bibasilar reticulonodular or micronodular infiltrates which may coalesce into an alveolar pattern (Solal-Celigny *et al.*, 1985; Grieco and Chinoy-Acharya, 1986; Lin *et al.*, 1988). Honeycombing may be seen in up to one third of patients. Hilar adenopathy and pleural effusion are uncommon in adults (White and Matthay, 1989). In children, similar infiltrates are seen, often associated with mediastinal widening and hilar enlargement, which correlate pathologically with pulmonary lymphoid hyperplasia (Rubinstein, 1986). Computerized tomography may reveal the additional presence of bronchiectasis (Amorosa *et al.*, 1992; McGuiness *et al.*, 1993).

Pulmonary function testing usually demonstrates restriction with a reduced or normal diffusion capacity, although severe obstructive airways disease has also been reported. Arterial blood gas measurement may reveal a normal pO_2 or profound hypoxemia and there may be an increased alveolar to arterial oxygen gradient. These findings may be helpful in assessing the severity of illness in some instances, but are non-specific and do not aid the clinician in diagnosis (Solal-Celigny *et al.*, 1985; Grieco and Chinoy-Acharya, 1986; Back, 1987; Lin *et al.*, 1988; Itescu *et al.*, 1990).

Laboratory testing generally reveals polyclonal hypergammaglobulinemia, although hypogammaglobulinemia has also been reported. Although hypergammaglobulinemia is found in 50–75% of all HIV patients, it is nearly universal among those with LIP. In the pediatric LIP population elevated LDH (300–500 IU/L, about half the range seen in *Pneumocystis carinii* pneumonia or PCP) is often found. In adults LDH has been infrequently reported and consequently this constitutes inconclusive data (White and Matthay, 1989).

The diagnosis of LIP is definitively made by histopathologic examination of transbronchial or open lung biopsy specimens. Transbronchial biopsy can generally provide a diagnosis, but open lung biopsy may be required in the face of non-specific findings (White and Matthay, 1989).

LIP is characterized by alveolar septal and intra-alveolar infiltration by small, mature, non-cleaved polyclonal lymphocytes and plasma cells; lymphoid follicles or micronodules may also be present. The bronchiolar submucosa is thickened, often causing significant airway narrowing and mucus impaction. Infiltration is not associated with intrapulmonary lymphadenopathy, vasculitis, or necrosis. However, there may be areas of extensive interstitial fibrosis. Even non-caseating granulomata have been reported (Teirstein and Rosen, 1988; White and Matthay, 1989).

The infiltrating lymphocytes are in adults largely CD8$^+$ T cells (Solal-Celigny *et al.*, 1985; Guillon *et al.*, 1987; Itescu *et al.*, 1990). Both CD4 and CD8 cell predominance have been reported in children (Broaddus *et al.*, 1985). Another report from the pediatric HIV population noted significant numbers of B cells in the infiltrating lymphocytes (Joshi *et al.*, 1985).

Extrapulmonary visceral lymphocytic infiltration in LIP patients has also been confirmed histologically. Involved organs included kidneys, liver, stomach, meninges, cranial nerves, motor neurons, parotid and other salivary and lacrimal glands, nasopharynx, bone marrow, spleen, colon, duodenum, thymus, and uvea (Solal-Celigny *et al.*, 1985; Morris *et al.*, 1987; Couderç *et al.*, 1987; Itescu *et al.*, 1990).

The histopathologic differential diagnosis includes lymphoproliferative disorders previously identified in HIV-infected patients: that is, lymphoma and angioimmunoblastic lymphadenopathy (Lin *et al.*, 1988). Therefore, the clinician and pathologist should correlate clinical and histologic findings and determine if adequate tissue has been obtained.

Treatment

In symptomatic patients with LIP, corticosteroids are usually the initial treatment. Improvement has been noted in most cases (Solal-Celigny *et al.*, 1985; Morris *et al.*, 1987; Lin *et al.*, 1988; Itescu *et al.*, 1990). Complications of treatment have not been well documented, and the occurrence of opportunistic infections in patients with advanced HIV disease may be difficult to interpret. Length of treatment has varied from weeks to chronic suppressive treatment (Solal-Celigny *et al.*, 1985; Morris *et al.*, 1987; Lin *et al.*, 1988; Itescu *et al.*, 1990). Chlorambucil has been used in one patient with reported improvement (Itescu *et al.*, 1990). Zidovudine has been used in three patients with LIP, two of whom improved (Bach, 1987); the third patient, more advanced in the stage of HIV infection, did not improve (Helbert, 1987).

NON-SPECIFIC INTERSTITIAL PNEUMONIA

The clinician caring for HIV patients with respiratory illness may encounter the clinicopathologic entity of non-specific interstitial pneumonitis (NSIP). It has been previously recognized that immunocompromised individuals may have evidence of chronic lung injury related to such insults as infection, chemotherapy,

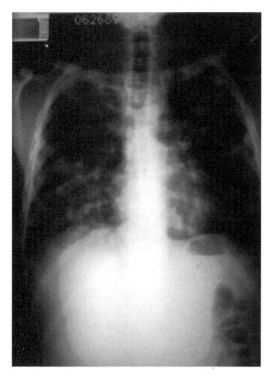

Fig. 21.5 Chest radiograph of an HIV-infected individual with significant hypoxemia and found to have DAD.

oxygen toxicity and radiation therapy (Katzenstein, Bloor and Leibow, 1976). Commonly, the lung histopathology in these instances reveals one or more phases of diffuse alveolar damage (DAD) (Figures 21.5 and 21.6), ranging from early injury to repair. Similar lesions have been found in HIV-infected individuals without definitive etiologic agents. The pathologic lesion of NSIP is sufficiently different from that of LIP and similar to that of DAD seen in other immunocompromised patients that an additional insult seems likely in triggering this process.

Clinical features

NSIP is a common finding in HIV-infected individuals. In a study of 110 AIDS patients, 41 (38%) were found to have non-specific

interstitial pneumonitis on lung biopsy. Of these 41 patients, 28 had concurrent pulmonary Kaposi's sarcoma, a history of PCP, a history of drug abuse, or had received previous experimental therapies, while 13 had no other risk factors for pulmonary injury (Suffredini *et al.*, 1987). Transbronchial biopsies of 24 HIV patients without pulmonary symptoms and with normal chest radiographs demonstrated NSIP in 11 individuals (48%, Ognibene *et al.*, 1988). This subclinical pneumonitis appears to constitute a more subtle, indolent form of NSIP, recently dubbed chronic NSIP (Mayaud and Cadranel, 1993).

Most patients have mild symptoms including cough, usually non-productive, exertional dyspnea, and fever (Suffredini *et al.*, 1987); occasionally, an accelerated course may be seen (Ramaswamy, Jagadha and Tchetkoff, 1985). Râles are usually heard in symptomatic patients (Ramaswamy, Jagadha and Tchetkoff, 1985).

Etiology and pathogenesis

The pathologic findings of this entity may be induced by a wide variety of insults to the lung, including previous infection, drug abuse, pulmonary tumors, radiation, oxygen toxicity, and chemotherapy (Katzenstein, Bloor and Leibow, 1976; Ramaswamy, Jagadha and Tchetkoff, 1985). Lung biopsies of patients with active or previous PCP may show diffuse alveolar damage similar to that seen in NSIP (Nash and Fligiel, 1984; Ramaswamy, Jagadha and Tchetkoff, 1985). Viral infections, notably with cytomegalovirus (CMV), adenovirus, and influenza virus, appear to be associated with DAD in non-HIV patients (Ramaswamy, Jagadha and Tchetkoff, 1985). Many patients with HIV-associated NSIP have serologic evidence of CMV infection, but characteristic inclusion bodies have been reported in only a few patients (Suffredini *et al.*, 1987). It is unclear whether CMV is an epiphenomenon

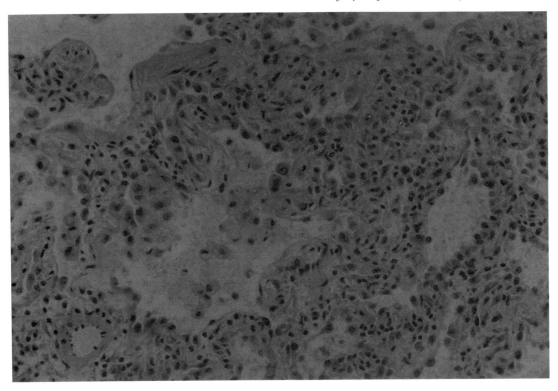

Fig. 21.6 Histopathologic section demonstrating marked type II cell hyperplasia, interstitial fibrosis, and minimal mononuclear cell infiltrate in an open lung biopsy specimen obtained from the patient whose chest radiograph is shown in Fig. 21.5. (Courtesy of Dr John Hayes, Department of Pathology, Boston Veterans' Administration Medical Center.)

or an etiologic agent in some cases of HIV-associated NSIP. As with other immunocompromised patients, it is suspected that a variety of infectious and non-infectious insults can trigger the development of DAD in HIV-infected patients.

Recently it has been suggested that these triggering factors may amplify ongoing subclinical pulmonary injury due to HIV-induced local immune dysregulation (Mayaud and Cadranel, 1993). According to this hypothesis, subclinical pneumonitis may be induced by pulmonary macrophages, lymphocytes and neutrophils activated by overexpressed cytokines including TNF-α, IL-1, IL-2, and granulocyte-macrophage-colony stimulating factor (GM-CSF). Ac-

tivated macrophages, targets for HIV-specific cytotoxic T cells, may release free radicals and proteases which may cause injury to the alveolocapillary barrier. Cytotoxic T cells themselves may also contribute to parenchymal injury (Meignan *et al.*, 1990). This process may be amplified by infection or other insults to the lung which enhance inflammatory cytokine expression, activating potentially injurious leukocytes (Mayaud and Cadranel, 1993).

Natural history

NSIP often resolves spontaneously, but may persist, resulting in chronic fibrosis (Suffredini *et al.*, 1987). Some patients who develop acute respiratory distress with NSIP require supportive care or further intervention. The outcome of these episodes has not been clearly reported in the literature.

Diagnosis

The chest radiograph most commonly demonstrates the presence of bilateral reticulonodular or interstitial infiltrates (Ramaswamy, Jagadha and Tchetkoff, 1985; Suffredini *et al.*, 1987). Bronchiectasis may be evident on computerized tomographic images (McGuiness *et al.*, 1993).

Arterial blood gas measurement may be helpful in selected patients since hypoxemia may be present (Suffredini *et al.*, 1987). Pulmonary function testing in HIV patients may reveal progressive small reductions in diffusion capacity even in the face of a normal chest radiograph and the absence of respiratory symptoms (Shaw *et al.*, 1988; Nieman *et al.*, 1992). Whether these findings are related to NSIP, lymphocytic aveolitis or other processes is not clear.

Both transbronchial biopsy and open lung biopsy have been used to diagnose NSIP. Histopathologic findings include mild mononuclear interstitial infiltration and patchy areas of fibrosis. It is distinguishable from LIP less by the degree of cellular infiltration than by the presence of hyaline membranes, alveolar cell hyperplasia, and interstitial edema. The term DAD encompasses these findings and is the most common finding. All phases of DAD may be present on the lung section. The **early exudative phase** of DAD is characterized by interstitial edema and hemorrhage, alveolar exudation and hemorrhage, hyaline membrane formation, minimal alveolar septal thickening, and type I pneumocyte necrosis. This stage is followed by the **proliferative phase** in which alveolar septal thickening is pronounced due to marked fibroblast and tortuous capillary proliferation. Vascular intimal thickening is also seen.

Type II pneumocyte hyperplasia is also a prominent feature of this phase. Findings in the alveoli include hemosiderin-laden macrophages and focal areas of exudative DAD. The resolution of this process is the **fibrotic phase**, in which interstitial fibrosis is present along with marked vascular medial hypertrophy and occlusive intimal thickening (Ramaswamy, Jagadha and Tchetkoff, 1985).

Treatment

Most symptomatic cases of NSIP spontaneously resolve or stabilize (Suffredini *et al.*, 1987). However, in a series of severely compromised individuals with NSIP, it is unclear what clinical interventions were provided (Ramaswamy, Jagadha and Tchetkoff, 1985). Corticosteroids have been employed by some clinicians for severely symptomatic patients (White and Matthay, 1989).

REFERENCES

Agostini, C., Trentin, L., Zambello, R. *et al.* (1993) HIV-1 and the lung: infectivity, pathogenic mechanisms, and cellular immune responses taking place in the lower respiratory tract. *American Review of Respiratory Disease*, **147**, 1038–49.

Amorosa, J., Miller, R., Laraya-Cuasay, L. *et al.* (1992) Bronchiectasis in children with lymphocytic interstitial pneumonia and acquired immune deficiency syndrome: Plain film and CT observations. *Pediatric Radiology*, **22**, 603–6.

Andiman, W., Eastman, R., Martin, K. *et al.* (1985) Opportunistic lymphoproliferations associated with Epstein-Barr viral DNA in infants and children with AIDS. *Lancet*, **2**, 1390–93.

Bach, M. (1987) Zidovudine for lymphocytic interstitial pneumonia associated with AIDS. *Lancet*, **2**, 655–61.

Banerjee, D. and Ahmed, D. (1982) Malignant lymphoma complicating lymphocytic interstitial pneumonia. *Human Pathology*, **13**, 780–82.

Broaddus, C., Dake, M., Stulbarg, M. *et al.* (1985) Bronchoalveolar lavage and transbronchial biopsy for the diagnosis of pulmonary infections in the acquired immunodeficiency syndrome. *Annals of Internal Medicine*, **102**, 747–52.

Carrington, C. and Liebow, A. (1966) Lymphocytic interstitial pneumonia (abstr.). *American Journal of Pathology*, **48**, 36a.

Centers for Disease Control (CDC) (1985) Revision of case definitions of AIDS for national reporting – US. *Morbidity and Mortality Weekly Report*, **34**, 373–5.

Chayt, K., Harper, M., Marsell, L. *et al.* (1986) Detection of HTLV-111 RNA in lungs of patients with AIDS and pulmonary involvement. *JAMA*, **256**, 2356–59.

Clerici, M., Hakim, F., Venzon, D. *et al.* (1993) Changes in IL-2 and IL-4 production in asymptomatic HIV-infected individuals. *Journal of Clinical Investigation*, **91**, 759–65.

Couderç, L., D'Agay, M., Danon, F. *et al.* (1987) Sicca complex and infection with human immunodeficiency virus. *Archives of Internal Medicine*, **147**, 898–901.

Dean, N., Golden, J., Evans, L. *et al.* (1988) Human immunodeficiency virus recovery from bronchoalveolar lavage fluid in patients with AIDS. *Chest*, **93**, 1176–79.

DeCoteau, W., Tourville, D., Ambrus, J. *et al.* (1974) Lymphoid interstitial pneumonia and autoerythrocyte sensitization syndrome. *Archives of Internal Medicine*, **134**, 519–22.

DeMartini, J., Brodie, S., Concha-Bermejillo, A. *et al.* (1993) Pathogenesis of lymphoid interstitial pneumonia in natural and experimental ovine lentivirus infection. *Clinical Infectious Diseases*, **17** (Supplement 1), S236–42.

Essig, L., Tumms, E., Aancock, E. *et al.* (1974) Plasma cell interstitial pneumonia and macroglobulinemia: a response to corticosteroid and cyclophosphamide therapy. *American Journal of Medicine*, **56**, 398–405.

Gordon, J., Golbus, J., Kurtides, E. (1984) Chronic lymphadenopathy and Sjögren's syndrome in a homosexual man. *New England Journal of Medicine*, **311**, 1441–42.

Greenberg, S., Haley, M., Jenkins, D. *et al.* (1973) Lymphoplasmacytic pneumonia with accompanying dysproteinemia. *Archives of Pathology*, **96**, 73–80.

Grieco, M. and Chinoy-Acharya, P. (1986) Lymphocytic interstitial pneumonia associated with the acquired immune deficiency syndrome. *American Review of Respiratory Disease*, **131**, 952–55.

Guillon, J., Fouret, P., Mayaud, C. *et al.* (1987) Extensive T8+ lymphocytic visceral infiltrates in a homosexual man. *American Journal of Medicine*, **82**, 655–61.

Guillon, J., Autran, B., Denis, M. *et al.* (1988) Human immunodeficiency virus-related lymphocytic alveolitis. *Chest*, **94**, 1264–70.

Helbert, M. (1987) Zidovudine for lymphocytic interstitial pneumonia in AIDS (letter). *Lancet*, **2**, 1390–93.

Helman, C., Keeton, G. and Benatar, S. (1977) Lymphoid interstitial pneumonia with associated chronic active hepatitis and renal tubular acidosis. *American Review of Respiratory Disease*, **115**, 161–64.

Itescu, S., Brancato, L., Buxbaum, J. *et al.* (1990) A diffuse infiltrative CD8 lymphocytosis syndrome in HIV infection: a host immune response associated with HLADR5. *Annals of Internal Medicine*, **112**, 3–10.

Itescu, S., Dalton, J., Zhang, H. *et al.* (1993) Tissue infiltration in a CD8 lymphocytosis syndrome associated with human immunodeficiency virus-1 infection has the phenotypic appearance of an antigenically driven response. *Journal of Clinical Investigation*, **91**, 2216–25.

Jason, J., Stehr-Green, J., Holman, R. *et al.* (1988) HIV infection in hemophiliac children. *Pediatrics*, **82**, 565–70.

Joshi, V., Oleske, J., Minnefor, A. *et al.* (1987) Pathology of suspected AIDS in children. *Pediatric Pathology*, **2**, 71–87.

Kaufman, S. and Long, J. (1977) Parotid mass and pulmonary nodules in a 36 year old woman. *New England Journal of Medicine*, **297**, 652–60.

Kamholz, S., Sher, A., Barland, P. *et al.* (1987) Sjögren's syndrome: severe upper airways obstruction due to primary malignant tracheal lymphoma developing during successful treatment of LIP. *Journal of Rheumatology*, **14**, 588–94.

Katz, B.Z., Berkman, A. and Shapiro, E. (1992) Serologic evidence of active Epstein-Barr virus infection in Epstein-Barr virus-associated lymphoproliferative disorders of children with acquired immunodeficiency syndrome. *Journal of Pediatrics*, **120**, 228–32.

Katzenstein, A., Leibow, A. and Bloor, C. (1976) Diffuse alveolar damage: role of oxygen, shock, and related factors. *American Journal of Clinical Pathology*, **85**, 210–24.

Kradin, R. and Mark, E. (1983) Benign lymphoid disorders of the lung with a theory regarding their development. *Human Pathology*, **14**, 857–67.

Kramer, M., Saldana, M., Ramos, M. *et al.* (1992) High titers of Epstein-Barr virus antibodies in adult patients with lymphocytic interstitial pneumonitis associated with AIDS. *Respiratory Medicine*, **86**, 49–52.

Lairmore, M., Rosadio, R., DeMartini, J. *et al.* (1986) Ovine lentivirus lymphoid interstitial pneumonia: rapid induction in neonatal lambs. *American Journal of Pathology*, **125**, 173–81.

Levinson, A., Hopewell, P., Stites, D. *et al.* (1976) Coexistent lymphoid interstitial pneumonia, pernicious anemia, and agammaglobulinemia; comment on autoimmune pathogenesis. *Archives of Internal Medicine*, **136**, 213–16.

Liebow, A. and Carrington, C. (1973) Diffuse pulmonary lymphoreticular infiltration associated with dysproteinemia. *Medical Clinics of North America*, **57**, 809–43.

Lin, R., Gruber, P., Saunders, R. *et al.* (1988) Lymphocytic interstitial pneumonitis in adult HIV infection. *New York State Journal of Medicine*, **88**, 273–76.

Linneman, C., Baughman, R., Frame, P. *et al.* (1989) Recovery of human immunodeficiency virus and detection of p24 antigen in bronchoalveolar lavage fluid from adult patients with AIDS. *Chest*, **96**, 64–7.

Marchevsky, A., Rosen, M., Chrystal, G. *et al.* (1985) Pulmonary complications of AIDS: a clinicopathologic study of 70 cases. *Human Pathology*, **16**, 659–70.

Mayaud, C. and Cadranel, J. (1993) HIV in the lung: guilty or not guilty? *Thorax*, **48**, 1191–95.

McFarlane, A. and Davies, D. (1973) Diffuse lymphoid interstitial pneumonia. *Thorax*, **28**, 768–76.

McGuiness, G., Naidich, D., Garay, S. *et al.* (1993) AIDS associated bronchiectasis: CT features. *Journal of Computer Assisted Tomography*, **17**, 260–66.

Meignan, M., Guillon, J.M., Denis, M. *et al.* (1990) Increased lung epithelial permeability in HIV-infected patients with isolated cytotoxic T lymphocyte alveolitis. *American Review of Respiratory Disease*, **141**, 1241–8.

Montes, M., Tomasi, T., Noehren, T. (1968) Lymphoid interstitial pneumonia with monoclonal gammopathy. *American Review of Respiratory Disease*, **98**, 277–80.

Morris, J., Rosen, M., Marchevsky, A. *et al.* (1987)

Lymphocytic interstitial pneumonia in patients at risk for AIDS. *Chest*, **91**, 63–7.

Nash, G. and Fligiel, S. (1984) Pathologic features of the lung in the acquired immune deficiency syndrome (AIDS): an autopsy study of seventeen homosexual males. *American Journal of Clinical Pathology*, **81**, 6–12.

Nieman, R., Fleming, J., Coler, R. *et al.* (1992) Reduced carbon monoxide transfer factor (T_{LCO}) in human immunodeficiency virus type I (HIV-1) infection as a predictor for faster progression to AIDS. *Thorax*, **48**, 481–85.

Ognibene, F., Masur, H., Rogers, P. *et al.* (1987) Nonspecific interstitial pneumonitis without evidence of *Pneumocystis carinii* in asymptomatic patients infected with human immunodeficiency virus (HIV). *Annals of Internal Medicine*, **109**, 874–9.

Oleske, J., Minnefor, A., Cooper, R. *et al.* (1983) Immune deficiency syndrome in children. *JAMA*, **249**, 2345–49.

Pahwa, S., Kaplan, M., Fikrig, S. *et al.* (1986) Spectrum of human T-cell lymphotropic virus type III infection in children. Recognition of symptomatic, asymptomatic and seronegative patients. *JAMA*, **255**, 2299–310.

Pantaleo, G., Koenig, S. and Baseler, H. (1990) Defective clonogenic potential of CD8$^+$ T lymphocytes in patients with AIDS. *Journal of Immunology*, **144**, 1696–704.

Popa, V. (1988) Lymphocytic interstitial pneumonitis of common variable immunodeficiency. *Annals of Allergy*, **60**, 203–6.

Ramaswamy, G., Jagadha, V. and Tchertkoff, V. (1985) Diffuse alveolar damage and interstitial fibrosis in AIDS patients without concurrent pulmonary infection. *Archives of Pathology and Laboratory Medicine*, **109**, 408–12.

Rubinstein, A., Sicklick, M., Gupta, A. *et al.* (1986) Acquired immune deficiency with reversed T4/T8 ratios in infants born to promiscuous and drug-addicted mothers. *JAMA*, **249**, 2350–56.

Saldana, M., Montes, J., Buck, B. (1983) Lymphoid interstitial pneumonia in Haitian residents of Florida (abstr.). *Chest*, **84**, 347.

Scott, G., Buch, B., Leterman, J. *et al.* (1984) Acquired immune deficiency syndrome in infants. *New England Journal of Medicine*, **310**, 76–81.

Semenzato, G. and Agostini, C. (1989) Human retroviruses and lung involvement. *American Review of Respiratory Disease*, **139**, 1317–22.

Setoguchi, Y., Takahashi, G. and Nokwa, K. (1991) Detection of human T-cell leukemia virus-

1 related antibodies in patients with lymphocytic interstitial pneumonia. *American Review of Respiratory Disease*, **144**, 1361–65.

Shaw, R., Roussak, C., Forster, S. *et al.* (1988) Lung function abnormalities in patients infected with the human immunodeficiency virus with and without overt pneumonitis. *Thorax*, **43**, 436–40.

Solal-Celigny, P., Couderç, L., Herman, D. *et al.* (1985) Lymphoid interstitial pneumonitis in acquired immunodeficiency syndrome-related complex. *American Review of Respiratory Disease*, **131**, 956–60.

Spain, B., Soliman, D. and Twigg, H. (1994) Enhanced interleukin-2 production by lymphocytes from HIV-infected patients with lymphocytic alveolitis is compartmentalized within the lung. *American Journal of Respiratory and Critical Care Medicine*, **149**, A2640.

Strimlan, C., Rosenow, E., Divertie, M. *et al.* (1976) Pulmonary manifestation of Sjögren's syndrome. *Chest*, **70**, 354–61.

Strimlan, C., Rosenow, E., Weiland, L. *et al.* (1978) Lymphocytic interstitial pneumonitis: a review of 13 cases. *Annals of Internal Medicine*, **88**, 616–21.

Suffredini, A., Ognibene, F., Lack, E. *et al.* (1987) Nonspecific interstitial pneumonitis: a common cause of pulmonary disease in the acquired immunodeficiency syndrome. *Annals of Internal Medicine*, **107**, 7–13.

Sugimoto, M., Nakashima, H., Matsumoto, M. *et al.* (1989) Pulmonary involvement in patients with HTLV-1-associated myelopathy: increased soluble IL-2 receptors in bronchoalveolar lavage fluid. *American Review of Respiratory Disease*, **139**, 1329–35.

Sugimoto, M., Mita, S., Tokunaga, M. *et al.* (1993) Pulmonary involvement in human T cell lymphotropic virus type-1 uveitis: T lymphocytosis and high proviral DNA load in bronchoalveolar lavage fluid. *European Respiratory Journal*, **6**, 938–43.

Teirstein, A. and Rosen, M. (1988) Lymphocytic interstitial pneumonia. *Clinics in Chest Medicine*, **9**, 467–71.

Travis, W., Fox, C., Devaney, K. *et al.* (1992) Lymphoid pneumonitis in 50 adult patients infected with the human immunodeficiency virus: lymphocytic interstitial pneumonitis versus non-specific interstitial pneumonitis. *Human Pathology*, **23**, 529–41.

White, D.A. and Matthay, R.A. (1989) Noninfectious pulmonary complications of infection with the human immunodeficiency virus. *American Review of Respiratory Disease*, **140**, 1763–87.

Yodoi, J. and Uchiyama, T. (1992) Diseases associated with HTLV-1: virus, IL-2 receptor dysregulation, and redox regulation. *Immunology Today*, **13**, 405–10.

Yoshioka, M., Yamaguchi, K., Yoshinaga, T. *et al.* (1985) Pulmonary complications in patients with adult T cell leukemia. *Cancer*, **35**, 2491–5.

Ziza, J., Brun-Vezinet, F., Venet, A. *et al.* (1985) Lymphadenopathy-associated virus isolated from bronchoalveolar lavage fluid in AIDS-related complex with lymphocytic interstitial pneumonia. *New England Journal of Medicine*, **313**, 183.

Alimuddin Zumla and Robert F. Miller

INCIDENCE OF SINUSITIS

While there is extensive literature describing lower respiratory tract infections in HIV-infected individuals, comparatively little is known about infection of the upper respiratory tract and paranasal sinuses. Although the percentage of patients with symptoms specifically localized to the nose and paranasal sinuses is not known precisely, clinical impressions are that a large majority of HIV-infected patients will develop sinusitis. Prospective studies of patients infected with HIV describe a 30% to 68% prevalence of sinusitis (Rubin and Honigberg, 1990; Spech, Rehm and Longworth, 1988). Wallace *et al.* (1993) determined the incidence of each respiratory diagnosis in a large prospective study of 1353 homosexual or bisexual men, intravenous drug users, and female partners of HIV-infected men from centers located in 6 US cities (San Francisco, Los Angeles, Detroit, Chicago, Newark, and New York City) over an 18-month period. This study examined types of respiratory disorders which occurred over the full range of HIV disease from the very mild to severely immunocompromised. The most frequent conditions seen were: upper respiratory infection (33.4%); acute bronchitis (16%); acute sinusitis (5.3%); bacterial pneumonia (4.8%); and *Pneumocystis carinii* pneumonia (3.9%). Nasal and paranasal sinus manifestations appear to be among the more common presentations of respiratory infection in individuals infected with HIV.

CLINICAL FEATURES

The entire spectrum of sinonasal inflammatory disease may be present, including acute sinusitis, recurrent acute sinusitis, chronic sinusitis with mucosal thickening, or chronic rhinitis indicated by nasal congestion and thick mucopurulent postnasal discharge (Table 22.1). Presenting symptoms and signs include fever, headache, nasal stuffiness, nasal blockage, other localizing symptoms, and mucopurulent discharge at the sinus ostia. Not all patients have localizing signs and symptoms (Godofsky *et al.*, 1992; Grant *et al.*, 1993; Mofensen *et al.*, 1995). In a retrospective review of 1461 consecutive admissions of 667 patients to the Johns Hopkins Hospital HIV Unit, in Baltimore, Maryland, USA, sinusitis was identified in 72 patients, predominantly in those with a CD4 T lymphocyte count of less than 200/mm^3 (Godofsky *et al.*, 1992). Although nasal congestion and postnasal discharge were found in the majority of these patients, the diagnosis was incidental in 28 patients. Grant *et al.* (1993) in a retrospective review of case

AIDS and Respiratory Medicine. Edited by A. Zumla, M.A. Johnson and R.F. Miller. Published in 1997 by Chapman & Hall, London. ISBN 0 412 60140 0

Table 22.1 Spectrum of sinonasal inflammatory disease in HIV infection

---

Acute sinusitis
Recurrent acute sinusitis
Chronic sinusitis with mucosal thickening
Chronic rhinitis
Sinusitis with abscesses

---

notes and radiological records of 476 patients admitted to the HIV-dedicated inpatient unit at the Middlesex Hospital, London, UK, over a three-and-a-half year period found that 30 patients (6.3%) had radiological evidence of paranasal sinus disease. At time of admission, sinusitis was the diagnosis in only 12 of the 30 patients with 13 having an admission diagnosis of meningitis.

In a retrospective study by Zurlo *et al.* (1992) of 145 HIV-infected patients who had imaging of the sinuses by plain radiography, CT or MRI scans at the National Institutes of Health Clinical Center over a 7-year period (1982–1989), 89 patients had radiographic evidence of sinusitis. Acute sinusitis was seen in 10 patients (13%) while 75 patients had mucosal thickening indicative of chronic sinusitis. 50 patients (67%) were symptomatic, with fever, nasal congestion, or discharge and headache being the most common symptoms. 19 patients were asymptomatic when their radiographs showed active disease. The mean CD4 count for the group was 276 cells/mm^3 while 32 (43%) had CD4 counts ≤100 cells/mm^3.

Information on sinusitis in HIV-infected children is scanty. Mofenson and colleagues (1995) studied 95 episodes of sinusitis in 60 HIV-positive children. Sinusitis episodes were commonly associated with non-specific chronic symptoms such as persistent nasal discharge (67.4%), or nocturnal or persistent cough (54.7%), whereas symptoms specific to acute sinusitis were less frequent and included headache or facial pain (17.9%), periorbital swelling (9.5%), temperature of >102°F (25.3%), total white blood cell count of ≥15 000/mm^3. The sinuses primarily involved were the maxillary sinus (85.9%) and the ethmoidal sinus (42.3%) with 36% of episodes involved two or more sinuses. CD4$^+$ lymphocyte counts in children with and without sinusitis did not differ significantly.

MICROBIOLOGY OF SINUSITIS

Recognized pathogens as well as opportunistic organisms have been associated with sinusitis in HIV-infected patients (Table 22.2). The bacteriology of acute sinusitis in this population includes the same organisms normally considered in the immunocompetent patient, namely *Streptococcus pneumoniae* and *Haemophilus influenzae*. *Staphylococcus aureus* and *Pseudomonas aeruginosa* have also been described in

Table 22.2 Microbiology of sinusitis in HIV infection

Classification	Specific organism
Bacteria	*Streptococcus pneumoniae*
	Streptococcus viridans
	Haemophilus influenzae
	Staphylococcus aureus
	Pseudomonas aeruginosa
	Legionella pneumophila
	Listeria monocytogenes
	Branhamella catarrhalis
	Anaerobes
Fungi	*Aspergillus* spp
	Alternaria alternata
	Pseudoallescheria boydii
	Cryptococcus neoformans
	Candida albicans
Viruses	Cytomegalovirus
	Herpes simplex virus
Protozoa	*Acanthamoebae castellani*
	Microsporidia spp

acute sinusitis but are more commonly associated with chronic sinusitis, often in association with anaerobic bacteria (Sooy, 1987). In a retrospective study (Milgrim *et al.*, 1994) of sinus cultures from 41 HIV-infected patients the most common isolates were *Streptococcus pneumoniae* (19%), *Streptococcus viridans* (19%), and *Pseudomonas aeruginosa* (17%). Occasionally atypical infections can present primarily in the nose or paranasal sinuses. Fungal sinusitis has been reported with *Alternaria alternata*, *Aspergillus* spp., *Pseudoallescheria boydii*, *Cryptococcus neoformans*, and *Candida albicans* (Carranzana, Rossitch and Morris, 1991; Choi, Lawson and Buttone, 1988; Meiteles and Lucente, 1990; Sooy, 1987; Milgrim *et al.*, 1994). Severe rhinosinusitis resulting from primary cytomegalovirus infection has been reported (Brillhart, Gath and Piot, 1991) and unusual reports of sinusitis caused by *Acanthamoebae castellani* (Gonzalez *et al.*, 1986), *Listeria monocytogenes* (Milgrim *et al.*, 1994), *Legionella pneumophila* (Schlanger, Lutwick and Kurzman, 1984), and *Microsporidia* spp (Lacey *et al.*, 1992; Weber *et al.*, 1994) suggest that an aggressive approach to diagnosis and treatment must be considered for all patients who fail empiric antibiotic therapy. Antral lavage (or a sinus drainage procedure for other sinuses) is indicated for both diagnostic and therapeutic reasons if symptoms persist following initial medical therapy.

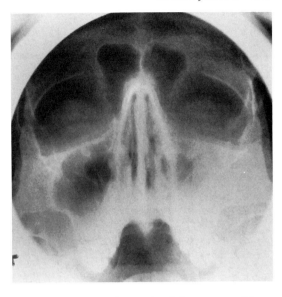

Fig. 22.1 Plain radiograph of the sinuses. There is marked mucosal thickening throughout the left antrum. The right antrum and frontal sinuses are clear.

Chong *et al.*, 1993; Zurlo *et al.*, 1992). The number of radiologically abnormal sinuses also tends to correlate inversely with the CD4 count (Godowsky *et al.*, 1992; Chong *et al.*, 1993). Nasal endoscopic evaluation of the middle meatus region and posterior choana is also a valuable tool in diagnosing sinusitis as well as in evaluating therapeutic response (Tami and Wawrose, 1992).

INVESTIGATIONS

Although plain sinus radiographs (Figure 22.1) can be useful in the evaluation and management of patients, CT scanning more clearly defines the extent of sinus abnormalities. Magnetic resonance imaging (Figure 22.2) or computed tomography appears significantly more sensitive than plain radiography in defining the extent of the disease, particularly with posterior sinus involvement (Godowski *et al.*, 1992; Grant *et al.*, 1993;

MANAGEMENT

Standard outpatient therapy for acute sinusitis is often effective. A two-pronged approach consisting of an antibiotic as well as a decongestant arm should be employed (Tami and Wawrose, 1992, 1995; Meiteles and Lucente, 1990; Rubin and Honigberg, 1990; Godowsky *et al.*, 1992). Although amoxicillin or sulfamethoxazole/trimethoprim are reasonable antibiotics for primary therapy of acute sinusitis, amoxycillin with clavulanate (Augmentin/AmoxiClav) or an

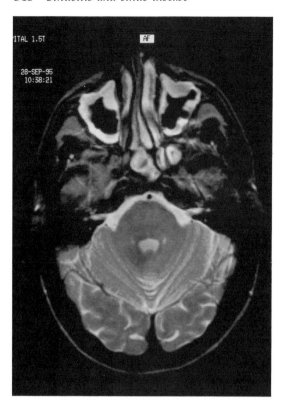

ITAL 1.5T   AF

28-SEP-95
10:38:21

Fig. 22.2 MRI scan of the head (transverse T2 weighted image). There is thickened mucosa indicative of marked paranasal sinus disease.

oral cephalosporin are effective alternatives. Outpatient antibiotic therapy should be continued for at least 3 weeks. In cases resistant to this therapy and in those with signs of impending complications, hospital admission for intravenous antibiotics or surgical drainage is imperative. Decongestant therapy is as important as antibiotic therapy. Systemic decongestants (usually pseudoephidrine 120 mg every 12 hours) is used throughout the 3 weeks of therapy. Topical decongestant sprays are recommended for the first 5 days of therapy only in order to avoid rebound nasal congestion. In a double-blind randomized trial which compared Guaifenesin 1200 mg every 12 hours to placebo as an adjunct to standard

3-week therapy for acute sinusitis, nasal secretions were considerably thinner and nasal congestion significantly decreased in the group receiving Guaifenesin (Tami and Wawrose, 1992).

While many patients respond well to antibiotic therapy, recurrent acute sinusitis is common, severe and difficult to treat. Patients with CD4 counts less than 200/mm^3 are prone to disease which involves multiple sinuses and which responds incompletely to antibiotic therapy, often resulting in chronic sinusitis. Unlike the situation in the immunocompetent host, the majority of HIV-infected patients with advanced immunodeficiency develop posterior sinus disease. As the CD4 count decreases and the patient becomes more immunocompromised, sinusitis often becomes chronic and recurrent. Patients with CD4 counts below 200/mm^3 seem particularly resistant to standard therapy for acute sinusitis. In these patients antibiotic coverage must be extended to cover *S. aureus*, anerobic bacteria and *P. aeruginosa*. Culture-directed antibiotic coverage is prudent. Ciprofloxacin plus metronidazole or Augmentin with metronidazole or clindamycin are rational choices. Because of the chronic, resistant nature of these infections, treatment is usually continued for 5 to 6 weeks to optimize chances of success. Decongestants are also used for chronic sinusitis. Topical sprays should be avoided. Recurrent episodes of sinusitis occur commonly in patients with HIV infection (Rubin and Honigberg, 1990; Slavit, Yocum and Kern, 1990; Schrager, 1988; Godowsky *et al.*, 1992). When medical measures fail to control the sinusitis, surgery may be necessary to enhance drainage as well as to obtain culture material to identify or exclude fungal, mycobacterial and other opportunistic infections. Although traditional surgical procedures such as bilateral antral washouts or antrostomy are employed, in many cases endoscopic sinus surgery (ESS) appears to be effective.

COMPLICATIONS OF SINUSITIS

When complications of sinusitis occur in HIV-infected patients the clinical course appears fulminant and response to therapy impaired. Data detailing the incidence of orbital and intracranial complications are not available. Severe periorbital, epidural and brain abscesses have been described.

MISCELLANEOUS SINONASAL CONDITIONS IN HIV INFECTION

Other sinonasal conditions which have been described in HIV-infected individuals include: mucocutaneous lesions (Kaposi's sarcoma, herpes simplex, herpes zoster, rhinosporidiosis, seborrheic dermatitis); nasal obstruction (adenoidal hypertrophy, allergic rhinitis, nasal polyposis, chronic sinusitis, and neoplasms of the paranasal sinuses or nasopharynx (Kaposi's sarcoma and non Hodgkin's lymphoma).

CONCLUSIONS

Sinonasal disease is an extremely common manifestation of infection with HIV. Sinusitis is an understudied manifestation of HIV infection and several areas require further study. These include the relative contribution of infection and allergy in the pathogenesis of the condition, the establishment of optimal diagnostic methods, and the appropriate use of antibiotics for therapy and prophylaxis.

REFERENCES

Brillhart, T., Grath, J. Jr. and Piot D. (1991) Symptomatic cytomegaloviral rhinosinusitis in patients with AIDS (abstract M.B.2182). In VIIth International Conference on AIDS, Florence, Italy, 227.

Carranzana, E.J., Rossitch, E. and Morris, J. (1991) Isolated central nervous system aspergillosis in the acquired immunodeficiency syndrome. *Clin. Neurol. Neurosurg.*, **93**, 227–30.

Choi, S.S., Lawson, W. and Buttone, E.J. (1988) Cryptococcal sinusitis: A case report and review of literature. *Otolaryngol. Head Neck Surg.*, **99**, 414–18.

Chong, W.K., Hall-Craggs, M.A., Wilkinson, I.D. *et al.* (1993) The prevalence of paranasal sinus disease in HIV infection and AIDS on cranial MR imaging. *Clin. Radiol.*, **47**, 166–9.

Godofsky, E.W., Zinreich, J., Armstrong, M. *et al.* (1992) Sinusitis in HIV-infected patients: A clinical and radiographic review. *Am. J. Med.*, **93**, 163–70.

Colmero, C., Monur, A., Valencia, E. and Castro, A. (1990) Successfully treated Candida sinusitis in an AIDS patient. *J. Cranio. Maxillofac. Surg.*, **18**, 175–8.

Gonzalez, M.M., Gould, E., Dickinson, G. *et al.* (1986) Acquired immunodeficiency syndrome associated with Acanthamoeba infection and other opportunistic organisms. *Arch. Pathol. Lab. Med.*, **110**, 749–51.

Grant, A., von Schoenberg, M., Grant, H.R. and Miller, R.F. (1993) Paranasal sinus disease in HIV antibody positive patients. *Genitourin. Med.*, **69**, 208–12.

Hoover, D.R., Graham, N.M., Bacellar, H. *et al.* (1991) Epidemiologic patterns of upper respiratory illness and *Pneumocystis carinii* pneumonia in homosexual men. *Am. Rev. Respir. Dis*, **144**, 756–59.

Lacey, C.J.N., Clarke, A.M.T. and Fraser, P. (1992) Chronic microsporidian infection of the nasal mucosae, sinuses and conjunctivae in HIV disease. *Genitourin. Med.*, **68**, 179–81.

Meiteles, L.Z. and Lucente, F.E. (1990) Sinusitis and nasal manifestations of the acquired immunodeficiency syndrome. *Ear Nose Throat J*, **69**, 454–9.

Meyer, R.D., Gaultier, C.R., Yamashita, J.T. *et al.* (1994) Fungal sinusitis in patients with AIDS: report of 4 cases and review of literature. *Medicine-Baltimore*, **73**, 69–78.

Milgrim, L.M., Rubin, J.S., Rosenstreich, D.L. and Small, C.B. (1994) Sinusitis in human immunodeficiency virus infection: typical and atypical organisms. *J. Otolaryngol.*, **23**, 450–3.

Mofenson, L.M., Korelitz, J., Pelton, S. *et al.* (1995) Sinusitis in children infected with human immunodeficiency virus: clinical characteristics, risk factors and prophylaxis. *Clin. Infect. Dis*, **21**, 1175–81.

Rubin, J.S. and Honigberg, R. (1990) Sinusitis in

patients with the acquired immunodeficiency syndrome. *Ear Nose Throat J.*, **69**, 460–3.

Schrager, L.K. (1988) Bacterial infections in AIDS patients. *AIDS*, (suppl. 1), S183–S185.

Schlanger, G., Lutwick, L. and Kurzman, M. (1984) Sinusitis caused by *Legionella pneumophila*: A patient with the acquired immune deficiency syndrome. *Am. J. Med.*, **77**, 957–60.

Slavit, D.H., Yocum, M.W. and Kern, E.B. (1990) Chronic sinusitis and dyspnea: Could this be AIDS? *Otolaryngol. Head Neck Surg*, **103**, 650–54.

Sooy, C.D. (1987) The impact of AIDS on otolaryngology–head and neck surgery. *Adv. Otolaryngol. Head Neck Surg.*, **1**, 1–28.

Spech, T.J., Rehm, S.J. and Longworth, D.L. (1988) Frequency of sinusitis in AIDS patients in IVth International Conference on AIDS. Abstracts. Stockholm, International Fairs, 399.

Tami, T.A. and Wawrose, M.S. (1992) Diseases of the nose and paranasal sinuses in the human immunodeficiency virus-infected population. *Otololaryngol. Clin. N. Am.*, **25**, 6, 1199–210.

Tami, T.A. (1995) The management of sinusitis in patients infected with the human immunodeficiency virus (HIV). *Ear Nose Throat J.*, **74**, 5, 360–63.

Verghese, A., Al-Samman, M., Nabhan, D. *et al.* (1994) Bacterial bronchitis and bronchiectasis in human immunodeficiency virus infection. *Arch. Intern. Med.*, **154**, 2086–91.

Wallace, J.M., Rao, A.V., Glassroth, J. *et al.* (1993) Respiratory illness in persons with human immunodeficiency virus infection. The pulmonary complications of HIV infection study group. *Am. Rev. Respir. Dis.*, **148**, 1523–9.

Weber, R., Bryan, R.T., Schwartz, D.A. and Owen, R.L. (1994) Human microsporidial infections. *Clin. Micro. Rev.*, **7**, 4, 426–55.

Zurlo, J.J., Feuerstein, I.M., Lebovics, R. and Lane, H.C. (1992) Sinusitis in HIV-1 infection. *Am. J. Med.*, **93**, 157–62.

23

PULMONARY DISEASE IN PEDIATRIC HIV INFECTION

Mike Sharland and Diane Gibb

INTRODUCTION

EPIDEMIOLOGY OF PEDIATRIC HIV INFECTION

Heterosexual transmission of HIV is resulting in a dramatic increase in the number of women infected worldwide. By the year 2000 the World Health Organization estimates that nearly 90% of all new HIV infections will be transmitted heterosexually, with 50% of all new infections occurring in women (Chin, 1990). The WHO also predicts that over 10 million children worldwide will be infected with HIV by the year 2000 (Chin, 1991). Although the great majority of these children will be born in Africa, India, SE Asia and South America, the numbers of infected children in North America and Europe are also steadily increasing. By 1993, over 4000 children under 13 years of age had been reported with AIDS in the USA. AIDS is now among the top five causes of childhood death in some American states. Over 3000 children have been reported with AIDS in Europe. HIV is transmitted to children perinatally from their infected mother (vertical transmission). Among children with AIDS reported in the USA in 1992, 90% acquired their infection vertically.

Worldwide pediatric acquisition of HIV through infected blood products is now almost completely eradicated in countries that can afford screening programs. The reported rates of vertical transmission vary between 15–20% in Europe, between 16–30% in USA, and 25–35% in Africa (Newell and Peckham, 1993). The greatest numbers of children with HIV infection and AIDS in Europe have been reported from France, Spain, and Italy, where intravenous drug use (IVDU) is an important risk factor, and Romania, where transmission via infected needles and blood products occurred. In other North European countries (e.g. UK, Belgium and France), HIV infection in women has commonly been acquired heterosexually in families who are refugees from highly endemic areas (e.g. Sub-Sahara Africa) (Keenlyside, Johnson and Mabey, 1993). Women in the USA have mainly acquired their infection through IVDU, although heterosexual transmission is increasing (Rogers *et al.*, 1993).

Children with HIV infection often come from disrupted families living in relative poverty in inner city areas. In one study, of over 1500 children born to HIV-infected mothers, only 55% were living with a natural parent (Caldwell, 1992). There are important

AIDS and Respiratory Medicine. Edited by A. Zumla, M.A. Johnson and R.F. Miller. Published in 1997 by Chapman & Hall, London. ISBN 0 412 60140 0

influences of family structure, poverty, and origin of maternal disease on pulmonary infections in children with HIV infection.

NATURAL HISTORY OF PEDIATRIC HIV INFECTION

It is now recognized that children with vertically acquired HIV infection fall into two groups. One group of 'rapid progressors' or short-term survivors usually present in the first year of life with opportunistic infections, and severe encephalopathy. The outlook for this group is poor. In a French study of 94 infected children, only 32% of the rapid progressors survived to 3 years of age (Duliege, 1992). However children without early progressive disease had a 97% survival rate at 3 years of age. The prospective European Collaborative Study (ECS) has documented an overall infant mortality rate of 15%, and an under 5 mortality rate of 28% (ECS, 1994). The Italian collaborative study has confirmed the improved survival prospects in a group of 1325 infected children prospectively followed from birth, who had a survival of 68% at 6.5 years (Italian Register, 1994). In the Italian collaborative study lymphocytic interstitial pneumonitis was a sign of intermediate disease, while *Pneumocystis carinii* pneumonia, and disseminated cytomegalovirus infection, were significant and independent negative predictors of survival (Tovo, 1992). In general, the type of pulmonary disease and the age at presentation are highly predictive of the child's outcome.

ETIOLOGY OF RESPIRATORY DISEASE

In 1983, the first clinical descriptions of children with AIDS were published. The original reports were from New York (Rubinstein *et al.*, 1983) and New Jersey (Oleske *et al.*, 1983), while Scott *et al.* (Scott *et al.*, 1984) presented details of 14 infants from Miami. Failure to thrive,

hepatosplenomegaly and a chronic intestinal pneumonitis were originally regarded as cardinal features of the syndrome.

Further experience has led to the recognition that pulmonary disease is the major cause of morbidity and mortality in children infected with HIV, occurring in over 80% of all cases (Hauger, 1991; CDC, 1986). Many different pathological processes may lead to pulmonary disease, including pneumonia due to bacterial, viral, or opportunistic infections, the pulmonary lymphoid hyperplasia/lymphocytic interstitial pneumonitis complex, and rarer noninfectious causes (Table 23.1).

PNEUMOCYSTIS CARINII PNEUMONIA

BACKGROUND

Pneumocystis carinii, now classified as a fungus (Edman, 1988), is believed to be transmitted by droplet spread from human to human. The cycle of asexual reproduction is from mature cysts forming eight sporozoites, transforming into trophozoites which subsequently mature into cysts. This cycle of reproduction is thought to take place in the alveolar air sacs and surrounding epithelial cells. The majority of children mount an immune response to *Pneumocystis carinii* in early childhood, suggesting early acquisition of asymptomatic infection is common (Pifer *et al.*, 1978).

In the 1950s, *Pneumocystis carinii* was recognized as a cause of the interstitial plasma cell pneumonia frequently reported across Europe over the preceding 20 years. The pneumonia was commonest in malnourished and premature infants (Gajdusek, 1957) from 6 weeks to 4 months of age. The majority of the cases reported were seen during outbreaks in institutions, with an estimated incubation period of between 1–2 months. In later years, *Pneumocystis carinii* was recognized as a common cause of pneumonia in infants and children with

Table 23.1 Reported causes of respiratory disease in pediatric HIV infection

Pneumocystis carinii pneumonia

Lymphocytic interstitial pneumonitis complex

Bacterial pneumonia
  Streptococcus pneumoniae, Haemophilus influenzae, Staphylococcus aureus,
  Pseudomonas aeruginosa, Mycoplasma pneumoniae, Chlamydia pneumoniae,
  Mycobacterium tuberculosis, and avium complex

Viral pneumonia
  Cytomegalovirus, measles, adenovirus, parainfluenza, influenza, respiratory syncytial virus,
  varicella, Herpes simplex

Fungal infections
  Aspergillosis, histoplasmosis

Congestive cardiac failure
  cardiomyopathy/cor pulmonale

Malignancy
  Kaposi's sarcoma, leiomyoma and leiomyosarcoma, lymphoma

primary immunodeficiencies (Walzer *et al.*, 1973) and those receiving immunosuppressive chemotherapy (Hughes *et al.*, 1973). It is assumed that the infection in infancy represents a primary infection with late childhood and adult disease caused by a resurgence of a previously acquired dormant infection. Failure of T-cell function appears to be of primary importance in the development of PCP (Sanders-Laufer, De Bruin and Edelson, 1991).

The pathology of the original reports of *Pneumocystis carinii* pneumonia (PCP) in debilitated infants revealed a mononuclear cell infiltration of the alveolar septa, compressing and collapsing the alveolar air spaces and ducts, with occasional dilatation of alveoli leading to emphysema and pneumothorax. A foamy exudate containing organisms filled the alveoli (Gajdusek, 1957), an appearance similar to that documented in infants dying with PCP and AIDS (Joshi, Oleske and Minnefor, 1985).

PCP is one of the commonest AIDS-defining diagnoses, occurring in about 40–50% of children reported (CDC, a, b, 1991) (Rogers *et al.*, 1987; Gibb *et al.*, 1994). PCP is more common in children aged less than 1 year (72%) compared to those aged over 1 (38%) (Vernon *et al.*, 1988). A recent British study of vertically infected HIV children documented a median age at PCP diagnosis of 4.1 (1.4–27.3) months (Gibb *et al.*, 1994).

CLINICAL FEATURES

The classical tetrad of clinical features of PCP are tachypnea, dyspnea, cough and fever. The onset may be insidious over 1–2 weeks with slowly increasing tachypnea. Coughing is not usually prominent until the full clinical picture develops with severe dyspnea. Physical findings are usually limited to fine crepitations. Fever is often low grade throughout the illness. Hypoxia is common, with one study finding all children

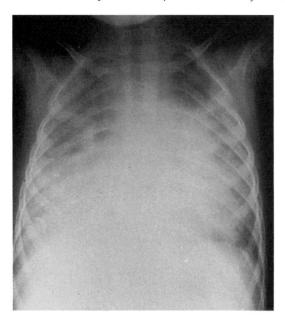

Fig. 23.1 A 1-year-old infant with *Pneumocystis carinii* pneumonia.

original method of diagnosing PCP in many of the early reports of children with HIV infection (Scott *et al.*, 1984; Shannon and Amman, 1985; Marolda *et al.*, 1991) but less invasive methods are now more widely used. In infants the diagnosis can often be obtained from a nasopharyngeal aspirate (Gibb, Davison and Holland, 1994), which should be tried first. Bronchoscopy with bronchoalveolar lavage (BAL) is now frequently used for diagnosing PCP in children (Birriel, Adams and Saldana, 1991). In a study by de Blic and colleagues (de Blic *et al.*, 1989), *Pneumocystis carinii* was identified using this method in 14/22 children with acute interstitial pneumonitis, with one-third of the children in the study being less than 1 year of age. A similar study of 105 bronchoscopies with BAL diagnosed PCP in 22% of specimens, with serious complications of the procedure occurring in less than 1% (Abadco *et al.*, 1992). Bronchoalveolar lavage can be performed safely without bronchoscopy using an 8F nasogastric feeding tube in intubated children who may not tolerate bronchoscopy, and provides a significantly improved yield in comparison to tracheal suctioning alone (Amaro-Galvez, Rao and Abadco, 1991). The use of methenamine silver, toluidine, immunofluorescent antibody or other stains depends on local availability, preference and experience. Increased levels of lactate dehydrogenase (LDH) have been reported in children with PCP but the overlap of values with other pulmonary disorders precludes its usefulness. As PCP is an AIDS-defining diagnosis with an especially poor outlook, it is very important to make a definitive diagnosis even after commencing treatment.

with PCP having an alveolar–arterial oxygen gradient greater than 30 mmHg (Bernstein, Byre and Rubinstein, 1989). A rapidly progressive course of disease leading to respiratory failure in a few days has also been described (Rubinstein *et al.*, 1986).

The chest X-ray may be normal early in the disease, but there is usually rapid development of complete opacification with air bronchograms (Figure 23.1). The alveolar infiltrates progress peripherally with late apical sparing (Hughes, 1991) and small pleural effusions have been reported. Occasionally bullae, cysts, and pneumothoraxes may be seen (Berdon, Mellins and Abramson, 1993). Without treatment, the clinical course is one of progressive respiratory failure.

Diagnosis

In adults and older children, the diagnosis of PCP is usually based on an induced sputum, but this is less sensitive and practical in younger children. Open lung biopsy was the

MANAGEMENT

Treatment

The recommended initial treatment of PCP is trimethoprim, 20 mg/kg/day–sulphamethazole 100 mg/kg/day (TMP/SMX), given in 4 divided doses infused over 1 hour. It is not unusual for the child to clinically deteriorate for a few days after commencing therapy, then significantly improve by 1 week. The course is 21 days and the trimethoprim/sulphamethoxazole should be given intravenously for at least 1 week. Side effects from TMP/SMX are not frequent, an erythematous rash being the commonest which responds to temporarily stopping the drug. An urticarial rash or signs of Stevens–Johnson syndrome requires immediate discontinuation of the drug. Gastrointestinal disturbance and bone marrow suppression also occur.

If there is failure to respond to TMP/SMX or an allergic reaction to the drug, the treatment should be changed to slow intravenous pentamidine isethionate (once daily, 4 mg/kg/day) for 3 weeks. Side effects include neutropenia, thrombocytopenia, hepatitis, renal impairment, and early hypoglycemia with late development of insulin dependent diabetes. Adult studies have demonstrated a reduced morbidity in PCP with early use of corticosteroids. Although data are lacking in children, methylprednisolone should be added when a diagnosis of PCP has been made. The recommended regime for methylprednisolone is 0.5 mg/kg/dose, 4 times a day for 5 days, twice daily for 3 days and once daily for 2 days (Van Dyke, 1993). This may be changed to oral prednisolone in the same doses. One retrospective case review provides some evidence for the use of steroids in children with PCP (McLaughlin, 1995). Nutritional support is extremely important, and a goal of 150 cal/kg/day should be aimed for (Sanders-Laufer, De Bruin and Edelson, 1991). Failure to respond to TMP/SMX alone should raise the possibility of a second treatable infection and repeat BAL or lung biopsy should be considered. CMV is frequently found at BAL in PCP infection, but its role in the pathogenesis of the lung disease is not clear. In one small study the outcome for children

with PCP was not significantly different whether or not CMV was detected at BAL (Glaser *et al.*, 1992). The use of ganciclovir should be considered in a child with PCP and CMV, if the child is not responding to standard PCP therapy.

The role of aggressive ventilatory support in children with HIV and PCP is controversial. In one study of children with AIDS and PCP, 60% required ventilation and only 22% were alive after a year (Bernstein, Byre and Rubinstein, 1989). This mortality rate has been confirmed by other studies (Vernon *et al.*, 1988; Connor *et al.*, 1991). In a recent British review, 79% of the children who required ventilation died, with some children dying after being ventilated for over a month. Although children are often ventilated prior to the diagnosis of PCP being made, these results do raise the issue as to whether reventilation for a relapse is appropriate therapy for young children with AIDS and PCP. There seems to be a high rate of severe encephalopathy in PCP survivors.

Prevention

For a newborn HIV-infected child the risk of having PCP is estimated to be 8% during the first year (Hughes, 1991), with a subsequent risk of about 6 cases/100 HIV infected child years (Van Dyke, 1993). In adults, clearly defined guidelines for PCP prophylaxis are well established. Unfortunately, it became clear in the pediatric epidemic that children could develop PCP with CD counts >500/mm^3 (Scott *et al.*, 1984). A further study of 39 children with PCP and AIDS noted that 26% had CD4 counts over 500/mm^3 at presentation, but in infants under 1 year only 10% had a CD4 count of over 1500/mm^3 at diagnosis (Kovacs *et al.*, 1990) and 10% of uninfected children under 1 year of age will have a CD4 count <1500/mm^3. Although North American guidelines have now been published for commencing PCP prophylaxis in children based on age adjusted CD4 values

(CDC, 1991), a further difficulty in the prophylaxis of children is deciding whether the child is definitely infected with HIV, which can take from 6–18 months. Because of the overlap between normal and abnormal CD4 counts in infants, and the observed variation of CD4 counts in children, many centers are giving PCP prophylaxis to all children born to HIV-positive women until the child is shown to be uninfected (ECS, 1994). As PCP has been reported in a 19-day-old infant with HIV, prophylaxis should begin at 4–6 weeks of age (Beach *et al.*, 1991).

In a prophylactic dosage of 150 mg trimethoprim/750 mg sulfamethoxazole/m²/day 3 days a week, TMP/SMX is generally well tolerated. For the child who is persistently intolerant to TMP/SMX other forms of prophylaxis are available. Dapsone (1 mg/kg/day) is well tolerated, early safety and efficacy data are available for children with HIV infection, but significant breakthrough is documented (Stavola and Noel, 1993). Adequate lung deposition of nebulized pentamidine has been demonstrated in children aged over 8 years (O'Doherty, Thomas and Gibb, 1993), and monthly doses of 300 mg via a Respirgard II nebulizer, for children with heights >160 cm and 150 mg for those with a height of 130–160 cm are used. There are few pediatric data available on prophylactic efficacy or safety.

LYMPHOCYTIC INTERSTITIAL PNEUMONITIS

BACKGROUND

The first studies of children with HIV infection reported CXR changes of a chronic interstitial pneumonitis. Frequently a characteristic lymphocytic infiltrate was described that proved to be histologically identical to lymphocytic interstitial pneumonia (LIP). This disease had first been des-

cribed in adults by Carrington and Liebnow (Carrington and Liebnow, 1966). Before the association of LIP with HIV had been recognized, the condition has been reported in autoimmune diseases (Sjögren's syndrome, thyroiditis, myasthenia, etc.).

Epidemiology

The diagnosis of LIP is most frequently made on a routine CXR in an asymptomatic child in the second year of life. The median age of presentation in one series of 42 children was 12 months (range 5–81 months) (Scott *et al.*, 1989), although in the absence of severe symptoms, some children are presenting much older (Persaud *et al.*, 1992). Between 30–50% of vertically infected children develop LIP (Pitt, 1991). In Europe LIP represented 24% of the AIDS diagnoses (ECS, 1994). In a cohort of vertically infected children being followed in London, a clinical and radiological diagnosis of LIP had been made in 33% of 82 children, the diagnosis was seen more frequently in children from a Black African ethnic background (Sharland, Davison and Davies, 1994).

Pathology

In a detailed study of the pulmonary pathological findings of AIDS, Joshi and colleagues (Joshi, Oleske and Minnefor, 1985; Joshi and Oleske, 1986) described children with diffuse alveolar damage due to oxygen therapy and ventilation, a pneumonitis associated with PCP, and the pulmonary lymphoid hyperplasia (PLH)/lymphocytic interstitial pneumonitis (LIP) complex. A peribronchiolar nodular hyperplasia with or without germinal centers was characteristic of PLH, while in cases of LIP, a diffuse lymphocytic infiltration of the interalveolar septa was present. Bronchial associated lymphoid tissue (BALT) is normally seen as nodules of lymphoid tissue at the origin of lymphatic channels, usually occurring at the bifurcation of bronchioles, and draining to intrapulmonary and hilar lymph nodes. The spectrum of PLH and LIP is characterized by an absence of cells within the airway lumen, and an absence of vasculitis and necrosis (Connor *et al.*, 1991). In some children, LIP can progress to the more widespread and histologically more aggressive looking polyclonal B cell lymphoproliferative disorder (PBLD), with hyperplastic lymphoid lesions apparent throughout the body (Joshi *et al.*, 1987). One child with LIP has been reported progressing to disseminated Burkitt's lymphoma (Young and Crocker, 1991). Other cases of non Hodgkin's lymphoma (NHL) have been reported in children with HIV infection, with a peak in adolescence (Serraino *et al.*, 1992). Whether the predominantly young children now seen with PLH/LIP/PBLD will have an increased incidence of NHL when older is not yet known. At a cellular level, the lymphoid infiltrate is polyclonal (Joshi and Oleske, 1986), with B cells predominating. Few pathological studies have been performed, as increased reliance on transbronchial diagnostic techniques has led to fewer lung biopsies being performed (Bonfils-Roberts, Nickodem and Nealen, 1990; Whitehead *et al.*, 1992).

Etiology

The exact cause of LIP has still not been clearly defined. The two principal hypotheses are that LIP represents an abnormal lymphoproliferative response, either to the HIV virus alone, or due to the co-infection of HIV and a herpesvirus. It is known that a clinical and pathologically similar picture to LIP can be seen in animal models infected with lentiviruses (retrovirus family), with complex interactions between antigen presenting cells and lymphocytes via the cytokine pathways documented (Mornex, 1990). The highest serum levels of tumor necrosis factor (TNF) and interleukin-1 in children with HIV infection are seen in those

with LIP (Arditi, Kabat and Yogev, 1991; Ellaurie and Rubinstein, 1992), as are very high serum levels of polyclonal IgG, providing further evidence for the idea that LIP represents an abnormal response of the child's developing immune system to HIV infection. Germinal centers and lymphoid tissue have been demonstrated to contain high concentrations of free HIV (Fox *et al.*, 1991).

The other principal hypothesis of the etiology of LIP is that it may be caused by an abnormal response to primary infection by a herpesvirus, particularly Epstein–Barr virus (EBV). Pathological studies have demonstrated EBV DNA significantly more frequently in the lungs of children with LIP compared to controls (Andiman *et al.*, 1985), and children with LIP have serological evidence of active EBV infection significantly more frequently than controls (Katz, Berkman and Shapiro, 1992). EBV has been recognized for a long time as a potent agent of B cell proliferation. The studies of EBV and LIP are small; documenting EBV genome in pathological samples is not proof of causation, and it is possible that the serological findings are part of the polyclonal gammopathy seen in children with LIP. Larger prospective studies directly linking EBV acquisition to the onset of LIP are required to prove causation.

CLINICAL FEATURES

The onset of LIP is usually slow, characterized by a chronic cough in children usually with evidence of generalized lymphadenopathy, parotid enlargement, and hepatosplenomegaly (Teirstein and Rosen, 1988). Many children are asymptomatic initially, and the diagnosis is most frequently made on a routine CXR (Figure 23.2). The main clinical problem is an increased frequency of acute lower respiratory tract infection (ALRTI). Analysis of the London cohort demonstrated that admission with

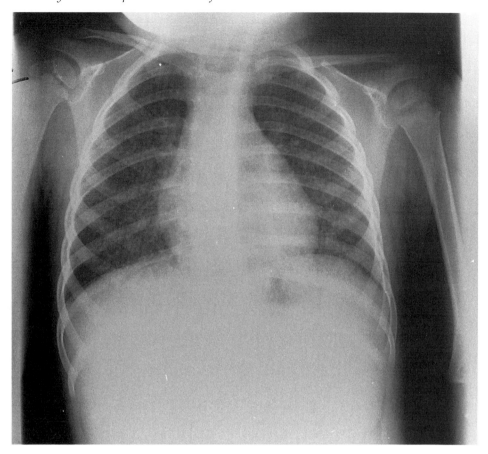

Fig. 23.2   Typical appearances of LIP seen on a routine CXR in an asymptomatic 2-year-old child.

ALRTI was twice as common in children with LIP compared to children with HIV but no LIP. Positive pathology in these children was identified in only 33% of admissions, with *Streptococcus pneumoniae* and *Haemophilus influenzae* being the commonest organisms. Progressive restrictive pattern respiratory disease can lead to the development of persistent chest signs, and tachypnea, occasionally with wheezing. Clubbing is seen and lower lobe bronchiectasis can develop (Amorosa *et al.*,1992), with chronic hypoxia.

Although a definitive diagnosis of LIP requires a lung biopsy, fewer biopsies are now being performed. The presence of reticulonodular shadowing in a well child, with or without hilar lymphadenopathy, persisting on a CXR for greater than 2 months, which does not respond to antibiotic treatment, can be considered as presumptive evidence for LIP. It is not possible to diagnose LIP with certainty on a CXR alone (Zimmerman *et al.*, 1987), and CMV pneumonitis, fungal infections, PCP, and in particular tuberculosis should be considered. Figures 23.3 and 4 demonstrate a typical CXR of moderately severe LIP, and the child's lung biopsy. Figure 23.5 demonstrates the CXR of a child with LIP and bronchiectasis after recurrent ALRTI. The nodules are usually between 1–5 mm in diameter (Rubinstein *et*

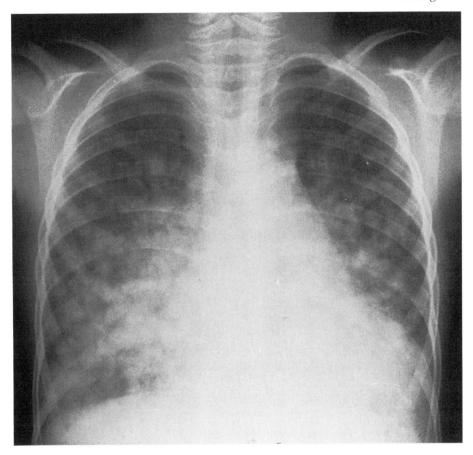

Fig. 23.3 Moderately severe LIP in a 6-year-old boy.

al., 1986), and a scoring system has been devised based on nodular size, and the presence of reticular shadowing (Oldham *et al.*, 1989). Other imaging techniques (gallium scans, chest CT) are rarely helpful (Conner and Andiman, 1994). Rapid respiratory deterioration is unusual, and broncho-alveolar lavage or lung biopsy should be considered.

MANAGEMENT

The frequent bacterial superinfections, with slow progression to clubbing, bronchiectasis and respiratory failure, are familiar to pediatricians caring for children with cystic fibrosis, and there are similarities in the management strategies of the two conditions.

Vaccination against *Streptococcus pneumoniae* (Pneumovax) and *Haemophilus influenzae* (Hib) and influenza are recommended (Connor and Andiman, 1994). Recognition of the increased frequency of ALRTI requires aggressive treatment of any acute infection, with early use of intravenous antibiotics. In children with frequent recurrent infections, prophylactic antibiotics (daily co-trimoxazole or amoxycillin) may be useful. Corticosteroids have been reported to be of benefit to children with LIP (Rubinstein *et al.*, 1988), particularly when chronic lung disease or hypoxia has developed. A dose of 2 mg/kg/day of pred-

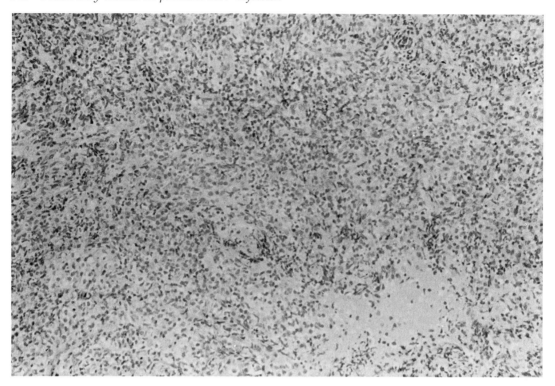

Fig. 23.4 The lung biopsy of the child in Figure 23.3, demonstrating the characteristic lymphocytic infiltration.

nisolone is used for 1–2 months, followed by a reduction based on response to therapy. A low dose maintenance alternate day dosage can then be continued, with short high dose pulses given during intercurrent infections. Bronchodilators, inhaled steroids, regular physiotherapy and oxygen can also be helpful in symptom control. In end stage LIP, right-heart failure may need treatment (Connor and Andiman, 1994). LIP is not an AIDS-defining diagnosis by Centers for Disease Control (CDC) criteria. There are anecdotal reports of successful treatment with zidovudine (Bach, 1987; Gibb, personal communication), but no controlled trials. The frequency of LIP in pediatric AIDS appears to be declining in the USA and one factor in this reduction could be increasing zidovudine usage (Connor and Andiman, 1994).

The prognosis of LIP is considerably better than other HIV-related diseases. Growth is often normal, with surprisingly little clinical or radiological progression of LIP for many years. Many children do eventually progress to chronic lung disease, but there is increasing evidence that, in a few children, clinical and radiological remission occurs. This is often associated with the failure of a child's immune system (Marquis, Berman and Oleske, 1993). The rate of late malignancies has yet to be determined.

BACTERIAL INFECTIONS

NON-MYCOBACTERIAL

Background

Many studies have documented the increased frequency of bacterial infections in

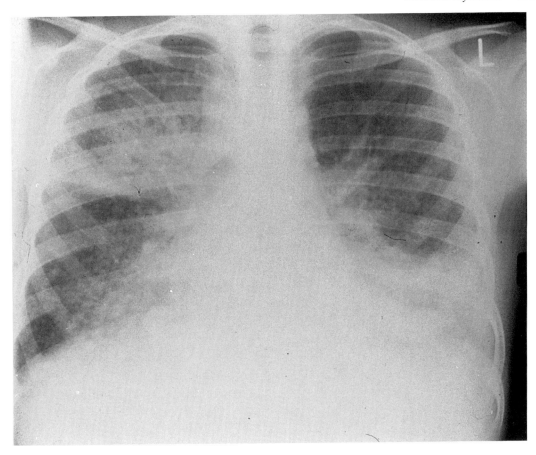

Fig. 23.5 An 8-year-old boy with severe LIP and bronchiectasis.

children with HIV infection. In a study of 71 HIV infected children, Krasinski and colleagues reported proven serious bacterial infections (SBI) in 38% of all children over a 3.5 year period (Krasinski *et al.*, 1988). Bacterial pneumonia was seen in 19%. A more recent retrospective review of 105 children reported that 61% experienced a bacterial infection in 3 years, and although soft tissue infections and bacteremia were most common, pneumonia was seen in 13% (Roilides *et al.*, 1991a, b). The National Institute of Child Health and Human Development intravenous immunoglobulin (NICHD IVIG) trial, on 376 enrolled children with 545 patient years of follow up, docu-

mented in the placebo arm approximately one SBI in each patient every 2 years, over 6 times the rate seen in healthy pre-school children. The commonest clinically diagnosed infection was acute pneumonia, occurring on average once in every 4 patient/years. Primary bacteremias (74%) were more common than pneumonia (22%) as laboratory proven infections (Mofenson and Moya, 1993; NICHD IVIG Study Group, 1991). The frequency of bacterial infection apparently increases with HIV disease progression. Marolda and colleagues reported 30% of children with AIDS developed bacterial pneumonia over a 6-year period (Marolda *et al.*, 1991). The increased risk of bacterial pneumonia for children with LIP has previously been discussed. Clinically, persistence of a lobar bacterial pneumonia despite an apparently adequate treatment course is a common problem. Greater use of parenteral antibiotics, with longer treatment regimes, is often required.

The cause of the increased susceptibility to SBI (including pneumonia) in children with HIV infection is multifactorial. One of the earliest manifestations of HIV infection is a polyclonal hypergammaglobulinemia which masks a functional defect in humoral immunity (Bernstein, Ocks and Wedgewood, 1985). IgG subclass deficiencies are reported in children with HIV infection (particularly IgG$_2$), but quantitative deficiencies of specific subclasses do not relate to the frequency of SBI (Roilides *et al.*, 1991b). *In vitro* studies have demonstrated defects in neutrophil chemotaxis and bactericidal activity in symptomatic HIV-infected children (Roilides *et al.*, 1990). Other *in vitro* studies of T-helper cell function demonstrate that a loss of the response to recall antigens appeared to be associated with an increased rate of bacterial infection (Roilides *et al.*, 1991a). The commonest organisms identified in all the studies are the encapsulated *Streptococcus pneumoniae* and *Haemophilus influenzae*. *Staphylococcus aureus* and Gram-negative infections, especially *Pseudomonas aeruginosa*, are also important.

CLINICAL FEATURES

The clinical presentation of acute bacterial pneumonia in children with early HIV infection is similar to non-infected children (Figure 23.6). The clinical signs may be less obvious in children with AIDS. Because of the difficulties of obtaining sputum in younger children, it is always important to obtain blood cultures, despite the poor yield.

The importance of upper respiratory tract infections in children with HIV infection must be recognized. Ear infections, sinusitis, and throat infections are very common, and cause considerable morbidity. Weight loss due to a reduced appetite is a particular problem in chronic ENT infections.

MANAGEMENT

Many clinicians will initially treat ALRTI empirically with a broad spectrum antibiotic (for example, Augmentin, or a cephalosporin). The choice of oral or intravenous antibiotic depends on the child's clinical condition. Failure to respond rapidly within 48 hours is an indication for bronchoalveolar lavage, as this may significantly improve the diagnostic yield (de Blic *et al.*, 1989; Birriel, Adams and Saldana, 1991).

Immunization

The importance of *Streptococcus pneumoniae* in causing both bacteremia and pneumonia has been discussed and immunization with a polyvalent pneumococcal vaccine is recommended in all children over the age of 1 year. Data are available to show immunogenicity, but efficacy studies have not been performed. Although a less common cause of disease, all children should also receive conjugate *Haemophilus influenzae* type B vaccine.

IVIG

The NICHD IVIG trial was a double-blind placebo-controlled study determining whether IVIG given intravenously at a dose of 0.4 g/kg every 28 days would reduce the risk of SBI in vertically infected HIV-positive children. A total of 376 children were divided into 2 groups on the basis of a CD4 count greater or less than 200/mm^3. In the IVIG treated children who entered the trial with a CD4 count >200/mm^3, treatment significantly increased the time free from SBI.

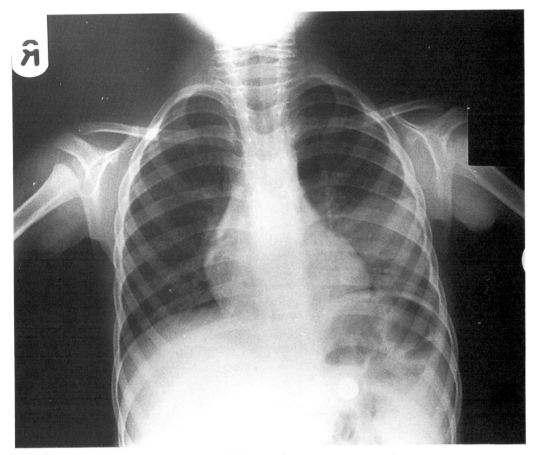

Fig. 23.6 Lobar pneumonia in a 2-year-old due to *Streptococcus pneumoniae*.

There was a 53% reduction in the rate of clinically diagnosed acute pneumonia for IVIG recipients with entry CD4 counts >200/mm³ (Mofenson and Moya, 1993). No effect of IVIG was seen in the smaller group of children with CD4 counts <200/mm³. There was no overall difference in mortality between the two groups. The effect on morbidity was also delayed, with many children staying well for years before developing their first SBI. A second placebo-controlled IVIG study in children already taking zidovudine (with many children on TMP/SMX) also demonstrated no effect on progression to AIDS or survival (Spector, 1993). A smaller effect on the frequency of bacterial infections was noted, with no benefit seen in the subgroup taking regular TMP/SMX.

On the basis of the above studies, because of the difficulties for the child and family that occur with monthly infusions, and the long lag time for many children from diagnosis to first SBI, and the observed lack of any effect on disease progression, it is our current practice to consider IVIG in children having recurrent bacterial infections despite taking regular TMP/SMX for PCP prophylaxis. Other possible treatment options that are used but not fully evaluated include daily TMP/SMX or other antibiotic (amoxycillin/azithromycin) for prophylaxis. They can be particularly useful in chronic ENT infections.

MYCOBACTERIAL DISEASE

MYCOBACTERIUM TUBERCULOSIS

Background

Tuberculosis is still one of the most important infections in childhood worldwide. Current WHO estimates suggest that there are about 1.5 million clinical infections in childhood due to tuberculosis every year (Kochi, 1991). The last 5–10 years has seen a reversal in many countries of the steady post-war decline in new TB cases. In the US in 1991, 1656 cases of childhood TB were reported to CDC, a 39% increase from 1987 (Jacobs and Starke, 1993), with 60% of the cases occurring in infants and children under 5. This childhood increase continued in 1992 and 1993 (MMWR, 1994). The great majority of cases were reported from large cities in the seven states with the highest rates of HIV infection. No such association is apparent as yet in the UK (Davies, 1993).

Over three quarters of the 4 million people estimated by the WHO to be co-infected with TB and HIV live in Sub-Saharan Africa. A high HIV seroprevalence has been reported in studies of adults with tuberculosis in Africa (De Cock *et al.*, 1991) ranging from 20–60%. In comparison to adults there is little information available on rates of HIV infection in children with TB. In a study of 60 vertically infected children in Kinshasa, Zaire, 90% of the children had lung disease, which was diagnosed as TB in 30% (Muganga, Nkuadiolandu and Mashaka, 1991). In Lusaka, Zambia, a case-control study of 237 hospitalized children with TB and 242 controls demonstrated an overall HIV seroprevalence rate in patients with TB of 37% compared to 10.7% in controls. The HIV seroprevalence rate was highest in children aged 12–18 months (53%). The risk of TB attributable to HIV infection was 27% (Chintu, 1993a).

Young children are recognized as being highly susceptible to tuberculosis infection acquired from adults in the family. Preliminary estimates have revealed that symptomatic HIV infected children have a rate of TB that is 10 times higher than other children in New York (Bakshi *et al.*, 1993). A study of 60 families of children with HIV infection in New York diagnosed TB in 7 children and 6/7 children had a history of exposure to tuberculosis in an HIV-infected parent who was either an intravenous drug user, homeless, and/or non-compliant with antituberculous chemotherapy (Bakshi *et al.*, 1993). Adults with HIV and tuberculosis seem to be as infectious as HIV-negative patients (Githui *et al.*, 1992). Most cases of active tuberculosis in people infected with HIV are thought to occur due to reactivation of a previously suppressed infection (Selwyn *et al.*, 1989). As the number of co-infected adults with HIV and TB increases, it is likely that the number of children with vertically acquired HIV and postnatal acquired TB infection will increase.

CLINICAL FEATURES

The diagnosis of TB in children remains difficult whether or not they are infected with HIV. The incubation period in children can be up to 6 months, and many children remain asymptomatic. Fever, weight loss and night sweats are unusual and symptoms range from a persistent cough to apathy and lethargy in disseminated disease. CXR signs include hilar lymphadenopathy, segmented or lobar disease, atelectasis, effusions or miliary shadowing. Surprisingly, the clinical reports published suggest that extra-pulmonary disease is unusual in children with TB and HIV co-infection. In the Zambian study, pulmonary disease was present in 90% of the HIV-positive children and 85% of the HIV-negative (Chintu *et al.*, 1993a). Severe cavitating pulmonary TB has been reported in a child with AIDS (Varteresian-Karanfil *et al.*, 1988). Mantoux test interpretation in the

HIV-infected child is complex. Factors that need to be taken into account in interpreting a positive reaction are the stage of HIV disease, infectious contact, country of origin, and age (Jacobs and Starke, 1993).

If the child has had BCG as an infant, a reactive Mantoux >10 mm by 3–5 years may be taken as indicating possible infection with tuberculosis requiring further investigation (American Thoracic Society, 1990). There are no good studies of the effect of HIV on the Mantoux test in children. Culture is still the gold standard for TB diagnosis, allowing drug sensitivity patterns to be established, but culture positive rates of only 30–50% are usual. Gastric lavage may be more sensitive than broncho-alveolar lavage (Jacobs and Starke, 1993). Diagnostic scoring systems have been used (Bhat *et al.*, 1993) but need local evaluation to be reliable.

MANAGEMENT

Recommended treatment regimes for tuberculosis in children are published (AAP, 1992; Ormerod, 1990). There are no controlled trials of tuberculosis treatment in HIV-infected children. Current practice is to extend the standard requirement to 9–12 months, depending on clinical response and state of immunosuppression. In the USA, where BCG is not widely used, it is standard in asymptomatic Mantoux-positive children to treat with isoniazid monotherapy for 12 months. There have been reports of multidrug resistant TB (MDR) in children (Van Dyke, 1993). If a child does have MDR TB, then a combination of drugs should be started based on susceptibility data. Because of severe cutaneous hypersensitivity reactions, thiacetazone should be avoided if at all possible in the treatment of the HIV-infected child (Chintu *et al.*, 1993b).

The WHO Special Programme on AIDS (Global Programme on AIDS) and Expanded Programme on Immunization recommends BCG vaccination only in asymptomatic HIV-infected children where the prevalence of tuberculosis in the community is high (Tarantola and Mann, 1987). Disseminated BCG-osis and fistula formation have been reported after immunization of children with rapidly progressive HIV disease (Besnard *et al.*, 1993). In the only study performed so far, analyzing the protective efficacy of BCG in children with TB and HIV infection, there was a 59% protective effect (OR 0.41; 95% CI, 0.18, 0.92) in HIV-negative children, but no protective effect in HIV-positive children (OR 1.0 95% CI, 0.2, 4.6). In a recent study, the median survival time after TB diagnosis was 20 months (Khouri, Mastrucci and Hutto, 1992).

Non-tuberculous mycobacterial disease

Disseminated non-tuberculous mycobacterial disease (DNTM) is the commonest bacterial infection of adults with AIDS, occurring in nearly 25%. It is associated with severe immunosuppression, and a CD4 count <50/mm^3 (Horsburgh, 1991). In the USA, between 1981 and 1991, DNTM was diagnosed in nearly 6% of children with AIDS. Nearly 90% of cases were due to *Mycobacterium avium*-intracellulare complex (MAC) and 70% of the cases were in children with a CD4 count <50/mm^3 (Horsburgh, Caldwell and Simonds, 1993). The median age at diagnosis for the vertically infected children was 3.3 years. The median survival of children from the date of diagnosis was 6 months (95%, CI, 4 to 7 months). The clinical features usually include prolonged fever, weight loss and chronic GI symptoms (Rutstein *et al.*, 1993). In patients with DNTM, MAC may be isolated from the lungs (Abadco *et al.*, 1992). Radiological presentation can occur with enlarged hilar lymph nodes (Berdon, Mellins and Abramson, 1993). Treatment involves a complex multidrug regime. Prophylaxis for all children with

HIV and CD4 counts $<100/mm^3$ has been recommended (Van Dyke, 1993).

VIRAL INFECTIONS

CYTOMEGALOVIRUS

In contrast to adults, disseminated rather than focal cytomegalovirus (CMV) infection is the important AIDS-defining diagnosis in HIV-infected children. In the Italian collaborative study disseminated CMV infection was the second commonest cause of death in HIV-infected children, and was of particular importance in children under 1 year (Tovo *et al.*, 1992). In a study of the use of bronchoalveolar lavage in 85 children with AIDS and respiratory distress, cytomegalovirus was the commonest isolate, seen in over two-thirds of all positive cultures (Abadco *et al.*, 1992). However, one or more co-existing pathogens was always identified in the specimens, and how frequently the CMV isolated was the principal cause of the pneumonitis was not clear. In a study of children with PCP infection, the concurrent isolation of CMV at BAL had no effect on disease outcome (Glaser *et al.*, 1992). In a prospective study of CMV acquisition in 38 HIV-infected children, the prevalence of active CMV infection in symptomatic children was 45%. CMV was identified in only 4 of 14 children who survived, and in 7 out of 10 children who died (Frenkel *et al.*, 1990). In this study, 3 out of the 24 CMV-infected patients had evidence of CMV pneumonia. Although CMV can be asymptomatically shed in secretions and be cultured on BAL, patients with disseminated CMV disease are viremic, and often have radiological evidence of CMV pneumonia (Figure 23.7). Patients with proven disseminated disease are treated with ganciclovir (a nucleoside analog). A two-week induction phase of 5 mg/kg every 12 hours intravenously is followed by a prolonged maintenance phase of 5 mg/kg/day given 3–7 days/week (Mustafa, 1994). In older children an adult pattern of CMV disease is seen.

OTHER VIRAL INFECTIONS

There are very few data available on the importance of other viral infections in pediatric HIV disease. Viruses remain the most important cause of upper respiratory tract infections. Asymptomatic and symptomatic HIV-infected children usually have a normal clinical course with the common viral infections of childhood. Many of the reports of serious morbidity and mortality due to viral infections in children with AIDS are because of secondary bacterial infections.

Respiratory syncytial virus (RSV) infection is a well recognized cause of respiratory distress in children with HIV infection (Rubenstein *et al.*, 1988). In one study of 10 HIV-infected children with RSV, two children died. Both of the deaths were in infants with severely reduced CD4 counts and, in both, *Pseudomonas aeruginosa* was detected at postmortem, despite negative BALs (Chandwani *et al.*, 1990). The clinical course in children with reasonable immunity is similar to that seen in non-immunosuppressed infants. Ribavirin should be given to all infants known to be HIV-positive who develop RSV bronchiolitis. Prolonged shedding of the RSV is common.

A severe measles pneumonitis has been reported in the absence of a rash and may be fatal (Joshi and Oleske, 1986). Pneumonia was not reported in 13 children with vertically acquired HIV infection who developed chickenpox (Kelley *et al.*, 1994). Only 3 of these children had CD4 counts $<500/mm^3$ and acyclovir therapy was started promptly. In a previous report of 8 children (5 with AIDS), pneumonia and severe secondary bacterial infections were common (Jura, 1989). At present, all children with chickenpox contact should be given varicella zoster immune globulin (VZIG), and intra-

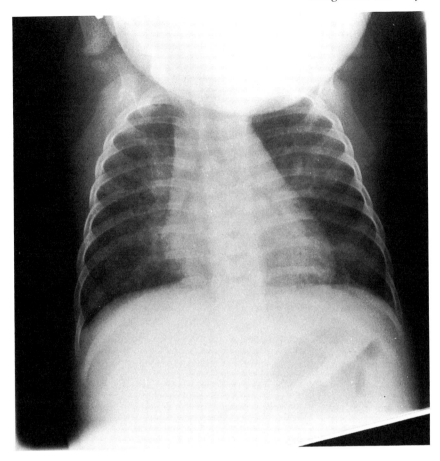

Fig. 23.7 A 1-year-old child with CMV pneumonitis.

venous acyclovir should be given promptly to children with chickenpox disease and severe immunosuppression.

Some small studies have suggested that children with HIV infection appear to be more susceptible to acute upper respiratory tract viral infections, with higher rates of respiratory viral isolation found compared to controls, with prolonged virus excretion documented (Josephs *et al.*, 1988; Hague *et al.*, 1992). Other viruses that have been isolated from the respiratory tract include:

- parainfluenza;
- influenza;
- adenoviruses;

- rhinoviruses;
- herpes simplex;
- enterovirus.

Although the response to vaccine is poor in children with AIDS (Chadwick, 1994), at present, it is recommended that all HIV-infected children should be considered for influenza vaccine each winter.

FUNGAL AND OTHER INFECTIONS

There have been very few cases reported of children with HIV infection and pulmonary fungal disease. Wright and colleagues (Wright, Fikrig and Holder, 1993) reported one case of pulmonary aspergillosis. Two hemophiliac children with AIDS and pulmonary disease were reported in a series of 18 cases of invasive aspergillosis (Minamoto, Barlam and Vander Els, 1992). The condition was associated with previous underlying lung disease and prolonged courses of broad spectrum antibiotics. The diagnosis was difficult, frequently being made at postmortem. Treatment was not successful, with all patients dying within a few months of the diagnosis.

Other infections that have been reported in HIV-infected children include mycoplasma, chlamydia, and legionella (Rubinstein *et al.*, 1988), but there are few available data on their varying clinical presentations. As HIV infection spreads worldwide, tropical and parasitic lung infections are being recognized in association with HIV disease. These include melioidosis, paracoccidioidomycosis, paragonomiasis, and strongyloidiasis (Iralu and Maguire, 1991).

MALIGNANT DISEASE

NON HODGKIN'S LYMPHOMA

Non Hodgkin's lymphoma (NHL) is one of the commonest malignancies associated with HIV infection. Aggressive B cell lymphomas usually present in the central nervous system, bone marrow, and GI tract. One peak of NHL presentation occurs in the 10-19 year age group (Serraino *et al.*, 1992) and, although unusual, pulmonary presentation does occur (Joshi, 1993).

Kaposi's sarcoma

Cutaneous lesions of Kaposi's sarcoma (KS) in children are rare. Visceral involvement predominates, occurring in 85% of cases, mainly in children from Africa and Haiti. Widespread lesions of KS can occur in the lungs without skin involvement, presenting with respiratory distress (Orlow *et al.*, 1993).

Smooth muscle tumors

Both leiomyomas and leiomyosarcomas have been reported in pediatric HIV infection, with most of the tumors arising in the viscera. Smooth muscle tumors are thought to be the second commonest neoplastic disorder in pediatric AIDS after NHL and can present as mass lesions in the lung (Chadwick *et al.*, 1990), which are often multiple (Berdon, Mellins and Abramson, 1993).

CARDIOMYOPATHY

The etiology of the dilated cardiomyopathy seen in pediatric HIV infection is unknown. The pathology is T lymphocytic infiltration of a focal myocarditis (Joshi, 1993). Clinically, ventricular dilatation, hypertrophy, myocarditis, pericarditis, and pericardial effusions have been noted (Mast *et al.*, 1992). There may be significant cardiac disease with a normal heart size on CXR. Pulmonary edema can occur secondary to either primary HIV cardiomyopathy, or to cor pulmonale following chronic lung disease, usually associated with LIP. Diuretics and inotropic agents may be required to treat the cardiac failure. The role of antiretroviral drugs in treating HIV-related cardiomyopathy has yet to be determined.

RESPIRATORY FAILURE

Early in the HIV epidemic, it was noted that the progression to acute respiratory failure (ARF) can be very rapid in the HIV-infected child, and that ARF was the commonest reason for admission to the pediatric intensive care unit for the child with AIDS (Wilkinson and Greenwold, 1988). A number of recent studies have audited the outcome of respiratory failure requiring ventilation in children with AIDS. Abadco and colleagues studying 23 children managed to wean 50% from ventilation (Abadco *et al.*, 1992). Vernon and colleagues, in a study of 33 children, noted only 5 (16%) survived to be discharged from intensive care, with a further 3 children dying within 6 months (Vernon, 1988). Marolda and colleagues reviewed 18 children, successfully weaned 8 (44%) but noted that 4 of the 8 died within 6 months (Marolda *et al.*, 1989). Notterman and colleagues reviewed 22 pediatric AIDS patients requiring 27 episodes of ventilation. Sixteen of the children were admitted with ARF (50% PCP) (Notterman *et al.*, 1990). The non ARF patients required short-term ventilation following diagnostic procedures (BAL, lung biopsy, endoscopy, central line insertion). For patients with ARF, the ICU mortality was 81%, with an in-hospital mortality of 91% and no 1 year survivors. For non ARF patients, the mortality was 9% (Notterman *et al.*, 1990). These studies indicate that severely ill children cope well with invasive procedures, but the outlook for a child with AIDS and progressive respiratory failure is at present still poor.

CONCLUSIONS

Because the outlook for respiratory failure is poor, active prevention of respiratory disease in HIV-infected children assumes even greater importance. PCP prophylaxis with TMP/SMX is remarkably safe and well tolerated. The recent ACTG 076 trial reporting a two-thirds reduction in the maternal HIV transmission rate following the use of perinatal zidovudine is likely to encourage prenatal HIV testing, and therefore increase the proportion of infected infants taking PCP prophylaxis (Anonymous, 1994). Improved recognition of LIP is leading to prompt treatment of the associated bacterial infections, and other treatment strategies are being evaluated. Active case finding and control measures should decrease the numbers of HIV families infected with tuberculosis, at least in developed countries. There is increased awareness that recurrent and persistent bacterial pneumonia should be

aggressively treated to prevent progression to bronchiectasis.

There has been a steady improvement in the recognition and treatment of opportunistic infections in pediatric HIV infection, leading to considerably improved life expectancy (Italian Register, 1994). As children with HIV live longer one of the major causes of morbidity will be chronic lung disease. Management of these children is going to require the expertise of respiratory teams (especially physiotherapists), and the introduction of management regimes which have so successfully improved the outlook for children with chronic lung disease not caused by HIV infection.

REFERENCES

Abadco, D.L., Amaro-Galvez, R., Rao, M. *et al.* (1992) Experience with flexible flbreoptic bronchoscopy with bronchoalveolar lavage as a diagnostic tool in children with AIDS. *AJDC*, **146**, 1056–9.

Amaro-Galvez, R., Rao, M. and Abadco, D. (1991) Non bronchoscopic bronchoalveolar lavage in ventilated children with acquired immunodeficiency syndrome: a simple and effective diagnostic method for *Pneumocystis carinii* infection. *Pediatr. Infect. Dis. J.*, **10**, 473–75.

American Thoracic Society (1992) Diagnostic standards and classification of tuberculosis. *Am. Rev. Respir. Dis.*, **142**, 725–35.

American Academy of Pediatrics (1992) Chemotherapy for tuberculosis in infants and children. *Pediatrics*, **89**, 161–5.

Amorosa, J.K., Miller, R.W., Laraya-Cuasay, L. *et al.* (1992) Bronchiectasis in children with LIP and AIDS. *Pediatr. Radiol.*, **22**, 603–7.

Andiman, W.A., Eastman, R., Martin, K. *et al.* (1985) Opportunistic lymphoproliferations associated with Epstein-Barr viral DNA in infants and children with AIDS. *Lancet*, **ii**, 1390–3.

Anonymous (1994) Trial halted after drug cuts maternal HIV transmission rates by two thirds [news]. *JAMA*, **271**, 807.

Arditi, M., Kabat, W., Yogev, R. (1991) Serum tumour necrosis factor-alpha, interleukin-1 beta, p24 antigen concentrations and CD4+ cells at various stages of human immunodeficiency virus-1 infection in children. *Pediatr. Infect. Dis. J.*, **10**, 450–5.

Bach, M.C. (1987) Zidovudine for lymphocytic interstitial pneumonia associated with AIDS. *Lancet*, **ii**, 656–61.

Bakshi, S.S., Alvarez, D., Hilfer, C.L., *et al.* (1993) Tuberculosis in human immunodeficiency virus infected children. A family infection. *AJDC*, **147**, 320–4.

Beach, R.S., Garcia, E.R., Sosa, R. *et al.* (1991) *Pneumocystis carinii* pneumonia in a human immunodeficiency virus-1 infected neonate with meconium aspiration. *Pediatr. Infect. Dis. J*, **10**, 953–4.

Berdon, W.E., Mellins, R.B. and Abramson, S.J. (1993) Pediatric HIV infection in its second decade – the changing pattern of lung involvement. *Radiol. Clin. N. Am.*, **31**, 453–63.

Bernstein, L.J., Byre, M.R. and Rubinstein, A. (1989) Prognostic factors and life expectancy in children with acquired immunodeficiency syndrome and *Pneumocystis carinii* pneumonia. *Am. J. Dis. Child.*, **143**, 775–8.

Bernstein, L.J., Ocks, H.D. and Wedgewood, R.J. (1985) Defective humoral immunity in pediatric acquired immunodeficiency syndrome. *J. Pediatr.*, **107**, 352–7.

Besnard, M., Sauvion, S., Offredo, C. *et al.* (1993) Bacillus Calmette-Guérin infection after vaccination of human immunodeficiency virus-infected children. *Pediatr. Infect. Dis. J.*, **12**, 993–7.

Bhat, G.J., Diwan, V.K., Chintu, C. *et al.* (1993) HIV, BCG and TB in children: a case control study in Lusaka, Zambia. *J. Trop. Paediatr.*, **39**, 218–23.

Birriel, J.A., Adams, J.A. and Saldana, M.A. (1991) Role of flexible bronchoscopy and bronchoalveolar lavage in the diagnosis of paediatric acquired immunodeficiency syndrome related pulmonary disease. *Pediatrics*, **87**, 897–9.

Bonfils-Roberts, B.A., Nickodem, A. and Nealen, T.F. Jr. (1990) Retrospective analysis of the efficacy of open lung biopsy in acquired immunodeficiency syndrome. *Ann. Thorac. Surg.*, **49**, 115–7.

Caldwell, M.B., Mascola, L., Smith, W. *et al.* (1992) Biologic, foster, and adoptive parents: care givers of children exposed perinatally to human immunodeficiency virus in the United States. *Pediatrics*, **90**, 603–7.

Carrington, C. and Liebow, A. (1966) Lymphocytic interstitial pneumonitis (abstr). *Am. J. Pathol.*, **42**, 36a.

Centers for Disease Control (1986). Update: Acquired immunodeficiency syndrome – United States. *MMWR*, **35**, 757–9.

Centers for Disease Control (1991a). Guidelines for prophylaxis against *Pneumocystis carinii* pneumonia for children infected with human immunodeficiency virus. *JAMA*, **265**, 1637–44.

Centers for Disease Control (1991b). Guidelines for prophylaxis against *Pneumocystis carinii* pneumonia for children infected with human immunodeficiency virus. *MMWR*, **40** (No.RR-2), 1–13.

Chadwick, E.G., Connor, E.J., Hanson, I.C. *et al.* (1990) Tumours of smooth muscle origin in HIV-infected children. *JAMA*, **263**, 3182–4.

Chadwick, E.G., Chang, G., Decker, M.D., *et al.* (1994) Serologic response to standard inactivated influenza vaccine in human immunodeficiency virus infected children. *Pediatr. Infect. Dis. J.*, **13**, 206–11.

Chandwani, S., Borkowsky, W., Krasinski, K. *et al.* (1990) Respiratory syncitial virus infection in human immunodeficiency virus infected children. *J. Pediatr.*, **117**, 251–4.

Chin, J. (1990a) Global estimates of HIV infection and AIDS cases. *AIDS*, **5**, (Suppl), S57–61.

Chin, J. (1990b). Current and future dimensions of the HIV/AIDS pandemic in women and children. *Lancet*, **336**, 221–4.

Chintu, C., Bhat, G., Luo, C. *et al.* (1993a) Seroprevalence of human immunodeficiency virus type 1 infection in Zambian children with tuberculosis. *Pediatr. Infect. Dis. J.*, **12**, 499–504.

Chintu, C., Luo, C., Bhat, G. *et al.* (1993b) Cutaneous hypersensitivity reaction due to thiacetazone in the treatment of Zambian children infected with HIV-1. *Arch. Dis. Child*, **68**, 665–8.

Connor, E., Bagarazzi, M., McSherry, G. *et al.* (1991) Clinical and laboratory correlates of *Pneumocystis carinii* pneumonia in children infected with HIV. *JAMA*, **265**, 1693–7.

Connor E.M. and Andiman, W.A. (1994) Lymphoid interstitial pneumonitis, in *Pediatric AIDS: the challenge of HIV infections in infants, children and adolescents*, 2nd edn (eds P.A. Pizzo and C.M. Wilfert) Williams and Wilkins, Baltimore, MD.

Connor, E.M. and Marquis, J., Oleske, M. (1991) Lymphoid interstitial pneumonitis, in *Pediatric AIDS: the challenge of HIV infection in infants, children and adolescents*, 2nd edn (eds P.A. Pizzo and C.M. Wilfert) Williams and Wilkins, Baltimore, MD, pp. 343–54.

Davies, P.D.O. (1993) Tuberculosis and HIV: blind mans buff. *Thorax*, **48**, 193–4.

de Blic, J., Blanche, S., Danel, C. *et al.* (1989) Bronchoalveolar lavage in HIV infected patients with interstitial pneumonitis. *Arch. Dis. Child*, **64**, 1246–50.

De Cock, K.M., Gnaore, E., Braun, M. *et al.* (1991) Risk of tuberculosis in patients with HIV-I and HIV-II infection in Abidjan, Ivory Coast. *Br. Med. J.*, **302**, 496–99.

Duliege, A.M., Messiah, A. Blanche, S. (1992) Natural history of human immunodeficiency virus type-1 infection in children: prognostic value and laboratory tests on the bimodal progression of disease. *Pediatr. Infect. J*, **II**, 630–35.

Edman, J.C., Kovacs, J.A., Masur, H. *et al.* (1988) Ribosomal RNA sequence shows *Pneumocystis carinii* to be a member of the fungi. *Nature*, **334**, 519.

Ellaurie, M. and Rubinstein, A. (1992) Tumour necrosis factor α in paediatric HIV infection. *AIDS*, **6**, 1265–8.

European Collaborative Study (1994) The natural history of vertically acquired HIV-1 infection. *J. Pediatr.* In press.

Fox, C.H., Tenner-Racz, K., Racz, P. *et al.* (1991) Lymphoid germinal centres are reservoirs of human immunodeficiency virus type 1 RNA. *J. Infect. Dis.*, **164**. 1051–7.

Frenkel, L.D., Gaur, S., Tsolia, M. *et al.* (1990) Cytomegalovirus infection in children with AIDS. *Rev. Infect. Dis.*, **12**, (Suppl 7), S820–826.

Gajdusek, D.C. (1957) *Pneumocystis carinii* – aetiologic agent of interstitial plasma cell pneumonia of premature and young infants. *Pediatrics*, **19**, 543–65.

Gibb, D.M., Davison, C.F., Holland, F.J. *et al.* (1994) *Pneumocystis carinii* pneumonia in vertically acquired HIV infection in the British Isles. *Arch. Dis. Child*, **70**. 241–4.

Githui, W., Nunn, P. Juma, E. *et al.* (1992) Cohort study of HIV positive and HIV negative tuberculosis, Nairobi, Kenya: Comparison of bacteriological results. *Tuberc. Lung. Dis.*, **73**, 203–9.

Glaser, J.H., Schuval, S., Burstein, O. *et al.* (1992) Cytomegalovirus and *Pneumocystis carinii* pneumonia in children with acquired immunodeficiency syndrome. *J. Pediatr.*, **120**, 929–31.

Hague, R.A., Burns, S.E., Hargreaves, F.D. *et al.* (1992) Viral infections of the respiratory tract in HIV infected children. *J. Infect.*, **24**, 31–6.

Hauger, S.B. (1991) Approach to the paediatric patient with HIV infection and pulmonary symptoms. *J. Pediatr.*, **119**. S25–33.

Horsburgh, C.R. (1991) *Mycobacterium avium* complex infection in the acquired immunodeficiency syndrome. *N. Engl. J. Med.*, **324**, 1332–8.

Horsburgh, C.R., Caldwell, M.B. and Simonds, R.J. (1993) Epidemiology of disseminated non-tuberculous mycobacterial disease in children with acquired immunodeficiency syndrome. *Pediatr. Infect. Dis. J.*, **12**, 219–22.

Hughes, W.T., Price, R.A., Kim, H.Y. *et al.* (1973) *Pneumocystis carinii* pneumonia. *J. Pediatr.*, **82**, 404.

Hughes, W.T. (1991) *Pneumocystis carinii* pneumonia: new approaches to diagnosis, treatment and prevention. *Pediatr. Infect. Dis. J.*, **10**, 391–9.

Iralu, J.V. and Maguire, J.H. (1991) Pulmonary infections in immigrants and refugees. *Sem. Respir. Infect.*, **6**, 235–46.

Italian register for HIV infection in children. (1994) Features of children perinatally infected with HIV-1 surviving longer than 5 years. *Lancet*, **343**, 191–5.

Jacobs, R.F. and Starke, J.R. (1993) Tuberculosis in children. *Med. Clin. N. Am.*, **77**, 1335-15.

Josephs, S., Kim, H.W., Brandt, C.D. *et al.* (1983) Parainfluenza 3 virus and other common respiratory pathogens in children with human immunodeficiency virus infection. *Pediatr. Infect. Dis. J.*, **7**, 207–9.

Joshi, V.V. (1993) Pathology of pediatric AIDS. Overview, update and future directions. *Ann. NY Acad. Sci.*, **693**, 71–92.

Joshi, V.V., Kaufman, S., Oleske, J.M. *et al.* (1987) Polyclonal polymorphic B cell lymphoproliferative disorder with prominent pulmonary involvement in children with acquired immunodeficiency syndrome. *Cancer*, **59**, 1455–62.

Joshi, V.V., Oleske, J.M. and Minnefor, A.B. (1985) Pathologic pulmonary findings in children with acquired immune deficiency syndrome – a study of ten cases. *Hum. Pathol.*, **16**, 241–6.

Joshi, V.V. and Oleske, J.M. (1986) Pulmonary lesions in children with the acquired immunodeficiency syndrome: a re-appraisal based on data in additional cases and follow-up study of previously reported cases. *Hum. Pathol.*, **17**, 641–2.

Jura, E., Chadwick, E., Josephs, S. *et al.* (1989) Varicella zoster virus infections in children infected with human immunodeficiency virus. *Pediatr. Infect. Dis. J*, **8**, 586–90.

Katz, B.Z., Berkman, A.B. and Shapiro, E.D. (1992) Serologic evidence of active Epstein-Barr virus infection in Epstein-Barr virus associated lymphoproliferative disorders of children with acquired immunodeficiency syndrome. *J. Pediatr.*, **120**, 228–32.

Keenlyside, R.A., Johnson, A.M. and Mabey, D.E.W. (1993) The epidemiology of HIV-1 infection and AIDS in women. *AIDS*, **7**, (Suppl 1), S83–S90.

Kelley, R., Mancao, M., Lee, F. *et al.* (1994) Varicella in children with perinatally acquired human immunodeficiency virus infection. *J. Pediatr.*, **124**, 271–3.

Khouri, Y.F., Mastrucci, M.T. and Hutto, C. (1992) *Mycobacterium tuberculosis* in children with human immunodeficiency type 1 infection. *Pediatr. Infect. Dis. J.*, **11**, 950–5.

Kochi, A. (1991) The global tuberculosis situation and the new control strategy of the World Health Organisation. *Tubercule.*, **72**, 1–6.

Kovacs, A., Church, J., Mascola, L. *et al.* (1990) CD4 counts as predictors of *Pneumocystis carinii* pneumonia in infants and children with HIV infection. (Abstract FB 24), in 6th International Conference on AIDS, San Francisco.

Krasinski, K., Borkowsky, W., Bonk, S. *et al.* (1988) Bacterial infections in human immunodeficiency virus infected children. *Pediatr. Infect. Dis. J.*, **7**, 323–8.

Marolda, J., Pace, B., Bonforte, R.J. *et al.* (1989) Outcome of mechanical ventilation of children with acquired immunodeficiency syndrome. *Pediatr. Pulmonol.*, **7**, 230–4.

Marolda, J., Pace, B., Bonforte, R.J. *et al.* (1991) Pulmonary manifestations of HIV infection in children. *Pediatr. Pulmonol.*, **10**, 231–5.

Marquis, J.R., Berman, C.Z. and Oleske, J.M. (1993) Radiographic patterns of PLH/LIP in HIV positive children. *Pediatr. Radiol.*, **23**, 328–30.

Mast, H.L., Heller, J.D., Schiller, M.S. *et al.* (1992) Pericardial effusion and its relationship to cardiac disease in children with acquired immunodeficiency syndrome. *Pediatr. Radiol.*, **22**, 548–51.

McLaughlin, G.E., Virdee, S.S., Schlelen, C.L. *et al.* (1995) Effect of corticosteroids on survival of children with acquired immunodeficiency syndrome and *Pneumocystis carinii* related respiratory failure. *J. Pediatr.*, **126**, 821–4.

Minamoto, G.Y., Barlam, T.F. and Vander Els, N.J. (1992) Invasive aspergillosis in patients with AIDS. *Clin. Infect. Dis.*, **14**, 66–74.

MMWR (1994) Expanded tuberculosis surveillance and tuberculosis United States – 1993. *MMWR*, **43**, 361–6.

Mofenson, L.M. and Moya, J. (1993) Intravenous immune globulin for the prevention of infection in children with symptomatic human immunodeficiency virus infection. *Pediatr. Res.*, **33** (Suppl), S80–89.

Mornex, J.F., Ecochard, D., Greenland, T. *et al.* (1990) Diffuse interstitial pneumopathies caused by lentivirus in humans and animals. *Rev. Malad. Resp.*, **7**, 517–28.

Muganga, N., Nkuadiolandu, and A. Mashaka, L.M. (1991) [Clinical manifestations of AIDS in children in Kinshasa]. *Pediatrie*, **46**, 825–9.

Mustafa, M.M. (1994) Cytomegalovirus infection and disease in the immunocompromised host. *Pediatr. Infect. Dis. J.*, **13**, 249–59.

National Institute of Child Health and Human Development Intravenous Immunoglobulin Study Group (1991) Intravenous immune globulin for the prevention of bacterial infections in children with symptomatic human immunodeficiency infection. *N. Engl. J. Med.*, **325**, 73–80.

Newell, M.N. and Peckham, C. (1993) Risk factors for vertical transmission of HIV-1 and early markers of HIV-1 infection in children. *AIDS*, **7**, (Suppl. 1), S91–97.

Notterman, D.A., Greenwold, B.M., Di Maio-Hunter, A. *et al.* (1990) Outcome after assisted ventilation in children with acquired immunodeficiency syndrome. *Crit. Care Med.*, **18**, 18–20.

O'Doherty, M.J., Thomas, S.H.L. and Gibb, D. (1993) Lung deposition of nebulised pentamidine in children. *Thorax*, **48**, 210–26.

Oldham, S.A.A., Castillo, M., Jacobson, F.L. *et al.* (1989) HIV associated lymphocytic interstitial pneumonia : radiological manifestations and pathogenic correlation. *Thoracic. Radiol.*, **170**, 83–7.

Oleske, J., Minnefor, A., Cooper, R. *et al.* (1983) Immune deficiency syndrome in children. *JAMA*, **249**, 2345–9.

Orlow, S.J., Cooper, D., Petrea, S. *et al.* (1993) AIDS associated Kaposi's sarcoma in Romanian children. *Am. Acad. Dermotol.*, **28**, 449–53.

Ormerod, L.P. (1990) Chemotherapy and management of tuberculosis in the United Kingdom. Recommendation of the Joint Tuberculosis Committee of the British Thoracic Society. *Thorax*, **45**, 403–8.

Persaud, D., Chadwani, S., Rigaud, M. *et al.* (1992) Delayed recognition of human immunodeficiency virus in pre-adolescent children. *Pediatrics*, **90**, 628–41.

Pifer, L.L., Hughes, W.T., Stagna, S. *et al.* (1978) *Pneumocystis carinii* infection: evidence of high prevalence in normal and immunosuppressed children. *Pediatrics*, **61**, 35–40.

Pitt, J. (1991) Lymphocytic interstitial pneumonia. *Pediatr. Clin. N. Am.*, **38**, 89–95.

Rogers, M.F., Thomas, P.A., Starcher, E.T. *et al.* (1987) Acquired immunodeficiency syndrome in children: report of the Centers for Disease Central National Surveillance 1982 to 1985. *Pediatrics*, **79**, 1003–14.

Rogers, M.F., Caldwell, M.B., Gwin, M.L. *et al.* (1993) Epidemiology of paediatric immunodeficiency virus infection in the United States. *Ann N. Y. Acad. Sci.*, **693**, 4–8.

Roilides, E., Mertins, S. Eddy, J. *et al.* (1990) Impairment of neutrophil chemotactic and bactericidal function in children infected with human immunodeficiency virus type 1 and partial reversal after *in vitro* exposure to granulocyte-macrophage colony stimulating factor. *J. Pediatr.*, **117**, 531–40.

Roilides, E., Clerici, M., De Palma, L. *et al.* (1991a) Helper T cell responses in children infected with human immunodeficiency virus type 1. *J. Pediatr.*, **118**, 724–30.

Roilides, E., Black, C., Raimer, C. *et al.* (1991b) Serum immunoglobulin G subclasses in children infected with human immunodeficiency virus type 1. *Pediatr. Infect. Dis. J.* **10**, 134–9.

Roilides, E., Marshall, P., Vernon, D. *et al.* (1991c) Bacterial infections in human immunodeficiency virus type 1 infected children: the impact of central venous catheters and antiretroviral agents. *Pediatr. Infect. Dis. J.*, **10**, 813–9.

Rubenstein, A., Sicklick, M., Gupta, A. *et al.* (1983) Acquired immunodeficiency with reversed T4/T8 ratios in infants born to promiscuous and drug addicted mothers. *JAMA*, **249**, 2350–6.

Rubinstein, A., Bernstein, L.J., Charyton, M. *et al.* (1988) Corticosteroid treatment for pulmonary lymphoid hyperplasia in children with acquired immunodeficiency syndrome. *Pediatr. Pulmon.*, **4**, 13–17.

Rubinstein, A., Moreckis, R., Silverman, B. *et al.* (1986) Pulmonary disease in children with acquired immunodeficiency syndrome and AIDS related complex. *J. Pediatr.*, **108**, 498–503.

Rutstein, R.M., Cobb, P., McGowan, K.L. *et al.* (1993) *Mycobacterium avium intracellulare* complex infection in HIV infected children. *AIDS*, **7**, 507–12.

Sanders-Laufer, D., De Bruin, W. and Edelson, P.J. (1991) *Pneumocystis carinii* infection in HIV infected children. *Pediatr. Clin. N. Am.*, **38**, 69–88.

Scott, G.B., Buck, B.E., Leberman, J.G. *et al.* (1984) Acquired immunodeficiency syndrome in infants. *N. Engl. J. Med.*, **310**, 76–81.

Scott, G.B., Hutto, C., Makuch, R.W. *et al.* (1989) Survival in children with perinatally acquired human immunodeficiency virus type 1 infection. *N. Engl. J. Med.*, **321**, 1791–6.

Selwyn, P.A., Hartel, D., Lewis, V.A. *et al.* (1989) A prospective study of the risk of tuberculosis among intravenous drug users with human immunodeficiency virus infection. *N. Engl. J. Med.*, **320**, 545–50.

Serraino, D., Salamina, G., Franceshi, S. *et al.* (1992) The epidemiology of AIDS associated non-Hodgkin's lymphoma in the World Health Organisation European Region. *Br. J. Cancer*, **66**, 912–16.

Shannon, K.M. and Amman, A.J. (1985) Acquired immunodeficiency syndrome in childhood. *J. Pediatr.*, **106**, 332–42.

Sharland, M., Davison, C. and Davies, E.G. (1994) Mortality due to non PCP respiratory disease in paediatric HIV infection. Proceedings BPA Annual Meeting. **66**, 44.

Stavola, J.J. and Noel, G.T. (1993) Efficacy and safety of dapsone prophylaxis against a *Pneumocystis carinii* pneumonia in human immunodeficiency virus infected children. *Pediatr. Infect. Dis. J.*, **12**, 644–7.

Tarantola, O. and Mann, J.M. (1987) Acquired immunodeficiency syndrome (AIDS) and expanded programme in immunisation. Special programme on AIDS, World Health Organisation, Geneva.

Teirstein, A.S. and Rosen, M.J. (1988) Lymphocytic interstitial pneumonia. *Clin. Chest. Med.*, **9**, 467–71.

Tovo, P.A., De Martino, M., Galiano, C. *et al.*

(1992). Prognostic factors and survival in children with perinatal HIV-1 infection. *Lancet*, **339**, 1249–53.

Van Dyke, R.B. (1993) Opportunistic infections in paediatric HIV disease. *Ann. N. Y. Acad. Sci.*, **693**, 158–65.

Varteresian-Karanfil, L., Josephson, A., Fikrig, S. *et al.* (1988) Pulmonary infection and cavity formation caused by *Mycobacterium tuberculosis* in a child with AIDS. *N. Engl. J. Med.*, **319**, 1018–19.

Vernon, D.D., Holzman, B.H., Lewis, P. *et al.* (1988) Respiratory failure in children with acquired immunodeficiency syndrome and acquired immunodeficiency syndrome complex. *Pediatrics*, **82**, 223–8.

Walzer, P.D., Perl, D.P., Kragstad, D.J. *et al.* (1973) *Pneumocystis carinii* pneumonitis and primary immune deficiency diseases of infancy and childhood. *J. Pediatr.*, **82**, 416.

Whitehead, B., Scott, J.P., Helms, P. *et al.* (1992) Technique and use of transbronchial biopsy in children and adolescents. *Pediatr. Pulmon.*, **12**, 240–46.

Wilkinson, J.D. and Greenwold, B.M. (1988) The acquired immunodeficiency syndrome: impact on the paediatric intensive care unit. *Crit. Care Clin.*, **4**, 831–44.

Wright, M., Fikrig, S. and Holder, J.O. (1993). Aspergillosis in children with acquired immunodeficiency. *Pediatr. Radiol.*, **23**, 492–4.

Young, S.A. and Crocker, D.W. (1991) Burkitts lymphoma in a child with AIDS. *Pediatr. Pathol.*, **II**, 115–22.

Zimmerman, B.L., Haller, J.O., Price, A.P. *et al.* (1987) Children with AIDS: is pathologic diagnosis possible based on chest radiographs? *Pediatr. Radiol.*, **17**, 303–7.

24

POTENTIAL IMMUNOTHERAPY FOR TUBERCULOSIS AND FUTURE POTENTIAL FOR HIV

John L. Stanford and Graham A.W. Rook

Modern concepts of the immunopathology of tuberculosis disclose a series of parallels with HIV disease and some other conditions. These observations suggest that correcting the immune abnormality of tuberculosis could be a model for the correction of that of HIV. We review the history of immunotherapy for tuberculosis, and describe some new data supportive of such a view.

HISTORY OF IMMUNOTHERAPY FOR TUBERCULOSIS

Once the infectious nature of tuberculosis was firmly established by Villemin (Villemin, 1868), scientists of the day started to think of rational approaches to the treatment of the disease. Following the demonstration of tubercle bacilli by Robert Koch in 1882 (Koch, 1882), and their successful culture, bacterial products became available as potential therapeutics. Early experiments had shown that antisera alone did not promote cure in experimental animals, and therefore the use of bacterial products directly injected into man was the obvious approach. This was especially so after the discovery by Koch of what has become known as his phenomenon

(Koch, 1891). This is the ability of an already infected animal to cast off and heal small challenge doses of live tubercle bacilli injected intradermally. The same phenomenon occurs when proteinaceous extracts of tubercle bacilli, rather than live bacilli, are injected. It was an easy inference from this that treatment might be based on the promotion of this mechanism around all the tubercle bacilli in the body, and it was on this basis that Koch developed his immunotherapy.

KOCH'S IMMUNOTHERAPY

Koch demonstrated and described successful treatment for tuberculosis in guinea pigs in 1890 (Koch, 1890), and described the application of this treatment to man later in the same year. His initial work in guinea pigs showed that repeated injections of large doses of tuberculin could halt the progress of tuberculous disease, and even lead to cure. This was the first breakthrough in treating tuberculosis, and used with care in selected patients Koch, and some of those following his system, successfully treated a number of tuberculosis patients. However, it soon be-

AIDS and Respiratory Medicine. Edited by A. Zumla, M.A. Johnson and R.F. Miller. Published in 1997 by Chapman & Hall, London. ISBN 0 412 60140 0

came apparent that this treatment could kill as well as cure.

Providing lesions were superficial or small and in non-vital tissue, repeatedly injecting tuberculin – at first called Koch's brown fluid – resulted in their necrosis. Dead tissue plus live bacilli were sloughed from superficial lesions, and contaminated tissue in deep lesions became encapsulated, cutting off the oxygen supply to the bacilli and effectively returning them to a kind of persister state (Grange, 1992). The reaction producing this effect was considerable, with the patient developing a fever and sometimes going into shock leading to death within a few hours of the first injection (Anonymous, 1890). These unwanted phenomena, the tuberculin shock syndrome, were presumably due to release of excessive amounts of tumor necrosis factor (TNFα) and other cytokines in persons primed for their toxicity (Hernandez-Pando and Rook, 1994). Local reaction around deep lesions could also lead to death through organ failure. Since Koch produced his tuberculin from heat-sterilized culture medium, it was rich in heat-stable secreted substances, focusing attention for the first time on the importance of secreted antigens of tubercle bacilli, a concept to which mycobacteriology has recently returned. Although generally successful in Koch's own hands, his immunotherapy was too uncertain a tool for most clinicians and by the beginning of this century its use was abandoned. Modern explanation of the mechanism of Koch's treatment suggests that it depended on a process related to the Shwartzman reaction in which the endothelium of vasculature within the infected tissue is necrosed in response to local sensitization to circulating TNFα, secondarily leading to death of the infected tissue (Rook, 1991). (It is remarkable that in New York in the very same year, 1891, Coley introduced his toxin prepared from bacterial products for the treatment of certain cancers (Starnes, 1992). We have suggested elsewhere that the mechanism by

which it worked was probably similar to the mechanism of Koch's treatment (Grange, Stanford and Rook, 1995).)

During the years following Koch's first efforts, immunotherapy was extensively investigated for leprosy, and many generally unsubstantiated claims for its efficacy in treating various forms of this disease can be found in the literature. One of the difficulties in their interpretation was the lack of a conceptual framework for the immunopathology of the disease – still a problem today.

FRIEDMANN AND THE SCHILDKROTENTUBERKELBAZILLUS

Felix Friedmann, working in Berlin in 1903, isolated the cause of tuberculosis in captive sea turtles in the Berlin Zoo (Friedmann, 1903). He recognized that treatment of tuberculosis required the antigens shared by all species of mycobacteria rather than those specific to the tubercle bacillus itself. Thus Friedmann was the first person to recognize the importance of what we now know as the group i, common mycobacterial, antigens (Figure 24.1). However, Friedmann still followed the dogma that the therapeutic organism had to be alive and give rise to a limited form of tuberculous disease before it could be effective. Rather remarkably, Friedmann's preparation is still available for use in the treatment of a number of diseases under the registered name of Anningzochen (Laves-Arzeimittel GmbH, Barbarastrasse 14, 3003 Ronnenberg, Germany). This organism has now been established as *Mycobacterium chelonae*, at first thought to be non-pathogenic for man, but now known to cause injection abscesses (Inman *et al.*, 1969) which can be life-threatening in the immunosuppressed. In Friedmann's later years he recognized the non-specific value of his agent and advocated its use in asthma, psoriasis, rheumatoid arthritis and undoubtedly he would have seen its potential for HIV.

In 1922 Debré and Bonnet (Debré and

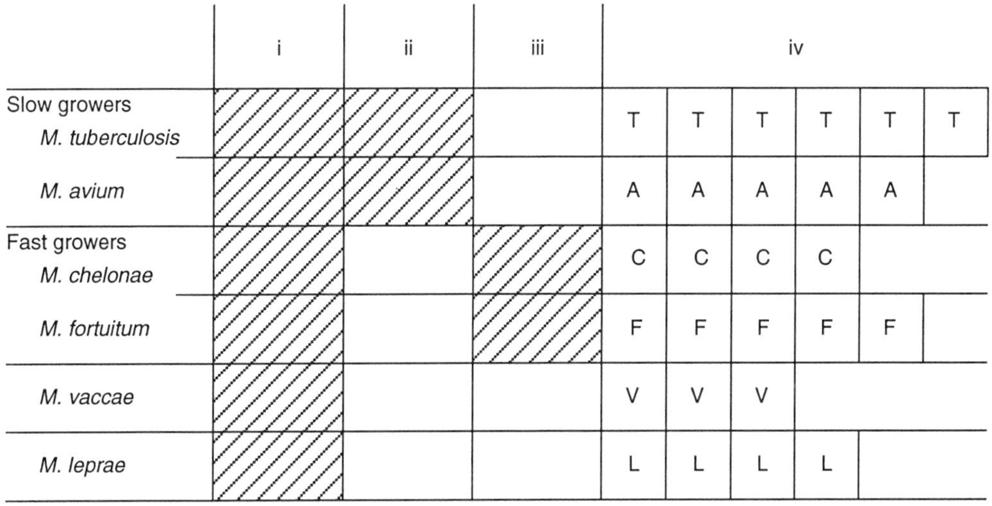

Fig. 24.1 Diagram illustrating the sharing of antigens between mycobacterial species. Group i antigens are common to all species of the genus, and include the stress proteins which share considerable homology with their human counterparts, yet also contain species-specific epitopes. Group ii antigens are shared between tubercle bacilli and other slow-growing species. Group iii antigens are shared by most fast-growing species and also by nocardiae. *M. vaccae* and *M. leprae* appear to be unique in their lack of group ii and iii antigens. The group iv antigens are almost exclusive to individual species. It is important to appreciate that many large molecules incorporate epitopes of several levels of specificity.

Bonnet, 1922) recognized that there were two distinct cellular responses seen in animals challenged with mycobacteria. Responses following injection of Friedmann's reagent, cross-reactive with *M. tuberculosis* only via the common antigens, did not produce the necrosis, fever and shock associated with the use of Koch's treatment, but it was not realized that the difference might reflect the observations of Debré and Bonnet until the development of *M. vaccae* as an immunotherapeutic 70 years later (Stanford *et al.*, 1990).

SPAHLINGER'S TREATMENTS

The next major steps forward were taken by Henry Spahlinger in Geneva, with the development of his 'vaccine' and 'serum' therapies (Macassey, 1934). Spahlinger believed that therapeutic agents should be prepared from tubercle bacilli grown on media made as similar as possible to those pertaining in the host tissues. Thus if the preparations were for human disease the medium should be enriched with human sera, and if for tuberculosis of cattle the bacilli should be grown on media enriched with bovine serum. In order not to damage the 'toxins' produced by any mechanism of killing the bacilli, Spahlinger incubated his cultures for long periods and then left them hermetically sealed at room temperature in the dark for a year or more. If subcultures then showed no growth, the material was considered ready for direct injection into patients, or for use in the production of antisera. In Spahlinger's time the ability of organisms to go into a stationary phase, but without producing spores, had not been described. Thus it is likely that many of his patients were injected with live, though dormant bacilli. Nonetheless, remarkable results were recorded.

Spahlinger describes heat stressing tubercle bacilli during their incubation with a view to stimulate synthesis of relevant antigens (Spahlinger, 1992) in immunotherapeutics particularly for use in 'surgical' tuberculosis. Thus he could be considered the first person to have appreciated the importance of heat-shock proteins from mycobacteria, and of stationary phase products, albeit without recognizing them, nearly 70 years before the rest of us!

Spahlinger also believed in 'serum' therapy for tuberculosis for which he raised antisera in black Irish hunters (horses) that he favored for this purpose. He produced several different 'partial' or 'complete' sera for treatment of different forms of tuberculosis, prepared by immunizing the horses with tubercle bacilli grown under various conditions. In retrospect his treatments seem to have been highly successful, although some of his ideas sound strange today, and in direct conflict with the misconception that antibodies play no part in immunity to tuberculosis. It is true that antibody is not sufficient, but there are no data to prove that antibody does not play an essential role by neutralizing bacterial products that have the ability to disturb the cell-mediated pathways. However as emphasized below, we must distinguish between pathways that are helpful in treating established disease, and those that confer resistance to infection.

AFTER SPAHLINGER

After Spahlinger came the practice, no doubt influenced by his ideas, of injecting patients with their own sputum, either fresh or heat-inactivated. But all was swept aside by the development of the first drugs effective against tubercle bacilli in the tissues, streptomycin, para amino salicylic acid and isoniazid. But immunotherapy is needed again for the treatment of tuberculosis.

THE MODERN PROBLEM OF TUBERCULOSIS

Modern short-course chemotherapy for tuberculosis is potentially very effective with a possible cure rate in excess of 98%. Nonetheless, the World Health Organisation has declared tuberculosis to be a global emergency, with a third of the world's population infected with the bacilli, 8–10 million new clinical cases arising each year, and about 3 million deaths from the disease occurring annually. The causes for this are multiple, including inadequate prescription by doctors, non-compliance with treatment by patients, lack of funds for drugs and supervision, increasing numbers of infections with drug-resistant bacilli and co-affliction with HIV seropositivity. These troubles are largely due to the capacity of the tubercle bacillus to be held in the tissues by the immune system in a live, but very slowly metabolizing state as persisters – perhaps paralleling bacilli in the vaccine preparations of Spahlinger. This makes them unavailable to the bactericidal action of antituberculosis drugs. To overcome the problem treatment has to be for a long period, currently six months for an optimum cure rate (Figure 24.2a). With the unlikelihood of drugs being developed that can kill resting bacilli, their recognition and effective removal by the immune system would be highly desirable, yet we can hardly return to the double-edged sword of the Koch phenomenon.

MODERN IMMUNOTHERAPY FOR TUBERCULOSIS

Much has been learned since the days of Koch and Spahlinger about both immunology and mycobacterial infections. The idea of there being two pathways of cell-mediated response to mycobacteria has become estab-

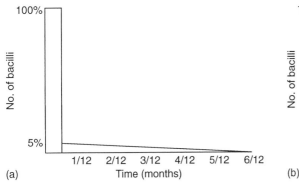
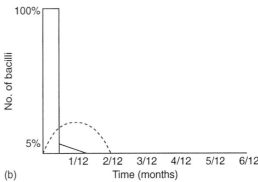

Fig. 24.2 (a) Graph illustrating the disappearance of tubercle bacilli from a patient with pulmonary tuberculosis during treatment with short-course chemotherapy. The left-hand block represents the great majority of bacilli that are killed by the early bactericidal action (EBA) of the drugs, and the decreasing tail represents the slow removal of slowly metabolizing, intracellular bacilli by the sterilizing action of the drugs. (b) Graph illustrating the disappearance of tubercle bacilli from a patient with pulmonary tuberculosis during treatment with chemotherapy **plus** an injection of *M. vaccae* (IT) on the first day of treatment. The left-hand block represents the great majority of bacilli that are killed by the early bactericidal action (EBA) of the drugs, and the short decreasing tail represents the rapid removal of slowly metabolizing, intracellular bacilli following their recognition by the immune system. The period of maximal immunotherapeutic effect is indicated by the broken line.

lished, and the separation between antibacterial immunity and allergy has been expanded. Investigations using a complicated series of skin tests separated the two response types and were used to identify mycobacterial species capable of regulating out the Koch phenomenon and replacing it with non-necrotizing antibacterial mechanisms.

Introduction of an immunotherapeutic capable of switching off the necrotizing action of the Koch phenomenon and replacing it with restored antibacterial immunity would be extremely valuable (Stanford, 1991). Given during the first few days of chemotherapy when drugs are exerting their early bactericidal activity, immune mechanisms could be directed to eradicate antigenically recognizable, but drug insusceptible persisters. Such an action should allow a major reduction in the period of chemotherapy, perhaps to just a few weeks (Figure 24.2b).

THE RELEVANCE TO HIV AND AIDS

SIMILARITIES BETWEEN TUBERCULOSIS AND HIV DISEASE

Studies on a series of situations including tuberculosis, leprosy, Chagas' disease, rheumatoid arthritis and HIV seropositivity show a number of significant parallels as outlined below.

1. *Not everyone infected by the etiological agent develops the disease*: the results of skin tests clearly demonstrate that far more people overcome challenges with tubercle or leprosy bacilli than succumb to clinical disease. Far more children are exposed to *Trypanosoma cruzi* than develop long-lasting seropositivity to the parasite. Spouses of rheumatoid arthritis patients show similar increases of agalactosyl immunoglobulin (see below) in their sera to those of their afflicted partners, but without developing the disease. Some persons at risk of developing HIV disease

register their infection by T cell recognition of HIV-specific antigens, rather than by seropositivity to the virus, and do not go on to disease (Clerici and Shearer, 1993). Thus HIV disease, like those others mentioned above, and many more, does not always follow infection. In view of this, it has to be asked whether the mechanism by which infection is overcome is the same as that responsible for its immunopathology? In tuberculosis these are clearly distinct mechanisms (discussed below) and it seems probable that the same is true for HIV.

2. *Except in the special conditions of tuberculoid leprosy, patients with mycobacterial infections lack skin test responses to common mycobacterial antigens*: these common mycobacterial antigens include, amongst others, the mycobacterial stress proteins, which share considerable sequence homology with their human homologues. A loss of skin-test responsiveness to the common mycobacterial antigens must therefore encompass a loss or dysregulation of Th1 response to stress proteins. Similar reduced skin-test responsiveness to these antigens is seen in tuberculosis (Kardjito *et al.*, 1986), multibacillary leprosy, rheumatoid arthritis (Bahr *et al.*, 1987), Chagas' seropositivity (Bottasso *et al.*, 1994) and HIV seropositivity (Khoo *et al.*, 1996) (Table 24.1).

3. *Despite persistence of high titers of antibodies, disease progresses, and indeed these antibodies may constitute part of the immunopathology in each case*: production of antibodies, at least of IgG class, is promoted by Th2 matured helper cells (Romagnani, 1991), and with a return to Th1 maturation, antibody titers fall. Antibodies may be powerless in destroying tubercle bacilli whose cell envelope can withstand the effects of complement, but their contribution to host cell destruction may be considerable. Similarly, in HIV disease, the antibodies specific to the virus may not have the right specificity to neutralize the virus, but may play a major role in host cell destruction or in facilitating entry into susceptible cell

types (Amadori and Chieco-Bianchi, 1990).

4. *Each disease is associated with tissue destruction, and autoimmune manifestations*: these diseases in which skin-test responses to common mycobacterial antigens (and heat-shock proteins) are lost, are all accompanied by autoimmune manifestations. The lung in pulmonary tuberculosis, skin, joint and nerve in the erythema nodosum leprosum of leprosy, synovium and cartilage in rheumatoid arthritis, nerve and heart in Chagas' disease and $CD4^+$ cells in HIV, may all be destroyed in part by auto-immune cellular mechanisms. It may be relevant that destruction of tissue or blood cells can occur by the action of $CD8^+$ cytotoxic cells recognizing stress protein epitopes of parasitic or even of human origin, presented on the surfaces of cells (Koga *et al.*, 1989). This may reflect the dysregulation of the response to stress proteins.

A further interesting correlate of T-cell-mediated tissue destructive diseases associated with autoimmunity is a rise in the proportion of agalactosyl IgG (Gal[0]). This is raised in tuberculosis (Rook *et al.*, 1994), leprosy during ENL reactions (Filley *et al.*, 1989), rheumatoid arthritis (Parekh *et al.*, 1985), and HIV disease (Hernandez-Munoz and Stanford, 1996), and is discussed further below.

5. *Loss of circulating $CD4^+$ T cells in tuberculosis and HIV disease, an important parallel*: it is frequently forgotten that depletion of $CD4^+$ T cells occurs to some extent in tuberculosis (Swanson-Beck *et al.*, 1985; Singhal *et al.*, 1989) as well as in HIV disease, so, to explain it, a mechanism is required that is not entirely dependent on the HIV virus itself. Elsewhere we have suggested an endocrinological mechanism (Rook, Onyebujoh and Stanford, 1993), but apoptosis of T cells may be triggered by the immune response itself. The increase in $CD4^+$ counts seen after successful treatment of tuberculosis in patients unafflicted or co-afflicted with HIV may be due to compensation for this destructive mechanism.

Table 24.1 Diseases showing reduced responses to common mycobacterial antigens

Patient group	Category 1 responders (responders to common mycobacterial antigens)
Controls	55/78 (71%) data from G. Bahr (Kuwait)
	$p < 0.0001$
Tuberculosis patients	17/111 (15%)
Controls	55/78 (71%) data from G. Bahr (Kuwait)
	$p < 0.0001$
Rheumatoid arthritics	13/46 (28%)
Controls	7/37 (19%) data from O. Bottasso (Argentina)
	$p = 0.006$
T. cruzi seropositives	0/37
Controls	18/67 (27%) data from S. Khoo (UK)
	$p < 0.0001$
HIV seropositives	0/51[a]

[a]These comprise 27 patients with $CD4^+$ counts above 400 amongst whom there is a normal distribution (11/27) of responsiveness to species-specific antigens of mycobacteria, and 24 patients with $CD4^+$ counts below 400, none of whom was responsive to either common or species-specific mycobacterial antigens.

6. *Relationship of susceptibility to pre-existing anti-mycobacterial immunity?*: although more speculative, each of these conditions may predominantly occur in persons whose immune system is primed to make an immunopathological rather than a protective response. Thus data recently obtained comparing persons at risk with those recently recognized as HIV seropositive show that there are serological differences in their levels of Gal[0] and in their responses to different antigens of *M. avium* serotypes (Hernandez-Munoz and Stanford, 1996) (see below). Admittedly, this may be indicative of a different capacity to respond to challenge resulting from established HIV seropositivity, although the combination with lack of skin test responsiveness to common mycobacterial antigens, mentioned above (Khoo *et al.*, 1996), suggests that it may be a persisting predisposing factor.

MATURATION OF T CELLS: TH1 AND TH2

Demonstration of at least two types of helper T cell in mice (Mossman *et al.*, 1986) was followed by proof of a similar dichotomy in man (Romagnani, 1991). These helper T cells, together with other cell types, give rise to patterns of cytokine release known as Type 1 (typically gamma interferon, IL-2 and IL-12) and Type 2 (IL-4, IL-5 and IL-10) (Salgame *et al.*, 1991) that may hold the key to the immunopathology and the treatment of HIV disease and tuberculosis.

TYPE 1 AND TYPE 2 RESPONSES AND HIV DISEASE

Data summarized in a number of of papers (Clerici and Shearer, 1993, 1994), and now supported by some other groups (Goetz and Sreedharan, 1992), show that there are two different types of response made to infectious challenge with HIV. In one of these, high titers of antibody to the virus develop, and the well-known pattern begins in which gradual loss of immunity leads to AIDS and death in most cases. In the other, T-cell mediated responses to certain viral antigens develop, but without seropositivity or the development of disease. For instance study of more than 100 seronegative homosexuals, drug users, 'needlestick' health care workers, and seronegative babies born to seropositive mothers, has confirmed that many of them have indeed been exposed to the virus because peptides from gp 160 stimulate IL-2 (a Th1 cytokine) release from their peripheral blood lymphocytes. These data, together with reports of very long-term seronegativity amongst certain prostitutes, constitute the best evidence that protective immunity may be possible (although an alternative explanation is congenital lack of a chemokine receptor involved in entry of HIV into T cells; Dragic *et al.*, 1996). If this is correct (Clerici and Shearer, 1993), protective immunity is quite different from the response seen in the seropositive group, and seems to be characterized by the presence of Th1-like cells able to recognize HIV-derived peptides, in the absence of antibody production. It seems that cytotoxic T cells are also desirable, and these secrete IFN-γ, and constitute part of the 'Type 1' (Salgame *et al.*, 1991) pattern of response in both CD4$^+$ and CD8$^+$ T cells. They are probably crucial in resistance to tuberculosis as well, since MHC Class 1 is essential for immunity to this disease in mice (Flynn *et al.*, 1992).

The clear concept that a Th1 response without antibody correlates with protection from HIV disease has been clouded by a dispute about whether a progressive shift from Th1 towards Th2 can be shown to accompany AIDS or tuberculosis. This is probably not the right question to ask. In neither early AIDS nor tuberculosis is the Th1 response entirely lost, but there is a superimposed Th2 component that is clearly inappropriate. HIV-exposed people who resist progressive infection appear to have no detectable antibody, whereas seropositivity and IL-4 expression in the periphery accompany an inexorable progression towards death. In tuberculosis the inappropriate Th2 component is manifested as IgE antibody (Yong *et al.*, 1989), high levels of IgG antibody, and peripheral blood lymphocytes that express IL-4 (Schauf *et al.*, 1993; Surcel, Troye-Blomberg and Paulie, 1994). Thus their Th1 response may be maintained (Barnes *et al.*, 1990), but there is a Th2 response superimposed upon it. In a mouse model this Th1 + Th2 situation leads to cytokine-mediated tissue damage (Hernandez-Pando and Rook, 1994).

In other words, the basic pattern of response required for immunity to HIV is similar to that required for immunity to tuberculosis. Salk and others (Salk *et al.*, 1993) propose that a vaccine promoting type 1 maturation of T-cells, and an immunotherapeutic capable of switching from Th2 towards Th1 are the requirements for prevention and treatment of HIV disease.

These requirements were precisely those that our group had been defining for tuberculosis over a number of years, and at the time Clerici's and Shearer's ideas were published, we had obtained data that suggested that in patients co-afflicted with tuberculosis and HIV seropositivity, immunotherapy for their tuberculosis might have other important effects (Stanford *et al.*, 1993).

ENVIRONMENTAL INFLUENCES

Fundamental to the immune response to infectious challenge is the ability to overcome the pathogen and to prevent the spread of disease. The mechanisms by which these can be achieved may be different, reflecting the different needs of the person in the process of being challenged, and the person in whom disease has become established. Some organisms depend for their pathogenicity on perturbing the host's optimal response, and there is no doubt that the nature of the response can be predetermined, both for better or for worse, by previous contact with related environmental organisms (Stanford, Shield and Rook, 1981; Fine *et al.*, 1994). Such organisms may lack virulence, but nonetheless they undermine immunity to challenge with more virulent organisms. The organism predetermining the response may be quite dissimilar to the eventual pathogen, the unity of responsivity being directed towards commonly shared epitopes, such as those of the stress proteins (Young, 1992). Thus the response evoked to highly conserved antigens such as stress proteins through contacting an environmental mycobacterium such as *M. avium* may predetermine the nature of the response that will subsequently be directed towards cells presenting epitopes from autologous stress proteins as a result of invasion by HIV (Hernandez-Munoz and Stanford, 1996; Khoo *et al.*, 1996).

If this is true, priming an effectively antimycobacterial pattern of response against shared (such as heat-shock protein) epitopes might enhance immunity to HIV. Thus a vaccine protective against HIV disease may not need be directed towards the antigens of HIV itself, but rather towards epitopes evoked by the virus on the parasitized cell. Attempts to produce a vaccine from components of HIV itself have not met with success.

THE DEVELOPMENT OF *MYCOBACTERIUM VACCAE* FOR IMMUNOTHERAPY OF TUBERCULOSIS

Mycobacterium vaccae strain NCTC 11659 is a stable rough variant of an organism grown from the environment in Uganda (Stanford and Paul, 1973) where BCG vaccine had been shown to be effective against leprosy (Brown,

Stone and Sutherland, 1966). As such, *M. vaccae* was found to be one of the environmental influences priming the population for successful vaccination. It was subsequently demonstrated that prior feeding of mice with this strain resulted in accentuation of their footpad responses to tuberculin of a type thought to signify increased protective immunity, after vaccination with BCG (Stanford, Shield and Rook, 1981). The same effect could be achieved by adding killed *M. vaccae* to the BCG vaccine (Stanford *et al.*, 1989).

In early studies of the way that immunization with killed *M. vaccae* worked, it was shown that the effect was dose related. From the extensive studies of Shepard and colleagues (Shepard *et al.*, 1980), and others such as Rees, Gaugas and their colleagues, it was established that normal mice require an injection of about 10^6 live leprosy bacilli to develop cellular immunity, and that lesser doses multiply up to this number, before the mice control bacillary replication. Using this model, groups of mice were vaccinated with 10^5, 10^6, 10^7, 10^8 or 10^9 killed *M. vaccae* 3 months before challenge with 10^4 leprosy bacilli. A month later all the mice were footpad tested with Leprosin A (a soluble preparation of sonicated leprosy bacilli from armadillos) (Stanford, Shield and Rook, 1979). The greatest response was found in mice primed with 10^7 *M. vaccae*, and this was taken as the starting dose for work in man (Stanford *et al.*, 1990).

As an additive to BCG vaccine, 10^7 killed *M. vaccae* was found to improve significantly the ability of children living in close or casual contact with leprosy patients to develop skin-test positivity to Leprosin A (Stanford *et al.*, 1981, 1989; Ganapeti *et al.*, 1989). In children negative to Leprosin A, but unsuitable for BCG vaccination because of prior tuberculin positivity or a scar of earlier BCG vaccination, an injection of 10^8 killed *M. vaccae* alone produced a similar result to that achieved by the BCG + *M. vaccae* combination (Stanford *et al.*, 1989).

Table 24.2 Determination of the optimal doses of *M. vaccae* for immunotherapy of leprosy and tuberculosis

Leprosy (Fontilles, Spain)
Leprosin A conversion in long-treated lepromatous patients

Saline control	1/47 (2%)
10^7 irradiated *M. vaccae*	3/29 (10%)
10^8 irradiated *M. vaccae*	0/6
10^9 irradiated *M. vaccae*	13/34 (38%)
10^9 irradiated *M. vaccae* plus Tuberculin	15/30 (50%)[a,b]

Tuberculosis (Kuwait)
Recognition of common mycobacterial antigens in LTT

Saline control	5/49 (11%)
10^8 irradiated *M. vaccae*	2/8
10^9 irradiated *M. vaccae*	11/38 (29%)
10^9 irradiated *M. vaccae* plus Tuberculin	5/19 (26%)
10^9 irradiated *M. vaccae* plus Murabutide	1/18 (6%)
10^9 irradiated *M. vaccae* plus T plus M	9/25 (36%)
10^9 autoclaved *M. vaccae*	10/22 (45%)[a,c]

[a]Significantly different from values for saline groups.
[b]$p < 0.00001$.
[c]$p < 0.002$.

To be clinically useful in the control of leprosy reactions, or in treatment of tuberculosis, a reagent was needed that could switch off the Koch phenomenon and restore protective, antibacterial immunity (Stanford, 1991). The Th1 pathway of T helper cell maturation needed to be encouraged at the expense of the Th2 pathway – Th1 adjuvanticity. This was thought to be the mechanism by which contact with environmental mycobacterial species predetermines the variable efficacy of BCG vaccination in different geographical environments. In other words, certain environmental species can prime a Th1 response to the common epitopes. A search for organisms with this property began.

The method used was to mix tuberculins prepared from different species and look for regulation of response to some antigens by the presence of others (Stanford *et al.*, 1981; Nye *et al.*, 1983; Morton *et al.*, 1984). This was then extended to studies of the mixtures injected in one arm on the response to single reagents injected in the other. In this way it was found that the antigens of some species could regulate response to those of other species. Skin-test responses signifying Koch responsiveness tend to be necrotic and so differ subjectively from those signifying protective immunity, and these can be distinguished with experience, though with a degree of error (Stanford, Shield and Rook, 1979). Thus the skin test correlate of the Koch phenomenon (Th1 plus Th2; Hernandez-Pando and Rook, 1994) to antigens of slow-growing species injected on one arm could be regulated to the skin-test correlate of protective immunity (Th1) by mixing the antigens of certain fast-growing species with the same preparation of the slow-growers and injecting the mixture on the other arm. Extracts of other fast-growers could limit reactivity at the site of injection of the mixture, but did not effect distant responses. Early fractionation experiments showed that the substances responsible for distant control differed from those responsible for local suppression of reaction (Nye *et al.*, 1986). Organisms found to have both local and distant effects included *M. chitae*, *M. nonchromogenicum* and *M. vaccae*.

The doses of 10^7 and 10^8 *M. vaccae* selected from the vaccine studies were then used as the starting point for studies of immunotherapy of patients with lepromatous leprosy in an attempt to induce positivity to Leprosin A, as distinct from Mitsuda positivity to lepromin. In fact these doses were too small to have a significant effect in patients, but when increased to 10^9, and especially when a low dose of tuberculin was added, significant Leprosin A conversion was achieved (Table 24.2) (Stanford *et al.*, 1987).

This information, in its turn, became the starting point for investigation of *M. vaccae* as an immunotherapeutic for tuberculosis. Following a pilot study designed to investigate the influence of an injection of 10^9 *M. vaccae* on the subjective responsiveness to tuberculin in patients undergoing chemotherapy for tuberculosis in London (Pozniak *et al.*, 1987), comprehensive studies of *M. vaccae* as an immunotherapeutic started in Kuwait (Bahr *et al.*, 1990a).

As in leprosy, 10^7 and 10^8 *M. vaccae* were found to be without significant effect, but 10^9 produced laboratory markers of what were considered to be beneficial reactions (Stanford *et al.*, 1990). Further investigation showed that addition of tuberculin or of murabutide (a water-soluble adjuvant) made little difference unless added together, and that bacilli killed by autoclaving were more effective than those killed by exposure to 2.5 Mrads from a ^{60}Co source (Bahr *et al.*, 1990b).

PILOT TRIALS OF *M. VACCAE* IN THE IMMUNOTHERAPY OF TUBERCULOSIS

A number of randomized and variably blinded comparisons between an injection of saline and immunotherapy with 10^9 killed *M. vaccae* NCTC 11659 have been carried out. In a study in the Gambia, patients received irradiation-killed *M. vaccae* plus tuberculin, or saline placebo, 6 weeks after starting chemotherapy. This consisted of either standard 18-month daily streptomycin, isoniazid and thiacetazone for 2 months, followed by isoniazid and thiacetazone for 16 months, or a 6-month regimen of rifampicin, isoniazid, ethambutol and pyrazinamide for 2 months, followed by rifampicin and isoniazid 3 times weekly for 4 months.

Two studies were carried out in Vietnam comparing placebo with autoclaved *M. vaccae* given 1 to 5 weeks after starting short-course chemotherapy. In one center this consisted of daily streptomycin, isoniazid, rifampicin and pyrazinamide for 2 months followed by isoniazid and ethambutol for 6 months. In the other center it consisted of daily streptomycin, isoniazid and pyrazinamide for 3 months followed by twice weekly streptomycin and isoniazid for 6 months.

The combined results of the Gambian and Vietnamese studies showed that immunotherapy reduced the numbers of deaths occurring during chemotherapy and reduced the number of treatment failures by half (Table 24.3).

A randomized study was carried out in Kano, Nigeria, under conditions of very poor chemotherapy (Onyebujoh *et al.*, 1995). Free drugs were almost unavailable, and most had to bought by the patient at high price from private dispensaries. Much of the purchased drug was of low quality, either being long out of date, or counterfeit. This resulted in few patients being able to comply with prescribed treatment, and results of chemotherapy alone were little better than those recorded in the days before the discovery of streptomycin. A single dose of 10^9 autoclaved *M. vaccae* was given to patients randomized to receive it, between 1 and 4 weeks after starting chemotherapy. *M. vaccae* or

Table 24.3   Data pooled from 3 randomized and blinded studies in which patients undertook complete courses of chemotherapy

	Cure[a]	*Deaths*
Placebo group	171/218 (78%)	17/218 (8%)
	$p < 0.005$	$p < 0.03$
Immunotherapy group	179/202 (89%)	6/202 (3%)

[a]Cure signifies bacteriological and clinical cure at the end of a course of chemotherapy.

saline was injected after 1 to 3 weeks of chemotherapy. Thereafter patients took chemotherapy according to what they could afford and how well they felt. At follow-up, recipients of immunotherapy reported buying chemotherapy for a mean of 3.2 months, and survivors in the placebo group bought drugs for a mean of 6.8 months.

Follow-up was between 10 and 12 months after immunotherapy was given. Under conditions of such poor chemotherapy, immunotherapy had striking effects both in reducing deaths and improving cure rate (Table 24.4). Unfortunately, for a variety of reasons, the numbers followed up were much fewer than had been hoped, reducing the value of the study.

Immunotherapy for drug-susceptible tuberculosis

A study has been completed in Romania in which the drug susceptibility patterns are known for the bacilli causing disease in most patients. A single injection of 10^9 autoclaved *M. vaccae* given after 1 month of a 6-month chemotherapy regimen improved the rate at which sputum became smear-negative and culture-negative for acid-fast bacilli. This was accompanied by improved weight regain, ESR and chest X-ray appearances. However, the immunotherapy did not significantly improve the eventual cure rate in this group (Corlan *et al.*, 1996a).

IMMUNOTHERAPY FOR MULTIDRUG-RESISTANT AND CHRONIC TUBERCULOSIS

The results of poor prescription or poor compliance with potentially good therapy in many countries, chronic treatment failures and multidrug resistant bacilli have become an increasing problem. Depending on quite different criteria of efficacy, immunotherapy with *M. vaccae* should have a major part to play in the treatment of these difficult cases. Studies are progressing with such patients and the data from that in Mashad, Iran, have already been published (Farid *et al.*, 1994). This study employed up to 4 injections of the immunotherapeutic and demonstrated a number of important features:

1. Immunotherapy could be effective even when the only drugs being given were those to which the organism was resistant.
2. Patients with treatment histories of 2 years or less could be successfully treated with a single injection of *M. vaccae*, whatever the pattern of drug resistance.
3. A proportion of patients with chronic disease and treatment histories of 3 years or more responded to multiple injections of *M. vaccae*.
4. Two months is a suitable time-gap between doses of *M. vaccae*.

The overall result of the study was that 11/41 patients were cured with im-

Table 24.4 Results of a randomized study of immunotherapy with *M. vaccae* and saline (placebo), in patients with pulmonary tuberculosis receiving poor-quality chemotherapy. A study carried out by Dr P. Onyebujoh in Kano, Nigeria, where the standard of chemotherapy was very poor

	Immunotherapy group		*Placebo group*
Numbers entering the study	90		90
Follow-up after 10–12 months			
Mortality	0/34	$p < 0.00001$	19/47
Sputum −ve for AFB	21/34	$p < 0.0001$	4/28
Weight gain of survivors	$7.9 \pm 1.0\,\text{kg}$	$p < 0.001$	$2.00 \pm 1.7\,\text{kg}$
Mean fall in ESR	$41.8 \pm 7.9\,\text{mm}$	$p < 0.00$	$115.0 \pm 8.5\,\text{mm}$

munotherapy plus chemotherapy, in comparison with a historical control of only 1 success in more than 100 patients with the available chemotherapy alone ($p<0.00001$). Subsequently, similar data have come from 2 studies in Vietnam, and 1 in the Philippines.

The study completed in Romania shows the significant deleterious effect of even single drug resistance on treatment with chemotherapy alone (Stanford *et al.*, 1994). Yet treatment including an injection of *M. vaccae* is just as effective in such patients as it is in the treatment of fully drug susceptible infections (Corlan *et al.*, 1996b).

IMMUNOTHERAPY WITH *M. VACCAE* IN TUBERCULOSIS PATIENTS CO-AFFLICTED WITH HIV SEROPOSITIVITY

Amongst the patients entering the study in the Gambia were 11 patients seropositive for HIV-2, 6 receiving immunotherapy and 5 in the control group. Three of these patients (1 receiving immunotherapy) died during the period of chemotherapy. Unfortunately no further follow-up data are available. Amongst those studied in Nigeria were 17 patients seropositive for HIV-1, 8 receiving *M. vaccae* and 9 placebo. The fates of these patients were followed with considerable interest, and have been published (Stanford *et al.*, 1993). Surprisingly, immunotherapy

had a dramatic effect; all 8 recipients of *M. vaccae* survived for at least 2 years, whereas at least 8 of those receiving placebo died during this time (Table 24.5). At the 10–12 month follow-up after intervention the 8 immunotherapy recipients were clinically cured of tuberculosis, although one still had visible acid-fast bacilli in the sputum. The generalized lymphadenopathy present at diagnosis in 5 patients had resolved. Of the 3 patients surviving to the 10–12 month follow-up in the placebo group, all had advanced tuberculosis, AFB in the sputum, and generalized lymphadenopathy. Most remarkable of all were the serological results on the sera obtained from 2 out of each group of patients at the 10–12 month follow-up. Those from the placebo recipients were HIV-1 seropositive by 2 ELISA techniques and Western blotting, whereas the 2 from the *M. vaccae* recipient group had apparently converted to seronegativity by these tests. Autoantibody profiles on these 2 sera were the same as on the initial samples, suggesting that they really were from the same patients.

A single patient co-afflicted with HIV seropositivity and drug resistant tuberculosis has been successfully treated with *M. vaccae* in the United Kingdom. Two injections of *M. vaccae* were given, 2 months apart, and this patient made a good recovery from tuberculosis. Six months later he remained clini-

Table 24.5 Results from Kano, Nigeria, for patients entering the study of immunotherapy of pulmonary tuberculosis and found to be co-infected with HIV-1 in retrospect

	Immunotherapy group		Placebo group
Initial data			
HIV-1 seropositive			
patients followed up	8/42 (19%)		9/47 (19%)
Lymphadenopathy	5/8 (63%)		7/9 (78%)
10–12-month follow-up data			
Survival	8/8	$p < 0.01$	3/9
Sputum still +ve for AFB	1/8	$p < 0.03$	3/3
Clinically improved	8/8	$p < 0.001$	0/3
Lymphadenopathy	0/8	$p < 0.001$	3/3
Still HIV-1 seropositive	0/2		2/2
Two-year follow-up data			
Survival	8/8	$p < 0.001$	?1/9

Note: Patients were HIV-1 seropositive by 2 different ELISA systems, and Western blots. All 3 tests showed reversion to seronegativity, and correct allocation of sera to individuals who were initially seropositive was suggested by their patterns of low-titer auto-antibodies.

cally well but was still seropositive for HIV. Further serum samples will be studied.

At first sight it seems surprising that immunotherapy should still work against tuberculosis in the presence of HIV seropositivity. It seems even more surprising that immunotherapy based on a mycobacterium and designed for tuberculosis might hold promise for the treatment of HIV disease itself, and the rest of this chapter is devoted to this possibility.

RESPONSES TO MYCOBACTERIAL ANTIGENS OF HIV SEROPOSITIVE PERSONS

As mentioned above, people who develop seropositivity to HIV and progress to HIV-related disease differ from HIV seronegative persons in their responses to mycobacterial antigens. This can be seen both in serological tests (Hernandez-Munoz, 1996) and in tests of cellular immunity such as skin tests with tuberculins (Khoo *et al.*, 1996).

GALACTOSYLATION OF IgG

During the production of (? T cell dependent) IgG antibody the terminal *N*-acetyl glucosamine on sugar chains attached in the conserved region of antibody heavy chains is galactosylated by the enzyme galactosyl transferase. Terminating with galactose the sugar chain is bound to a galactose-specific lectin-like site on the same heavy chain; thus the sugar chain forms a loop bound by both ends to the heavy chain (Parekh *et al.*, 1988). Failure to galactosylate results in sugar chains terminating with *N*-acetylglucosamine – a bacteriomimetic sugar rarely exposed on mammalian molecules. Such agalactosyl IgG (Gal[0]) is always present to some extent in human sera and there is an age-curve for its presence (Parekh *et al.*, 1988). In patients with certain diseases the proportion of Gal[0] is markedly increased, and it is thought that this might have some immunoregulatory role associated with the exposed sugar since it seems to occur in situations where chronic

T-cell-mediated tissue damage is occurring (Rook and Stanford, 1995). Such conditions include tuberculosis, certain forms of leprosy, rheumatoid arthritis and Crohn's disease; it has now been shown to be associated both with HIV seropositivity (Hernandez-Munoz and Stanford, 1996) and with lentivirus infection of goats (McCulloch *et al.*, 1994). Patients with AIDS who develop infection with *M. avium* serotypes show an additional increase in Gal[0] similar to that seen in HIV-seronegative persons when they develop tuberculosis. It is interesting that regulation of galactosylation is still operative in patients with such advanced immune deficiency.

IgA AND IgG ANTIBODIES TO *M. AVIUM*

Recent studies in our department (Hernandez-Munoz and Stanford, 1996) show differences between HIV seronegative and seropositive people in the ratios of IgA to IgG against sonicate and secreted antigens of *M. avium* serotypes 4 and 8. These serotypes were selected for special study since they are involved in infection (aviumosis) in patients with AIDS to different degrees in the UK (serotype 4 is incriminated in 70% of cases and serotype 8 in 20% of cases). Unless recent development of HIV seropositivity is associated with subtle regulatory effects on antibodies to different *M. avium* specificities, this balance is likely to reflect the situation prior to development of HIV seropositivity. An interpretation of this might be that it reflects the T helper cell maturation pattern imposed by environmental contact with *M. avium*, and that this might differently predispose to the outcome of HIV challenge.

SKIN TEST RESPONSES TO TUBERCULINS

Quadruple skin testing with new tuberculins allows groups of individuals to be divided into a number of responder categories according to their ability to produce skin reactions to common (group i) or species specific (group iv) antigens of mycobacteria. A study performed by Khoo and colleagues in Manchester, UK (Khoo *et al.*, 1996) showed that HIV-seropositive persons, even with high CD4$^+$ cell counts, did not respond to the common mycobacterial antigens. Their study also showed that the distribution of responses to tuberculins prepared from *M. avium* of serotypes 4 and 8 were similar to the distribution of these serotypes in causation of AIDS-associated aviumosis. This too suggested that fate related to HIV is predetermined before challenge occurs. If susceptibility can be predetermined, why not protective immunity?

'FALSE POSITIVE' TESTS FOR HIV ANTIBODY IN LEPROSY AND TUBERCULOSIS

Recently reports have appeared in the literature of apparently falsely positive HIV ELISA tests in some patients with leprosy (Schechter *et al.*, 1991) or tuberculosis (Werneck-Barroso *et al.*, 1994). These have been considered false because the HIV antibodies seem to disappear with effective treatment of the mycobacterial disease.

There are undoubtedly shared epitopes between all living things, and several years ago it was noted in India that certain *M. avium* strains possessed antigenic epitopes shared with HIV. It was suggested that the slow onset of the HIV epidemic in India might be due to protection afforded by naturally occurring immune reactions to these antigens in response to such *M. avium* strains in the Indian environment. The recent work outlined above from our group showing surprising changes in antibody to *M. avium* in HIV seropositive patients may be associated with the observations from India.

The reports of 'false positive' HIV serology in tuberculosis and leprosy patients may have an explanation other than that initially proposed, especially since the observations have been made in HIV-endemic countries. This might be that the patients had dual infection, but that the changes in immune regulation occasionally occurring during treatment of mycobacterioses has resulted in spontaneous 'cure' of HIV seropositivity. If so, then this might be maximized by immunotherapy with *M. vaccae*. This would be in accord with our preliminary observations of simultaneous efficacy of *M. vaccae* against both tuberculosis and HIV seropositivity in Kano (Stanford *et al.*, 1993). Whatever the true explanation it is essential that it is fully investigated since the observations may offer a clue to both vaccination against HIV and effective immunotherapy for HIV-related disease.

SUMMARY

The immunological similarities and relationships between tuberculosis and HIV infection are considerable. In both diseases there is a CD4 lymphopenia and an inappropriate Th2 component to the immune response that appears irrelevant to immunity, and may contribute to immunopathology. Thus in both diseases protective immunity differs from the mechanism of immunopathology in similar ways. The prophesies of Salk, Clerici, Shearer, and their colleagues that a Th1 adjuvant might both treat and prevent HIV infection appear to have been borne out by our chance, and at present anecdotal, findings. Intensive investigation of this possibility has begun.

Immunotherapy with killed *Mycobacterium vaccae* is a simple, and potentially very cheap, adjunct to chemotherapy that could revolutionize the treatment of tuberculosis. In newly diagnosed patients it can reduce mortality and improve cure rate. By opening the possibility for a major shortening of regimens it may overcome the problem of non-compliance with treatment, although this still has to be proven. It may also offer hope for chronic treatment-failure patients

and for those infected with multi-drug-resistant bacilli. It is just as effective in patients co-infected with HIV, and the part it may play in the treatment of HIV infection itself offers an exciting prospect.

Stable for at least a year at +4°C, its distribution in the developing world should not pose a problem greater than that already faced by the Expanded Programme of Immunization (EPI). If the trials currently progressing lead to regulatory acceptance of its use, the balance of control of tuberculosis should swing definitively in favor of mankind. Lastly, its investigation should lead to even better Th1 adjuvants, and new prospects of treatment for a series of diseases, including HIV, currently defying cure.

REFERENCES

Amadori, A. and Chieco-Bianchi, L. (1990) B-cell activation and HIV-1 infection: deeds and misdeeds. *Immunol. Today*, **11**, 374–9.

Anonymous (1890) Professor Koch's remedy for tuberculosis; Austria. *Br. Med. J.*, **2**, 1490.

Bahr, G.M., Sattar, I., Stanford, J.L. *et al.* (1987) HLA-DR and tuberculin tests in rheumatoid arthritis and tuberculosis. *Ann. Rheum. Dis.*, **48**, 63–8.

Bahr, G.M., Stanford, J.L., Chugh, T.D. *et al.* (1990a) An investigation of patients with pulmonary tuberculosis in Kuwait in preparation for studies of immunotherapy with *Mycobacterium vaccae*. *Tubercle*, **71**, 77–86.

Bahr, G.M., Shaaban, M.A, Gabriel, M. *et al.* (1990b) Improved immunotherapy for pulmonary tuberculosis with *Mycobacterium vaccae*. *Tubercle*, **71**, 259–66.

Barnes, P.F., Fong, S.J., Brennan, P.J. *et al.* (1990) Local production of tumor necrosis factor and IFN-gamma in tuberculous pleuritis. *J. Immunol.*, **145**, 149–54.

Bottasso, O.A., Ingledew, N., Keni, M. *et al.* (1994) Cellular immune response to common mycobacterial antigens in subjects seropositive for *Trypanosoma cruzi*. *Lancet*, **344**, 1540–1.

Brown, J.A.K., Stone, M.M. and Sutherland, I. (1966) BCG vaccination of children against leprosy in Uganda. *Br. Med. J.*, **1**, 7–14.

Clerici, M. and Shearer, G.M. (1993) A TH1 to TH2

switch is a critical step in the etiology of HIV infection. *Immunol. Today*, **14**, 107–11.

Clerici, M. and Shearer, G.M. The Th1-Th2 hypothesis of HIV infection: new insights. *Immunol. Today*, **15**, 575–81.

Corlan, E., Marica, C., Macavei, C. *et al.* (1996a) Immunotherapy with *Mycobacterium vaccae* in the treatment of newly diagnosed pulmonary tuberculosis in Romania. *Respir. Med.*, in press

Corlan, E., Marica, C., Macavei, C. *et al.* (1996b) Immunotherapy with *Mycobacterium vaccae* in the treatment of chronic or relapsed tuberculosis in Romania. *Respir. Med.*, in press.

Debré, R. and Bonnet, H. (1922) Surinfection du cobaye tuberculeux après l'établissement de l'état allergique. *C.R. Soc. Biol.*, **87**, 449–68.

Dragic, T., Litwin, V., Allaway, G. P. *et al.* (1996) HIV-1 entry into CD4$^+$ cells is mediated by the chemokine receptor CC-CKR-5. *Nature*, **381**, 667–73

Farid, R., Etemadi, A., Stanford, J.L. *et al.* (1994) *Mycobacterium vaccae* immunotherapy in the treatment of multi-drug-resistant tuberculosis: a preliminary report. *Iran. J. Med. Sci.*, **19**, 37–9.

Filley, E., Andreoli, A., Steele, J. *et al.* (1989) A transient rise in agalactosyl IgG correlating with free IL-2 receptors during episodes of erythema nodosum leprosum. *Clin. Exp. Immunol.*, **76**, 343–7.

Fine, P.E., Sterne, J.A.C., Ponnighaus, J.M. and Rees, R.J.W. (1994) Delayed type hypersensitivity, mycobacterial vaccines and protective immunity. *Lancet*, **344**, 1245–9.

Flynn, J.L., Goldstein, M.M., Triebold, K.J. *et al.* (1992) Major histocompatibility complex class I-restricted T cells are required for resistance to *Mycobacterium tuberculosis* infection. *Proc. Natl. Acad. Sci. U.S.A.*, **89**, 12013–17.

Friedmann, F.F. (1903) Spontane Lungen-tuberkulose bei Schildkroten und die Stellung des Tuberkelbazillus im System. *Zeitschrift für Tuberkulose*, **4**, 439–57.

Ganapati, R., Revankar, C.R., Lockwood, D.N.J. *et al.* (1989) A pilot study of three potential vaccines for leprosy in Bombay. *Int. J. Lepr.*, **57**, 33–7.

Ghazi-Saidi, K., Stanford, J.L., Stanford, C.A. *et al.* (1989) Vaccination and skin test studies on children living in villages with differing endemicity for leprosy and tuberculosis. *Int. J. Lepr. Other Mycobact. Dis.*, **57**, 45–53.

Goetzl, E.J. and Sreedharan, S.P. (1992) Mediators of communication and adaptation in the neuroendocrine and immune systems. *FASEB. J.*, **6**, 2646–52.

Grange, J.M. (1992) The mystery of the mycobacterial persister. *Tubercle Lung Dis.*, **73**, 249–51.

Grange, J.M., Stanford, J.L. and Rook, G.A.W. (1995) Tuberculosis and cancer; parallels in host responses and therapeutic approaches. *Lancet*, **345**, 1350–2.

Hernandez-Munoz, H.E. and Stanford, J.L. (1996) IgA and IgG antibodies to distinct serotypes of *Mycobacterium avium* in HIV seropositivity and AIDS. *J. Med. Microbiol.*, **44**, 1–5.

Hernandez-Pando, R. and Rook, G.A.W. (1994) The role of TNFα in T cell-mediated inflammation depends on the Th1/Th2 cytokine balance. *Immunology*, **82**, 591–5.

Inman, P.M., Beck, A., Brown, A.E. and Stanford, J.L. (1969) Outbreak of injection abscesses due to *Mycobacterium abscessus*. *Arch. Derm.*, **100**, 141–7.

Kardjito, T., Beck, J.S., Grange, J.M. and Stanford, J.L. (1986) A comparison of the responsiveness to four new tuberculins among Indonesian patients with pulmonary tuberculosis and healthy subjects. *Eur. J. Respir. Dis.*, **69**, 142–5.

Khoo, S.H., Wilkins, E.G.L., Fraser, I., *et al.* (1996) Lack of skin test reactivity to common mycobacterial antigens in human immunodeficiency virus infected individuals with high CD counts. *Thorax*, **51**, 932–5.

Koch, R. (1882) Die Aetiologie der Tuberculose. *Berliner Klinische Wochenschrift*, **19**, 221.

Koch, R. (1890) An address on bacteriological research delivered before the International Medical Congress held in Berlin, August 1890. *Br. Med. J.*, **2**, 380–3.

Koch, R. (1891) Fortsetzung über ein Heilmittel gegen Tuberculose. *Deutsch. Med. Wochenschr.*, **17**, 101–2.

Koga, T., Wand-Wurttenberger, A., DeBruyn, J. *et al.* (1989) T cells against a bacterial heat shock protein recognise stressed macrophages. *Science*, **245**, 1112–15.

Macassey, L. and Saleeby, C.W. (1934) *Spahlinger contra tuberculosis 1908–1934*. An international tribute. In: Macassey L. Saleeby, C.W., ed. London: John Bale and Sons and Danielsson Ltd.

McCulloch, J., Zang, Y.W., Dawson, M. *et al.* (1994) Glycosylation of IgG during potentially arthritogenic lentiviral infections. *Rheumatol. Int.*, **14**, 243–8.

Morton, A., Nye, P., Rook, G.A. *et al.* (1984) A further investigation of skin-test responsiveness and suppression in leprosy patients and healthy school children in Nepal. *Lepr. Rev.*, **55**, 273–81.

Mossman, T.R., Cherwinski, H., Bond, M.W. *et al.* (1986) Two types of murine helper T cell clone. 1) Definition according to profiles of lymphokine activities and secreted proteins. *J. Immunol.*, **136**, 2348–57.

Nye, P.M., Price, J.E., Revankar, C.R. *et al.* (1983) The demonstration of two types of suppressor mechanism in leprosy patients and their contacts by quadruple skin-testing with mycobacterial reagent mixtures. *Lepr. Rev.*, **54**, 9–18.

Nye, P.M., Stanford, J.L., Rook, G.A. *et al.* (1986) Suppressor determinants of mycobacteria and their potential relevance to leprosy. *Lepr. Rev.*, **57**, 147–57.

Onyebujoh, P.C., Abdulmumini, T., Robinson, S. *et al.* (1995) Immunotherapy for tuberculosis in African conditions. *Respir. Med.*, **89**, 199–207.

Parekh, R.B., Dwek, R.A., Sutton, B.J. *et al.* (1985) Association of rheumatoid arthritis and primary osteoarthritis with changes in the glycosylation pattern of total serum IgG. *Nature*, **316**, 452–7.

Parekh, R., Roitt, I., Isenberg, D. *et al.* (1988) Age-related galactosylation of the N-linked oligosaccharides of human serum IgG. *J. Exp. Med.*, **167**, 1731–6.

Pozniak, A., Stanford, J.L., Johnson, N.M. and Rooke, G.A.W. (1987) Preliminary studies of immunotherapy of tuberculosis in man. Proceedings of the International Tuberculosis Congress, Singapore, 1986. *Bull. Int. Union. Tub.*, **62**, 39–40.

Romagnani, S. (1991) Human TH1 and TH2 subsets: doubt no more. *Immunol. Today*, **12**, 256–7.

Rook, G.A.W. and Al Attiyah, R. (1991) Cytokines and the Koch phenomenon. *Tubercle*, **72**, 13–20.

Rook, G.A.W., Onyebujoh, P. and Stanford, J.L. (1993) TH1 → TH2 switch and loss of CD4 cells in chronic infections; an immuno-endocrinological hypothesis not exclusive to HIV. *Immunol. Today*, **14**, 568–9.

Rook, G.A.W., Onyebujoh, P., Wilkins, E. *et al.* (1994) A longitudinal study of % agalactosyl IgG in tuberculosis patients receiving chemotherapy, with or without immunotherapy. *Immunol.*, **81**, 149–54.

Rook, G.A.W. and Stanford, J.L. (1995) Adjuvants, endocrines and conserved epitopes; factors to consider when designing "Therapeutic Vaccines". *Int. J. Immunpharmac.*, **17**, 91–102.

Salgame, P.R., Abrams, J.S., Clayberger, C. *et al.* (1991) Differing lymphokine profiles of functional subsets of human CD4 and CD8 T cell clones. *Science*, **254**, 279.

Salk, J., Bretscher, P.A., Salk, P.L. *et al.* (1993) A strategy of prophylactic vaccination against HIV. *Science*, **260**, 1270–2.

Schauf, V., Rom, W.N., Smith, K.A. *et al.* (1993) Cytokine gene activation and modified responsiveness to interleukin-2 in the blood of tuberculosis patients. *J. Infect. Dis.*, **168**, 1056–9.

Schechter, M., Andrade, V.L., Avelleira, J.C. *et al.* (1991) Leprosy as a cause of false-positive results in serological assays for the detection of antibodies to HIV-1. *Int. J. Lepr.*, **59**, 125–6.

Shepard, C.C., Minagawa, F., Van Landingham, R. and Walker, L. (1980) Foot-pad enlargement as a measure of induced immunity to *Mycobacterium leprae*. *Int. J. Lepr.*, **48**, 371–81.

Singhal, M., Banavalikar, J.N., Sharma, S. and Saha, K. (1989) Peripheral blood T lymphocyte subpopulations in patients with tuberculosis and the effect of chemotherapy. *Tubercle*, **70**, 171–8.

Spahlinger, H. (1922) Note on the treatment of tuberculosis. *Lancet*, **i**, 5–8.

Stanford, J.L. and Paul, R.C. (1973) A preliminary report of some studies of environmental mycobacteria from Uganda. *Ann. Soc. Belge. Med. Trop.*, **53**, 389–93.

Stanford, J.L., Shield, M.J. and Rook, G.A.W. (1978) *Mycobacterium leprae*, other mycobacteria and a possible vaccine in Latapi, F., Saul, A., Rodriguez, O., Malacara, M., Browne, S.G., ed. Proceedings of the XI International Leprosy Congress. Mexico City, Elsevier, Amsterdam, 102–7.

Stanford, J.L., Shield, M.J. and Rook, G.A. (1981a) How environmental mycobacteria may predetermine the protective efficacy of BCG. *Tubercle*, **62**, 55–62.

Stanford, J.L., Nye, P.M., Rook, G.A. *et al.* (1981b) A preliminary investigation of the responsiveness or otherwise of patients and staff of a leprosy hospital to groups of shared or species antigens of mycobacteria. *Lepr. Rev.*, **52**, 321–7.

Stanford, J.L., Terencio de Las Aguas, J., Torres, P. *et al.* (1987) Studies on the effects of a potential immunotherapeutic agent in leprosy patients. *Quaderni di Cooperazione Sanitaria*, **7**, 201–6.

Stanford, J.L., Rook. G.A.W., Bahr, G.M. *et al.*, (1990) *Mycobacterium vaccae* in immunoprophylaxis and immunotherapy of leprosy and tuberculosis. *Vaccine*, **8**, 525–30.

Stanford, J.L., Stanford, C.A., Ghazi-Saidi, K. *et al.* (1989) Vaccination and skin test studies on the children of leprosy patients (published erratum appears in *Int J Lepr Other Mycobact Dis* 1989 Dec; **57**(4):following 927). *Int. J. Lepr. Other Mycobact. Dis.*, **57**, 38–44.

Stanford, J.L., Bahr, G.M., Rook, G.A. *et al.* (1990) Immunotherapy with *Mycobacterium vaccae* as an adjunct to chemotherapy in the treatment of pulmonary tuberculosis. *Tubercle*, **71**, 87–93.

Stanford, J.L. (1991) Koch's phenomenon: can it be corrected? *Tubercle*, **72**, 13–20.

Stanford, J.L., Onyebujoh, P.C., Rook, G.A.W. *et al.* (1993) Old plague, new plague and a treatment for both? *AIDS*, **7**, 1275–7.

Stanford, J.L., Stanford, C.A., Etemadi, A. *et al.* (1994) Immunotherapy for multidrug-resistant tuberculosis. *Proceedings of 4th WPCCID, supplement to JAMA Southeast Asia* (1994); December: 42–6.

Starnes, C.O. (1992) Coley's toxins in perspective. *Nature*, **357**, 11–12.

Surcel, H.M., Troye-Blomberg, M., Paulie, S. *et al.* (1994) Th1/Th2 profiles in tuberculosis based on proliferation and cytokine response of peripheral blood lymphocytes to mycobacterial antigens. *Immunology*, **81**, 171–6.

Swanson-Beck, J., Potts, R.C., Kardjito, T. and Grange, J.M. (1985) T4 lymphopenia in patients with active pulmonary tuberculosis. *Clin. Exp. Immunol.*, **60**, 49–54.

Villemin, J.A. *Ètudes expérimentales et cliniques sur tuberculose*, Ballière et fils, Paris.

Werneck-Barroso, E., Kritski, A.L., Ma, V. *et al.* (1994) Tuberculosis as a cause of false-positive results in HIV screening tests. *Tuber. Lung Dis.*, **75**, 394–8.

Yong, A.J., Grange, J.M., Tee, R.D. *et al.* (1989) Total and anti-mycobacterial IgE levels in serum from patients with tuberculosis and leprosy. *Tubercle*, **70**, 273–9.

Young, D.B. (1992) Heat-shock proteins: immunity and autoimmunity. *Curr. Opin. Immunol.*, **4**, 396–400.

RESEARCH PRIORITIES FOR THE COMMON HIV-RELATED RESPIRATORY INFECTIONS

25

Adam S. Malin and Keith P.W.J. McAdam

INTRODUCTION

Pneumocystis carinii pneumonia (PCP) is the major respiratory pathogen affecting HIV-infected individuals in the industrialized world. Clear advances have been made in prevention and treatment. This has resulted in a reduction in disease incidence and morbidity. Co-trimoxazole is still the drug of choice for prophylaxis and treatment. However, drug toxicity is a serious problem and the alternatives available, although of lower toxicity, are less efficacious. Thus, the search for an alternative agent is of key importance.

In terms of its frequency of presentation, tuberculosis can be considered counterpart in the developing world to PCP. However, there the similarity ends. Poorer countries are predicted to experience an increase in tuberculosis of mammoth proportions. Disease does not preclude those who are immunocompetent. Treatment regimens are lengthy and expensive and compliance remains a major hurdle. The specter of multiple drug resistance overshadows developing world control programs.

Pneumococcal disease, like tuberculosis, affects asymptomatic HIV-infected in-dividuals with relatively high $CD4^+$ T cell counts. In particular, invasive disease is more common among the HIV-infected and this contributes significantly to overall mortality. The present vaccine fails to immunize asymptomatic HIV-infected individuals adequately. Moreover, multiple drug resistance may well become a significant problem.

This chapter will describe the research priorities pertaining to these three major infections. These priorities have been summarized in tables in the relevant sections (see pp. 397–411) below. However, it must be remembered that the importance for any given research programme varies according to the needs of individual countries and these tables only give a general overview. WHO has declared tuberculosis a global emergency. For this reason the tuberculosis section (below) is given particular emphasis.

TUBERCULOSIS

PUBLIC HEALTH ISSUES

In 1992, the Tuberculosis (TB) Programme of the World Health Organization estimated that 1.7 billion people were latently infected

AIDS and Respiratory Medicine. Edited by A. Zumla, M.A. Johnson and R.F. Miller. Published in 1997 by Chapman & Hall, London. ISBN 0 412 60140 0

with *Mycobacterium tuberculosis* (MTB). Eight million cases of active disease annually resulted in 2.9 million deaths (Narain, Raviglione and Kochi, 1992b). This makes tuberculosis a bigger killer than all other infectious pathogens. Moreover, HIV infection is the most potent risk factor for the development of TB, with a relative risk of 6–100 when compared with HIV-negative individuals (Nunn, 1994). HIV infection is increasing throughout the developing world with the burden residing in Sub-Saharan Africa. WHO estimated that over 9 million adults were infected by the end of 1993. Africa is experiencing a major resurgence in tuberculosis, mainly as a consequence of the overlap between high levels of latent TB infection and a very high level of HIV infection. For example, TB accounted for 40% of all HIV-infected deaths found at post-mortem in Abidjan compared with only 4% in HIV-negative deaths (Abouya, 1992). Despite endeavors to control the spread of TB, WHO estimate an increase from 7.5 million cases in 1990 to 10.2 million in 2000. Overall, forecasts for this decade estimate 88 million new cases of TB globally of which 8 million will be attributable to HIV infection. Thirty million of these TB cases will die including the 2.9 million who are dually infected with HIV and TB (Dolin, 1994).

There are now over 4 million people co-infected with TB and HIV worldwide. Mathematical modeling predicts a 6–10 fold increase in many urban areas in the developing world by the year 2000 (Schulzer *et al.*, 1992). Particularly worrying is the fact that only one tenth of the world's tuberculous infected population reside in Africa; a further billion live in Asia and the western Pacific. As spreads into these countries, this devastating 'cruel duet' will ensue.

Compounding the problem of TB-HIV co-infection, multidrug resistant TB (MDR-TB) has emerged as a major problem along the eastern seaboard of the United States (Bennett and Watson, 1994; Iseman, 1993). Whilst this has been limited to specific cities in the US, there are worrying trends to suggest that the problem may develop in other parts of the world (Kochi, Vareldzis and Styblo, 1993). The ingredients for such an epidemic already exist: namely, overburdened national TB control programs plus increasing HIV prevalence on a background of high latent TB infection.

A list of TB research priorities is given in Table 25.1 and these topics are described in the section that follows. No specific ranking is given within the list. Suffice it to say that no single means of tuberculosis control is likely to solve this global emergency. The only rational approach is a multifaceted one (WHO, 1995).

Defining those at risk

Only 5% of exposed non-HIV infected individuals will develop tuberculosis within 1 year followed by a further lifetime risk of reactivation of about 5%. HIV-infected individuals are more susceptible to TB and the course of infection is more compressed (Elliott *et al.*, 1993; Narain, Raviglione and Kochi, 1992a). They are particularly likely to progress directly from the initial TB infection to overt disease. For example, 37% of HIV-infected intravenous drug users (IVDU) exposed to MTB developed active disease within 15 weeks of exposure (Daley *et al.*, 1992). Contact study data suggest that the infectiousness of TB is not affected by the presence of HIV. This is supported by the observation that HIV-infected TB patients secrete fewer bacilli (Brindle, 1992). Nevertheless, atypical presentation of TB is common and this may delay diagnosis and thus prolong exposure to contacts. Surveillance data are essential to quantify the extent of the problem and to monitor the impact made by TB control programs and specific interventions. Such surveillance data should also argue for appropriate allocation of funds, particularly to support drug purchase where

Table 25.1 Research priorities for tuberculosis

Define those at risk
    surveillance data on size and spread of TB and HIV/AIDS
    surveillance data on multiple-drug-resistant tuberculosis (MDR-TB)
    DNA fingerprinting to distinguish new infections from reactivation/relapse
    identify health professionals at risk and requirements for effective containment
    identify genetic susceptibility

Develop rapid, low cost, broadly applicable and robust tests
    improve diagnosis of clinical specimens
    improve susceptibility testing e.g. luciferase reporter phages
    identify markers of immunity and active disease including simple skin tests (search for highly specific peptide epitopes) and serology

Optimize tuberculosis control programs
    improve control program management
    assess novel methods for improving compliance e.g. refundable deposit, blister packs
    operational studies to assess different drug regimens and delivery systems
        intermittent versus daily; directly observed versus self-medication; and
        hospital-based specialist center versus local clinic or home therapy

Assess old and new drugs
    optimize short course regimens
    define best regimens for MDR-TB
    develop slow release formulations e.g. depot preparations
    assess role for corticosteroids and need for long-term maintenance therapy in the context of HIV
    develop improved animal and *in vitro* models to assess drug activity
    assess role for long-acting drugs e.g. rifapentine

Role of chemoprophylaxis
    isoniazid alone versus combined short course regimens
    assess intermittent, supervised courses to improve compliance

Role of vaccination and immunotherapy
    role of BCG in HIV-infected adults and children and protection against the development of MDR-TB
M. vaccae immunotherapy
    develop novel vaccines e.g. genetically manipulated BCG, attenuated *M. tuberculosis* and non-replicating viral vectors expressing tuberculous immunodominant antigens
    assess novel routes for administration e.g. inhaled immunization

Characterize host immune response
    define T cell repertoire (relative roles of CD4$^+$ T cell subsets and CD8$^+$ T cells)
    define cellular and cytokine components involved in immunity, tissue damage and memory
    assess roles of secretory and heat shock proteins in protection and regulation of inflammation
    develop longitudinal studies of protective immunity in immunocompetent/deficient individuals

Characterize molecular mechanisms controlling virulence and dormancy
    define genetic and phenotypic differences distinguishing virulent and avirulent strains
    elucidate the genetic basis of dormancy and persistence

Define biochemical structure relevant for the development of new drugs
    elucidate key biosynthetic pathways e.g. cell wall structure
    investigate access of drugs to sites of action
    define action of key enzymes involved in envelope and cell wall physiology and permeability

poor countries are opting for less efficacious regimens.

Nosocomial outbreaks

Most outbreaks are the consequence of poor infection control. Patients and health care workers are exposed to the source case because of (1) failure to diagnose disease; (2) failure to confine untreated active TB (or those on treatment for less than 2 days); and (3) failure to recognize drug-resistant TB (Bennett and Watson, 1994). Such a problem has been well exemplified at a London hospital (Kent *et al.*, 1994). US guidelines issued from the Centers for Disease Control and Prevention (CDC) in 1990 indicated need to limit exposure from infectious droplet nuclei with use of negative pressure isolation, 6 air changes an hour and air disinfection using ultraviolet light. Some authorities also advocated the use of respirator masks. Revised CDC guidelines from 1994 include the addition of high-efficiency particulate air (HEPA) filters. However, there is little evidence to support the benefits of these expensive devices and such control measures require field evaluation (Soeiro and Segal-Maurer, 1994). Adequate control measures should include isolation of the smear-positive source case during the first 2 weeks of treatment, ideally with a commode, an ante-room and negative pressure ventilation to the outside.

Multiple drug resistant tuberculosis (MDR-TB)

CDC reported 3% of new cases and 6.9% of recurrent cases in the US which were resistant to both rifampicin and isoniazid. Moreover, there have been 22 institutional outbreaks between 1990 and 1992 and the majority of cases were HIV positive. Those without HIV have a 50% treatment failure rate within 18–24 months (Bennett and Watson, 1994). For those with HIV, prognosis is particularly poor, with a mortality of 70–80% within 1–4 months of diagnosis (Benson, 1994). Whilst the majority of MDR-TB has occurred in pockets throughout North America, there is some evidence that rifampicin resistance may be increasing in Thailand and Tanzania (Kochi, Vareldzis and Styblo, 1993). High rates of MDR-TB have been recorded in West and Central Africa, with greater than 30% primary isoniazid resistance. However, drug resistance in East Africa prior to HIV was stable at 7% isoniazid resistance for over 30 years. Data from a cohort in Kenya show no evidence of a subsequent increase (Nunn, Elliott and McAdam, 1994).

Factors contributing to the development of MDR-TB include the following:

1. poor compliance;
2. a failing host immune system unable to contain disease;
3. inadequate infection control measures;
4. delays in recognition of resistance and request for susceptibility testing;
5. delays in changing to an appropriate regime; and
6. adding another drug when a case is not responding to conventional therapy.

Given the potential increases in both HIV and TB throughout the developing world, an increase in MDR-TB in poorer countries poses a major threat to tuberculosis control. Moreover, availability of drugs becomes a major issue for impoverished control programs. It is a research priority to survey meaningfully both initial and acquired drug resistance in control programs throughout the world (Vareldzis *et al.*, 1994).

A number of specific questions remain unsolved. Whilst superinfection with MDR-TB has been recognized in some HIV-infected TB patients, it is not known whether previous infection with MTB or BCG vaccination would offer some protection against MDR–

TB. Knowledge of this may have an important impact on the role of immunization in HIV-infected individuals. Nor is it known what chemoprophylactic regimen should be used to those individuals exposed to MDR-TB. Intriguing preliminary data have emerged on the use of *M. vaccae* to treat MDR-TB (*M. vaccae* is a heat-killed mycobacterium used as adjunctive immunotherapy for TB – see below) (Stanford and Grange, 1993). The most compelling data come from Romania where immunotherapy was used in the re-treatment of chemotherapy failures. Sputum culture positivity was reduced from 47% in the control group to 8% in the immunotherapy group 6 months after infection ($p<0.005$) (Stanford and Grange, 1993; Stanford, personal communication).

Genetic susceptibility of host

To date, there has been no clear identification of HLA genes encoding resistance or susceptibility to TB in humans. Several twin studies of tuberculosis have favored some genetic factors but these remain poorly characterized. Larger family studies assessing HLA co-segregation may identity susceptibility or resistance genes. This will have significant implications for epitope mapping by permitting their identification with the use of predicted peptide motifs (Hill *et al.*, 1991). Ultimately this will assist in vaccine development.

PATHOGENESIS

Virulence factors – host intracellular killing and organism survival strategies

The macrophage utilizes several intracellular mechanisms to inhibit or kill intracellular MTB (Kaufmann, 1993). These include: phagosome acidification; phagolysosomal fusion; and development of reactive nitrogen and oxygen intermediates. MTB manages to survive by: neutralization of phagosomal pH; inhibition of phagolysosomal fusion; and resistance to lysosomal enzymes. The relative importance of reactive oxygen and nitrogen intermediates is a moot point. However, some experimental evidence suggests that they may induce tuberculostasis. The induction of heat shock in the organism may help inhibit the effects of these intermediates (Kaufmann, 1993). Macrophages are a heterogeneous group of cells and their ability to prevent MTB replication may depend on activation by interferon-γ. Further characterization of macrophage killing and intracellular survival strategies may result in the development of novel chemotherapeutic agents capable of undermining organism survival. Furthermore, knowledge concerning factors leading to enhanced macrophage activation may direct the development of cytokine therapy. For example, exogenous site-specific interleukin-12 could play a role in refractory serosal disease (Zhang *et al.*, 1991).

Other virulence factors

As well as displaying elegant intracellular survival strategies, virulent strains of MTB demonstrate other distinguishing qualities which set them apart from their avirulent siblings. These include macrophage adherence; ability to invade cells; and augmentation of macrophage phagocytosis. Both the complement component receptor, CR3, and mannose receptors appear to be important in adherence and subsequent phagocytosis. Cloning strategies have defined further virulence factors. Loci encoding enhanced macrophage invasion, phagocytosis, survival and contact-dependent cytolytic activity have been identified and these activities have been induced in *E. coli* (Bennett and Watson, 1994). Studies are required to further screen plasmid gene bank libraries for genetic differences distinguishing virulent from avirulent strains.

Mycobacterial structural studies to assist in drug development

Many of the effects of antimicrobial drugs are mediated by inhibiting synthesis or function of enzymatic and structural proteins. Microorganisms have developed strategies to overcome such inhibition. These include destruction of the antimicrobial agents, development of alternative metabolic pathways and prevention of access of drugs to their site of action. Mycobacterial structural studies are important to characterize potential drugs and enable the development of interventions that circumvent drug resistance. Priorities that should facilitate such understanding are as follows:

1. knowledge concerning the mode of action of key enzymes involved in cell wall physiology and permeability;
2. analysis of functional macromolecules;
3. investigation of access of drugs to sites of action; and
4. elucidation of key biosynthetic pathways.

Genetic basis of dormancy and persistence

M. tuberculosis has the ability to alter its physiological state and become metabolically inactive and undetectable by the host immune system. In about 5% of infected immunocompetent individuals such 'persister' organisms then reactivate to cause disease, usually many years later. Why this occurs and what genetic switch initiates such 'waking up' is not known. One could also postulate that recrudescence might occur as a consequence of waning immunity. For example, memory T cells could be performing an immune surveillance role and curb the growth of metabolically reactivated organisms released from otherwise dormant tuberculous foci. This would explain the high rates of tuberculous reactivation in immunocompromised individuals but not in otherwise healthy adults. It would be very useful to know the genetic mechanism underlying dormancy, particularly as this may lead to the development of inhibiting such persistence. Understanding dormancy and persistence is a major priority if we are to challenge the organism's ability to evade both a seemingly adequate immune response and chemotherapy given for courses shorter than 6 months. Development of an animal model of dormancy would be especially useful.

Evidence that HIV enhances susceptibility to TB

Human $CD4^+$ T cell depletion appears to enhance the risk of primary progression and reactivation of latent TB. Specifically, $CD4^+$ cytotoxic-T lymphocyte (CTL) activity is impaired and the degree of impairment correlates with $CD4^+$ lymphocyte depletion (Forte *et al.*, 1992). HIV is known to infect macrophages and this may also contribute to impairment of anti-mycobacterial function.

Evidence that TB enhances HIV replication

Blood monocytes from HIV-negative TB patients show an enhanced *in vitro* susceptibility to productive HIV infection (Toossi *et al.*, 1993). Indirect evidence from Uganda is also suggested by the enhanced release of TNF-α and β-2-microglobulin from both T cells and macrophages derived from dually infected Ugandans. Levels were lower in three control groups including: treated HIV-infected TB patients, HIV-infected individuals without TB and TB patients without HIV (Wallis *et al.*, 1993). TNF-α is a pro-inflammatory cytokine which is known to increase HIV replication. β-2-microglobulin reflects immune activation and acts as a surrogate marker for disease progression. The results of further studies which are under way in the Gambia will specifically assess viral load and may confirm this association. A small but important clinical trial demonstrated a reduction in disease progression and death in a group of HIV-infected Haitians latently infected with TB who were given isoniazid prophylaxis for 12 months (Pape *et al.*, 1993). This requires further verification in larger controlled studies and such studies are under way in Africa.

T cell contribution to immunity

Human immunity to tuberculosis is poorly understood. In mice, there is good evidence for genetically mediated host resistance. Moreover, lymphokine-activated mouse macrophages can effectively kill MTB. However, in this case, mice and men differ and MTB seems relatively resistant to killing by interferon-γ-activated human macrophages (Rook *et al.*, 1986). Evidence from mouse cellular kinetic studies suggests a complex set of events characterizing initial protection, induction of memory, delayed-type hypersensitivity (DTH) and memory. Phenotypically and functionally distinct T cell sub-populations emerge and disappear during the course of infection (Orme, Andersen and Boom, 1993). A CD4$^+$ Th1-type subset of T cells (interferon-γ secreting) is thought to occur early in the infection and is associated with activation of tissue macrophages, induction of both memory T cells and DTH, and the development of granulomas. A CD4$^+$ Th2-type T cell subset (IL-4 and IL-10 secreting) follows and this is thought to be associated with downregulation of the inflammatory response within granuloma. T cells may also contribute to macrophage lysis and immune regulation. Others have not found such clear patterns of cytokine release (Bennett and Watson, 1994). Moreover, evidence from human *in vitro* work suggests a role for CD4$^+$ CTL either in lysis of functionally incapacitated macro-

phages or perhaps immune tissue damage (Forte *et al.*, 1992). In addition, a finding by Flynn and colleagues demonstrated the importance murine of CD8$^+$ T cells which were previously considered non-essential. β-2-microglobulin gene-disrupted mice (lacking functional CD8$^+$ T cells) died of overwhelming tuberculosis but were unaffected by BCG (Flynn *et al.*, 1992). These studies represent important breakthroughs in the understanding of the complex cellular and cytokine events occurring in the immune response against tuberculosis. Nevertheless, mouse studies are limited. In order to confirm or refute the relative roles played by immune cell populations identified in mice, it is necessary to define the immune repertoire in humans.

Immunoendocrine aspects of TB – regulation of the Th1/Th2 balance

It has long been recognized that there is two-way interaction between the immune system and the hypothalamic–pituitary–adrenal axis (HPA). Specific pathways permitting this 'cross-talk' have been identified. For example, glucocorticoids bias the immune response in favor of a Th2-type response (antibody production and down-regulation of cell-mediated responses) and dehydroepiandrosterone (DHEA), acting as a antiglucocorticoid, promotes a Th1-type response. Thus, the Th1/Th2 balance is determined, in part, by the balance of steroid hormones in the lymphoid microenvironment (Rook, Hernandez-Pando and Lightman, 1994). This is supported by evidence implicating a shift from a Th1–type to a Th2-type response in both HIV infection and TB. This shift is associated with a fall in both DHEA levels and the DHEA-cortisol ratio (Rook, Onyebujoh and Stanford, 1993). A clearer understanding of these complicated immunoendocrine pathways may permit intervention – perhaps with adjuvants with potent Th1-inducing properties or hormone analogs.

Viral constructs to dissect the human immune response

Utilizing viral vectors expressing recombinant mycobacterial proteins offers one method for dissection of the human immune response. Both vaccinia and adenovirus constructs could be used to expand human CTL precursors and infect target cells for assessment in a CTL assay. They would be of particular value in assessing the role of $CD8^+$ T cells and cytosolic antigen processing: a cell population found to be essential in protection in mice. Such recombinants would also be beneficial in mouse protection studies and offer a means to assess promising immunodominant antigens.

Immunodominant or 'oligodominant'?

It is important to define antigens capable of inducing protective immunity prior to the development of a vaccine. A group of 33 tuberculous proteins can be categorized by their property of being exported out of the bacillus. Such secretory proteins are only found in live, actively metabolizing organisms and immunization with several of them appear to confer both protection and memory early in the course of disease (Orme, Andersen and Boom, 1993). Whilst no one protein appears to be immunodominant and thus suitable for the development of a single antigen vaccine, a group of 'oligodominant' antigens may well confer protection within a heterogeneous human population. Studies are required to define which antigens are important. To date, some of the likely candidates include the antigen 85 complex (30–32 kDa), a small 6 kDa protein, a 12 kDa heat-shock protein, a 25 kDa superoxide dismutase protein and a 38 kDa phosphate-binding protein (Orme, Andersen and Boom, 1993).

Vaccine design – what vehicle?

Vaccine design not only requires a suitable repertoire of antigens: the vehicle or adjuvant accompanying the antigen also contributes to antigen processing and immunogenicity. Silva and Lowrie demonstrated mouse protection utilizing mycobacterial hsp 60 expressed as a recombinant in a macrophage-like cell line (Silva and Lowrie, 1994). Both MHC Class I and Class II antigen presentation were identified. Thus, this live cellular vehicle was able to induce both $CD4^+$ and $CD8^+$ T cell immunity – a likely prerequisite for the induction of immunity. Further studies must address the issue of using live vehicles for vaccination, with consideration given to induction of more than one T cell subset. Non-replicating pox and adenoviruses represent one means of achieving some of these goals without the risk of disseminated vaccine infection in an immunocompromised host. BCG is limited in effect in that it only appears to prevent blood-borne dissemination (miliary disease or childhood meningitis). Its major failing is that it is unable to induce pulmonary mucosal immunity, the mucosa being the main site of infection. Vaccine studies should address this issue with studies utilizing aerosolized vaccination. Genetically manipulated BCG and MTB may be suitable 'vehicles' for induction of immunity. Modification of BCG may require the addition of missing genetic elements required for full immunogenesis. Approaches specifically to attenuate MTB may also be beneficial.

Immunopathogenesis and the Koch phenomenon – a role for *Mycobacterium vaccae*?

Tissue damage is in part mediated by the host immune response. Some individuals develop an excessive and necrotizing inflammatory response (the Koch phenomenon) associated with very high levels of pro-inflammatory cytokines such as TNF-α and IL-6 (Rook and al Attiyah, 1991). Inability to downregulate inflammation may represent one extreme end of a continuum between Th1-mediated macrophage activation and Th2-mediated control of excessive immune damage. Whilst macrophage activation is essential in order to contain and kill MTB, exaggerated inflammation may be detrimental and result in marked caseous necrosis, fibrosis and persistence of metabolically inactive organisms within the necrotic debris. Adjunctive immunotherapy with killed *M. vaccae*, one of the environmental mycobacteria, may induce a switch from an inappropriate immune response (Koch-type) to an appropriate one (Listeria-type) (Stanford *et al.*, 1990). Evidence to date is encouraging but mostly anecdotal. A large placebo-controlled trial, underway in South Africa, should clarify its role both for those dually infected with TB and HIV and those singly infected with TB.

Reassessment of corticosteroids in the context of HIV

Indications for the use of corticosteroids as an adjunct in treating tuberculosis remain unclear and there are a number of theoretical reasons against their use (Rook, Onyebujoh and Stanford, 1993; Rook, Hernandez-Pendo and Lightman, 1994). However, many authorities would argue for their use in tuberculous pericarditis, meningitis and critically enlarging lymphadenitis. These drugs are recognized immunosuppressive agents and will exacerbate herpes, candida and bacterial infections. Nevertheless, tuberculosis causes chronic immune activation with a concomitant increase in HIV replication. Combining corticosteroids with effective anti-tuberculous chemotherapy may inhibit progression of HIV disease. It is impossible to say whether such an intervention will be deleterious or beneficial. Carefully controlled trials are required to answer this question.

DIAGNOSIS

Tuberculin testing

Whilst skin testing plays an important epidemiological role, it has only limited value for individual diagnosis (Bennett and Watson, 1994). A positive test in BCG-negative contacts remains a useful marker for infection and thus identifies the need for prophylaxis. Research into identifying alternative DTH-inducing antigens such as highly specific peptides may improve positive and negative prediction by distinguishing BCG vaccinees or environmental exposure from active or past infection. However, anergy will always hamper the value of skin testing in immunocompromised individuals.

Microbial identification

The likely diagnosis is rapidly achieved when a clinical sample stains positive for acid-fast bacilli (AFB). Smear positivity rates can be improved with cytocentrifugation (Saceanu, Pfeiffer and McLean, 1993). However, whilst a useful indicator for initial management, a number of problems remain outstanding: such as (1) increasing immune depression is associated with a higher incidence of smear-negative disease; (2) the presence of AFB does not exclude atypical mycobacteria, such as *Mycobacterium avium-intracellulare* (MAI) complex (although this latter diagnosis is unlikely in Africa); and (3) drug susceptibility cannot be deduced.

Species identification and drug susceptibility have been very slow. In sophisticated laboratories, rapid diagnosis and susceptibility testing can be achieved within 10–21 days using radiometric culture, nucleic acid probes and high performance liquid chromatography of mycolic acids. This is in contrast to the usual 6–10 weeks required with standard laboratory practice (Hopewell, 1992). However, such facilities are not available to the developing world and, without dramatic modification, nor are they likely to be.

Polymerase chain reaction (PCR) – research tool or routine test?

Several assay refinements and modifications have established PCR as a useful research tool used in both identification and strain-specific fingerprinting. However, it remains in its infancy as a tool for routine diagnosis with high specificity but poor sensitivity due to the presence of inhibitors in sputum (Clarridge *et al.*, 1993). Several groups have assessed its clinical applicability. Problems include false positives from PCR carryover; specimen contamination; or inability to distinguish active disease from those with prior or inactive disease. The IS6110 sequence, unique to MTB, produces highly sensitive and specific results for smear positive samples but sensitivity is poor when smear-negative, culture-positive samples are included. Once the problem of false positive results is minimized, PCR may be useful for culture-negative clinical specimens and more rapid diagnosis of smear-negative specimens (Wilson *et al.*, 1993).

Given the urgency for rapid diagnosis of tuberculosis, there is a need for a universal and robust PCR procedure which is translatable into routine public health laboratories. Ideally, this should include efficient recovery of organism, isolation of DNA, internal controls to detect presence of inhibitor and assess efficiency of amplification, and perhaps a two-step procedure, one to identify mycobacterial species and another to identify MTB. A simpler amplicon detection system utilizing an ELISA format would also be more applicable for the developing world.

DNA fingerprinting and molecular epidemiology

The unique repetitive insertion sequence, IS6110, permits generation of strain-speci-

fic fingerprints using restriction fragment length polymorphism (RFLP). Thus the specific transfer of infection, including multidrug-resistant (MDR) strains, can be monitored within a population. It can also assist in assessing the impact of various prophylaxis interventions by distinguishing relapse from new infection, i.e. failure of prophylaxis to sterilize, or reinfection occurring after the prophylaxis has finished. Some Indian isolates lack or have very few copies of IS6110. However, fingerprinting can be successfully performed using either a polymorphic GC-rich repetitive sequence or 36 base pair direct repeat element (van Soolingen *et al.*, 1993). Conventional RFLP requires 1–2 weeks of culture to obtain enough DNA, thus limiting its use when monitoring an outbreak. The addition of PCR to the assay saves time. Again, cost and labor intensity limit its use in routine clinical laboratories and there is need to develop simple, robust and less costly methods.

Novel molecular techniques

An intriguing technique may permit very rapid detection of both organism and susceptibility testing. Viable mycobacteria can be infected with reporter phages expressing the firefly luciferase gene resulting in photon release in only the live organisms. Moreover, the light goes out with the addition of an anti-tuberculous drug to drug-sensitive strain of MTB (Jacobs Jr, *et al.*, 1993). Jacobs and colleagues hope to produce a phage that will work with the small number of cells found in sputum samples. Variations of this theme are predicted since reporter phages are not always effective at colonizing all mycobacterial strains.

Up until now species identification has depended on the use of several nucleic acid probes identifying only a narrow range of species. A well grown culture is also required. However, a direct sequence determination from PCR product of a hypervariable region within the 16s ribosome has permitted speciation of clinical isolates.

TREATMENT

In the USA, the Advisory Council on the Elimination of Tuberculosis (ACET) has advocated a 9-month regimen for HIV-infected TB patients. The initial 8-week induction should include 4 drugs: isoniazid (H), rifampicin (R), pyrazinamide (Z) and either ethambutol (E) or streptomycin (S) daily or directly observed twice/thrice weekly. Susceptibility testing should be done for all initial isolates. The continuation phase requires drug susceptibility results before a change can be made to rifampicin and isoniazid given alone for 7 months (WHO notation; 2HRZE, 7HR) plus conversion to culture-negative for at least 6 months. Where drug susceptibility testing is not available, either streptomycin or ethambutol should be added to the continuation phase. This regimen is similar in all but duration to those who are HIV-negative. Greater than 95% of US TB patients will receive at least two drugs which will be effective against their strain (Centers for Disease Control, 1993).

Whilst this regimen approaches the council of perfection, developing countries are unable to implement such guidelines; particularly with regard to HIV testing of all patients and performing, universal drug susceptibility testing. Previously, the International Union against Tuberculosis and Lung Disease have advocated a cheaper, modified short-course regimen applicable to the developing world. Rifampicin was only given during the induction phase and thiacetazone (T) was added to isoniazid for a longer, 6-month continuation phase (2SHRZ/6TH). Thiacetazone has since been associated with an unacceptably high level of severe and often fatal side effects in adults and children (Chintu *et al.*, 1993; Nunn, Elliott and McAdam, 1994) and WHO no

longer advocates its use in HIV-infected TB patients. But it is still a very cheap drug and it may not be viable to dispense with it completely. Streptomycin should also be avoided given the potential for parenteral transmission of HIV and HBV (Raviglione, Narain and Kochi, 1922).

Studies are required on three levels: (1) to assess modified short course regimens not using rifampicin during the continuation phase; (2) to define those at low-risk to thiacetazone-induced skin reactions, particularly where this drug is being selected for economic reasons; and (3) to compare daily with intermittent regimens, particularly with respect to the use of longer half-life rifamycins such as rifapentine. Such studies should judge adverse effects, compliance, mortality rates, time taken to culture-negativity and relapse rates.

Treatment of MDR-TB

Initially, HIV-positive patients with proven or suspected MDR-TB should receive 5–6 drugs when (1) the strain is known to be multiply resistant; (2) TB was contracted in the setting of other cases of MDR-TB; or (3) where the patient had previously been treated with antituberculous drugs (Centers for Disease Control, 1993; Iseman, 1993). If the sensitivity is known, at least 3 sensitive drugs should be given for 18–24 months plus greater than 12 months from culture conversion. The mortality is high despite these measures and approaches 80% within 4 months. This poor prognosis is partly a consequence of (1) delay in diagnosis (presentation may be atypical); (2) disease in an already immunocompromised host; and (3) failure to recognize drug resistance requiring a change to the most aggressive MDR regimen. However, prognosis in HIV-infected patients with susceptible MTB is considerably better. Thus, the only hope is to limit both the development of MDR-TB and produce new and effective agents.

Poor compliance

From a public health perspective, a patient who has no treatment is better than one who completes only weeks of treatment. The development of secondary drug resistance in poorly compliant patients represents a major hurdle to effective control both in terms of reducing transmission and the development of MDR-TB. However, the patient cannot always be blamed. Many countries lack a regular supply of antituberculous therapy and treatment facilities are extremely pressurized. This results in poor patient supervision, premature hospital discharge of smear-positive cases and inadequate patient education. Research is needed into ways to increase compliance. Such studies should take into account social, cultural, economic and behavioral factors. Several strategies have been employed successfully in different countries. These include intermittent, locally based, directly observed therapy where non-medically trained supervisors such as store owners would monitor therapy given twice weekly (Wilkinson, 1994). Other examples include daily home-based therapy in Botswana and a system of paying back an initial deposit when the patient completes their regimen in Bangladesh. The administration of tablets to patients in blister packs may further aid self-medication. However, without financial backing to maintain a basic standard of case finding and treatment, a program designed to improve compliance will have no value.

Case finding and treatment

Prior to HIV, incidence of tuberculosis appeared to be on the wane. With adequate drugs and effective public health measures it was felt that this disease might effectively disappear. Thus, research and funding diminished and public health services shrank. Since the unexpected upsurge with the confounding problem of MDR-TB, it has become even more essential to break the cycle of transmission. This requires case finding, treatment and case holding. It is not known why patients with diagnosed disease fail to attend or why health care workers fail to diagnose disease. As discussed above, factors concerning compliance are poorly understood.

PREVENTION

Prevention can be achieved by improving living standards, case-finding and treatment, chemoprophylaxis and vaccination. The first of these appears, sadly, to be the most difficult to achieve. Case control has been discussed above. The relative contribution to prevention by drug prophylaxis and vaccination is hotly debated, particularly in non-industrialized countries where control programs may be overstretched and heavy water-borne and other environmental mycobacterial exposure occurs from birth and may strongly impinge on the benefit of BCG.

Chemoprophylaxis

The policy in the USA is clear. People who are HIV-positive, have not had previous BCG (most of the population of North America), and have a positive skin test, should receive preventative therapy. Moreover, additional recipients should include those contacts who are anergic and any HIV-infected individual from an area where TB is endemic despite a negative skin test (Moreno *et al.*, 1993). Pape and colleagues showed reduction in incidence of TB measured at 5 years in HIV-infected PPD-positive Haitian individuals given 12 months of daily isoniazid (Pape *et al.*, 1993).

It is questionable whether this is a realistic proposition in the developing world. Cost benefit analysis is essential to assess the potential savings made in both monetary and human terms. There are major logistical, financial and political problems associated with nationwide application. Controlled trials are needed to solve these issues. Two large studies are underway in Kenya and Zambia; the latter study compares six months' isoniazid with three months of combined rifampicin and pyrazinamide. The results could advocate a role for selected prophylaxis for sites such as HIV clinics, self-referral centers, commercial organizations or highly motivated workforces such as the military, police or health care workers. However, a place for massive community prophylaxis might be viable, particularly if long-duration rifamycins, such as rifapentine, could be shown to sterilize infected individuals, together with a low side-effect profile and minimal risk of inducing drug resistance. A further problem includes reinfection which may occur after the prophylactic regimen. DNA fingerprinting can be used to assess the proportion of reactivation from failed sterilization or new infections.

There has been no published prospective study for the effect of prophylaxis on those exposed to drug-resistant MTB. The following regimens have been suggested but remain unproven until the results of trials are available. These include rifampicin alone; rifampicin and pyrazinamide; rifampicin combined with ethambutol; pyrazinamide combined with ethambutol; or pyrazinamide combined with a fluoroquinolone. It would also be valuable to assess rifapentine, a longer acting rifamycin.

Vaccination – efficacy of BCG

Over 3 billion doses of BCG have been given, making it the most widely distributed vaccine known. However, the effectiveness of BCG against tuberculosis is in doubt (Ponnighaus *et al.*, 1992). It seems likely that the main efficacy is in reducing bacillemia, resulting in both less miliary and childhood meningitis. Thus, BCG does not prevent infection but limits the initial spread. It is not particularly effective in preventing primary complexes, local extension into the lung parenchyma or lymphadenopathy.

There has been no randomized control study of BCG on HIV-positive individuals and the Immunization Practices Advisory Committee (ACIP) of the United States Public Health Service state that BCG should not be given to HIV-positive individuals. WHO advises that BCG can be given to asymptomatic HIV-positive individuals in areas with high risk of TB infection (Weltman and Rose, 1993). There are over 15 studies underway to assess its benefit in infants born to HIV-infected mothers in Africa (Weltman and Rose, 1993). Whilst there is no clear role for a booster, vaccination may be more effective at 3 months, both in terms of immunogenicity and increased uptake, as many mothers deliver at home, away from health care services. The expanded program of immunization could more readily target 3-month-old infants as part of their program. Operational studies are required to assess this possibility.

There is no proven benefit from BCG in the HIV-infected; there is a potential risk of local or disseminated BCG disease; and there is also the potential risk of enhanced HIV replication from vaccine-induced CD4$^+$ T cell activation. However, there is no *in vivo* evidence of accelerated HIV immunosuppression from other vaccinations. Moreover, in a review of case reports of HIV-positive BCG complications, regardless of severity, the outcomes were generally favorable (Weltman and Rose, 1993). In studies with denominator data (4 prospective cohort studies) there was no obvious increase in rates of BCG complications. However, such studies are not conclusive. In some cases, there was a problem with inadequate controls, no record of type of BCG strain was recorded, and details such as dose and route of inoculum were often lacking. Also it was not clear whether infants were HIV-infected or only serologically positive. BCG-related abscess formation with lymph node involvement was a consequence of a change to the more virulent Pasteur strain of BCG and not HIV-positivity (Weltman and Rose, 1993). Overall, no clear problems have been identified with BCG vaccination in asymptomatic HIV-positive individuals (Reichman, 1989). It is possible that cases are occurring but not being identified and reported and that these will increase as greater numbers of HIV-positive BCG vaccinees become more immunosuppressed or, alternatively, cases do not occur at higher rates in those who are HIV-infected. BCG-related illness is a rare event. Case reports, therefore, must be interpreted with caution (Weltman and Rose, 1993). Controlled studies of adequate size and duration are needed to confirm association and quantify risk. Whilst cohort or case-control data could provide information on the more common local problems (abscess formation and lymph node involvement), only a case-control study would be feasible to assess rarer disseminated disease. This would need to be derived from surveillance data covering 10 000 vaccinees and an effective reference laboratory able to distinguish TB from BCG.

PNEUMOCYSTIS CARINII PNEUMONIA (PCP)

Research priorities for *Pneumocystis carinii* infection are summarized in Table 25.2. A fuller discussion of these priorities is given below.

EPIDEMIOLOGY

There has been a significant reduction in both the morbidity and mortality of PCP as a consequence of early recognition, rapid diagnostic confirmation and aggressive treatment. Furthermore, in countries where PCP is common, primary and secondary prophylaxis have brought about a decline in incidence (Decker and Masur, 1994). How-

ever, PCP will continue to remain a problem among those individuals who are unaware of being HIV-infected, have poor access to health care or who opt not to take prophylaxis. In most parts of the industrialized world, PCP still remains the case defining illness for the majority of patients presenting with AIDS. If further improvements are desired, then it will be necessary to provide an environment to encourage healthy, high-risk individuals to test for HIV infection. The main argument for such testing is to enable commencement of PCP prophylaxis when CD4$^+$T cell counts drop below 200 cells/μl. It is also necessary to improve compliance and convince skeptics of the value of PCP prophylaxis. Given the recognized toxicity of co-trimoxazole, readiness to accept primary prophylaxis would be particularly facilitated by the discovery of an equally effective but less toxic alternative.

PCP in Africa – improve diagnosis or a clinical algorithm

Interestingly, PCP is relatively uncommon in Africa. For example, only 9% of deaths from a respiratory ward, in a postmortem study in Abidjan, Côte d'Ivoire, were due to PCP (Abouya *et al.*, 1992). The organism appears to be generally ubiquitous and thus it is hard to explain the apparent rarity in Africa (Atzori *et al.*, 1993; Daley, 1994; Machiels and Urban, 1992). One possible interpretation is that AIDS patients in Africa die of other HIV-related problems such as tuberculosis before the CD4$^+$T cell count drops to the level associated with PCP. This argument is flawed by the fact that cryptococcal meningitis is particularly common in Africa and is associated with a similar degree of immune suppression. In any event, PCP does occur in Africa, albeit relatively infrequently. Diagnosis of interstitial pneumonia remains a significant problem. There are particular difficulties in distinguishing PCP from bacterial

Table 25.2 Research priorities for *Pneumocystis carinii* infection

Define the problem in developing countries
   morbidity and mortality
   seasonality

Improve patient education
   encourage early diagnosis permitting wider primary prophylaxis coverage
   assess non-compliance and address methods for improvement

Improve diagnosis and management
   develop non-invasive, universally applicable and cheap tests
   optimize management algorithms for where diagnosis is unavailable

Identify improved anti-*Pneumocystis* agents
   make better use of available drugs
      reformulate atovaquone to improve bioavailability
      role for drug assay during treatment to minimize toxicity
   assess existing alternative drugs
   design new drugs
      based on molecular studies defining metabolic pathways unique to *Pneumocystis*

Optimize use of adjunctive steroids
   best regimen
   assess role in mild PCP ($PaO_2 > 90\,mmHg$)
   assess role in children

pneumonia, tuberculosis and Kaposi's sarcoma. Lack of fiberoptic bronchoscopy and an adequate pathology service contribute to the problem (Decker and Masur, 1994). WHO proposes an algorithmic approach to management (Piot *et al.*, 1992). In principle, this offers an excellent solution to the problems of inadequate facilities for diagnosis. However, clinical studies are required to evaluate the local applicability of an algorithm. The results of such research will permit this approach to be tailored to the needs of individual countries. Nevertheless, the long-term goal should be to ascertain the diagnosis. Immunofluorescence and polymerase chain reaction of induced sputum improve diagnostic yield but are, as yet, too expensive for the developing world. Research into a cheap and simple diagnostic test would greatly benefit resource-poor centers where PCP is a problem.

Co-trimoxazole remains the most effective drug

Despite many studies assessing the efficacy and side-effect profile of numerous agents, co-trimoxazole remains the most effective for both treatment and prophylaxis (Girard and Feinberg, 1994). It is clear that it is a more effective prophylactic agent than aerosolized pentamidine. In a European trial of primary prophylaxis, 11% of HIV-infected individuals developed PCP in the pentamidine arm (300 mg monthly) compared with none in two co-trimoxazole arms (one double-strength or one single-strength tablet daily). However, toxicity requiring discontinuation in the pentamidine group was very low (2 out of 71) compared with the other groups (17 out of 71 for low dose and 18 out of 71 for high dose co-trimoxazole) (Schneider *et al.*, 1992). Co-trimoxazole has the same pattern of high efficacy but significant toxicity for both secondary prophylaxis (Decker and Masur, 1994) and treatment (Girard and Feinberg, 1994). Seen favorably, the drug is a cheap oral preparation readily available throughout the world. Moreover, it is more likely to protect against disseminated PCP than aerosolized pentamidine and it may confer protection against toxoplasmosis, *Streptococcus pneumoniae*, *Salmonella* spp., *Staphylococcus aureus* and nocardiosis. However, approximately 25% of patients will be unable to tolerate it (Schneider *et al.*, 1992). Most adverse effects are mild and can be managed either symptomatically or with a switch to an alternative agent. But severe skin exfoliation or bone-marrow suppression are not uncommon and an equally effective but less toxic alternative is required.

Prophylactic alternatives to co-trimoxazole

Pentamidine has limited efficacy, it is expensive and there are significant logistic problems associated with a location for administration (Decker and Masur, 1994). This latter problem is particularly pertinent following the recognized association with nosocomial transmission of MDR-TB (Soeiro and Segal-Maurer, 1994). A number of other oral agents have been assessed for use as prophylaxis. They include dapsone, dapsone-pyrimethamine, dapsone-trimethoprim, sulfadoxine-pyrimethamine (Fansidar), primaquine-clindamycin and atovaquone. Except for dapsone and dapsone-pyrimethamine, the evidence for their efficacy is limited and further data are required before they can be considered anything but third-line alternatives. The data for dapsone and its combination with pyrimethamine are variable and may depend on dose and frequency of administration.

Several studies suggest that these drugs are well tolerated, of similar efficacy to aerosolized pentamidine but less effective than co-trimoxazole (Decker and Masur,

1994). When the largest dose of dapsone is used (100 mg daily), it appears to produce similar efficacy to co-trimoxazole but no improvement in toxicity (Blum *et al.*, 1992). It is doubtful if any of these alternative drugs will supersede co-trimoxazole. However, there is a clear need for an alternative and research should be directed into assessing potential agents. Techniques in molecular biology may be able to define metabolic pathways unique to *P. carinii*. Progress in this direction would permit the development of novel agents able to interfere selectively with its life cycle with minimal toxicity to the host.

Treatment alternatives to co-trimoxazole

Atovaquone, although approved for use in mild to moderate PCP, is much less effective than co-trimoxazole. One large randomized, double-blind head-on comparison between the two regimens demonstrated 11 deaths out of 160 in the atovaquone arm and only 1 death out of 162 in the co-trimoxazole arm ($p<0.003$). The treatment failures and deaths were associated with diarrhea and low plasma levels of atovaquone (Hughes *et al.*, 1993). It would be valuable to reformulate this poorly absorbed drug as it has a powerful anti-pneumocystis effect in an animal model and it has a much lower side-effect profile than the sulfa-based alternative. For the time being, it should only be used for mild disease in those patients who are intolerant to co-trimoxazole and who do not have diarrhea or malabsorption. Moreover, whilst there are no comparative data, the alternative regimens such as intravenous pentamidine, trimethoprim-dapsone and clindamycin-primaquine would also appear to be more effective. It is not known which of these regimens should be used as a second-line intervention for co-trimoxazole treatment failure or toxicity. Nor is it known when a switch should be considered. Research is being directed into answering ques-

Table 25.3 Research priorities for *Pneumococcus* infection

Epidemiology
    monitor extent of problem and identify those at risk
    possible role for specific chemoprophylaxis in targeted groups
    influence of co-trimoxazole prophylaxis

Vaccine
    optimize immunization with existing 23-valent polysaccharide vaccine e.g. give with
      anti-retrovirals
    assess role of protein-conjugate vaccines
    identify optimal regimen for protein-conjugate vaccines e.g. role for booster

Drug resistance
    monitor pattern of spread: community versus nosocomial
    optimize antibiotic use
      local antibiotic policy
      rapid identification and susceptibility testing
      medical education – avoiding unnecessary use of broad spectrum agents

---

tions on the use of comparative treatment regimes (Safrin *et al.*, 1996).

Role of corticosteroids

Several studies have established the benefit of adjunctive prednisolone for moderate ($PaO_2 < 70$ mmHg) to severe adult PCP if given within 3 days of presentation with improvements in both morbidity and mortality (Masur, 1992). It would be useful to know if the same were true for children. A small study of 11 children suggested that it was so. Three out of four ventilated children receiving adjuvant corticosteroids recovered from acute infection, whilst all seven ventilated children receiving antimicrobial therapy alone died (Sleasman *et al.*, 1993). A larger study is required to assess the role of corticosteroids in moderate as well as severe PCP in children. Additionally, it would be useful to know what impact corticosteroids would have on those with mild PCP. Whilst the majority make a satisfactory recovery, a small number continue to deteriorate despite seemingly adequate antimicrobial therapy. The potential toxicity related to corticosteroids has not been seen to be a problem.

A small placebo-controlled study assessing corticosteroids in mild PCP suggested that morbidity was significantly improved. This even included exercise tolerance on day 30 in those who received immediate as opposed to deferred prednisolone introduced 3 days later (Montaner *et al.*, 1993). Whilst the results are encouraging, the power of the study was too low to detect a difference in mortality or less common adverse effects. A larger study would be useful.

PNEUMOCOCCAL DISEASE

Research priorities for *Pneumococcus* infection are summarized in Table 25.3. These priorities are discussed in detail below.

EPIDEMIOLOGY

Invasive pneumococcal pneumonia is the most common bacterial respiratory tract infection among people with HIV. Prior to the HIV era in Africa, bacterial pneumonia (mainly due to *Streptococcus pneumoniae*) was a common cause of acute adult admission to general hospitals in East Africa. Since the advent of HIV, cohort and case-control studies have shown an increase rate among HIV-infected individuals (Daley, 1994; Gilks, 1993). There are similar findings in San Francisco where the rate of pneumococcal bacteremia is 100-fold greater in AIDS patients than the rate reported in patients before the HIV epidemic arose (Redd *et al.*, 1990). Interestingly, more than half of all the episodes of pneumococcal bacteremia occurred in HIV-infected patients without AIDS. This tendency to develop pneumococcal disease may reflect deficiency of IgG_2 which has been noted in AIDS patients.

VACCINATION

Pneumococcal vaccination should be a cost-effective way of protecting against invasive disease. However, in a large case-control study of immunocompetent and immunocompromised adults, protective efficacy was only effectively achieved in the immunocompetent group (56% compared with 21%) (Butler *et al.*, 1993). Antibody response in HIV-infected individuals can be improved with concomitant administration of zidovudine but overall the results are less than satisfactory (Mufson, 1994).

Alternatives to the 23-valent capsular polysaccharide vaccine

Polysaccharide vaccines are less immunogenic than protein vaccines. This is particularly pertinent for immunocompromised individuals and children under five. Chemical binding of immunogenic protein to the capsular polysaccharide vaccine may improve immunogenicity (Mufson, 1994). Candidate protein-conjugates include tetanus toxoid, pertussis toxin and outer membrane protein complex from *Neisseria meningitidis* serogroup B. The latter protein has been linked to *Haemophilus influenzae* and has produced a highly effective *H. influenzae* vaccine which is now widely used. Animal studies of protein-conjugate pneumococcal vaccines have demonstrated several important characteristics which distinguish this group of immunogens. Initial vaccination may fail to induce antibody in neonatal mice; but re-immunization can induce protection (Peeters *et al.* 1992). Monovalent conjugate-vaccines can induce type-specific antibody responses in nude athymic mice (Vella *et al.*, 1992). Such a response suggests that this type of vaccine may be more effective in those with impaired T cell immunity. Field trials of two different heptavalent pneumococcal polysaccharide-protein conjugate vaccines are taking place.

ANTIBIOTIC RESISTANCE

The number of pneumococcal strains resistant to penicillin is increasing. Surveillance conducted in South Africa from 1979 to 1988 described an average rate of penicillin resistance to be just below 10%. In the following 2 years this climbed to 16.3% and 14.1% respectively (Koornhof, Wasas and Klugman, 1992). Similar observations have been seen in France and Spain (Mufson, 1994). However, this geographic clustering will become less distinct with time. Highly resistant strains (MICs 4–8 μg/mol) and multiply-resistant pneumococci are occurring more and more frequently throughout the world. For example, 22 multiply resistant strains of serotype 23F were recovered in the US (McDougal *et al.*, 1992). Using genotype and ribotype profiles and penicillin protein-binding patterns, the majority of these could be traced back to an original clone from Spain. Further, such examples of transcontinental travel can only be expected. In order to stem the spread of multiply-resistant strains, vigilant pursuit and identification of the organism is required. Specific narrow spectrum antimicrobials should be selected as soon as susceptibility data are available. Collecting and publishing surveillance data, establishment and adherence to hospital antibiotic policy and medical education will all help to limit the spread. Molecular epidemiological techniques will also permit the rapid recognition of likely local strains and thus permit decisions concerning choice of blind therapy prior to the availability of laboratory data.

REFERENCES

Abouya, Y.L., Beaumel, A., Lucas, S. *et al.* (1992) *Pneumocystis carinii* pneumonia. An uncommon cause of death in African patients with acquired immunodeficiency syndrome. *Am. Rev. Respir. Dis.*, **145**, 617–20.

Atzori, C., Bruno, A., Chichino, G. *et al.* (1993) *Pneumocystis carinii* pneumonia and tuberculosis in Tanzanian patients infected with HIV. *Trans. R. Soc. Trop. Med. Hyg*, **87**, 55–6.

Bennett, D., Watson, J. (1994) Tuberculosis in the immunocompetent patient. *Curr. Op. Infect. Dis.*, **7**, 184–91.

Benson, C.A. (1994) *Mycobacterium tuberculosis* and *Mycobacterium avium* complex disease in patients with HIV infection. *Curr. Op. Infect. Dis.*, **7**, 95–107.

Blum, R.N., Miller, L.A., Gaggini, L.C. *et al.* (1992) Comparative trial of dapsone versus trimethoprim/sulfamethoxazole for primary prophylaxis of *Pneumocystis carinii* pneumonia. *J. Acquir. Imm. Defic. Syndr.*, **5**, 341–7.

Brindle, R. (1992) Aspects of tuberculosis in Africa. 2. The value of microbiology in the management of tuberculosis in Nairobi, Kenya. *Trans. R. Soc. Trop. Med. Hyg.*, **86**, 470–1.

Butler, J.C., Breiman, R.F., Campbell, J.F. *et al.* (1993) Pneumococcal polysaccharide vaccine efficacy. An evaluation of current recommendations. *JAMA*, **270**, 1826–31.

Centers for Disease Control (1993) Initial therapy for tuberculosis in the era of multidrug resistance. Recommendations of the Advisory Council for the Elimination of Tuberculosis. *MMWR. Morb. Mortal Wkly. Rep.*, **42**, 1–8.

Chintu, C., Luo, C., Bhat, G. *et al.* (1993) Cutaneous hypersensitivity reactions due to thiacetazone in the treatment of tuberculosis in Zambian children infected with HIV-I. *Arch. Dis. Child*, **68**, 665–8.

Clarridge, J.E.I., Shawar, R.M., Shinnick, T.M. *et al.* (1993) Large-scale use of polymerase chain reaction for detection of *Mycobacterium tuberculosis* in a routine mycobacteriology laboratory. *J. Clin. Microbiol.*, **31**, 2049–56.

Daley, C.L. (1994) Pulmonary infections in the tropics: impact of HIV infection. *Thorax*, **49**, 370–8.

Daley, C.L., Small, P.M., Schecter, G.F. *et al.* (1992) An outbreak of tuberculosis with accelerated progression among persons infected with the human immunodeficiency virus. An analysis using restriction-fragment-length polymorphisms. *N. Engl. J. Med.*, **326**, 231–5.

Decker, C.F., Masur, H. (1994) Current status of prophylaxis for opportunistic infections in HIV-infected patients. *AIDS*, **8**, 11–20.

Dolin, P.J., Raviglione, M.C. and Kochi, A. (1994) Global tuberculosis incidence and mortality during 1990–2000. *Bull. World Health Organ.*, **72**, 213–20.

Elliott, A.M., Hayes, R.J., Halwiindi, B. *et al.* (1993) The impact of HIV on infectiousness of pulmonary tuberculosis: a community study in Zambia. *AIDS*, **7**, 981–7.

Flynn, J.L., Goldstein, M.M., Triebold, K.J. *et al.* (1992) Major histocompatibility complex class I-restricted T cells are required for resistance to *Mycobacterium tuberculosis* infection. *Proc. Natl. Acad. Sci. USA*, **89**, 12013–17.

Forte, M., Maartens, G., Rahelu, M. *et al.* (1992) Cytolytic T-cell activity against mycobacterial antigens in HIV. *AIDS*, **6**, 407–11.

Gilks, C. (1993) Pneumococcal disease and HIV infection. *Ann. Intern. Med.*, **118**, 393.

Girard, P.M. and Feinberg, J. (1994) Progress and problems in AIDS-associated opportunistic infections. *AIDS*, **8**, S249–S259.

Hill, A.V., Allsopp, C.E., Kwiatkowski, D. *et al.* (1991) Common West African HLA antigens are associated with protection from severe malaria (see comments). *Nature*, **352**, 595–600.

Hopewell, P.C. (1992) Impact of human immunodeficiency virus infection on the epidemiology, clinical features, management, and control of tuberculosis. *Clin. Infect. Dis.*, **15**, 540–47.

Hughes, W., Leoung, G., Kramer, F. *et al.* (1993) Comparison of atovaquone (566C80) with trimethoprim-sulfamethoxazole to treat *Pneumocystis carinii* pneumonia in patients with AIDS. *N. Engl. J. Med.*, **328**, 1521–7.

Iseman, M.D. (1993) Treatment of multidrug-resistant tuberculosis. *N. Engl. J Med.*, **329**, 784–91.

Jacobs Jr, W.R., Barletta, R.G., Udani, R. *et al.* (1993) Rapid assessment of drug susceptibilities of *Mycobacterium tuberculosis* by means of luciferase reporter phages (see comments). *Science*, **260**, 819–22.

Kaufmann, S.H.E. (1993) Immunity to intracellular bacteria. *Annu. Rev. Immunol.*, **11**, 129–63.

Kent, R.J., Uttley, A.H., Stoker, N.G. *et al.* (1994) Transmission of tuberculosis in British centre for patients infected with HIV. *Br. Med. J.*, **309**, 639–40.

Kochi, A., Vareldzis, B., and Styblo, K. (1993) Multidrug-resistant tuberculosis and its control. *Res. Microbiol.*, **144**, 104–10.

Koornhof, H.J., Wasas, A. and Klugman, K. (1992) Antimicrobial resistance in *Streptococcus pneumoniae*: a South African perspective. *Clin. Infect. Dis.*, **15**, 84–94.

Machiels, G. and Urban, M.I. (1992) *Pneumocystis carinii* as a cause of pneumonia in HIV-infected patients in Lusaka, Zambia. *Trans. R. Soc. Trop. Med. Hyg.*, **86**, 399–400.

Masur, H. (1992) Prevention and treatment of pneumocystis pneumonia (published erratum appears in *N. Engl J. Med* 1993 Apr 15;**328**(15):1136). *N. Engl. J. Med.*, **327**, 1853–60.

McDougal, L.K., Facklam, R., Reeves, M *et al.* (1992) Analysis of multiply antimicrobial-resistant isolates of *Streptococcus pneumoniae* from the United States. *Antimicrob. Agents Chemother.*, **36**, 2176–84.

Montaner, J. S., Guillemi, S., Quieffin, J. *et al.* (1993) Oral corticosteroids in patients with mild *Pneumocystis carinii* pneumonia and the acquired immune deficiency syndrome (AIDS). *Tuber. Lung Dis.*, **74**, 173–9.

Moreno, S., Baraia Etxaburu, J., Bouza, E. *et al.* (1993) Risk for developing tuberculosis among anergic patients infected with HIV (see comments). *Ann. Intern. Med.*, **119**, 194–8.

Mufson, M.A. (1994) Pneumococcal infection. *Curr. Op. Infect. Dis.*, **7**, 178–83.

Narain, J.P., Raviglione, M.C. and Kochi, A. (1992) HIV-associated tuberculosis in developing countries: epidemiology and strategies for prevention. *Tuber. Lung Dis.*, **73**, 311–21.

Nunn, P.P., Elliott, A.M. and McAdam, K.P.W.J. (1994) Impact of human immunodeficiency virus on tuberculosis in developing countries. *Thorax*, **49**, 511–18.

Orme, I.M., Andersen, P. and Boom, W.H. (1993) T cell response to *Mycobacterium tuberculosis*. *J.*

Infect. Dis., **167**, 1481–7.

Pape, J.W., Jean, S.S., Ho, J.L. *et al.* (1993) Effect of isoniazid prophylaxis on incidence of active tuberculosis and progression of HIV infection. *Lancet*, **342**, 268–72.

Peeters, C.C., Tenbergen Meekes, A.M., Poolman, J.T. *et al.* (1992) Immunogenicity of a *Streptococcus pneumoniae* type 4 polysaccharide– protein conjugate vaccine is decreased by admixture of high doses of free saccharide. *Vaccine*, **10**, 833–40.

Piot, P., Kapita, B.M., Ngugi, E.N. *et al.* (1992) *Aids in Africa: a manual for physicians*. World Health Organization, Geneva, pp. 87.

Ponnighaus, J.M., Fine, P.E., Sterne, J.A. *et al.* (1992) Efficacy of BCG vaccine against leprosy and tuberculosis in northern Malawi (see comments). *Lancet*, **339**, 636–9.

Raviglione, M.C., Narain, J.P. and Kochi, A. (1992) HIV-associated tuberculosis in developing countries: clinical features, diagnosis, and treatment. *Bull. World Health Organ.*, **70**, 515–26.

Redd, S.C., Rutherford, G.W., Sande, M.A. *et al.* (1990) The role of human immunodeficiency virus infection in pneumococcal bacteremia in San Francisco residents. *J. Infect. Dis.*, **162**, 1012–7.

Reichman, L.B. (1989) Why hasn't BCG proved dangerous in HIV-infected patients? (letter) (see comments). *JAMA*, **261**, 3246.

Rook, G.A.W., Hernandez-Pando, R. and Lightman, S.L. (1994) Hormones, peripherally activated prohormones and regulation of the Th1/Th2 balance. *Immunol. Today*, **15**, 301–3.

Rook, G.A. and al Attiyah, R. (1991) Cytokines and the Koch phenomenon. *Tubercle*, **72**, 13–20.

Rook, G.A., Onyebujoh, P. and Stanford, J.L. (1993) TH1/TH2 switching and loss of CD4+ T cells in chronic infections: an immunoendocrinological hypothesis not exclusive to HIV (letter). *Immunol. Today*, **14**, 568–9.

Rook, G.A., Steele, J., Ainsworth, M. *et al.* (1986) Activation of macrophages to inhibit proliferation of *Mycobacterium tuberculosis*: comparison of the effects of recombinant gamma-interferon on human monocytes and murine peritoneal macrophages. *Immunology*, **59**, 333–8.

Saceanu, C.A., Pfeiffer, N.C. and McLean, T. (1993) Evaluation of sputum smears concentrated by cytocentrifugation for detection of acid-fast bacilli. *J. Clin. Microbiol.*, **31**, 2371–4.

Safrin, A., Finkelstein, D.M., Feinberg, J. *et al.* (1996) Comparison of three regimens for treatment of mild to moderate *Pneumocystis carinii* pneumonia in patients with AIDS. *Ann. Intern. Med.*, **124**, 9, 792–802.

Schneider, M.M., Hoepelman, A.I., Eeftinck Schattenkerk, J.K. *et al.* (1992) A controlled trial of aerosolized pentamidine or trimethoprim-sulfamethoxazole as primary prophylaxis against *Pneumocystis carinii* pneumonia in patients with human immunodeficiency virus infection. The Dutch AIDS Treatment Group (see comments). *N. Engl. J. Med.*, **327**, 1836–41.

Schulzer, M., Fitzgerald, J.M., Enarson, D.A. *et al.* (1992) An estimate of the future size of the tuberculosis problem in Sub-Saharan Africa resulting from HIV infection (published erratum appears in *Tuber. Lung Dis.*, 1992 Aug;73(4):245-6). *Tuber. Lung Dis.*, **73**, 52–8.

Silva, C.L. and Lowrie, D.B. (1994) A single mycobacterial protein (hsp 65) expressed by a transgenic antigen-presenting cell vaccinates mice against tuberculosis. *Immunology*, **82**, 244–8.

Sleasman, J.W., Hemenway, C., Klein, A.S. *et al.* (1993) Corticosteroids improve survival of children with AIDS and *Pneumocystis carinii* pneumonia. *Am. J. Dis. Child*, **147**, 30–4.

Soeiro, R. and Segal-Maurer, S. (1994) Tuberculosis: nosocomial transmission and control of infection. *AIDS*, **8**, S239–S247.

Stanford, J.L. and Grange, J.M. (1993) New concepts for the control of tuberculosis in the twenty first century. *J. R. Coll. Phys. Lond.*, **27**, 218–23.

Stanford, J.L., Rook, G.A., Bahr, G. *et al.* (1990) *Mycobacterium vaccae* in immunoprophylaxis and immunotherapy of leprosy and tuberculosis. *Vaccine*, **8**, 525–30.

Toossi, Z., Sierra Madero, J.G., Blinkhorn, R.A. *et al.* (1993) Enhanced susceptibility of blood monocytes from patients with pulmonary tuberculosis to productive infection with human immunodeficiency virus type 1. *J. Exp. Med.*, **177**, 1511–6.

van Soolingen, D., de Haas, P.E., Hermans, P.W. *et al.* (1993) Comparison of various repetitive DNA elements as genetic markers for strain differentiation and epidemiology of *Mycobacterium tuberculosis*. *J. Clin. Microbiol.*, **31**, 1987–95.

Vareldzis, B.P., Grosset, J., de Kantor, *et al.* (1994) Drug-resistant tuberculosis: laboratory issues. *Tuber. Lung Dis.*, **75**, 1–7.

Vella, P.P., Marburg, S., Staub, J.M. *et al.* (1992) Immunogenicity of conjugate vaccines consisting of pneumococcal capsular polysaccharide types 6B, 14, I9F, and 23F and a meningococcal outer membrane protein complex. *Infect. Immun.*, **60**, 4977–83.

Wallis, R.S., Vjecha, M., Amir Tahmasseb, M. *et al.* (1993) Influence of tuberculosis on human immunodeficiency virus (HIV-1): enhanced cytokine expression and elevated beta 2-microglobulin in HIV-1-associated tuberculosis. *J. Infect. Dis.*, **167**, 43–8.

Weltman, A.C. and Rose, D.N. (1993) The safety of Bacille Calmette-Guérin vaccination in HIV infection and AIDS (editorial). *AIDS*, **7**, 149–57.

Wilkinson, D. (1994) High-compliance tuberculosis treatment programme in a rural community. *Lancet*, **343**, 647–8.

WHO (1995) *Tuberculosis and HIV Research: working Towards Solutions*. WHO/TB/95, 193.

Wilson, S.M., McNerney, R., Nye, P.M. *et al.* (1993) Progress toward a simplified polymerase chain reaction and its application to diagnosis of tuberculosis. *J. Clin. Microbiol.*, **31**, 776–82.

Zhang, Y., Lathigra, R., Garbe, T. *et al.* (1991) Genetic analysis of superoxide dismutase, the 23 kilodalton antigen of *Mycobacterium tuberculosis*. *Mol. Microbiol.*, **5**, 381–91.

INDEX

Page numbers appearing in **bold** refer to figures and page numbers in *italic* refer to tables. There is no main entry under AIDS; look for specific aspects of AIDS under the aspect itself. There are general entries under HIV and more specific entries under HIV-1 and HIV-2. Abbreviations: CMV=Cytomegalovirus; HIV=human immunodeficiency virus; KS=Kaposi's sarcoma; LIP=lymphocytic interstitial pneumonia; MAC=*Mycobacterium avium-intracellulare* complex; MAI=*Mycobacterium avium* infection; NSIP=nonspecific interstitial pneumonitis; PCP=*Pneumocystic carinii* pneumonia; TB=tuberculosis